MEDICAL LANGU OR

Medical Terminology
SIMPLIFIED

7TH EDITION

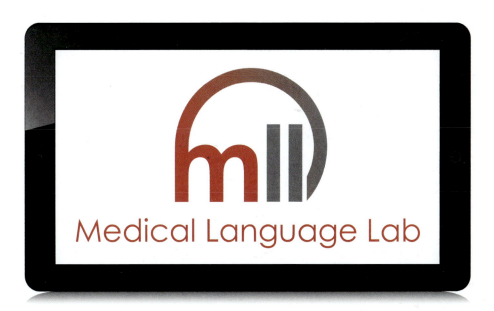

Medical Language Lab

Your journey to medical terminology
SUCCESS BEGINS HERE!

Medical Language Lab for Medical Terminology Simplified guides you step by step from basic through advanced levels of writing and speaking proficiency.

Don't miss everything that's waiting for you online to make learning less stressful and save you time. Follow the instructions on the inside front cover to use the access code to unlock your resources today.

STEP #1

LEARN
Build a solid foundation with your text.

Master the language of medicine frame by frame.
A programmed approach to learning breaks must-know content into small, student-friendly sections to make the information easier to master.

Build your vocabulary.
Word Elements tables develop your ability to recognize word parts and build new terms.

WORD ELEMENTS

This section introduces word elements related to the lymphatic system. Review the word elements and their meanings in the following table. Then, pronounce each term in the word analysis column, and place a ✓ in the box after you do so.

Word Element	Meaning	Word Analysis
Combining Forms		
aden/o	gland	**aden/o**/pathy (ă-dĕ-NŎP-ă-thē M): disease of a gland *-pathy:* disease
agglutin/o	clumping, gluing	**agglutin**/ation (ă-dĕ-NŎP-ă-thē M): process of cells clumping together *-ation:* process (of)
immun/o	immune, immunity, safe	**immun/o**/gen (ĭ-MŪ-nō-jĕn M): producing immunity *-gen:* forming, producing, origin *An immunogen is a substance capable of producing an immune response.*
lymph/o	lymph	**lymph/o**/poiesis (lĭm-fŏ-poy-Ē-sĭs M): formation of lymphocytes or of lymph tissue *-poiesis:* formation, production
lymphaden/o	lymph gland (node)	**lymphaden**/itis (lĭm-făd-ĕn-Ī-tĭs M): inflammation of a lymph gland (node) *-itis:* inflammation
lymphangi/o	lymph vessel	**lymphangi**/oma (lĭm-făn-jē-Ō-mă M): tumor composed of lymphatic vessels *-oma:* tumor

MEDICAL RECORD ACTIVITY 5-1

EMERGENCY DEPARTMENT REPORT: RULE OUT MYOCARDIAL INFARCTION

This activity contains an emergency department report on a patient who presents with chest pain. Read the emergency department report that follows, and underline the medical terms. Then complete the terminology and critical thinking exercises.

Prepare for practice.
Medical Record Activities feature case studies and critical-thinking exercises that illustrate how terminology is used in the real world in which you will practice, including activities for patient diagnosis and evaluation.

Blood Flow Through the Heart

5-35 Although general information on the circulatory system was discussed previously, this section covers in greater detail the specific structures involved in the flow of blood through the heart. The heart's double pump serves two distinct circulations: pulmonary circulation, which is the short loop of blood vessels that runs from the heart to the lungs and back to the heart, and systemic circulation, which routes blood through a long loop to all parts of the body before returning it to the heart.

Continue to label Figure 5-4 as you read the following information. The RA receives oxygen-poor blood from all tissues except those of the lungs. The blood from the head and arms is delivered to the RA through the (6) **superior vena cava** (SVC). The blood from the legs and torso is delivered to the RA through the (7) **inferior vena cava** (IVC).

superior inferior	**5-36** Refer to Figure 5-4 and use the words superior or inferior to complete this frame. The LA is _____ to the LV. The RV is _____ to the RA.
	5-37 Blood flows from the RA through the (8) **tricuspid valve** and into the RV. The leaflets (cusps) are shaped such that they form a one-way passage, which keeps the blood flowing in only one direction. Label the tricuspid valve in Figure 5-4.
tri/cuspid valve trī-KŪS-pĭd	**5-38** The prefix *tri-* means *three*. The valve that has three leaflets, or flaps, is the _____ / _____.
two	**5-39** The prefix *bi-* refers to *two*. A bi/cuspid valve has _____ leaflets, or flaps.

EMERGENCY DEPARTMENT REPORT

PATIENT NAME: Nichols, James
MEDICAL RECORD ID: 68-19347
DATE: May 1, 20xx

CHIEF COMPLAINT: Patient complains of chest pain.

PRESENT ILLNESS: Patient is a 22-year-old male, who states that he has had two previous myocardial infarctions related to his use of cocaine. The patient states he has not used cocaine for the last 3 months. He describes the pain as midsternal pain, a burning type sensation that lasted several seconds. The patient took one of his own nitroglycerin tablets without any relief. The patient became concerned and came into the emergency department. In the emergency department, the patient states that his pain is a 3 on a scale of 1 to 10. He feels much more comfortable. He denies any shortness of breath or dizziness and states that the pain feels unlike the pain of his myocardial infarction. The patient has no other complaints at this time.

PAST HISTORY: The patient's past medical history is significant for status post myocardial infarction in January of 19xx and again in April of 19xx. Both were related to illegal use of cocaine.

ALLERGIES: None

MEDICATIONS: Nitroglycerin p.r.n.

PHYSICAL EXAMINATION

GENERAL: A well-developed, well-nourished, white male in no acute distress. He is alert, oriented x3, and lying comfortably on the bed. **VITAL SIGNS:** Temperature 98.2, blood pressure 138/80 mm Hg, pulse

---

Terminology 5-1

Terms listed in the following table come from the consultation letter Emergency Department Report: Rule Out Myocardial Infarction. *Use a medical dictionary, such as Taber's Cyclopedic Medical Dictionary; the appendices of this book; or other resources to define each term. Then, pronounce the term, and place a checkmark (✓) in the box after you do so.*

Term	Definition
auscultation aws-kŭl-TĀ-shŭn ☐	
electrocardiogram ē-lĕk-trō-KĂR-dē-ō-grăm ☐	

thrombi
THRŎM-bī

anti-

5-99 Anti/coagulants are agents that prevent or delay blood coagulation; they are used in the prevention and treatment of a thrombus.

The plural form of *thrombus* is _____.

The element in this frame that means *against* is _____.

5-100 Use *-genesis* to form a word that means *producing or forming a blood clot.*

_____ / _____ / _____

5-101 If the anti/coagulant does not dissolve the clot, it may be surgically removed. A thromb/ectomy is an excision of a blood _____.

5-102 To prevent blood coagulation, the physician uses an agent known as an _____ / _____.

Test yourself.
Use the **FREE bookmark** to cover the answers in the left-hand column as you respond to each question.

Check your progress.
Section Reviews assess your mastery and identify areas for additional study.

SECTION REVIEW 5-1

For the following medical terms, first, write the suffix and its meaning. Then, translate the meaning of the remaining elements, starting with the first part of the word. The first word is completed for you.

Term	Meaning
1. endo/cardi/um	-um: structure, thing; in, within; heart
2. cardi/o/megaly	
3. aort/o/stenosis	
4. tachy/cardia	
5. phleb/it is	
6. thromb/o/lysis	
7. vas/o/spasm	

Critical Thinking

Review *SOAP Note: Chronic Interstitial Lung Disease* to answer the following questions.

1. When did the patient notice dyspnea?

_____

_____

_____

2. Other than the respiratory system, what _____ illness?

_____

Develop your competencies.
Terminology and **Critical-Thinking** exercises build your skills.

Make the connections.
Full-color illustrations depicting human anatomy, physiology, pathology, and medical treatments make their associated medical terms easy to understand.

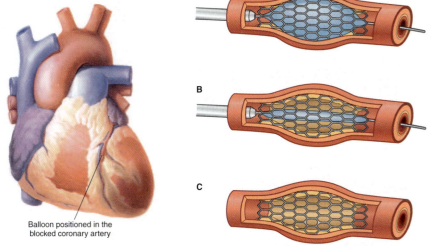

Balloon positioned in the blocked coronary artery

Figure 5-22 PTCA with stent placement. (A) Balloon inflated to widen the artery. (B) Deflated balloon. (C) Stent remains to hold artery open when catheter is removed.

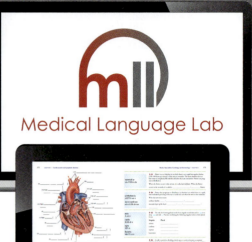

STEP #2

PRACTICE
Study smarter, not harder.

Study online. The integrated **eBook** with highlighting, note-taking, and bookmarking capabilities makes studying easy. Or download it for access wherever you are.

The pretest report indentifies areas that need attention based on your pretest results.

Lesson	Attention
1. Introduction to Programmed Learning and Medical Word Building	Slow
2. Body Structure	Stop
3. Integumentary System	Slow
4. Respiratory System	Slow
5. Cardiovascular and Lymphatic Systems	Slow
6. Digestive System	Stop
7. Urinary System	Slow
8. Reproductive Systems	Slow
9. Endocrine and Nervous Systems	Stop
10. Musculoskeletal System	Stop
11. Special Senses: Eyes and Ears	Stop

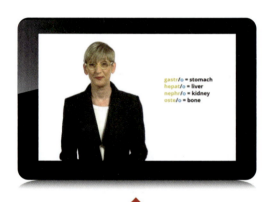

Watch & learn. Lecture videos present must-know concepts, while learning tips help you identify the ways you learn best.

Experience personalized learning. Take the **Pretest** to create your own Study Plan. You'll know exactly where to focus your time.

Improve your speaking skills. Pronunciation Guides let you listen to audio files linked to definitions from *Taber's*, the bestselling dictionary for health care students.

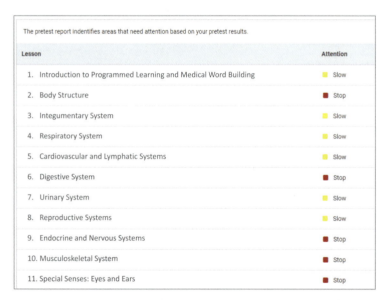

Pronunciation Guide   Return to Assignments

Medical Language Lab for Medical Terminology Simplified, 7th Edition

Lesson [Select All]   [Search Text]   [Search]

A B C D E F G H I J K L M N O P Q R S T U V W X Y Z All

Found in Taber's !
Click here to access definitions of the terms below in Glossary.

Term	Audio Pronunciation
abdominal	◄
abduction	◄
ablation	◄
abscess	◄
acoustic	◄

Listen to the audio recording below as many times as you need to in order to familiarize yourself with the content. When you are done listening, click the *Continue to Questions* button to view the questions associated with the audio. Please note that you will not be able to listen to the recording while you are answering the questions. Upon reviewing your results, you will be able to listen to the audio again and view excerpts of the key terminology in context.

▶ 00:00 / 00:45

CONTINUE TO QUESTIONS

Listen & respond. Audio recordings followed by questions develop your understanding of medical language as it's used in conversation.

Communicate like a health care professional. **Documenting health care activities** prepares you for professional practice. You'll apply your knowledge of medical terminology to the variety of administrative and clinical challenges you'll encounter in your future career.

Electronic Medical Record Workout Exercise ✕

Registered: 1315 hours		Samantha Nguyen, MD
Clinic Encounter		
Reynolds, Christian C. 10/15/1945		
File Edit Windows Actions New		
Tuesday, March 7, 2017		
1685 Smithtown Road Atlanta, GA 30080		**Encounter**
		●Encounters ●03/07/17 ●Medications ●03/07/17 ●Laboratory ●03/07/17 ●Medical Tests ●03/07/17
Allergies	**Problem List**	
Bees Sulfa	Joint inflammation Wrist pain Joint pain, fingers	
Other Sensitivities	**Routine Meds**	
		Assessment: 1. Arthritis
PMHX	**Referred By**	
Allergies Gastromegaly		**Plan:** Over-the-counter pain medication Return visit if not improved
Orders	**Insurance**	
	Medicare	
Chart Note		
Mr. Reynolds is here today because of joint pain. Examination reveals inflammation in the joints of his right index finger, right thumb, and left wrist. The inflammation is mild and can be managed with an over-the-counter medication. I instructed him to return if his symptoms worsen.		

1. Organ chamber or cavity that receives or holds fluid

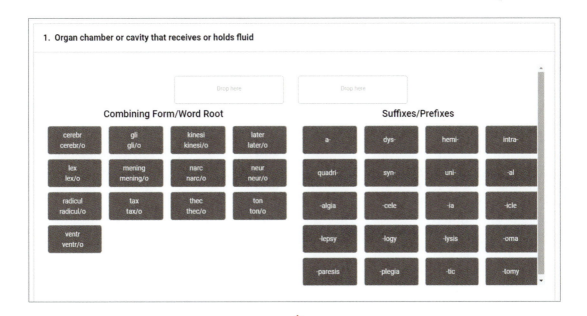

Drop here   Drop here

Combining Form/Word Root   **Suffixes/Prefixes**

cerebr cerebr/o	gli gli/o	kinesi kinesi/o	later later/o
lex lex/o	mening mening/o	narc narc/o	neur neur/o
radicul radicul/o	tax tax/o	thec thec/o	ton ton/o
ventr ventr/o			

a-	dys-	hemi-	intra-
quadri-	syn-	uni-	-al
-algia	-cele	-ia	-icle
-lepsy	-logy	-lysis	-oma
-paresis	-plegia	-tic	-tomy

Practice what you're learning. Complete the **exercises** to reinforce the lessons in the text and build your knowledge of medical terminology.

STEP #3

ASSESS
Build mastery. Attain fluency.

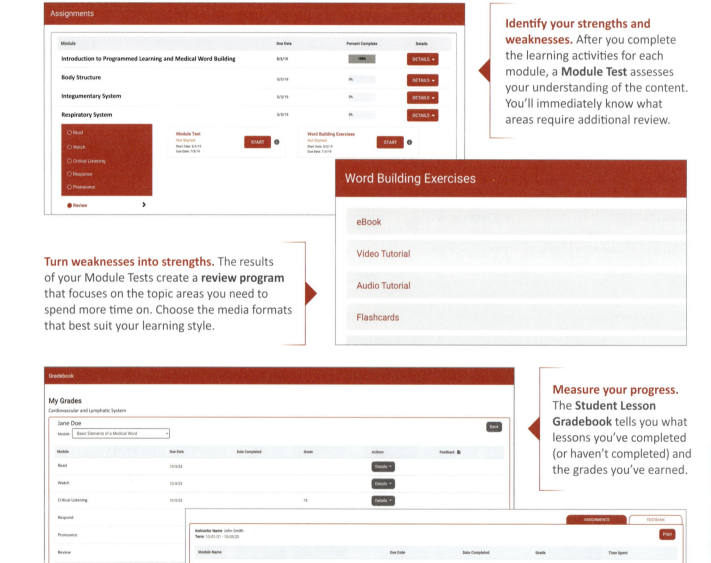

Identify your strengths and weaknesses. After you complete the learning activities for each module, a **Module Test** assesses your understanding of the content. You'll immediately know what areas require additional review.

Turn weaknesses into strengths. The results of your Module Tests create a **review program** that focuses on the topic areas you need to spend more time on. Choose the media formats that best suit your learning style.

Measure your progress. The **Student Lesson Gradebook** tells you what lessons you've completed (or haven't completed) and the grades you've earned.

Review your performance. The **Student Activity Gradebook** drills down to show you how you've performed on specific assignments and tracks how long it takes you to complete each one.

Online content subject to change upon publication

MEDICAL TERMINOLOGY
SIMPLIFIED

A Programmed Learning Approach by Body System

SEVENTH EDITION

Barbara A. Gylys (GĬL-ĭs), BS, MEd, CMA-A
Professor Emerita
College of Health and Human Services
University of Toledo
Toledo, Ohio

Regina M. Masters, BSN, MEd, RN, CMA
Adjunct Nursing Faculty
Lourdes University
Sylvania, Ohio

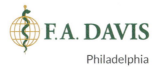

F.A. DAVIS

Philadelphia

F. A. Davis Company
1915 Arch Street
Philadelphia, PA 19103
www.fadavis.com

Printed in the United States of America

Last digit indicates print number: 10 9 8 7 6 5 4 3 2 1

Publisher: Quincy McDonald
Director of Content Development: George W. Lang
Content Project Manager: Julie Chase
Art and Design Manager: Carolyn O'Brien

As new scientific information becomes available through basic and clinical research, recommended treatments and drug therapies undergo changes. The author(s) and publisher have done everything possible to make this book accurate, up to date, and in accord with accepted standards at the time of publication. The author(s), editors, and publisher are not responsible for errors or omissions or for consequences from application of the book, and make no warranty, expressed or implied, in regard to the contents of the book. Any practice described in this book should be applied by the reader in accordance with professional standards of care used in regard to the unique circumstances that may apply in each situation. The reader is advised always to check product information (package inserts) for changes and new information regarding dose and contraindications before administering any drug. Caution is especially urged when using new or infrequently ordered drugs.

Library of Congress Cataloging-in-Publication Data

Names: Gylys, Barbara A., author. | Masters, Regina M., 1959- author.
Title: Medical terminology simplified : a programmed learning approach by
  body system / Barbara A. Gylys, Regina M. Masters.
Description: Seventh edition. | Philadelphia, PA : F.A. Davis Company,
  [2023] | Includes index.
Identifiers: LCCN 2022028403 (print) | LCCN 2022028404 (ebook) | ISBN
  9781719646161 (paperback) | ISBN 9781719648912 (ebook)
Subjects: MESH: Terminology as Topic | Programmed Instruction
Classification: LCC R123 (print) | LCC R123 (ebook) | NLM W 15 | DDC
  610.1/4--dc23/eng/20220829
LC record available at https://lccn.loc.gov/2022028403
LC ebook record available at https://lccn.loc.gov/2022028404

This Book is Dedicated with Love

to my best friend, colleague, and husband, Julius A. Gylys

and

to my children, Regina Maria and Julius A., II

and

to Andrew Masters, Dr. Julia Halm, Caitlin Masters, Anthony Bishop-Gylys, Matthew Bishop-Gylys, Liam Halm, Harrison Halm, and Emmett Halm

—BARBARA GYLYS

to my mother, best friend, mentor, and co-author, Barbara A. Gylys

and

to my father, Dr. Julius A. Gylys

and

to my husband, Bruce Masters, and my children Andrew, Dr. Julia, and Caitlin, all of whom have given me continuous encouragement and support, and to my grandsons Liam, Harrison, and Emmett, who bring me endless joy.

—REGINA MASTERS

Preface

Medical Terminology Simplified: A Programmed Learning Approach by Body System, 7th edition continuous to maintain its established track record of reflecting current trends and new approaches to teaching and learning medical terminology. Most importantly, instructors' feedback indicates that the didactic features of this book enhance their students' ability to readily learn the language of medicine. This workbook-text is designed for interactive engagement by students. Throughout each chapter, students engage in a new and exciting learning experience by interactively completing section reviews, labeling anatomical structures and diagrams, and answering questions to validate their understanding of the material discussed. Included in this edition are newly developed illustrations and innovative features to make studying the language of medicine a more encompassing and rewarding experience. The emphasis in this edition continues to reflect current trends and new approaches to teaching and learning medical terminology with numerous ancillaries accessible on the internet. The design and flexibility of *Simplified,* 7th edition, enable its use as a self-instructional book, an eBook, or as a text in traditional lecture and classroom environments. The organization and pedagogical devices are structured to help instructors teach and students learn medical terminology easily and quickly. When instructors and students utilize the available ancillary resources summarized in the preface, they will find the suggested approach of teaching and learning the language of medicine is greatly enhanced. With this approach, instructors will be successful in helping their students develop skills in using medical terminology that they can readily apply in the clinical field.

The 7th edition continues to present eponyms without showing the possessive form, such as *Alzheimer disease, Down syndrome,* and *Parkinson disease.* Medical dictionaries, as well as the American Association for Medical Transcription and the American Medical Association, support these changes. A newly designed summary of ICD-10-PCS replacement terms for discontinued eponyms are summarized in the Instructor's Guide. The ICD summary includes the page numbers in *Simplified,* 7th edition, on which the terms are discussed. In this edition, the medical records sections focus on helping students understand the transition of the paper medical chart to a digital version, the electronic medical record. Beginning in Chapter 2, the medical record sections emphasize the role of the electronic medical record (EMR) by providing authentically styled reports that are used in today's health-care settings. Included are various types of medical record activities to validate the student's proficiency with the terms and concepts presented in the medical records. Lastly, in Appendix D, drug classifications are enhanced and include the pronunciations of all listed drugs.

CHAPTERS

We have enhanced the popular, effective features found in the previous edition, so the learner can easily apply and process the language of medicine correctly in the workplace. The main focus of this edition is to improve retention of medical terms and demonstrate their applications in the clinical setting. Here is a brief summary of chapter content:

- Chapter 1 introduces the programmed learning, medical word-building approach. It also includes summaries and activities to reinforce retention of common suffixes and prefixes used in medical word building.
- Chapter 2 discusses the structural organization of the human body.
- Chapters 3 to 11 are organized according to specific body systems and may be taught in any sequence. These chapters include key anatomical and physiological terms; anatomy and physiology; combining forms, suffixes, and prefixes; terms related to signs, symptoms, and diseases as well as diagnostic, surgical and medical procedures; and abbreviations. Included are section reviews and medical record activities. All activities allow self-assessment and evaluation of competency.

APPENDICES

The appendices offer learning tools to help reinforce the information presented in the chapters. Your students will also find the appendices useful for study, review, and reference as they begin their careers in the allied health field:

- Appendix A: Glossary of Medical Word Elements
- Appendix B: Answer Key
- Appendix C: Index of Diagnostic, Medical, and Surgical Procedures
- Appendix D: Drug Classifications
- Appendix E: Abbreviations, Discontinued Abbreviations, and Common Symbols
- Appendix F: Medical Specialties
- Appendix G: Glossary of English-to-Spanish Translations

LEARNING STYLES

All enhancements in the 7th edition are designed to improve retention and make the study of medical terminology more enjoyable and engaging. As more and more students identify themselves as visual learners, the authors met this challenge by ensuring that the illustrations in the text and ancillary products are as helpful to students as possible. Many newly developed figures depict the toughest topics for students to grasp; alteration of figures from the previous edition add clarity for ease of understanding. Thus, one of the most extraordinary features of this edition is the collection of visually outstanding, full-color illustrations. These illustrations are extremely useful as students learn the association of medical terms to anatomy, physiology, pathology, and medical treatments of the human body. All of the artwork presents precise depictions of medical terms in action. Full-color figures enable students to see a true representation of the body system, pathological condition, or operative procedure.

Programmed Learning Approach

The programmed learning approach presents a word-building method for developing a medical vocabulary in an effective, interesting manner. The book is designed to help students learn skills that will enable them to analyze medical terms by breaking them down into their basic components. By learning and reinforcing this technique, students will master the terms in this book and learn to decipher new medical terms that they encounter in the workplace. It is not a book in which the student simply memorizes a list of vocabulary terms. In addition, the text can be used in a traditional classroom setting or with guidance from an instructor for independent study. The workbook text format is designed to guide the student through exercises that teach and reinforce medical terminology.

The programmed-learning technique makes use of frames, or isolated pieces of information that, together, give the student the building blocks of learning medical terminology. The frames, each numbered with the chapter number and then the frame number within that chapter, allow students to learn at their own pace and in their own way. Each frame contains not only information about terminology, but also fill-in lines students can use to reinforce understanding of the information. The student can find the answer to each fill-in line in the frame's answer box, located in the column at the left of the page.

The key to using frames wisely is the bookmark included with every book. Students should use it to cover the answer column to verify their understanding of the content provided in the frame. The frame answer boxes also include pronunciation keys for all medical words. Newly designed pronunciation guides in each chapter help students pronounce medical terms correctly. In addition, the F.A. Davis Online Resource Center includes an audio component that helps students learn to pronounce numerous medical terms they may encounter in the clinical setting. The audio components are designed as an interactive engagement of learning how to pronounce medical terms correctly.

TEACHING AND LEARNING PACKAGE

Numerous teaching aids are available free of charge to instructors who adopt *Medical Terminology Simplified: A Programmed Learning Approach by Body System,* 7th edition. These teaching aids contain an abundance of information and activities to help students retain what they have learned in a given chapter. Various types of electronic resources are designed to enhance course content and ensure a program of excellence in a medical terminology curriculum. These resources will also help you plan course work and provide you with various types of presentations to reinforce the learning process. These teaching aids include the web-based Medical Language Lab and the F.A. Davis Online Resource Center for students, and the Instructor's Online Resource Center for instructors.

Medical Language Lab

Included in every new copy of *Medical Terminology Simplified: A Programmed Learning Approach by Body System,* 7th edition, is access to the ultimate online medical terminology resource for students. The Medical Language Lab is a rich learning environment using proven language development methods to help students become effective users of medical language. To access the Medical Language Lab, students simply go to *http://www.medicallanguagelab.com* and register using the access code provided in their new copies of *Medical Terminology Simplified: A Programmed Learning Approach by Body System,* 7th edition.

Each lesson in the Medical Language Lab enables the student to develop skills to listen critically for important terms, respond to others using medical terminology, and generate their own terminology-rich writing and speech. By following the activities in each lesson, students graduate from simple memorization to becoming stronger users of the medical language.

Designed to work seamlessly with *Medical Terminology Simplified: A Programmed Learning Approach by Body System*, 7th edition, each activity in the Medical Language Lab has been crafted with content specific to the textbook. Every chapter in the textbook has a corresponding lesson in the Medical Language Lab. A designated icon found within the chapters tells students when it is most advantageous to integrate the activities on the Medical Language Lab into their studies. Students can be confident that every activity in the Medical Language Lab is relevant to the language of medicine and helps facilitate the learning process.

Some of the activities in the Medical Language Lab include:

- interactive audio activities that expose students to the use of medical terminology in clinical settings
- flash-card activities for preview and practice to reinforce word elements presented in the chapter
- lecture videos and full pronunciation guide that further enhance understanding of each chapter
- labelling activities that build understanding of anatomical terms
- automatically-graded pronunciation activities which provide instant feedback down to the phoneme level
- personalized remediation suggestions with corresponding practice quizzes
- short definitions of selected terms from *Taber's Cyclopedic Medical Dictionary*, 24th edition, the most trusted medical dictionary in the world

F.A. Davis Online Resource Center

The F.A. Davis web site, accessed at *https://fadavis.com/home,* is a study companion web site for *Simplified,* 7th edition. It provides activities to accelerate learning and reinforce information presented in each chapter. A designated icon found within the chapters tells students when it is most advantageous to integrate the activities on the F.A. Davis web site into their studies. All online exercises provide instructions for completing the various activities.

The Student Resource Center on FADavis.com include:

- audio exercises of pronunciations and meanings of newly introduced medical terms from the word elements tables (Chapters 1 through 11), designed to strengthen spelling, pronunciation, and meanings of selected medical terms and develop medical transcription skills
- medical record exercises (Chapters 3 through 11) that allow students to click highlighted terms in the medical record and hear their correct pronunciations and meanings to strengthen understanding of medical terms
- animations, such as exploration of the pathology of gastroesophageal reflux disease (GERD) or the various stages of pregnancy and delivery, to help students better understand complex processes and procedures
- study questions for Chapters 1 to 11, which the student can answer after completing a chapter to determine their competency level of the chapter and understand how the multiple choice questions are constructed in the electronic test bank and on accreditation examinations
- Medical Language Lab (MLL), the interactive, online program that helps the student master the language of medicine, which can also be accessed from the F.A. Davis site

Instructor's Online Resource Center

The Instructor's Online Resource Center provides an abundance of updated, innovative supplemental teaching aids. These teaching aids are designed to help instructors plan course work, enhance presentations, and make teaching medical terminology easier and more effective. Instructors can use these teaching tools in various educational settings, including the traditional classroom, distance learning, or independent studies. When the instructor integrates them into course content, they will provide a sound foundation for developing an extensive medical vocabulary and guarantee a full program of medical terminology excellence for all students. The Instructor's Online Resource Center includes:

- Instructor's Guide with Lesson Plans
- PowerPoint Lecture Notes
- Image Bank Resource
- Electronic Test Bank (ETB)
- LMS Integration Resource Kits
- *eBook* powered by VitalSource

Instructor's Guide with Lesson Plans

The printable Instructor's Guide is a resource full of instructional support for using the textbook and ancillary products. The authors have broadened and enhanced it to meet the challenges of today's instructional needs.

It is available in PDF format on the Instructor's Online Resource Center. The seventh edition includes:

- *Course Outlines.* Suggested course outlines help the instructor determine a comfortable pace and plan the best method of covering the material presented in the textbook.
- *Lesson Plans with Teaching Tips.* Each chapter of the Instructor's Guide begins with Learning Objectives and Lesson Outlines. These lesson plans consist of extensive instructional aides are matched to every lecture in a medical terminology course. They include sample homework assignments, class activities as well as extensive lecture notes with suggested topic durations. When viewed electronically, the Instructor Guide also provides live hyperlinks to the instructor resources at FADavis.com. Each chapter's lessons are followed up with an Activity Pack that compliments the text, with student- and instructor-directed activities as well as an answer key.
- *Clinical Connection Activities.* These activities integrate clinical scenarios in each chapter as a solid reinforcement of content. Instructors should feel free to select activities they deem suitable for their course and decide whether the students should complete the activity independently, with peers, or as a group project.
- *Student- and Instructor-Directed Activities.* These updated teaching aids, with new ones added for this edition, offer a variety of activities for each body system chapter. Activities can serve as course requirements or supplemental material. In addition, instructors can assign them as individual or collaborative projects, with Peer Evaluation Forms provided for group projects.
- *Oral and Written Research Projects.* The research projects provide an opportunity for students to hone their research skills. The Community and Internet Resources section offers an updated list of technical journals, community organizations, and Internet sources that students can use to complete the oral and written projects. This section also includes an evaluation template for the oral and written research projects. These projects will add variety and interest to the course while reinforcing the learning process.
- *Anatomy Test Questions.* Instructors can use the anatomy test questions for anatomy review or as a testing device. These questions also include an illustration for each body system chapter. An answer key is also provided.
- *Supplemental Medical Record Activities.* As in the textbook, these medical record activities use common clinical scenarios to show how the student would use medical terminology in the clinical area to document patient care. Each medical record includes activities for terminology, pronunciation, and critical thinking exercises. In addition, each medical record focuses on a specific medical specialty. Instructors can use these records for group activities, oral reports, medical coding activities, or individual assignments. The medical records are designed to reinforce and enhance terminology presented in the textbook. An answer key is also provided.
- *Crossword Puzzles.* These fun, educational activities reinforce material covered in each body system chapter. Instructors can use them for an individual or group activity, an extra-credit opportunity, or just for fun. An answer key is included for each puzzle.
- *Anatomy Coloring Activities.* Anatomy coloring activities, included for each body-system chapter, help reinforce the positions of the main organs that compose a particular body system.
- *Terminology Answer Keys.* In response to requests from instructors, this section summarizes the answers to the Terminology tables in the medical records sections of the textbook. This added feature provides instructional support in using the textbook and assists instructors in correcting terminology assignments.

PowerPoint Lecture Notes

Simplified, 7th edition, contains a completely updated and expanded ADA compliant PowerPoint Lecture Notes package that instructors can easily integrate, modify, or enhance to meet their classroom needs. We have included the additional 1,327 slides, with 58 new slides for the previous edition. These include, but are not limited to, full-color illustrations with captions from the textbook and other sources. The PowerPoint Lecture Notes slides also contain pedagogical notes for each chapter (at the bottom of the slide) to reinforce comprehension and offer suggestions for a higher retention level for material discussed. In addition, instructors can also arrange to use the PowerPoint presentations for independent study purposes.

The PowerPoint Lecture Notes provide an outline-based presentation for each body system chapter. Each presentation contains a chapter overview; the structure and functions of each body system; and selected pathology, vocabulary, and diagnostic medical and surgical procedures for each body system chapter. In addition, various exercises, including clinically related exercises, are included to verify retention of the material presented.

Image Bank Resource

We have enhanced and expanded the Image Resource, a popular feature of the past edition, to meet the current demands of numerous instructors. The Image Resource is an electronic image bank that contains all illustrations from the textbook. It is fully searchable and allows users to zoom in and out and display a JPG image of an illustration that can be copied into a Microsoft Word document or PowerPoint presentation.

Electronic Test Bank

The electronic test bank is provided in two formats: QTI and Microsoft Word. QTI allows for easy import into your LMS. The test bank contains more than 1,300 test items, with 47 new test items from the previous edition. The test bank includes multiple-choice, matching, true-false, and medical word-building questions.

LMS Resource Kits

Learning Management Systems Resource Kit is available for Blackboard, Angel, Moodle, Canvass, and SCORM-compliant systems.

eBook

Adopters have access to the complete content of the text online in a searchable format that can be bookmarked and accessed wherever there is a browser with a live internet connection.

HOW TO USE THIS BOOK

This self-instructional book is designed to provide the student with skills to learn medical terminology easily and quickly. The book's design and flexibility enable its use as a self-instructional book or one that can be used in traditional lecture and classroom environments. The following distinctive features are included in this learning package:

- The programmed learning approach presents a word-building method for developing a medical vocabulary in an effective, interesting manner. It is designed for use in a traditional classroom setting or for independent study with an instructor.
- The workbook-text format is designed to guide you through exercises that teach and reinforce medical terminology.
- Numerous activities in each unit are designed to enable the student to be interactively involved in the learning process. Writing, reading, listening, visualizing, and keyboarding encompass the various learning styles employed in the book to help the student master medical terminology. With this method, the student will not only understand but also remember the significant concepts of medical word building.
- Students learn by active participation. In this book, students write answers in response to blocks of information, complete section review exercise, and analyze medical reports. If a student is not satisfied with the level of comprehension after the review exercises, reinforcement frames direct the student to go back and rework the corresponding informational frames.

- In this edition a designated MLL icon in each chapter directs the student to visit the Medical Language Lab for a flash-card review of word elements covered in the chapter.
- The audio exercises provide reinforcement of pronunciation, definitions, and spelling practice of medical terms. The terms are now available by visiting FADavis.com.
- Pronunciation keys for all medical words are included in the frame answer boxes and help the student pronounce each term correctly. Newly designed pronunciation guides in each chapter give students a more accurate understanding of the proper pronunciation of medical words.
- The appendices include many tools students can use as references when they begin working in the clinical field.

We hope the pedagogical and visual features of *Medical Terminology Simplified: A Programmed Learning Approach by Body System,* 7th edition, makes learning the language of medicine an exciting, rewarding process. We invite instructors and students to continue the tradition of sending their suggestions to F.A. Davis so that we can consider them for the next edition.

—BARBARA A. GYLYS
—REGINA M. MASTERS

Reviewers

MARY BARR, RN
Lancaster County CTC
Willow Street, Pennsylvania

CAROLE BERUBE, MA, MSN, BSN, RN
Professor Emerita in Nursing
Health Sciences
Bristol Community College
Fall River, Massachusetts

BRITTANY A. BRENNAN, MSN, RN
Practical Nursing Instructor
Department of Nursing
Lake Area Technical Institute
Watertown, South Dakota

ANGELA CARMICHAEL, MBA, RHIA, CCS, CCS-P
Director of HIM Compliance
AHIM approved ICD-10-CM/PCS Instructor
J.A. Thomas and Associates
Atlanta, Georgia

MARY C. CARRICO, MS Ed, RN
Professor of Nursing
West Kentucky Community and Technical College
Paducah, Kentucky

JULIA HALM, DO
Private Practice
Perrysburg, Ohio

ANDREW MASTERS, LISW-S
University of Toledo Medical Center
Toledo, Ohio

SUE POLITO, MSN, APN-C
Specialist Professor
Nursing and Health Studies
Monmouth University
West Long Branch, New Jersey

GEORGINA SAMPSON, RHIA
Program Director
Health Information Technology and Medical Coding
Anoka Technical College
Anoka, Minnesota

PAMELA M. SANBORN, CMA(AAMA), MEd
Program Director
Medical Assisting
Cabrillo College
Aptos, California

R. CRAIG SCHNELL, PhD, Provost
School of Pharmacy/College of Health Professions
North Dakota State University
Fargo, North Dakota

MICHELLE SHIPLEY, MS, RHIA, CCS
Chair and Program Director
Allied Health Department
Washburn University
Topeka, Kansas

Acknowledgments

The 7th edition of *Medical Terminology Simplified: A Programmed Learning Approach by Body System* was greatly improved by comments that the authors received from the many users of previous editions—both educators and students. Although there are too many people to acknowledge individually, we are deeply grateful to each one. As in the past, the editorial and production staffs at F. A. Davis have inspired, guided, and shaped this project. The authors would like to acknowledge the valuable contributions of F. A. Davis's editorial and production team who were responsible for this project:

- Quincy McDonald, Publisher, provided the overall design and layout for the 6th edition. He was instrumental in assisting the authors in designing a wide variety of state-of-the-art pedagogical products within the text to aid students in their learning activities and help instructors plan course work and presentations. These teaching aids are described in the Preface.
- Paul Marino, Senior Developmental Editor for Digital Products, patiently and enthusiastically addressed our numerous questions and background queries to ensure the textbook's ancillaries were appropriately updated and accurately revised.
- George W. Lang, Director of Content of Development, expertly guided the manuscript through the developmental and production phases of the process.
- Julie Chase, Content Project Manager, systematically and meticulously read the manuscript, helping it along at every stage of production.
- Margaret Biblis, Editor-in-Chief, once again provided her support and efforts for the quality of the finished product.

We also acknowledge and thank our exceptionally dedicated publishing partners who helped guide and shape this large project:

- **Michael Kern,** Editorial Departmental Associate
- **Bob Butler,** Production Manager
- **Daniel Domzalski,** Illustrations Coordinator
- **Carolyn O'Brien,** Art and Design Manager
- **Matt Craven,** Director of Digital Solutions

We also extend our sincerest gratitude to Neil Kelly, Executive Director of Sales, and his staff of sales representatives, whose continued efforts have undoubtedly contributed to the success of this textbook.

Contents at a Glance

CHAPTER 1   Introduction to Programmed Learning and Medical Word Building   *1*

CHAPTER 2   Body Structure   *31*

CHAPTER 3   Integumentary System   *65*

CHAPTER 4   Respiratory System   *113*

CHAPTER 5   Cardiovascular and Lymphatic Systems   *161*

CHAPTER 6   Digestive System   *229*

CHAPTER 7   Urinary System   *291*

CHAPTER 8   Reproductive Systems   *341*

CHAPTER 9   Endocrine and Nervous Systems   *405*

CHAPTER 10   Musculoskeletal System   *471*

CHAPTER 11   Special Senses: Eyes and Ears   *529*

APPENDICES

APPENDIX A   Glossary of Medical Word Elements   *575*

APPENDIX B   Answer Key   *585*

APPENDIX C   Index of Diagnostic, Medical, and Surgical Procedures   *621*

APPENDIX D   Drug Classifications   *625*

APPENDIX E   Abbreviations, Discontinued Abbreviations, and Common Symbols   *633*

APPENDIX F   Medical Specialties   *643*

APPENDIX G   Glossary of English-to-Spanish Translations   *645*

Index   *655*

Rules for Singular and Plural Suffixes   *672*

Pronunciation Guidelines   *Inside back cover*

Contents

CHAPTER 1   Introduction to Programmed Learning and Medical Word Building   *1*

Objectives   1

Instructions   2

Word Elements   3

Word Roots   4

Combining Forms   5

Suffixes   7

Prefixes   13

Defining Medical Words   15

Pronunciation Guidelines   16

Pronunciation Tools   16

Section Review 1-1   17

Common Suffixes   17

Surgical Suffixes   17

Diagnostic Suffixes   19

Pathological Suffixes   21

Plural Suffixes   24

Section Review 1-2   25

Common Prefixes   26

CHAPTER 2   Body Structure   *31*

Objectives   31

Levels of Organization   31

Word Elements   33

Section Review 2-1   35

Basic Units of Structure   35

Directional Terms   36

Section Review 2-2   43

Word Elements   44

Section Review 2-3   45

Body Planes   45

Body Cavities   48

Abdominopelvic Quadrants and Regions   49

 Abdominopelvic Quadrants   49

 Abdominopelvic Regions   51

 Section Review 2-4   53

Abbreviations   54

Additional Medical Terms   54

 Diseases and Conditions   54

 Diagnostic Procedures 55

 Medical and Surgical Procedures   59

Word Elements Review   60

Additional Medical Terms Review   61

Medical Record Activities   62

Body Structure Chapter Review   63

 Word Elements Summary   63

Quadrants and Regions Review   64

CHAPTER 3 **Integumentary System** *65*

Objectives   65

Medical Specialty: Dermatology   65

 Anatomy and Physiology Overview   66

Word Elements   67

 Section Review 3-1   69

Skin and Accessory Organs   69

 Skin   69

 Accessory Organs of the Skin   76

 Section Review 3-2   80

Combining Forms Denoting Color   81

 Skin   81

 Cells   81

 Section Review 3-3   86

Abbreviations   87

Additional Medical Terms   87

 Diseases and Conditions   87

 Diagnostic Procedures   94

Medical and Surgical Procedures   95

Pharmacology   97

Word Elements Review   98

Additional Medical Terms Review   99

Primary and Secondary Lesions Review   100

Medical Record Activities   101

 Medical Record Activity 3-1—Consultation Letter: Skin Cancer Check   101

 Medical Record Activity 3-2—Progress Note: Psoriasis Vulgaris   105

 Medical Record Activity 3-3—Clinical Application   109

Integumentary System Chapter Review   110
   Word Elements Summary   110
   Vocabulary Review   111

CHAPTER 4   Respiratory System   *113*
Objectives   113
Medical Specialty: Pulmonology   113
   Anatomy and Physiology Overview   114
Word Elements   115
   Section Review 4-1   117
Respiratory System   117
   Upper Respiratory Tract   117
   Section Review 4-2   123
   Lower Respiratory Tract   124
   Section Review 4-3   136
Abbreviations   137
Additional Medical Terms   138
   Diseases and Conditions   138
   Diagnostic Procedures   143
   Medical and Surgical Procedures   146
Pharmacology   147
Word Elements Review   148
Additional Medical Terms Review   149
Medical Record Activities   150
   Medical Record Activity 4-1—Referral Letter: Allergic Rhinitis   150
   Medical Record Activity 4-2—Pulmonary Function Report   154
   Medical Record Activity 4-3—Clinical Application   157
Respiratory System Chapter Review   158
   Word Elements Summary   158
   Vocabulary Review   160

CHAPTER 5   Cardiovascular and Lymphatic Systems   *161*
Objectives   161
Medical Specialties: Cardiology and Immunology   162
   Cardiology   162
   Immunology   163
   Anatomy and Physiology Overview   163
Word Elements   165
   Section Review 5-1   167
Cardiovascular System   167
   Layers of the Heart Wall   167
   Circulation and Heart Structures   169
   Blood Flow Through the Heart   175
   Heart Valves   179
   Section Review 5-2   181

Conduction Pathway of the Heart 182

Cardiac Cycle and Heart Sounds 183

Lymphatic System 189

Word Elements 190

Section Review 5-3 191

Lymphatic Structures 191

Tonsil, Spleen, and Thymus 194

Section Review 5-4 196

Abbreviations 197

Additional Medical Terms 198

Diseases and Conditions 198

Lymphatic System 202

Diagnostic Procedures 204

Medical and Surgical Procedures 208

Pharmacology 213

Word Elements Review 214

Additional Medical Terms Review 215

Medical Record Activities 216

Medical Record Activity 5-1—Emergency Department Report: Rule Out

Myocardial Infarction 216

Medical Record Activity 5-2—Operative Report: Cardiac Catheterization 221

Medical Record Activity 5-3—Clinical Application 224

Cardiovascular and Lymphatic Systems Chapter Review 225

Word Elements Summary 225

Vocabulary Review 227

CHAPTER 6   **Digestive System** *229*

Objectives 229

Medical Specialty: Gastroenterology 229

Anatomy and Physiology Overview 230

Word Elements 231

Section Review 6-1 233

Upper Gastrointestinal Tract 233

Oral Cavity 233

Esophagus, Pharynx, and Stomach 238

Section Review 6-2 243

Word Elements 244

Section Review 6-3 246

Lower Gastrointestinal Tract 246

Small and Large Intestines 246

Rectum and Anus 251

Section Review 6-4 256

Word Elements 257

Section Review 6-5 258

Accessory Organs of Digestion   258

   Liver   259

   Gallbladder   260

   Pancreas   264

   Section Review 6-6   266

Abbreviations   267

Additional Medical Terms   267

   Diseases and Conditions   267

   Diagnostic Procedures   271

   Medical and Surgical Procedures   273

Pharmacology   276

Word Elements Review   277

Additional Medical Terms Review   278

Medical Record Activities   279

   Medical Record Activity 6-1—Progress Note: Rectal Bleeding   279

   Medical Record Activity 6-2—Operative Report: Esophageal Carcinoma   283

   Medical Record Activity 6-3—Clinical Application   286

Digestive System Chapter Review   287

   Word Elements Summary   287

   Vocabulary Review   289

CHAPTER 7 Urinary System *291*

Objectives   291

Medical Specialties: Urology and Nephrology   291

   Urology   291

   Nephrology   292

   Anatomy and Physiology Overview   292

Word Elements   294

   Section Review 7-1   296

Macroscopic Structures   296

   Kidneys   296

   Section Review 7-2   304

   Ureters, Bladder, and Urethra   304

   Section Review 7-3   311

Microscopic Structures   311

   Section Review 7-4   318

Abbreviations   319

Additional Medical Terms   319

   Diseases and Conditions   319

   Diagnostic Procedures   321

   Medical and Surgical Procedures   323

Pharmacology   326

Word Elements Review   327

Additional Medical Terms Review   328

Medical Record Activities   329

Medical Record Activity 7-1—Hospital Admission: Benign Prostatic Hypertrophy,
Carcinoma of the Colon   329

Medical Record Activity 7-2—Progress Note: Cystitis   333

Medical Record Activity 7-3—Clinical Application   336

Urinary System Chapter Review   337

Word Elements Summary   337

Vocabulary Review   339

CHAPTER 8   Reproductive Systems *341*

Objectives   341

Medical Specialties: Obstetrics, Gynecology, and Urology   341

Urology   342

Anatomy and Physiology Overview   342

Female Reproductive System   342

Word Elements   344

Section Review 8-1   346

Internal Structures   346

Section Review 8-2   355

External Structures   356

Breasts   358

Section Review 8-3   363

Male Reproductive System   364

Word Elements   364

Section Review 8-4   366

Section Review 8-5   374

Abbreviations   375

Additional Medical Terms   375

Diseases and Conditions   375

Diagnostic Procedures   381

Medical and Surgical Procedures   384

Pharmacology   389

Word Elements Review   390

Additional Medical Terms Review   391

Medical Record Activities   392

Medical Record Activity 8-1—Emergency Department Report: Pelvic
Inflammatory Disease   392

Medical Record Activity 8-2—Operative Report: Bilateral Vasectomy   397

Medical Record Activity 8-3—Clinical Application   400

Reproductive Systems Chapter Review   401

Word Elements Summary   401

Vocabulary Review   403

CHAPTER 9   Endocrine and Nervous Systems   *405*

Objectives   *405*
Medical Specialties: Endocrinology and Neurology   *405*
  Endocrinology   405
  Neurology   406
  Anatomy and Physiology Overview   406
  Endocrine System   406
Word Elements   *408*
  Section Review 9-1   410
  Hormones   410
  Pituitary Gland   412
  Table 9-1: Pituitary Hormones   416
  Thyroid Gland   418
  Table 9-2: Thyroid Hormones   419
  Section Review 9-2   422
  Parathyroid Glands   423
  Table 9-3: Parathyroid Hormone   423
  Adrenal Glands   424
  Table 9-4: Adrenal Hormones   425
  Pancreas (Islets of Langerhans)   425
  Table 9-5: Pancreatic Hormones   427
  Pineal and Thymus Glands   428
  Ovaries and Testes   428
  Section Review 9-3   429
Nervous System   *429*
Word Elements   *431*
  Section Review 9-4   432
  Brain   432
  Spinal Cord   434
  Mental Disorders   439
  Section Review 9-5   442
Abbreviations   *443*
Additional Medical Terms   *444*
  Diseases and Conditions   444
  Diagnostic Procedures   449
  Medical and Surgical Procedures   452
Pharmacology   *454*
Word Elements Review   *455*
Additional Medical Terms Review   *456*
Medical Record Activities   *458*
  Medical Record Activity 9-1—Discharge Summary: Diabetes Mellitus   458
  Medical Record Activity 9-2—Chart Note: Peripheral Neuropathy   462
  Medical Record Activity 9-3—Clinical Application   466

Endocrine and Nervous Systems Chapter Review   467
   Word Elements Summary   *467*
   Vocabulary Review   *469*

CHAPTER 10   Musculoskeletal System *471*
Objectives   471
Medical Specialties: Orthopedics, Rheumatology, and Chiropractic
Medicine   472
   Orthopedics and Rheumatology   *472*
   Chiropractic Medicine   *472*
   Anatomy and Physiology Overview   *473*
Word Elements   474
   Section Review 10-1   *476*
Muscles   476
   Section Review 10-2   *480*
Skeletal System   481
Word Elements   482
   Section Review 10-3   *485*
   Structure and Function of Bones   *485*
   Section Review 10-4   *492*
   Joints   *493*
   Combining Forms Related to Specific Bones   *495*
   Fractures and Repairs   *497*
   Vertebral Column   *500*
   Section Review 10-5   *505*
Abbreviations   506
Additional Medical Terms   506
   Diseases and Conditions   *506*
   Diagnostic Procedures   *512*
   Medical and Surgical Procedures   *513*
Pharmacology   514
Word Elements Review   515
Additional Medical Terms Review   516
Medical Record Activities   518
   Medical Record Activity 10-1—Radiology Report: Degenerative Intervertebral
   Disk Disease   *518*
   Medical Record Activity 10-2—Operative Report: Rotator Cuff Tear, Right
   Shoulder   *521*
   Medical Record Activity 10-3—Clinical Application   *525*
Musculoskeletal System Chapter Review   526
   Word Elements Summary   *526*
   Vocabulary Review   *528*

CHAPTER 11   Special Senses: Eyes and Ears   *529*
Objectives   529
Medical Specialties: Ophthalmology and Otolaryngology   529
   Ophthalmology   529
   Otolaryngology   530
   Anatomy and Physiology Overview   530
   Eyes   530
Word Elements   531
   Section Review 11-1   533
   Fibrous Tunic   533
   Vascular Tunic   534
   Sensory Tunic   534
Ears   540
Word Elements   541
   Section Review 11-2   542
   Section Review 11-3   547
Abbreviations   548
Additional Medical Terms   548
   Diseases and Conditions   548
   Diagnostic Procedures   554
   Medical and Surgical Procedures   556
Pharmacology   560
Word Elements Review   561
Additional Medical Terms Review   562
Medical Record Activities   563
   Medical Record Activity 11-1—Operative Report: Retinal Detachment Repair   563
   Medical Record Activity 11-2—SOAP Note: Otitis Media   567
   Medical Record Activity 11-3—Clinical Application   570
Special Senses: Eyes and Ears Chapter Review   571
   Word Elements Summary   571
   Vocabulary Review   573

APPENDICES

APPENDIX A   Glossary of Medical Word Elements   *575*

APPENDIX B   Answer Key   *585*

APPENDIX C   Index of Diagnostic, Medical, and Surgical Procedures   *621*

APPENDIX D   Drug Classifications   *625*

APPENDIX E   Abbreviations, Discontinued Abbreviations, and Common Symbols   *633*

APPENDIX F   Medical Specialties   *643*

APPENDIX G   Glossary of English-to-Spanish Translations   *645*

Index   *655*

Rules for Singular and Plural Suffixes   *672*

Pronunciation Guidelines   *Inside back cover*

Introduction to Programmed Learning and Medical Word Building

OBJECTIVES

Upon completion of this chapter, you will be able to:

- Learn medical terminology by using the programmed learning technique.
- Identify and define four elements used to build medical words.
- Analyze and define the various parts of a medical term.
- Apply the rules learned in this chapter to pronounce medical words correctly.
- Define and provide examples of surgical, diagnostic, pathological, and related suffixes.
- Define and provide examples of common prefixes and their meanings.
- Apply the rules learned in this chapter to construct singular and plural forms of medical words.
- Locate and apply guidelines for pluralizing medical terms.
- Practice pronouncing the medical terms presented in this chapter.
- Demonstrate your knowledge of this chapter by successfully completing the frames, reviews, and activities in the chapter.

Instructions

In the first few pages, you will learn the most efficient use of this self-instructional programmed learning approach.

First, remove the sliding card, and cover the left-hand-side answer column with it.

---

answer

1–1   This text is designed to help you learn medical terminology effectively. The principal technique used throughout the book is known *as programmed learning,* which consists of a series of teaching units called *frames.*

Each frame presents information and calls for an answer on your part. When you complete a sentence by writing an answer on the blank line, you are learning information by using the programmed learning technique.

A frame consists of a block of information and a blank line. The purpose of the blank line is to write an _____.

1–2   Slide the card down in the left column to see the correct answer. After you correct your answer, as needed, read the next frame.

---

answer

1–3   It is important to keep the left-hand-side answer column covered until you write your _____.

---

learning

1–4   This book employs several methods to help you master medical terminology, but the main technique used is called *programmed* _____.

---

answer(s)

1–5   After you write your answer, it is important to verify that it is correct. To do so, compare your answer with the one listed in the left-hand-side answer column.

To obtain immediate feedback on your responses, you must verify your

_____.

Study frames in sequence because each frame builds on the previous one. The book reviews and repeats words throughout to reinforce your learning. Consequently, you do not need to memorize every word presented.

---

one

1–6   The number of blank lines in a frame determines the number of words you write for your answer.

Review the number of blank lines in Frame 1–5. It has _____ blank line(s). Therefore, the answer requires one word.

---

two, lines

1–7   A frame that requires two answers will have _____ blank _____.

1–8   In some frames, you will be asked to write the answer in your own words. In these instances, there will be one or more blank lines across the entire frame.

List at least two reasons why you want to learn medical terminology. Keep these objectives in mind as you work through the book.

_____

_____

 Do not look at the answer column before you write your response, and do not move ahead in a chapter. Progress in developing a medical vocabulary depends on your ability to learn the material presented in each frame.

frame	**1–9** Completing one frame at a time is the most effective method of learning. To achieve your goal of learning medical terminology, complete one _____ at a time.
back	**1–10** Whenever you make an error, it is important to go back and review the previous frame(s). You need to determine why you wrote the wrong answer before proceeding to the next frame. You may always go _____ and review information you have forgotten. Just remember, do not look ahead.
correct, check, *or* **verify**	**1–11** Do not be afraid to make a mistake. In programmed learning, you will learn and profit by making mistakes, provided you correct them immediately. Always _____ your answer immediately after you write it.
answer	**1–12** Because accurate spelling is essential in medicine, correct all misspelled words immediately. Do so by comparing your answer with the one in the left-hand-side _____ column.
correctly *or* **accurately**	**1–13** In medicine, it is important to spell correctly. Correct spelling can be a crucial component in determining the validity of evidence presented in a malpractice lawsuit. A physician can lose a lawsuit because of misspelled words that result in misinterpretation of a medical record. To provide correct information, medical words must be spelled _____ in a medical record.

Word Elements

A medical word consists of some or all of the following elements:

- word root (WR)
- combining form (CF)
- suffix
- prefix

How you combine these elements and whether all or some of them are present in a medical word determine the meaning of a word. The purpose of this chapter is to help you learn to identify these elements and use them to form medical terms.

suffix, prefix	**1-14** The four elements used to build a medical word are the WR, CF, _____WR_____ , and _____CF_____ .

elements *or* **parts**	**1-15** Medical terminology is not difficult to learn when you understand how the elements are combined to form a word. To develop a medical vocabulary, you must understand the _____ that form medical words.

Word Roots

A word root (WR) is the main part, or foundation, of a word. All medical words have at least one WR.

teach	**1-16** In the words *teacher, teaches, teaching,* the WR is _____teach_____ .

read **spend** **play**	**1-17** Identify the roots in the following words: **Word**　　**Root** reader　　_____teach._____ spending　_____spend._____ playful　　_____play_____

A word root, also called a *root*, may be used alone or combined with other elements to form another word with a different meaning.

1-18 Review the following examples to see how roots are used alone or with other elements to form words. The meaning of each term in the right-hand-side column is also provided.

Root as a Complete Word	**Root as Part of a Word**
alcohol	**alcoholism** (condition marked by impaired control over alcohol use)
sperm	**spermicide** (agent that kills sperm)
thyroid	**thyroidectomy** (excision of the thyroid gland)

alcohol **dent** **lump** **insulin** **gastr**	**1-19** Throughout the book, a slash separates word elements, as shown in the following examples: Write the root in the right-hand-side column for each of these terms: alcohol/ic　_____alcohol_____ dent/ist　　_____dent_____ lump/ectomy _____lump._____ insulin/ism　_____insulin_____ gastr/itis　_____gastr_____

cardi	**1–20** In medical words, the root usually indicates a body part (anatomical structure). For example, the root in *cardi/al, cardi/ac,* and *cardi/o/gram* is ___*Cardi*___, and it means *heart*.
dent/al DĔN-tăl **pancreat/itis** păn-krē-ă-TĪ-tĭs **dermat/o/logist** dĕr-mă-TŎL-ō-jĭst	**1–21** You will find that the roots in medical words are usually derived from Greek or Latin words. Some examples include **dent** in the word dent/ist, **pancreat** in the word *pancreat/itis,* and **derma** in the word *dermat/o/logist*. Underline the roots in the following words: dent/al pancreat/itis dermat/o/logist
part	**1–22** In Frame 1–21, the root **dent** means *tooth,* **pancreat** means *pancreas,* and **dermat** means *skin*. All three roots indicate a body _____.

Combining Forms

A CF is created when a WR is combined with a vowel. This vowel is usually an *o*. The vowel has no meaning of its own, but enables the connection of two or more word elements. The difficulty of pronouncing certain combinations of WRs requires insertion of a vowel. For example, the WRs **gastr** (stomach) and **nephr** are difficult to pronounce, whereas their CFs **gastr/o** and **nephr/o** are easier to pronounce.

combining form	**1–23** Like the WR, the CF is the basic foundation on which other elements are added to build a complete word. In this text, a CF will be listed as *word root/vowel,* such as **gastr/o** and **nephr/o**. A WR + a vowel (usually an *o*) forms a new element known as a ___*Cf*___ _____.
gastr/o **nephr/o**	**1–24** The CF in *gastr/o/scope* is _____ / _____. The CF in *nephr/o/pathy* is _____ / _____.
combining form gastr, o	**1–25** *Gastr/o* is an example of the word element called a _____ _____. The root in **gastr/o** is _____; the combining vowel is _____.
o o o	**1–26** List the combining vowel in each of the following elements: arthr/o: _____ phleb/o: _____ lith/o: _____

therm/o **abdomin**/o **nephr**/o	**1–27** Underline the WR in the following CFs: therm/o abdomin/o nephr/o

1–28   Use the combining vowel *o* to change the following roots to CFs, and separate the elements with a slash.

cyst/o
arthr/o
leuk/o
gastr/o

Root	Combining Form (Root + Vowel)
cyst	_____
arthr	_____
leuk	_____
gastr	_____

1–29   Usually, the combining vowel is an *o*, although you may encounter other vowels occasionally.

o

The combining vowel is usually an _____.

chem/o/therapy
kē-mō-THĔR-ă-pē

dermat/o/logy
dĕr-mă-TŎL-ō-jē

encephal/o/graphy
ĕn-sĕf-ă-LŎG-ră-fē

neur/o/logy
nū-RŎL-ō-jē

therm/o/meter
thĕr-MŎM-ĕ-tĕr

1–30   Instead of joining the two elements *chem* and *-therapy* directly, the combining vowel *o* is attached to the root to form the word *chem/o/therapy*. The vowel has no meaning of its own but enables two elements to be connected to each other.

Use the combining vowel to build medical terms as follows. *Chem/o/therapy* is given as an example.

Word Root	Suffix		Medical Term
chem	therapy	*becomes*	*chem/o/therapy*
dermat	-logy	*becomes*	_____ / ____ / ____
encephal	-graphy	*becomes*	_____ / ____ / ____
neur	-logy	*becomes*	_____ / ____ / ____
therm	-meter	*becomes*	_____ / ____ / ____

1–31   The words in Frame 1–30 are easier to pronounce because the WRs are linked with the combining vowel *o*.

vowel

To make a word easier to pronounce, attach a combining _____ to the WR.

1–32   Although you may not know the meaning of all the words in this unit, you have already started to learn the word-building system by identifying the basic

elements *or* parts

_____ of a medical word.

1–33   Understanding the word-building system will help you decipher the meanings of medical terms.

medical

Using the word-building system to identify basic elements of a medical word will help you learn _____ terminology.

A combining vowel is used to link a root to another root to form a compound word. This rule holds true even if the next root begins with a vowel, as in gastr/o/enter/itis.

o	**1–34** In the word *gastr/o/enter/itis,* the roots gastr (stomach) and *enter* (intestine) are linked together with the combining vowel _____.
leuk, cyt **-penia**	**1–35** The roots in *leuk/o/cyt/o/penia* are ___*leuk*___ and ___*cyt*___. The suffix is ___*penia.*___
leuk/o, cyt/o	**1–36** Identify the CFs in *leuk/o/cyt/o/penia:* _____ / _____ and _____ / _____.
electr/o, cardi/o	**1–37** List the CFs in *electr/o/cardi/o/gram:* _____ / _____ and _____ / _____.
back	**1–38** You are now using the programmed learning method. If you are experiencing difficulty writing the correct answers, go back to Frame 1–1 and rework the frames. To master material that has been covered, you can always go ___*back*___ to review the frames.

 Throughout the textbook, all word roots and combining forms that stand alone are set in **boldface**.

Suffixes   *e.g penia.*

A suffix is a word element located at the end of a word. Substituting one suffix for another suffix changes the meaning of the word. In medical terminology, a suffix usually indicates a procedure, condition, disease, or part of speech. In this text, a suffix that stands alone is preceded by a hyphen and will be set in **boldface blue.**

suffix	**1–39** The element at the end of a word is called the _____.
play/er **read/er** **speak/er**	**1–40** *Play, read,* and *speak* are complete words and also roots. Add the suffix *-er-* (meaning *one who*) to each root to modify its meaning. Play *becomes* _____ / _____. Read *becomes* _____ / _____. Speak *becomes* _____ / _____.

one who one who one who	**1–41** By attaching the suffix *-er* (*one who*) to *play*, *read*, and *speak*, we create nouns that mean the following: Play/*er* means _____ _____ *plays.* Read/*er* means _____ _____ *reads.* Speak/*er* means _____ _____ *speaks.*

A word root links a suffix that begins with a vowel.

tonsill/itis tŏn-sĭl-Ī-tĭs **gastr/ectomy** găs-TRĔK-tō-mē **arthr/itis** ăr-THRĪ-tĭs	**1–42** Link the following roots with suffixes, each of which begins with a vowel. Then, practice pronouncing the terms aloud by referring to the pronunciations in the left-hand-side answer column.

Word Root	Suffix		Medical Term
tonsill	*-itis*	becomes	_____ / _____
gastr	*-ectomy*	becomes	_____ / _____
arthr	*-itis*	becomes	_____ / _____

root, suffix	**1–43** Changing the suffix modifies the meaning of the word. In the word *dent/al*, *dent* is the word _____ and *-al* is the _____.

- ist -al	**1–44** A *dent/ist* is a specialist in teeth. *Dent/al* means *pertaining to teeth.* Simply changing the suffix gives the word a new meaning. The suffix in *dent/ist* is _____. It means *specialist.* The suffix in *dent/al* is _____. It means *pertaining to.*

A combining form (root + **o**) links a suffix that begins with a consonant.

scler/o/derma sklĕr-ō-DĔR-mă **mast/o/dynia** măst-ō-DĬN-ē-ă **arthr/o/plasty** ĂR-thrō-plăs-tē	**1–45** Change the following roots to CFs, and link them with suffixes that begin with a consonant. Then, practice pronouncing the terms aloud by referring to the pronunciations in the left-hand-side answer column.

Word Root	Suffix		Medical Term
scler	*-derma*	becomes	_____ / _____ / _____
mast	*-dynia*	becomes	_____ / _____ / _____
arthr	*-plasty*	becomes	_____ / _____ / _____

hyphen	**1–46** Throughout the book, whenever a suffix stands alone, it will be preceded by a hyphen, as in *-oma* **(tumor).** The hyphen indicates that another element is needed to transform the suffix into a complete word. A suffix that stands alone will be preceded by a _____.

tonsilitis

 Pronouncing medical words correctly is crucial because mispronunciations can result in incorrect medical interpretations and treatments. In addition, misspelled terms in a medical report may become a legal issue. Learning how to pronounce and spell medical terms correctly is a matter of practice. To familiarize yourself with medical words, make it a habit to pronounce a word aloud each time you see the pronunciation listed in the answer column.

dent/ist DĔN-tĭst **arthr/o/centesis** ăr-thrō-sĕn-TĒ-sĭs **neur/algia** nū-RĂL-jē-ă **angi/oma** ăn-jē-Ō-mă **nephr/itis** nĕf-RĪ-tĭs **scler/o/derma** sklĕr-ō-DĔR-mă	**1–47** Underline the <u>suffixes</u> in the following words: dent/ist arthr/o/cent<u>esis</u> neur/algia angi/oma nephr/itis scler/o/derma
arthr/o, scler/o **dent, neur, angi, nephr**	**1–48** Elements preceding a suffix can be a WR or a CF. Review the medical terms in Frame 1–47 and list the CFs: <u>arthr</u> / <u>o</u> and <u>scler</u> / <u>o</u>. List the WRs: _____, _____, _____, and _____.

1–49   Analyze the following medical terms by identifying their elements. The first is completed as an example. The vowel has no meaning of its own but enables two elements to be connected. Refer to Appendix A: Glossary of Medical Word Elements, page 575, if needed.

Find answers to this frame in Appendix B: Answer Key, page 585.

Medical Term	Combining Form (root + o)	Word Root	Suffix
arthr/o/scop/ic ăr-thrōs-KŎP-ĭk	*arthr* / *o*	*scop*	*-ic*
erythr/o/cyt/osis ĕ-rĭth-rō-sī-TŌ-sĭs	_____ / ____	_____	_____
dermat/itis dĕr-mă-TĪ-tĭs	_____ / ____	_____	_____
gastr/o/enter/itis găs-trō-ĕn-tĕr-Ī-tĭs	_____ / ____	_____	_____
orth/o/ped/ic or-thō-PĒ-dĭk	_____ / ____	_____	_____
oste/o/arthr/itis ŏs-tē-ō-ăr-THRĪ-tĭs	_____ / ____	_____	_____

suffixes	**1–50** The examples in Frame 1–49 show how medical words can be formed by various combinations of CFs, WRs, and _____.

In addition to word roots and combining forms in **boldface**, in subsequent frames, all suffixes that stand alone will be set in **boldface blue.**

Three Rules of Word Building

There are three important rules of word building:
- **Rule 1:** A root links a suffix that begins with a vowel.
- **Rule 2:** A combining form (root + **o**) links a suffix that begins with a consonant.
- **Rule 3:** A combining form (root + **o**) links a root to another root to form a compound word. (This rule holds true even if the next root begins with a vowel.)

leuk/emia
loo-KĒ-mē-ă

cephal/algia
sĕf-ă-LĂL-jē-ă

gastr/itis
găs-TRĪ-tĭs

append/ectomy
ăp-ĕn-DĔK-tō-mē

1–51   Rule 1: In the following examples, use a WR to link suffixes that begin with a vowel.

Word Root	Suffix		Medical Word
leuk	*-emia*	becomes	_____ / _____
cephal	*-algia*	becomes	_____ / _____
gastr	*-itis*	becomes	_____ / _____
append	*-ectomy*	becomes	_____ / _____

gastr/o/scope
GĂS-trō-skōp

men/o/rrhea
mĕn-ō-RĒ-ă

angi/o/rrhexis
ăn-jē-ō-RĔK-sĭs

ureter/o/lith
ū-RĒ-tĕr-ō-lĭth

1–52   Rule 2: In the following examples, use a CF (root + *o*) to link the suffixes that begin with a consonant.

Word Root	Suffix		Medical Term
gastr	*-scope*	becomes	_____ / _____ / _____
men	*-rrhea*	becomes	_____ / _____ / _____
angi	*-rrhexis*	becomes	_____ / _____ / _____
ureter	*-lith*	becomes	_____ / _____ / _____

oste/o/chondr/itis
ŏs-tē-ō-kŏn-DRĪ-tĭs

oste/o/chondr/oma
ŏs-tē-ō-kŏn-DRŌ-mă

oste/o/arthr/itis
ŏs-tē-ō-ăr-THRĪ-tĭs

gastr/o/enter/itis
găs-trō-ĕn-tĕr-Ī-tĭs

1–53   Rule 3: In the following four examples, apply the rule, "Use a CF (root + o) to link a root to another root to form a compound word." (This rule holds true even if the next root begins with a vowel.)

oste + chondr + *-itis* becomes _____ / _____ / _____ / _____.

oste + chondr + *-oma* becomes _____ / _____ / _____ / _____.

oste + arthr + *-itis* becomes _____ / _____ / _____ / _____.

gastr + enter + *-itis* becomes _____ / _____ / _____ / _____.

word root	**1-54** Would you use a WR or a CF as a link to the following suffixes? *-algia, -edema,* and *-uria* _____ _____
cardi/o/gram KĂR-dē-ō-grăm **Rule 2: A CF (root + o) links a suffix that begins with a consonant.**	**1-55** Refer to the three rules of word building on page 10 to complete Frames 1–55 to 1–59. Form a word with ***cardi*** and *-gram:* _____ / ____ / _____ (root)(suffix) Summarize the rule that applies in this frame. *Rule 2:* _____ _____
carcin/oma kăr-sĭ-NŌ-mă **Rule 1: A WR links a suffix that begins with a vowel.**	**1-56** Form a word with ***carcin*** and *-oma:* _____ / _____ (root)(suffix) Summarize the rule that applies in this frame. *Rule 1:* _____ _____
enter/o/cyst/o/plasty ĕn-tĕr-ō-SĬS-tō-plăs-tē **Rule 3: A CF links a root to another root to form a compound word.** **Rule 2: A CF links a suffix that begins with a consonant.**	**1-57** Complete the following frames to reinforce the three rules of word building on page 10. Build a medical word with ***enter + cyst + -plasty:*** _____ / ____ / _____ / ____ / _____ Summarize the word-building rules that apply in forming the previous term. (Use *CF* to indicate combining form.) *Rule 3:* _____ _____ *Rule 2:* _____ _____
leuk/o/cyt/o/penia loo-kō-sī-tō-PĒ-nē-ă **Rule 3: CF links a root to another root to form a compound word.** **Rule 2: CF links a suffix that begins with a consonant.**	**1-58** Build a medical word with ***leuk + cyt + -penia:*** _____ / ____ / _____ / ____ / _____. Summarize the word-building rules that apply in forming the previous term. *Rule 3:* _____ _____ *Rule 2:* _____ _____

erythr/o/cyt/osis
ĕ-rĭth-rō-sī-TŌ-sĭs

Rule 3: CF links a root to another root to form a compound word.

Rule 1: AWR links a suffix that begins with a vowel.

1–59 Build a medical word with *erythr + cyt + -osis:*

_____ / _____ / _____ / _____.

Summarize the word-building rules that apply in forming the previous term.

Rule 3: _____

_____

Rule 1: _____

_____

1–60 Review Figure 1-1 that follows. It illustrates examples of common word elements. The terms reinforce the study of the "Three Rules of Word Building" summarized on page 10. First, analyze the word elements and their meanings in the illustration. Then, complete the subsequent word-building frames. This engaging method will help you analyze, build, and define medical terms. It also facilitates active involvement in the learning process.

Find answers in Appendix A: Glossary of Medical Word Elements.

1–61 The following suffixes are illustrated in Figure 1-1. Review the suffixes, and then write the meaning of each suffix in the right-hand-side column.

Suffix	Meaning
-itis	_____
-ectomy	_____
-megaly	_____
-scopy	_____

hepat/itis
hĕp-ă-TĪ-tĭs

pancreat/itis
păn-krē-ă-TĪ-tĭs

cholecyst/itis
kō-lē-sĭs-TĪ-tĭs

append/ectomy
ăp-ĕn-DĔK-tō-mē

1–62 Identify and then break down the medical terms shown in Figure 1-1 with the meanings listed as follows:

inflammation of the liver   _____ / _____

inflammation of the pancreas   _____ / _____

inflammation of the gallbladder   _____ / _____

excision of the appendix   _____ / _____

gastr/o/megaly
găs-trō-MĔG-ă-lē

splen/o/megaly
splē-nō-MĔG-ă-lē

colon/o/scopy
kō-lŏn-ŎS-kō-pē

1–63 The suffix *-megaly* means enlargement; the suffix *-scopy* means visual *examination*. Identify and then break down the medical terms in Figure 1-1 with the following meanings:

enlargement of the stomach   _____ /o/ _____

enlargement of the spleen   _____ /o/ _____

visual examination of the colon   _____ /o/ _____

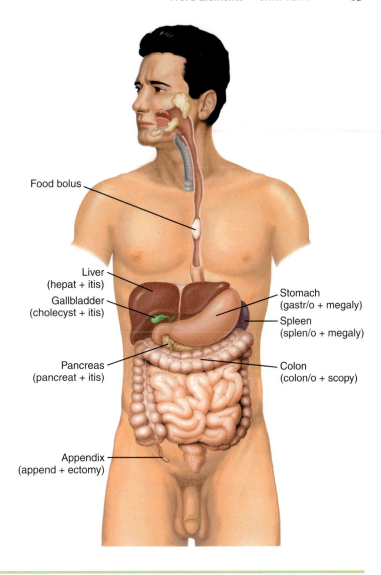

Food bolus

Liver
(hepat + itis)

Gallbladder
(cholecyst + itis)

Stomach
(gastr/o + megaly)

Spleen
(splen/o + megaly)

Pancreas
(pancreat + itis)

Colon
(colon/o + scopy)

Appendix
(append + ectomy)

Figure I-I Word elements of the digestive system.

 You are now beginning to learn various combinations of word elements discussed in this chapter. It is not necessary for you to know the meanings of all word elements yet because the terms and definitions will be reviewed again. At this time, it is important that you understand how to identify the component parts (word root, combining form, suffix of a word). If you can, you are ready to proceed, and congratulations as you begin your "study of medical terminology."

Prefixes

A prefix is a word element located at the beginning of a word. Substituting one prefix for another prefix changes the meaning of the word. A prefix usually indicates a number, time, position, or negation. Many prefixes found in medical terminology are also found in the English language. In this text, a prefix that stands alone is followed by a hyphen and will be set in boldface pink.

micro/cyte MĪ-krō-sīt	**I–64** In the term macro/*cyte, macro-* is a prefix that means *large; -cyte* is a suffix that means cell. A macro/cyte is a large *cell.* Form a new term meaning small cell by changing the prefix *macro-* to *micro-*: _____ / _____.

-al post- nat	**1-65** *Post/nat/al* refers to the period after birth. Identify the elements that mean *pertaining to:* _____. *after, behind:* _____. *birth:* _____.
pre/nat/al prē-NĀ-tl	**1-66** Use *pre-* (*before*) to build a word that means *pertaining to (the period) before* *birth:* _____ / _____ / _____.
beginning	**1-67** A prefix is a word element located at the _____ of a word.
intra- post- peri- pre-	**1-68** *Intra/muscul/ar, post/nat/al, peri/card/itis,* and *pre/operative* are medical terms that contain prefixes. Determine the prefix in this frame that means *in, within:* _____. *after:* _____. *around:* _____. *before, in front of:* _____.
prefix root suffix	**1-69** Whenever a prefix stands alone, it is identified with a hyphen after it, as in *hyper-*. When it is part of a word, the prefix is not highlighted, but a slash separates it from the next element, as in *hyper/tension.* Analyze *hyper/insulin/ism* by identifying the elements: *hyper-* is a _____. *insulin* is a _____. *-ism* is a _____.
prefixes	**1-70** *Hypo-, intra-, super-,* and *homo-* are examples of word elements called _____.
post/operative pōst-ŎP-ĕr-ă-tĭv after	**1-71** *Pre/operative* designates the time before a surgery. By changing the prefix, you alter the meaning of the word. Build a word that designates the time after surgery. _____ / _____. Can you remember what *post-* in post/operative means? _____.
post-, after after	**1-72** You will recognize many prefixes in medical terms because they are the same ones found in the English language. In the term *post/mortem,* the prefix is _____ and means _____. *Post/mortem* means _____ death.

pre-, before **before**	**1–73** In the term *pre/mature,* the prefix is _____ and means _____. *Pre/mature* means _____ maturity.

> In addition to word roots and combining forms in **boldface** and suffixes in **boldface blue,** in subsequent frames, all prefixes that stand alone will be set in **boldface pink** type.

Defining Medical Words

When defining a medical word, first, define the suffix; second, define the beginning of the word; and, finally, define the middle of the word. Here is an example using the term *osteoarthritis.*

oste/o/arthr/itis
(2)   (3)   (1)

1. Define the suffix first: *-itis* means inflammation.
2. Define the beginning of the word: *oste/o* means bone.
3. Define the middle of the word: *arthr* means joint.

Therefore, *oste/o/arthr/itis* is an inflammation of the bone and joint.

suffix **beginning** **last**	**1–74** The element that is defined first is the _____. The element that is defined next is the _____ of the word. The middle or rest of the word is defined _____.
-itis **gastr/o** **enter**	**1–75** Use the technique for defining medical words, described previously, to break the word *gastr/o/enter/itis* into its parts to define it. Write the element that is defined first: _____. Write the element that is defined next: _____ / _____. Write the element that is defined last: _____.
intestine (usually small)	**1–76** Appendix A: Glossary of Medical Word Elements on page 575 summarizes word elements and their meanings. Use this reference whenever you need to define an element. For example, look up the meaning of the CF *enter/o,* and write it here: _____
inflammation of the stomach and intestine (usually small intestine)	**1–77** Define gastr/o/enter/itis by using the technique for defining medical words as described previously. _____ _____

Pronunciation Guidelines

Although pronunciation of medical words usually follows the same rules that govern pronunciation of English words, you may have difficulty pronouncing some medical terms when you first encounter them. Phonetic pronunciation for selected terms in this book is included. In addition, you can find pronunciation guidelines on the inside back cover of this book. Use them whenever you need help with the pronunciation of medical words. Locate and study the pronunciation guidelines before proceeding with the pronunciation tools that follow.

Pronunciation Tools

At appropriate times in each chapter, you will be directed to use the following pronunciation tools:

- Visit the *Medical Terminology Simplified* online resource center at fadavis.com for an audio exercise of terms from the Word Elements tables. Other activities are also available to reinforce content.
- Visit the *Medical Terminology Simplified* online resource center at fadavis.com to hear the pronunciation and meaning of selected terms from the Medical Record Activities sections in Chapters 3-11.
- Visit the Medical Language Lab at *medicallanguagelab.com.* Use the "flash-card–word elements" exercises to reinforce your study of word elements. We recommend you complete the flash-card activity before starting the Word Elements Chapter Reviews.

SECTION REVIEW 1-1

Review the pronunciation guidelines (located on the inside back cover of this book). Use them as a reference, when needed. Then, in the following exercise, underline one of the items within parentheses to complete each sentence.

1. The diacritical mark ˘ is called a (breve, macron).

2. The diacritical mark ¯ is called a (breve, macron).

3. The macron (¯) above a vowel is used to indicate (short, long) vowel pronunciations.

4. The breve (˘) above a vowel is used to indicate the (short, long) vowel pronunciations.

5. When *pn* is in the middle of a word, pronounce (only *p, n, pn*). Examples are orthopnea and hyperpnea.

6. The letters c and g have a (hard, soft) sound before the letters *a* and *o.* Examples are cardiac, cast, gastric, and gonad.

7. When *pn* is at the beginning of a word, pronounce (only *p, n, pn*). Examples are *pn*eumonia and pneumotoxin.

8. When *i* is at the end of a word (to form a plural), it is pronounced like (*eye, ee*). Examples are bronchi, fung*i*, and nucle*i.*

9. For *ae* and *oe,* only the (first, second) vowel is pronounced. Examples are bursae, pleurae, and roentgen.

10. When *e* and es form the final letter or letters of a word, they are commonly pronounced as (combined, separate) syllables. Examples are syncope, systole, and appendices.

Competency Verification: Check your Answers in Appendix B: Answer Key, page 585. If you are not satisfied with your level of comprehension, review the pronunciation guidelines (on the inside back cover of this book), and retake the review.

Correct Answers _____ × 10 = _____ % Score

Common Suffixes

In previous frames, you learned that a CF is a WR + vowel and that the CF is the main part, or foundation, of a medical term. Examples of CFs are *gastr/o* (stomach), *dermat/o* (skin), and *nephr/o* (kidney). When you see *gastr/o* in a medical term, you will know that the term refers to the stomach. You also learned that a suffix is an element located at the end of a word. The following sections introduce common surgical, diagnostic, and pathological suffixes, as well as plural suffixes. Some of these elements have already been introduced in previous frames, but they are reinforced as follows.

Combinations of four elements are used to form medical words. These four elements are the WR, CF, suffix, and prefix. Some words may also be used as suffixes. Other words may consist of just a prefix and a WR.

Surgical Suffixes

Common suffixes associated with surgical procedures, their meanings, and an example of a related term are presented in the table that follows. First, study the suffix as well as its meaning. Then, pronounce the term, and place a ✓ in the box after you do so. Use the information to complete the meaning of the term. The first is completed for you. You may also refer to Appendix A: Glossary of Medical Word Elements, page 575. To build a working vocabulary of medical terms and understand how those terms are used in the health-care industry, it is important that you complete these exercises.

Suffix	Term	Meaning
-centesis surgical puncture	arthr/o/**centesis** ăr-thrō-DĒ-sĭs ☐ *arthr/o:* joint	*Surgical puncture of a joint (See Figure 1-2.)* *Arthrocentesis helps remove accumulated fluid or inject medications.*
-desis binding, fixation (of a bone or joint)	arthr/o/**desis** ăr-thrō-DĒ-sĭs ☐ *arthr/o:* joint	_____ _____ _____
-ectomy excision, removal	append/**ectomy** ăp-ĕn-DĔK-tō-mē ☐ *append:* appendix	_____ _____ _____
-lysis separation; destruction; loosening	thromb/o/**lysis** thrŏm-BŎL-ĭ-sĭs ☐ *thromb/o:* blood clot	_____ *Drug therapy for thrombosis usually helps dissolve the blood clot.*
-pexy fixation (of an organ)	mast/o/**pexy** MĂS-tō-pĕks-ē ☐ *mast/o:* breast	_____ *Mastopexy is performed to affix sagging breasts in a more elevated position, commonly improving their shape.*
-plasty surgical repair	rhin/o/**plasty** RĪ-nō-plăs-tē ☐ *rhin/o:* nose	_____ _____ _____
-rrhaphy suture	my/o/**rrhaphy** mī-OR-ă-fē ☐ *my/o:* muscle	_____ _____ _____
-stomy forming an opening (mouth)	trache/o/**stomy** tră-kē-ŎS-tō-mē ☐ *trache/o:* trachea (windpipe)	*Tracheostomy can help bypass an obstructed upper airway.*
-tome instrument to cut	oste/o/**tome** ŎS-tē-ō-tōm ☐ *oste/o:* bone	_____ _____
-tomy incision	trache/o/**tomy** tră-kē–ŎT-ō–mē ☐ *trache/o:* trachea (windpipe)	*Tracheotomy can help gain access to an airway below a blockage.*
-tripsy crushing	lith/o/**tripsy** LĬTH-ō-trĭp-sē ☐ *lith/o:* stone, calculus	_____ _____

Pronunciation Help	*Long Sound*	ā in rāte	ē in rēbirth	ī in īsle	ō in ōver	ū in ūnite
	Short Sound	ă in ălone	ĕ in ĕver	ĭ in ĭt	ŏ in nŏt	ŭ in cŭt

Competency Verification: Check your answers in Appendix B: Answer Key, page 586. If you are not satisfied with your level of comprehension, review the surgical suffixes and their meanings.

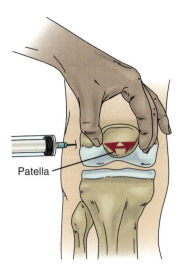

Patella

Figure 1-2 Arthrocentesis of the knee.

Diagnostic Suffixes

Common suffixes associated with diagnostic procedures, their meanings, and an example of a related term are presented in the table that follows. First, study the suffix as well as its meaning. Then pronounce the term, and place a ✓ in the box after you do so. Use the information to complete the meaning of the term. You may also refer to Appendix A: Glossary of Medical Word Elements, page 575. To build a working vocabulary of medical terms and understand how those terms are used in the health-care industry, it is important that you complete these exercises.

Suffix	Term	Meaning

-gram
 	
record, writing
	electr/o/cardi/o/**gram**
	ē-lĕk-trō-KĂR-dē-ō-grăm ☐
	  electr/o: electricity
	  cardi/o: heart
		_____
		
		An electrocardiogram allows for diagnosis of specific cardiac abnormalities. (See Figure 1-3.)

-graph
 	
instrument for recording
	electr/o/cardi/o/**graph**
	ē-lĕk-trō-KĂR-dē-ō-grăf ☐
	  electr/o: electricity
	  cardi/o: heart
		_____
		
		Interpretation of an output from the electrocardiograph includes heart rate and rhythm and identifying abnormalities in the shape of the electrical pattern produced on the graph paper. (See Figure 1-3.)

-graphy
 	
process of recording
	electr/o/cardi/o/**graphy**
	ē-lĕk-trō-kăr-dē-ŎG-ră-fē ☐
	  electr/o: electricity
	  cardi/o: heart
	  -graphy: process
	    of recording
		_____
		
		The electrocardiography (ECG) technician explains the procedure to the patient and attaches electrodes to perform the ECG (See Figure 1-3.)

Continued

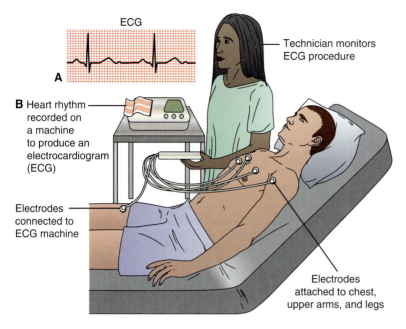

Figure I-3 Electrocardiography (ECG). The ECG technician attaches electrodes to the patient's chest (A) to produce an electrocardiogram (B).

Suffix	Term	Meaning
-meter	pelv/i/**meter***	_____
instrument for measuring	pĕl-VĬM-ĕ-tĕr ☐	_____
	pelv/i: pelvis	
-metry	pelv/i/**metry***	_____
act of measuring	pĕl-VĬM-ĕ-trē ☐	_____
	pelv/i: pelvis	
-scope	endo/**scope**	_____
instrument for examining	ĔN-dō-skōp ☐	_____
	endo-: in, within	
-scopy	endo/**scopy**	_____
visual examination	ĕn-DŎS-kō-pē ☐	_____
	endo-: in, within	

Pronunciation Help	Long Sound	ā in rāte	ē in rēbirth	ī in īsle	ō in ōver	ū in ūnite
	Short Sound	ă in ălone	ĕ in ĕver	ĭ in ĭt	ŏ in nŏt	ŭ in cŭt

*The *i* in *pelv/i/meter* is an exception to the rule of using the connecting vowel *o*.

Competency Verification: Check your answers in Appendix B: Answer Key, page 586. If you are not satisfied with your level of comprehension, review the diagnostic suffixes and their meanings.

Pathological Suffixes

Common suffixes associated with pathological (disease) conditions, their meanings, and an example of a related term are presented in the table that follows. First, study the suffix as well as its meaning. Then, pronounce the term, and place a ✓ in the box after you do so. Use the information to complete the meaning of the term. You may also refer to Appendix A: Glossary of Medical Word Elements, page 575. To build a working vocabulary of medical terms and understand how those terms are used in the health-care industry, it is important that you complete these exercises.

Suffix	Term	Meaning
-algia, -dynia pain	neur/**algia** nū-RĂL-jē-ă ☐ *neur:* nerve ot/o/**dynia** ō-tō-DĬN-ē-ă ☐ *ot/o:* ear	_____ _____ _____ _____
-cele hernia, swelling	hepat/o/**cele** hĕ-PĂT-ō-sēl ☐ *hepat/o:* liver	_____ _____
-ectasis dilation, expansion	bronchi/**ectasis** brŏng-kē-ĔK-tă-sĭs ☐ *bronchi:* bronchus (plural, bronchi)	_____ *Bronchiectasis is associated with various lung conditions and is commonly accompanied by chronic infection.*
-edema swelling	lymph/**edema** lĭmf-ĕ-DĒ-mă ☐ *lymph:* lymph	_____ _____ *Lymphedema may be caused by a blockage of the lymph vessels.*
-emesis vomiting	hyper/**emesis** hī-pĕr-ĔM-ĕ-sĭs ☐ *hyper-:* excessive, above normal	_____ _____
-emia blood condition	an/**emia** ă-NĒ-mē-ă ☐ *an-:* without, not	_____ *Iron deficiency anemia is a type of anemia caused by a lack of iron. (See Figure 1-4.)*
-iasis abnormal condition (produced by something specific)	chol/e/lith/**iasis*** kō-lē-lĭ-THĪ-ă-sĭs ☐ *chol/e:* bile, gall *lith:* stone, calculus	_____ _____
-itis inflammation	arthr/**itis** ăr-THRĪ-tĭs ☐ *arthr:* joint	_____ *Arthritis is commonly accompanied by pain, swelling, stiffness, and deformity. (See Figure 1-5.)*
-lith stone, calculus	chol/e/**lith*** KŌ-lē-lĭth ☐ *chol/e:* bile, gall	_____ _____

Continued

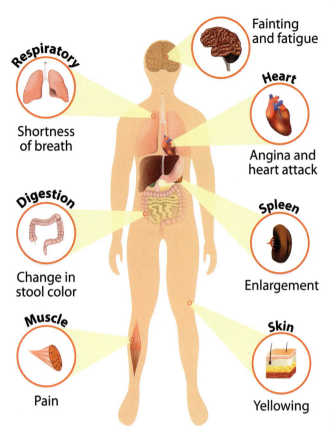

Fainting and fatigue

Respiratory
Shortness of breath

Heart
Angina and heart attack

Digestion
Change in stool color

Spleen
Enlargement

Muscle
Pain

Skin
Yellowing

Figure 1-4 Symptoms of iron deficiency anemia.

Suffix	Term	Meaning
-malacia softening	chondr/o/**malacia** kŏn-drō-mă-LĀ-shē-ă ☐ *chondr/o:* cartilage	_____ _____
-megaly enlargement	cardi/o/**megaly** kăr-dē-ō-MĔG-ă–lē ☐ *cardi/o:* heart	_____ _____
-oma tumor	neur/**oma** nū-RŌ-mă ☐ *neur:* nerve	_____ _____
-osis abnormal condition; increase (used primarily with blood cells)	cyan/**osis** sī-ă-NŌ-sĭs ☐ *cyan:* blue	_____ _____
-pathy disease	my/o/**pathy** mī-ŎP-ă-thē ☐ *my/o:* muscle	_____ _____
-penia decrease, deficiency	erythr/o/**penia** ĕ-rĭth-rō-PĒ-nē-ă ☐ *erythr/o:* red	_____ _____
-phobia fear	hem/o/**phobia** hē-mō-FŌ-bē-ă ☐ *hem/o:* blood	_____ _____

Suffix	Term	Meaning
-plegia paralysis	hemi/**plegia** hĕm-ē-PLĒ-jē-ă ☐ *hemi-:* one half	_____ _____ *Hemiplegia affects the right or left side of the body and is caused by a brain injury or stroke.*
-rrhage, -rrhagia bursting forth (of)	hem/o/**rrhage** HĔM-ĕ-rĭj ☐ *hem/o:* blood men/o/**rrhagia** mĕn-ō-RĀ-jē-ă ☐ *men/o:* menses, menstruation	_____ _____ _____ _____
-rrhea discharge, flow	dia/**rrhea** dī-ă-RĒ-ă ☐ *dia-:* through, across	_____ _____
-rrhexis rupture	arteri/o/**rrhexis** ăr-tē-rē-ō-RĔK-sĭs ☐ *arteri/o:* artery	_____ _____
-stenosis narrowing, stricture	arteri/o/**stenosis** ăr-tē-rē-ō-stĕ-NŌ-sĭs ☐ *arteri/o:* artery	_____ _____
toxic poison	hepat/o/**toxic** HĔP-ă-tō-tŏk-sĭk ☐ *hepat/o:* liver	_____ _____
-trophy nourishment, development	dys/**trophy** DĬS-trō-fē ☐ *dys-:* bad; painful; difficult	_____ _____

Pronunciation Help	Long Sound	ā in rāte	ē in rēbirth	ī in īsle	ō in ōver	ū in ūnite
	Short Sound	ă in ălone	ĕ in ĕver	ĭ in ĭt	ŏ in nŏt	ŭ in cŭt

*The e in *chol/e/lithiasis* and *chol/e/lith* is an exception to the rule of using the connecting vowel *o*.

Competency Verification: Check your answers in Appendix B: Answer Key, page pages 587 and 588. If you are not satisfied with your level of comprehension, review the pathological suffixes and their meanings.

 Visit the *Medical Terminology Simplified* online resource center at FADavis.com for an audio exercise of the terms in the Word Elements tables to help master pronunciations and meanings of the selected medical terms.

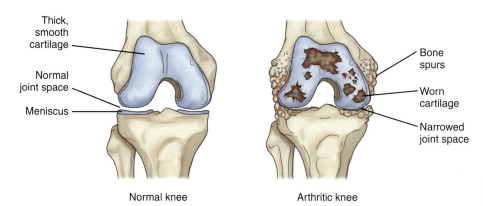

Thick, smooth cartilage

Normal joint space

Meniscus

Bone spurs

Worn cartilage

Narrowed joint space

Normal knee

Arthritic knee

Figure 1-5 (A) Normal knee. (B) Arthritis of the knee.

Plural Suffixes

Because many medical words have Greek or Latin origins, there are a few special rules you need to learn to change a singular word into its plural form. When you begin learning these rules, you will find that they are easy to apply. You will also find that some English word endings have been adopted for commonly used medical terms. When a word changes from the singular to the plural form, the suffix of the word is the part that changes. A summary of the rules for changing a singular word into its plural form is located on the page opposite the inside back cover of this book. Use it to complete Section Review 1–2 as follows and whenever you need help forming plural words.

SECTION REVIEW 1-2

Write the plural form for each of the following words, and state the rule that applies. The first word is completed for you.

Singular	Plural	Rule
sarcoma săr-KŌ-mă	*sarcomata*	*Retain the ma, and add ta.*
thrombus THRŎM-bŭs		
appendix ă-PĔN-dĭks		
diverticulum dī-vĕr-TĬK-ū-lŭm		
ovary Ō-vă-rē		
diagnosis dī-ăg-NŌ-sĭs		
lumen LŪ-mĕn		
vertebra VĔR-tĕ-bră		
thorax THŌ-răks		
spermatozoon spĕr-măt-ō-ZŌ-ŏn		

Competency Verification: Check your answers in Appendix B: Answer Key, page 588. If you are not satisfied with your level of comprehension, review the rules for changing a singular word into its plural form (on the page opposite the inside back cover of this book), and retake the review.

Correct Answers _____ × 10 = _____ % Score

Common Prefixes

Common prefixes, their meanings, and an example of a related term are presented in the table that follows. First, study the prefix as well as its meaning. Then, pronounce the term, and place a ✓ in the box after you do so. Use the information in the following table to complete the meaning of the term. You may also refer to Appendix A: Glossary of Medical Word Elements, page 575. To build a working vocabulary of medical terms and understand how those terms are used in the health-care industry, it is important that you complete these exercises.

Prefix	Term	Meaning
-a-*, an-* without, not	a/mast/ia ă-MĂS-tē-ă ☐ *mast:* breast *-ia:* condition	_____ _____ *Amastia may be the result of a congenital defect, an endocrine disorder, or mastectomy.*
	an/esthesia ăn-ĕs-THĒ-zē-ă ☐ *-esthesia:* feeling	_____ _____
auto- self, own	**auto**/graft AW-tō-grăft ☐ *-graft:* transplantation	_____ _____ *An example of an autograft is a transplant from the buttocks to the breast. (See Figure 1-6.)*

*The prefix *a-* is usually used before a consonant. **The prefix *an-* is usually used before a vowel.

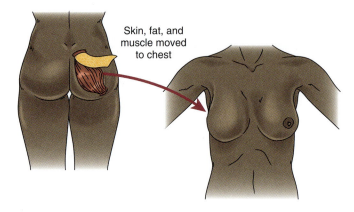

Skin, fat, and muscle moved to chest

Figure 1-6 Autograft in which tissue from the patient's buttocks is transplanted to her breast.

Prefix	Term	Meaning

circum-, peri-
around
	circum/duction
	sĕr-kŭm-DŬK-shŭn ☐
	    -duction: act of leading,
	                bringing, conducting
	
	peri/odont/al
	pĕr-ē-ō-DŎN-tăl ☐
	   odont: teeth
	    -al: pertaining to
		_____
		_____
		
		_____
		_____

dia-, trans-
through, across
	dia/rrhea
	dī-ă-RĒ-ă ☐
	   -rrhea: discharge, flow
	
	trans/vagin/al
	trăns-VĂJ-ĭn-ăl ☐
	   vagin: vagina
	    -al: pertaining to
		_____
		
		Diarrhea is a condition of abnormally frequent discharge or flow of fluid fecal matter from the bowel.
		
		_____
		_____

dipl-, diplo
double
	dipl/opia
	dĭp-LŌ-pē-ă ☐
	   -opia: vision
	
	diplo/bacteri/al
	dĭp-lō-băk-TĒR-ē-ăl ☐
	   bacteri: bacteria
	    -al: pertaining to
		_____
		_____
		
		_____
		
		Diplobacteria reproduce in such a manner that they are joined together in pairs.

endo-, intra-
in, within
	endo/crine
	ĔN-dō-krīn ☐
	   -crine: secrete
	
	intra/muscul/ar
	ĭn-tră-MŬS-kū-lăr ☐
	   muscul: muscle
	    -ar: pertaining to
		_____
		_____
		
		Endocrine refers to a gland that secretes directly into the bloodstream.
		
		_____
		_____

Continued

Prefix	Term	Meaning
hetero- different	**hetero**/graft HĔT-ĕ-rō-grăft ☐ *-graft:* transplantation	_____ _____ *A heterograft is also known as a xeno-graft. (See Figure 1-7.)*
homo-, homeo- same	**homo**/graft HŌ-mō-grăft ☐ *-graft:* transplantation **homeo**/plasia hō-mē-ō-PLĀ-zē-ă ☐ *-plasia:* formation, growth	_____ _____ *A homograft is called an allograft.* _____ _____
hypo- under, below, deficient	**hypo**/derm/ic hī-pō-DĔR-mĭk ☐ *derm:* skin *-ic:* pertaining to	_____ _____ *Hypodermic needles are used for injections and to take fluid samples from the body, for example, to take blood from a vein in venipuncture. (See Figure 1-8.)*

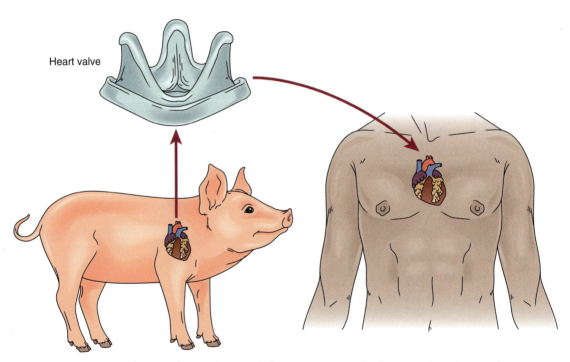

Heart valve

Figure I-7 Heterograft in which tissue (heart valve) from one species (pig) is transplanted to another species (human).

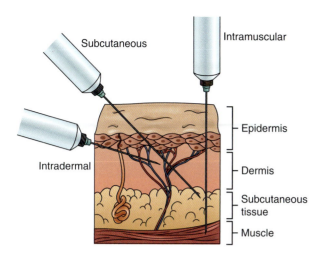

Subcutaneous

Intramuscular

Intradermal

- Epidermis

- Dermis

- Subcutaneous tissue

- Muscle

Figure I-8 Hypodermic needles inserted within the skin (intradermal), under the skin (subcutaneous), or within the muscular layer (intramuscular).

Prefix	Term	Meaning
macro- large	**macro**/cyte MĂK-rō-sīt ☐ -*cyte:* cell	_____ _____
micro- small	**micro**/scope MĬ-krō-skōp ☐ -*scope:* instrument for examining	_____ _____
mono-, uni- one	**mono**/cyte MŎN-ō-sīt ☐ -*cyte:* cell **uni**/nucle/ar ū-nĭ-NŪ-klē-ăr ☐ *nucle:* nucleus -*ar:* pertaining to	_____ _____ _____ _____
post- after, behind	**post**/nat/al pōst-NĀ-tăl ☐ *nat:* birth -*al:* pertaining to	_____ _____
pre-, pro- before, in front of	**pre**/nat/al prē-NĀ-tăl ☐ *nat:* birth -*al:* pertaining to **pro**/gnosis prŏg-NŌ-sĭs ☐ -*gnosis:* knowing	_____ _____ _____ _____
primi- first	**primi**/gravid prī-mĭ-GRĂV-ĭ-dă ☐ -*gravida:* pregnant woman	_____ _____

Continued

Prefix	Term	Meaning
retro- backward, behind	**retro**/version rĕt-rō-VĔR-shŭn ☐ *-version:* turning	_____ _____
super- upper, above	**super**/ior soo-PĒ-rē-or ☐ *-ior:* pertaining to	_____ _____

Pronunciation Help	Long Sound	ā in rāte	ē in rēbirth	ī in īsle	ō in ōver	ū in ūnite
	Short Sound	ă in ălone	ĕ in ĕver	ĭ in ĭt	ŏ in nŏt	ŭ in cŭt

Competency Verification: Check your answers in Appendix B: Answer Key, pages 588 and 589. If you are not satisfied with your level of comprehension, review the common prefixes tables. You may also visit the *medicallanguagelab.com* to review the chapter's flash-card exercises of suffixes and prefixes before proceeding to Chapter 2.

Visit the *Medical Terminology Simplified* online resource center at FADavis.com for an audio exercise of the terms in the Word Elements tables to help master pronunciations and meanings of the selected medical terms.

Body Structure

OBJECTIVES

Upon completion of this chapter, you will be able to:

- List and describe the basic structural units of the body.
- Describe the anatomical position of the body.
- Locate the body cavities and abdominopelvic regions of the body.
- Describe the terms related to the position, direction, and planes of the body and their applications during radiographic examinations.
- Describe the common diseases, conditions, and procedures related to several body systems.
- Recognize, define, pronounce, and spell terms correctly.
- Demonstrate your knowledge of this chapter by successfully completing the frames, reviews, and activities.

Levels of Organization

The human body consists of several structural and functional levels of organization. The complexity of each level increases from one to the next because the higher level incorporates the structures and functions of the previous level or levels. Eventually, all levels contribute to the structure and function of the entire organism. (See Figure 2-1.) The levels of organization from the least to the most complex are the:

- **cellular level,** the smallest structural and functional unit of the body.
- **tissue level,** groups of cells that perform a specialized function.
- **organ level,** groups of tissues that perform a specific function.
- **system level,** groups of organs that are interconnected or that have similar or interrelated functions.
- **organism level,** collection of body systems that make up the most complex level—a living human being.

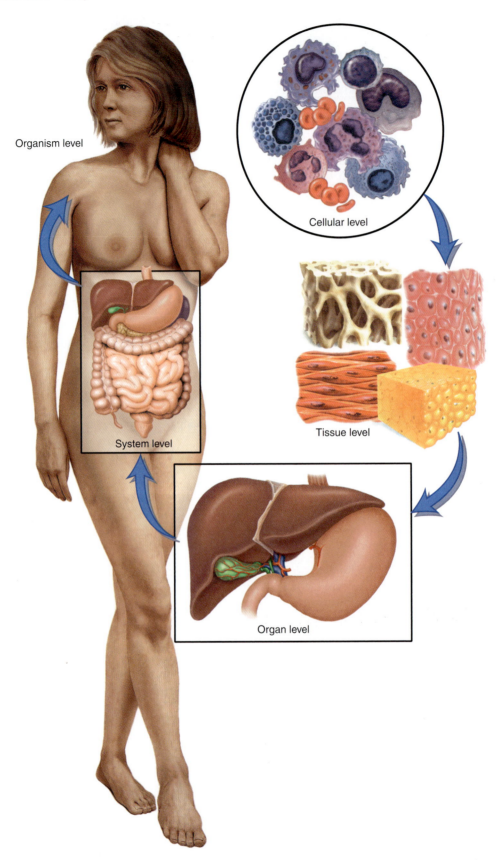

Figure 2-1 Levels of structural organization of the human body shown from the basic unit of structure, the cellular level, to the most complex, the organism level—a living human being. The body system illustrated is the digestive system.

WORD ELEMENTS

This section introduces word elements related to the basic structural units of the body and those that describe a particular location or direction in the body. Review the word elements and their meanings in the following table. Then, pronounce each term in the word analysis column and place a ✓ in the box after you do so.

Word Element	Meaning	Word Analysis
Combining Forms		
Basic Structural Units		
chondr/o	cartilage	**chondr**/oma (kŏn-DRŌ-mă ☐): - tumor composed of cartilage *-oma:* tumor
cyt/o	cell	**cyt/o**/meter (sī-TŎM-ĕ-ter ☐): instrument for counting and measuring cells *-meter:* instrument for measuring
hist/o	tissue	**hist/o**/lysis (hĭs-TŎL-ĭ-sĭs ☐): separation, destruction, or loosening of tissue *-lysis:* separation; destruction; loosening
nucle/o	nucleus	**nucle**/ar (NŪ-klē-ăr ☐): pertaining to the nucleus *-ar:* pertaining to
Directional		
anter/o	anterior, front	**anter**/ior (ăn-TĒ-rē-ōr ☐): pertaining to the front (of the body, organ, or structure) *-ior:* pertaining to
caud/o	**tail**	**caud**/ad (KAW-dăd ☐): toward the tail *-ad:* toward
dist/o	far, farthest	**dist**/al (DĬS-tăl ☐): pertaining to the farthest (point of attachment) *-al:* pertaining to
dors/o	back (of body)	**dors**/al (DŌR-săl ☐): pertaining to the back (of the body) *-al:* pertaining to
infer/o	lower, below	**infer**/ior (ĭn-FĒ-rē-or ☐): pertaining to below or lower (structure or surface) *-ior:* pertaining to
later/o	side, to one side	**later**/al (LĂT-ĕr-ăl ☐): pertaining to the side *-al:* pertaining to
medi/o	middle	**medi**/al (MĒ-dē-ăl ☐): pertaining to the middle *-al:* pertaining to
poster/o	back (of body), behind, posterior	**poster**/ior (pŏs-TĒ-rē-or ☐): pertaining to the back (of the body, organ, or structure) *-ior:* pertaining to
proxim/o	near, nearest	**proxim**/al (PRŎK-sĭm-ăl ☐): pertaining to the nearest (point of attachment) *-al:* pertaining to
super/o	upper, above	**super**/ior (soo-PĒ-rē-or ☐): pertaining to above or upper (part of the body, organ, or structure) *-ior:* pertaining to
ventr/o	belly, belly side	**ventr**/al (VĔN-trăl ☐): pertaining to the belly side (front of the body) *-al:* pertaining to

Continued

Word Element	Meaning	Word Analysis
Suffixes		
-ad	toward	medi/**ad** (MĒ-dē-ăd ☐) toward the middle or center *medi/o-:* middle
-logist	specialist in the study of	hist/o/**logist** (hĭs-TŎL-ō-jĭst ☐): specialist in the study of tissue *hist/o:* tissue
-logy	study of	cyt/o/**logy** (sī-TŎL-ō-jē ☐): study of cells *cyt/o:* cell
-lysis	separation; destruction; loosening	cyt/o/**lysis** (sī-TŎL-ĭ-sĭs ☐): destruction, dissolution, or separation of a cell *cyt/o:* cell
Pronunciation Help	*Long Sound* *Short Sound*	ā in rāte ē in rēbirth ī in īsle ō in ōver ū in ūnite ă in ălone ĕ in ĕver ĭ in ĭt ŏ in nŏt ŭ in cŭt

Visit the *Medical Terminology Simplified* online resource center at FADavis.com for an audio exercise of the terms in this table to help master pronunciations and meanings of the selected medical terms.

SECTION REVIEW 2-1

For the following medical terms, first write the suffix and its meaning. Then, translate the meaning of the remaining elements starting with the first part of the word. The first word is an example that is completed for you.

Term	Meaning
1. dist/al	–al: pertaining to*; far, farthest
2. poster/ior	
3. hist/o/logist	
4. dors/al	
5. anter/ior	
6. later/al	
7. medi/ad	
8. chondr/oma	
9. proxim/al	
10. ventr/al	

*Use the abbreviation PT to denote "pertaining to."

Competency Verification: Check your answers in Appendix B: Answer Key, page 590. If you are not satisfied with your level of comprehension, review the vocabulary, and retake the review.

Correct Answers _____ × 10 = _____ % Score

Basic Units of Structure

nucle/o

2-1   Cells are the smallest living units of structure and function in the human body. Every tissue and organ in the body is composed of cells. Review the illustration depicting the cellular level in Figure 2-1.

Note the nucleus, the darkened area in the center. The nucleus is the control center of the cell and is responsible for reproduction. This spherical unit contains genetic codes for maintaining life systems of the organism and for issuing commands for growth and reproduction.

The combining form (CF) for nucleus is _____ / _____.

-toxic

nucle/o

2-2   Any chemical substance, such as a drug, that interferes with or destroys the cellular reproductive process in the nucleus is referred to as a *nucle/o/toxic substance*. Examples of nucle/o/toxic drugs are those administered to patients with cancer during chemotherapy.

Identify the elements in this frame that mean

pertaining to poison: _____.

nucleus: _____ / _____.

cell	**2–3** Recall that *cyt/o* and *-cyte* are used to form words that refer to a _____.
cyt/o/logy sī-TŎL-ō-jē	**2–4** A cyt/o/logist is usually a biologist who specializes in the study of cells, especially one who uses cyt/o/log/ic techniques to diagnose neoplasms. Using *cyt/o,* build a word that means *study of cells:* _____ / _____ / _____.
cyt/o/logist sī-TŎL-ō-jĭst **cyt/o/meter** sī-TŎM- ĕ-ter	**2–5** Use *cyt/o* to form words that mean *specialist in the study of cells:* _____ / _____ / _____. *instrument for measuring cells (especially blood cells):* _____ / _____ / _____.
   -logist **hist/o**	**2–6** At the tissue level, the structural organization of the human body consists of groups of cells working together to carry out a specialized activity. (See Figure 2-1.) The medical scientist who specializes in the study of microscopic structures of tissues is called a hist/o/logist. Identify word elements *in hist/o/logist that mean* *specialist in the study of:* _____. *tissue:* _____ / _____.

 When defining a medical word, first define the suffix. Second, define the beginning of the word; finally, define the middle of the word. Here is an example of the term:

super/medi/al
(2)   (3)   (1)

1. Define the suffix first: *-al* means pertaining to.
2. Define the beginning of the word: *super-* means upper, above.
3. Define the middle of the word: *medi* means *middle.*

Directional Terms

The following frames introduce terms that describe regions of the body. Included are directional terms that describe a structure in relation to some defined center or reference point.

dors/al DŌR-săl **later/al** LĂT-ĕr-ăl **ventr/al** VĔN-trăl	**2–7** The suffixes *-ac, -al, -ar, -iac, -ic,* and *-ior* are adjective endings that mean pertaining to. You will find them used throughout this book. These suffixes help describe position, direction, body divisions, and body structures. Use the adjective ending *-al* to form words that mean *pertaining to the* *back (of body): dors* / _____. *side, to one side: later* / _____. *belly, belly side: ventr* / _____.

dors/al DŌR-săl **later/al** LĂT-ĕr-ăl **ventr/al** VĔN-trăl	**2-8** Practice building medical terms with *dors/o, later/o,* and *ventr/o.* Form medical terms that mean *pertaining to the* back (of body): ___dors___ / ___al___ . side, to one side: ___later___ / ___ac___ . belly, belly side: ___ventr___ / ___al___ .

2-9 Frame 2–7 reviews six adjective suffixes that mean pertaining to. Four additional adjective suffixes meaning pertaining to that are common in medical terms are *-ary, -eal, -ous,* and *-tic.* You may want to summarize these suffixes on a 5″×3″ index card and keep it in your book as a reference until you commit all of them to memory. However, if you are in doubt about meanings of any word elements, refer to Appendix A: Glossary of Medical Word Elements.

List in alphabetical order 10 adjective suffixes that mean pertaining to.

-ac

-al

-ar

-ary

-eal

-iac

-ic

-ior

-ous ✓

-tic

_____

_____

_____

_____

_____

_____

_____

_____

_____

_____

2-10 The human body is capable of being in many different positions, such as standing, kneeling, and lying down. To guarantee consistency in descriptions of location, the anatomic/al position is a reference point to describe the location or direction of a body structure. In anatomic/al position, the body is erect and the eyes are looking forward. The arms hang to the sides, with palms facing forward; the legs are parallel with the toes pointing straight ahead.

Review Figure 2-2, and study the terms to become acquainted with their usage in denoting positions of direction when the body is in the anatomic/al position. Refer to this figure to complete the following frames.

anatomic/al ăn-ă-TŎM-ĭk-ăl	**2-11** When a person is standing upright, facing forward, arms at his or her sides, palms facing forward, legs parallel, and feet slightly apart with the toes pointing forward, he or she is in the standard position called the _____ / _____ position.

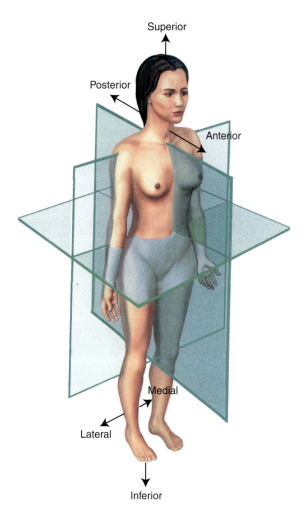

Figure 2-2 Directional terms. (Note the body is in the anatomical position.)

anter/ior, ventr/al ăn-TĒ-rē-or, VĔN-trăl **poster/ior, dors/al** pŏs-TĒ-rē-or, DŌR-săl	**2-12** Health-care professionals use a common language of special terms when referring to body structures and their functions. However, their descriptions of any region or part of the human body assume that it is in anatomic/al position. In anatomic/al position, the terms *anter/ior and ventr/al refer to the front of the body or the front of any body structure.* The terms *poster/ior and dors/al* refer to *the back of the body or the back of any body structure.* Identify the elements in this frame that refer to the *front of the body:* _____ / _____ *and* _____ / _____. *back of the body:* _____ / _____ *and* _____ / _____.
front **back**	**2-13** What position of the body do the terms *anter/ior* and *ventr/al* refer to? _____ (of the body) What position of the body do the terms *poster/ior* and *dors/al* refer to? _____ (of the body)

-ior **poster/o** **anter**	**2-14** *The term poster/o/anter/ior (PA) refers to the back and front of the body.* Identify the word elements in this frame that mean *pertaining to:* _____. *back:* _____ / _____. *front:* _____.
anterior or front ăn-TĒ-rē-or or **posterior *or* back** pŏs-TĒ-rē-or	**2-15** Directional terms are commonly used in radi/o/logy to describe the direction of the x-ray beam from its source and then its point of exit. A PA projection indicates that the path of the beam enters the body on the posterior side and exits anteriorly. (See Figure 2-3.) An anter/o/poster/ior (AP) projection indicates that the path of the beam enters the body on the _____ side and exits on the _____ side.
AP **PA**	**2-16** The chest x-ray (CXR) helps diagnose conditions affecting the chest, its contents, and nearby structures. It can be taken in either the AP or the PA position. The abbreviation that means *anter/o/poster/ior is* _____. *poster/o/anterior is* _____.
anter/ior ăn-TĒ-rē-or **poster/ior** pŏs-TĒ-rē-or	**2-17** Use *anter/ior* or *poster/ior* to complete the following statements, which refer to the position of body structures: The stomach is located on the ____anter____ / ____ior____ side of the body. The shoulder blades are located on the _____ / _____ side of the body.

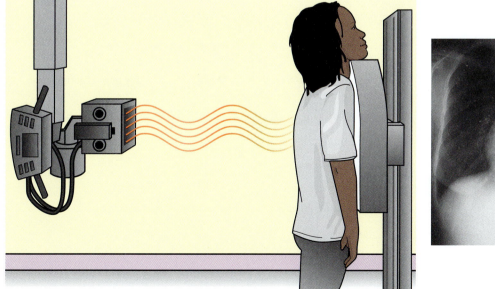
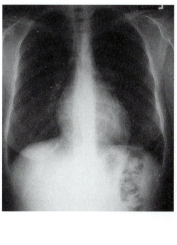

Figure 2-3 PA chest x-ray.

infer/ior ĭn-FĒ-rē-or	**2–18** The term *inferior* in the English language refers to something of little or no importance. However, when used in a medical report, it designates a position or direction meaning *lower, below*. Combine *infer/o* (lower, below) + *-ior* (pertaining to) to form a directional term that literally means *pertaining to lower or below*. _____ / _____
above	**2–19** In medical terms, the prefix *super-* designates an upper position. When you say "the head is superior to the stomach," you mean it is located above the stomach. When you say "the eyes are superior to the mouth," you mean they are located _____ the mouth.
side	**2–20** The word element *later/o* means **side, to one side.** A radiographic projection that enters through the left or right side of the body is referred to as a *later/al projection*. The term *later/al* position refers to the _____ (of the body).

> **Review the three basic rules for building medical words:**
> - **Rule 1:** The word root links a suffix that begins with a vowel.
> - **Rule 2:** The combining form (root + **o**) links a suffix that begins with a consonant.
> - **Rule 3:** The combining form (root + **o**) links a root to another root to form a compound word. (This rule holds true even if the next root begins with a vowel.)

later/al LĂT-ĕr-ăl **anter/o/later/al** ăn-tĕr-ō-LĂT-ĕr-ăl **poster/o/later/al** pŏs-tĕr-ō-LĂT-ĕr-ăl	**2–21** Following is a review of terms in radi/o/logy that specify the direction of the x-ray beam from its source to its exit surface before striking the film. Build directional terms that mean *pertaining to the side or to one side (of the body):* _____ / _____. *pertaining to the anterior, or front, and the side (of the body):* _____ / _____ / _____ / _____. *pertaining to the posterior, or back, and the side (of the body):* _____ / _____ / _____ / _____.
medi **-al**	**2–22** The term *medi/al* describes the midline of the body or a structure. The *medi/al* portion of the face contains the nose. From the term *medi/al,* determine the root that means *middle:* _____. suffix that means *pertaining to:* _____.
-ad, medi **medi/ad** MĒ-dē-ăd	**2–23** The suffix for *toward* is *-ad.* The word root for *middle* is _____. Combine *medi* + *-ad* to form a word that means *toward the middle.* _____ / _____

Pink indicates a prefix. Blue indicates a suffix. Boldface indicates a word root or combining form.

infer/ior ĭn-FĒ-rē-or **infer/ior** ĭn-FĒ-rē-or	**2-24** Anatomists and other health-care professionals use the *directional term* super/ior to refer to a body structure that is above another body structure or toward the head because the head is the most superior structure of the body. However, they use the term *infer/ior* to refer to a body structure located below another body structure or the lower part of a structure. For example, your chin is situated infer/ior to your mouth; and the rectum is the infer/ior portion of the colon. To indicate that a structure is below another structure, use the directional term _____ / _____ . To indicate the lower part of a structure, use the directional term _____ / _____ .
super/ior soo-PĒ-rē-or **infer/ior** ĭn-FĒ-rē-or **super/ior** soo-PĒ-rē-or	**2-25** Use *super/ior* or *infer/ior* to complete the following statements that refer to the relative position of one body structure to another body structure: The chest is _____ / _____ to the stomach. The stomach is _____ / _____ to the lungs. The head is _____ / _____ to the neck.
infer/ior ĭn-FĒ-rē-or **later/al** LĂT-ĕr-ăl	**2-26** Practice using the directional terms *later/al* and *infer/ior* to describe the following positions: The legs are _____ / _____ to the trunk. The eyes are _____ / _____ to the nose.
cephal/ad SĔF-ă-lăd	**2-27** *Cephal/ad* is a specific word that refers to the direction toward the head. When referring to the direction going toward the head, use the term _____ / _____ .
caud/al KAWD-ăl	**2-28** The CF *caud/o* means *tail.* In this sense, *tail* designates a position toward the end of the body, away from the head. In humans, it also refers to an infer/ior position in the body or within a structure. Combine *caud* + *al* to build a word that *means pertaining to the tail.* _____ / _____
proxim/al PRŎK-sĭm-ăl **dist/al** DĬS-tăl	**2-29** The terms *proxim/al* and *dist/al* are positional and directional terms. Proxim/al describes a structure as being nearest the point of attachment to the trunk or near the beginning of a structure. *Dist/al* describes a structure as being far from the point of attachment to the trunk or from the beginning of a structure. Identify the terms in this frame that mean *nearest the point of attachment:* _____ / _____ . *farthest from the point of attachment:* _____ / _____ .

proxim/al
PRŎK-sĭm-ăl

dist/al
DĬS-tăl

2-30   The directional element ***proxim/o*** means *near or nearest the point of attachment;* ***dist/o*** means *far or farthest from the point of attachment.* The knee is proxim/al to the foot; the palm is dist/al to the elbow.

To describe a structure nearest the point of attachment, use the directional term

_____ / _____.

To describe a structure as being farthest from the point of attachment, use the

directional term _____ / _____.

ad/duction
ă-DŬK-shŭn

2-31   Some directional terms, such as *ab/duction* and *ad/duction,* indicate movement away from the body and movement toward the body. (See Figure 2-4.)

The prefix *ab-* means *from, away from;* the suffix *-duction* means *act of leading, bringing, conducting.* Thus, *ab/duction means movement away from the body.*

Can you determine the directional term in this frame that means movement toward

the body? _____ / _____

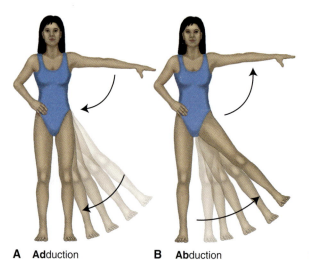

A   Adduction   **B   Ab**duction

Figure 2-4 (A) Adduction and (B) abduction.

SECTION REVIEW 2-2

Using the following table, write the CF or suffix that matches its definition in the space provided to the left of the definition. There may be more than one word element that matches a definition.

Combining Form

caud/o	later/o
cyt/o	medi/o
dist/o	proxim/o
hist/o	ventr/o
infer/o	

Suffix

-ad	-lysis
-al	-toxic
-ior	
-logist	
-logy	

1. _____ tissue

2. _____ pertaining to

3. _____ middle

4. _____ near, nearest

5. _____ study of

6. _____ cell

7. _____ belly, belly side

8. _____ poison

9. _____ toward

10. _____ tail

11. _____ specialist in study of

12. _____ far, farthest

13. _____ lower, below

14. _____ separation; destruction; loosening

15. _____ side, to one side

Competency Verification: Check your answers in Appendix B: Answer Key, page 590. If you are not satisfied with your level of comprehension, go back to Frame 2–1, and rework the frames.

Correct Answers _____ × 6.67 = _____ % Score

Frame **2–30** to Frame **2–31**

WORD ELEMENTS

This section introduces word elements that describe a body structure. When these elements are attached to positional prefixes or suffixes, they form words that describe a region or position in the body. Review the table, pronounce each term in the word analysis column, and place a ✓ in the box after you do so.

Word Element	Meaning	Word Analysis
Combining Forms		
abdomin/o	abdomen	**abdomin**/al (ăb-DŎM-ĭ-năl ☐): pertaining to the abdomen *-al:* pertaining to
cephal/o	head	**cephal**/ad (SĔF-ă-lăd ☐): toward the head *-ad:* toward
cervic/o	neck; cervix uteri (neck of uterus)	**cervic**/al (SĔR-vĭ-kăl ☐): pertaining to the neck of the body or the neck of the uterus *-al:* pertaining to
crani/o	cranium (skull)	**crani**/al (KRĀ-nē-ăl ☐): pertaining to the cranium or skull *-al:* pertaining to
gastr/o	stomach	**gastr**/ic (GĂS-trĭk ☐): pertaining to the stomach *-ic:* pertaining to
ili/o	ilium (lateral, flaring portion of hip bone)	**ili**/ac (ĬL-ē-ăk ☐): pertaining to the ilium *-ac:* pertaining to
inguin/o	groin	**inguin**/al (ĬNG-gwĭ-năl ☐): pertaining to the groin *-al:* pertaining to
lumb/o	loins (lower back)	**lumb**/ar (LŬM-băr ☐): pertaining to the loin area or lower back *-ar:* pertaining to
pelv/i*	pelvis	**pelv**/i/meter (pĕl-VĬM-ĕ-tĕr ☐): instrument for measuring the pelvis *-meter:* instrument for measuring
spin/o	spine	**spin**/al (SPĪ-năl ☐): pertaining to the spine or spinal column *-al:* pertaining to
thorac/o	chest	**thorac**/ic (thō-RĂS-ĭk ☐): pertaining to the chest *-ic:* pertaining to
umbilic/o	umbilicus, navel	peri/**umbilic**/al (pĕr-ē-ŭm-BĬL-ĭ-kăl ☐): pertaining to the area around the umbilicus *peri-:* around *-al:* pertaining to

Pronunciation Help						
	Long Sound	ā in rāte	ē in rēbirth	ī in īsle	ō in ōver	ū in ūnite
	Short Sound	ă in ălone	ĕ in ĕver	ĭ in ĭt	ŏ in nŏt	ŭ in cŭt

*The *i* in *pelv/i/meter* is an exception to the rule of using the connecting vowel *o*.

Visit the *Medical Terminology Simplified* online resource center at FADavis.com for an audio exercise of the terms in this table. It will help you master pronunciations and meanings of the selected medical terms.

Pink indicates a prefix. Blue indicates a suffix. Boldface indicates a word root or combining form.

SECTION REVIEW 2-3

For the following medical terms, first, write the suffix and its meaning. Then, translate the meaning of the remaining elements starting with the first part of the word. The first word is completed for you.

Term	Meaning
1. ili/ac	-ac: pertaining to; ilium (lateral, flaring portion of the hip bone)
2. abdomin/al	
3. inguin/al	
4. spin/al	
5. peri/umbilic/al	
6. cephal/ad	toward the head
7. gastr/ic	
8. thorac/ic	
9. cervic/al	
10. lumb/ar	

Competency Verification: Check your answers in Appendix B: Answer Key, page 590. If you are not satisfied with your level of comprehension, review the vocabulary, and retake the review.

Correct Answers _____ × 10 = _____ % Score

Body Planes

To visualize structural arrangements of various organs, the body may be sectioned (cut) according to planes of reference. The three major planes are the frontal, median, and horizontal planes, as shown in Figure 2-5.

2-32   Review the body planes illustrated in Figure 2-5 before proceeding. Use the figure to complete the following frames.

---

body plane

2-33   A body plane is an imaginary flat surface that divides the body into two sections. Different planes divide the body into different sections, such as front and back, left side and right side, and top and bottom. These planes serve as points of reference for describing the direction from which the body is being observed. Planes are particularly useful to describe views in which radiographic images are taken.

An imaginary flat surface that divides the body into two sections is a

_____ _____.

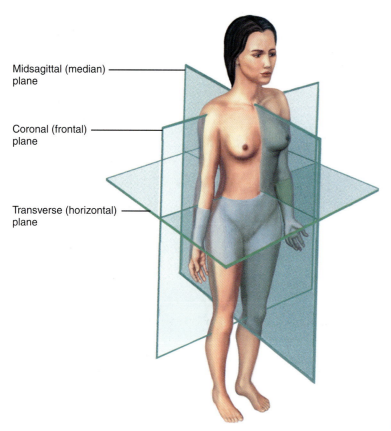

Midsagittal (median)
plane

Coronal (frontal)
plane

Transverse (horizontal)
plane

Figure 2-5 Body planes.

---

midsagittal (median)
mĭd-SĂJ-ĭ-tăl

coronal (frontal)
kŏ-rō-năl

transverse (horizontal)
trăns-VĔRS

2–34   Examine Figure 2-5 and list the three major planes of the body.

_____ (_____)

_____ (_____)

_____ (_____)

Competency Verification: When in doubt about the meaning of a word element, refer to Appendix A, page 575.

---

midsagittal
mĭd-SĂJ-ĭ-tăl

2–35   The median (midsagittal) plane lies exactly in the middle of the body and divides the body into two equal halves. (See Figure 2-5.)

When the chest is divided into equal right and left sides, it is divided by the median plane, also known as the _____ plane.

---

median

2–36   When the lungs are divided into equal right and left sides, they are divided by the midsagittal plane, also known as the _____ plane.

Pink indicates a prefix. Blue indicates a suffix. Boldface indicates a word root or combining form.

infer/ior, super/ior
ĭn-FĒ-rē-or, soo-PĒ-rē-or

2–37 The horizontal (transverse) plane runs across the body from the right side to the left side and divides the body into upper (superior) and lower (inferior) portions. Figure 2-5 shows the division of this plane.

Recall the term *super/ior*. It is a point of reference that refers to a structure above or oriented toward a higher place. For example, the head is superior to the heart. *Infer/ior* is a point of reference that refers to a structure situated below or oriented toward a lower place. For example, the feet are inferior to the legs.

Because the head is located superior to the heart, the heart is located

_____ / _____ to the head. Because the feet are located inferior to the

legs, the legs are located _____ / _____ to the feet.

transverse
trăns-VĔRS

2–38 The plane that divides the body into superior and inferior portions is the

horizontal plane. This plane is also called the _____ plane.

cross-sectional

2–39 Many different trans/verse planes exist at every possible level of the body, from head to foot. A trans/verse section is also called a *cross-sectional plane.* Some radiographic imaging devices produce cross-sectional images. Cross-sectioning of the body or of an organ along different planes results in different views.

In radiography, the horizontal, or trans/verse, plane is also known as the

_____ plane.

-graph

radi/o

trans-

-verse

2–40 A radi/o/graph of the liver along a trans/verse plane results in a different view than a radiograph along the frontal plane. That is why a series of x-rays commonly includes different planes. Views along different planes result in a comprehensive image of a body structure.

Identify the elements in this frame that mean

instrument for recording: _____.

radiation, x-ray; radius (lower arm bone on thumb side): _____ / _____.

through, across: _____.

turning: _____.

poster/ior
pŏs-TĒ-rē-or

2–41 The frontal (coronal) plane is commonly used to take anter/o/poster/ior (AP) chest radiographs, indicating that the x-ray beam enters the body on the

anterior side and exits the body on the _____ / _____ side. The radiograph produced shows a view from the front of the chest toward the back (of the body).

study of

2–42 In the previous frame, you learned that *anter/o/poster/ior* is used in radi/o/logy to describe the direction or path of an x-ray beam. The CF **radi/o** means *radiation; x-ray; radius (lower arm bone on thumb side).*

The suffix *-logy* means _____ _____.

radi/o/logy
rā-dē-ŎL-ō-jē

2–43 Use **radi/o** to form a word that means *study of radiation or x-rays:*

_____ / _____ / _____.

Body Cavities

Body cavities are hollow spaces within the body that contain, protect, and support internal organs. The cavities are also used as a point of reference to locate body structures within the cavities. There are four body cavities: two dors/al cavities, which are located in the back (posterior) part of the body, and two ventr/al cavities, which are located in the front (anterior) part of the body. (See Figure 2-6.)

2–44   The thorac/ic and abdominal cavities are separated by a muscular wall known as the diaphragm. Because the abdominal and pelvic cavities are not separated by a wall, they are commonly referred together as the abdominopelvic cavity. Review Figure 2-6 to study the location of the dors/al cavities.

crani/al
KRĀ-nē-ăl

spin/al
SPĪ-năl

2–45   The dors/al cavity is subdivided into the (1) **crani/al** and (2) **spin/al cav-ities.** The crani/al cavity is encased by the skull and contains the brain; the spin/al cavity contains the spinal cord.

Practice building words that refer to the body cavities by building a term that means

pertaining to the cranium (skull): _____ / _____.

pertaining to the spine: _____ / _____.

2–46   The (3) **diaphragm** is a dome-shaped muscle that plays an important role in breathing. It separates the thorac/ic cavity from the abdomin/o/pelv/ic cavity. Locate the diaphragm in Figure 2-6.

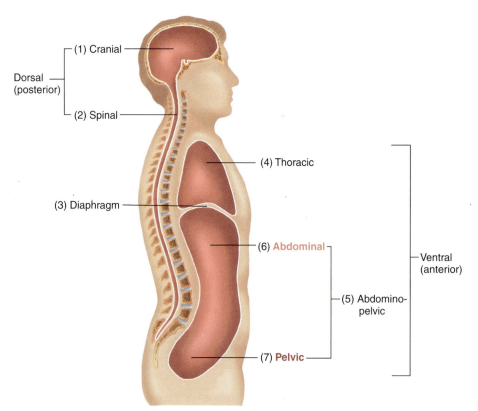

Dorsal (posterior)
(1) Cranial
(2) Spinal
(4) Thoracic
(3) Diaphragm
(6) Abdominal
Ventral (anterior)
(5) Abdomino-pelvic
(7) Pelvic

Figure 2-6 Body cavities.

Pink indicates a prefix. Blue indicates a suffix. Boldface indicates a word root or combining form.

pelv **thorac** **abdomin**	**2-47** Let us review some of the elements in the previous frame. Indicate the root that refers to the *pelvis:* _____. *chest:* _____. *abdomen:* _____.
	2-48 The major body cavities of the trunk are the thorac/ic and abdomin/o/pelv/ic cavities. The (4) **thoracic** cavity contains the heart and lungs, and the (5) **abdominopelvic** cavity contains the digestive and reproductive organs. The abdomin/o/pelv/ic cavity contains, by far, the greatest number of organs of any of the body cavities and is further subdivided into the (6) **abdominal** and (7) **pelvic** cavities. Locate these cavities in Figure 2-6.
ventr/al VĔN-trăl	**2-49** Review Figure 2-6 to identify the largest cavity in the body that incorporates the abdomin/o/pelv/ic and thorac/ic cavities: _____ / _____ cavity
super/ior soo-PĒ-rē-or **infer/ior** ĭn-FĒ-rē-or	**2-50** Medical personnel locate a structure of interest by referring to the body cavity in which it can be found. Use the terms *super/ior* and *infer/ior* to describe locations or positions of body cavities. The thoracic cavity is located _____ / _____ to the abdominopelvic cavity. The spinal cavity is located _____ / _____ to the cranial cavity.

Abdominopelvic Quadrants and Regions

The abdominopelvic cavity is further divided into quadrants and regions. (See Figure 2-7.)

Abdominopelvic Quadrants

	2-51 Because the abdomin/o/pelv/ic cavity is a large area and contains many organs, it is useful to divide it into smaller sections. One method divides the abdomin/o/pelv/ic cavity into quadrants. A second method divides the abdomin/o/pelv/ic cavity into regions. Physicians and other health-care professionals use quadrants or regions as a point of reference. The larger division of the abdomin/o/pelv/ic cavity consists of four quadrants: right upper quadrant (RUQ), left upper quadrant (LUQ), right lower quadrant (RLQ), and left lower quadrant (LLQ). Locate these quadrants in Figure 2-7A.
right upper quadrant **left upper quadrant** **right lower quadrant** **left lower quadrant**	**2-52** After you have located and reviewed the quadrants, determine the meaning of the following abbreviations. RUQ: _____ _____ _____ LUQ: _____ _____ _____ RLQ: _____ _____ _____ LLQ: _____ _____ _____

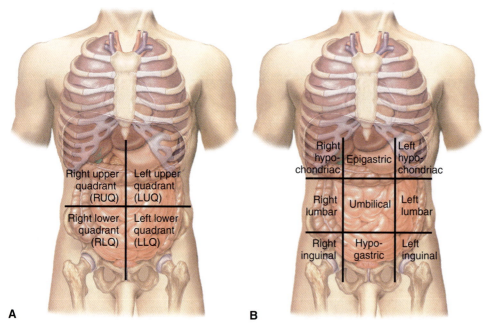

A   **B**

Figure 2-7 Abdominopelvic quadrants and regions. (A) Four quadrants of the abdomen.
(B) Nine regions of the abdomen showing the superficial organs.

RLQ	**2–53** Quadrants are useful in describing the location in the body where a surgical procedure will be performed. They are also useful in denoting incision sites or the location of abnormal masses, such as tumors. A tumor located in the right lower quadrant will most likely be denoted in the medical record with the abbreviation _____.
RLQ **LLQ**	**2–54** Quadrants may also describe the locations of the patients' symptoms. The physician may pinpoint a patient's abdominal pain in the RLQ. Such a finding could indicate a diagnosis of appendicitis because the appendix is located in that quadrant. Pain in another quadrant, such as the LLQ, would indicate a different diagnosis. *Identify the abbreviation for the* *right lower quadrant:* _____. *left lower quadrant:* _____.
left upper quadrant, **LUQ**	**2–55** Locate the quadrant that contains a major part of the stomach. This quadrant is the _____ _____ _____, and its abbreviation is _____.

Abdominopelvic Regions

2-56   Larger sections of the abdomin/o/pelv/ic cavity are divided into four quadrants, whereas the smaller sections are divided into nine regions, each of which corresponds to a region near a specific point in the body. As with quadrants, body region designation can also describe the location of internal organs and the origin of pain. Review Figure 2-7B to see the location of various organs within these regions.

hypo/chondr/iac
hī-pō-KŎN-drē-ăk

epi/gastr/ic
ĕp-ĭ-GĂS-trĭk

inguin/al
ĬNG-gwĭ-năl

lumb/ar
LŬM-băr

umbilic/al
ŭm-BĬL-ĭ-kăl

2-57   Now that you have examined the nine regions, let us review some of the terms within each region. These terms are commonly used to describe a location of organs within the abdominal cavity.

Although the CFs in the left-hand-side column of the table that follows denote a body structure, when attached to directional elements, they form terms denoting specific regions of the abdomen. Study the meaning of each regional term, and then divide each one in the right-hand-side column into its basic elements. The first term is completed for you.

Combining Form	Meaning	Regions of the Abdomen
chondr/o	cartilage	**hypo/chondr/iac***
gastr/o	stomach	**epigastric**
inguin/o	groin	**inguinal**
lumb/o	loins (lower back)	**lumbar**
umbilic/o	umbilicus, navel	**umbilical**

*Although *chondr/o* means *cartilage*, *hypo/chondr/iac* also refers to the right and left regions below the ribs.

hypo/gastr/ic
hī-pō-GĂS-trĭk

epi/gastr/ic
ĕp-ĭ-GĂS-trĭk

2-58   Use *gastr/o* to develop medical words that pertain to the area

under or below the stomach: _____ / _____ / _____.

above or on the stomach: _____ / _____ / _____.

epi/gastr/ic
ĕp-ĭ-GĂS-trĭk

2-59   The epi/gastr/ic region may be the location of "heartburn" pain. Pain in this area could be symptomatic of many abnormal conditions, including indigestion or heart attack.

The area of heartburn pain may be felt in the

_____ / _____ / _____ region.

Refer to Figure 2-7B to answer the following frames. If needed, use Appendix A: Glossary of Medical Word Elements, page 575.

loins (lower back)	**2–60** The lumbar regions consist of the middle right and middle left regions, located near the waistline of the body. *The term lumb/ar means pertaining to the* _____ (_____ _____).
umbilic/al ŭm-BĬL-ĭ-kăl	**2–61** The center of the umbilic/al region marks the point where the umbilic/al cord of the mother enters the fetus. This point is called the *navel* or, in layman's terms, the "belly button." The region that lies between the right and left lumbar regions is designated as the _____ / _____ region.
right inguin/al hernia ĬNG-gwĭ-năl HĔR-nē-ă	**2–62** Locate the right inguin/al region and the left inguin/al region in Figure 2-7B. A hernia on the right side of the groin is called a _____ _____ / _____ _____.
hypo/gastr/ic hī-pō-GĂS-trĭk	**2–63** The area between the right and left inguin/al regions is called the hypo/gastr/ic region. This region contains the large intestine (colon), which is involved in the removal of solid waste from the body. Identify the name of the region below the stomach that literally means *pertaining to below the stomach*. _____ / _____ / _____.

Pink indicates a prefix. Blue indicates a suffix. Boldface indicates a word root or combining form.

SECTION REVIEW 2-4

Using the following table, write the CF, suffix, or prefix that matches its definition in the space provided to the left of the definition. There may be more than one word element that matches a definition.

Combining Forms		Suffixes	Prefixes
abdomin/o	pelv/i, pelv/o	-ac	epi-
chondr/o	poster/o	-ad	hypo-
crani/o	spin/o	-al	
gastr/o	thorac/o	-ic	
inguin/o	umbilic/o	-ior	
lumb/o			

1. _____ad_____ toward

2. _____inguin/o_____ groin

3. _____gastr/o_____ stomach

4. _____pelv/o_____ pelvis

5. _____chondr/o_____ cartilage

6. _____epi/_____ above, on

7. _____al_____ pertaining to

8. _____lumb/o_____ loins (lower back)

9. _____thorac/o_____ chest

10. _____hypo-_____ under, below, deficient

11. _____crani/o_____ cranium (skull)

12. _____spin/o_____ spine

13. _____umbilic/o_____ umbilicus, navel

14. _____poster/o_____ back (of body), behind, posterior

15. _____abdomin/o_____ abdomen

Competency Verification: Check your answers in Appendix B: Answer Key, page 591. If you are not satisfied with your level of comprehension, go back to Frame 2–32, and rework the frames.

Correct Answers _____ × 6.67 = _____ % Score

Abbreviations

This section introduces abbreviations related to body structure and radiology.

Abbreviation	Meaning	Abbreviation	Meaning
Body Structure and Related			
AP	anteroposterior	LUQ	left upper quadrant
Bx, bx	biopsy	PA	posteroanterior; pernicious anemia; pulmonary artery; physician assistant
LAT, lat	lateral	RLQ	right lower quadrant
LLQ	left lower quadrant	RUQ	right upper quadrant
Radiology			
CT	computed tomography	PET	positron emission tomography
CXR	chest x-ray, chest radiograph	US	ultrasound; ultrasonography
MRI	magnetic resonance imaging	SPECT	single-photon emission computed tomography

Additional Medical Terms

The following are additional terms related to the structure of the body. Recognizing and learning these terms will help you understand the connection between a pathological condition, its diagnosis, and the rationale behind the method of treatment selected for a particular disorder.

Diseases and Conditions

adhesion
ăd-HĒ-zhŭn

Band of scarlike tissue that forms between two surfaces inside the body and causes them to stick together

Adhesions develop when the body's repair mechanisms respond to any tissue disturbance, such as surgery, infection, trauma, or radiation. Although adhesions can occur anywhere in the body, they form most commonly in the abdomen after abdominal surgery, inflammation, or injury (see Figure 2-8).

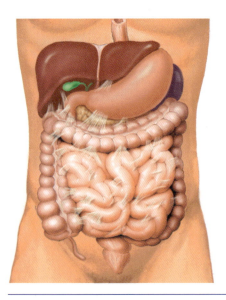

Figure 2-8 Abdominal adhesions.

edema ĕ-DĒ-mă **pitting**	Swelling caused by an abnormal accumulation of fluid in cells, tissues, or cavities of the body *Body parts swell from injury or inflammation. Edema can affect a small area or the entire body.* Edema caused by fluid accumulation that may be demonstrated by applying pressure to the swollen area (e.g., by depressing the skin with a finger). (See Figure 2-9.)

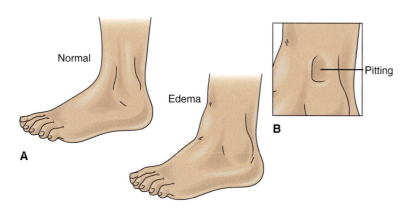

Figure 2-9 Normal foot. (A) Edema. (B) Pitting edema.

inflammation ĭn-flă-MĀ-shun	Protective response of body tissues to irritation, infection, or allergy *Signs of inflammation include redness, swelling, heat, and pain, commonly accompanied by loss of function.*

septicemia sĕp-tĭ-SĒ-mē-ă *septic:* infection *-emia:* blood	Systemic disease caused by infection with microorganisms and their toxins in circulating blood; also called sepsis and blood poisoning *If a patient becomes "septic," he or she will likely have low blood pressure leading to poor circulation. Septicemia can develop as a result of the body's own defense system or from toxic substances made by the infecting agent (e.g., a bacterium, virus, or fungus).*

Diagnostic Procedures

culture and sensitivity (C&S)	Laboratory test of a body fluid placed on a culture medium to identify the cause of an infection (usually a bacterium) and a sensitivity test that determines which antibiotic drug will work best to treat the infection *A C&S test may be done on many different body fluids, such as urine, mucus, blood, pus, saliva, spinal fluid, or discharge from the vagina or the penis. (See Figure 2-10.)*

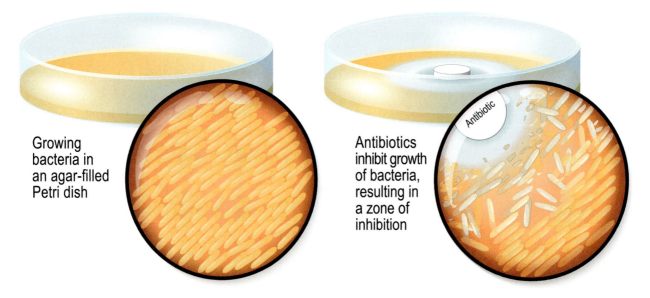

Growing bacteria in an agar-filled Petri dish

Antibiotics inhibit growth of bacteria, resulting in a zone of inhibition

Antibiotic

Figure 2-10: Culture and Sensitivity (C&S) Laboratory Test.

---

endoscopy

ĕn-DŎS-kō-pē

endo-: in, within
-scopy: visual
         examination

Visual examination of the interior of organs and cavities with a specialized lighted instrument called an endoscope

Endoscopy can also help obtain tissue samples for biopsy, perform surgery, and monitor the course of a disease, as in the assessment of the healing of gastric ulcers. The cavity or organ examined dictates the name of the endoscopic procedure, such as gastroscopy and bronchoscopy. Use of a camera and video recorder is common to provide a permanent record. (See Figure 2-11.)

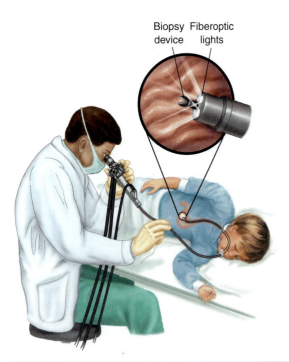

Biopsy   Fiberoptic
device   lights

Figure 2-11 Endoscopy of the stomach.

fluoroscopy floo-or-ŎS-kō-pē *fluor/o:* luminous, fluorescence *-scopy:* visual examination	Radiographic procedure that uses a fluorescent screen instead of a photographic plate to produce a visual image from x-rays that pass through the patient, resulting in continuous imaging of the motion of internal structures and immediate serial images *Fluoroscopy is invaluable in diagnostic and clinical procedures. It permits the radiographer to observe organs, such as the digestive tract and heart, in motion. It is also used during intrauterine fetal transfusion, biopsy, nasogastric tube placement, and cardiac catheterization.*
magnetic resonance imaging (MRI) măg-NĔT-ĭc RĔZ-ĕn-ăns ĬM-ĭj-ĭng	Radiographic procedure that uses electromagnetic energy to produce multiplanar cross-sectional images of the body *MRI does not require a contrast medium; however, one may be used to enhance visualization of internal structures. (See Figure 2-12E.) MRI is considered superior to CT for most abnormalities of the central nervous system (particularly of the brainstem and spinal cord), the musculoskeletal system, and the pelvic area.*
nuclear scan NŪ-klē-ăr	Radiographic procedure that produces images of an organ or area of the body by introducing a radionuclide substance (tracer or radiopharmaceutical) that releases a low level of radiation; also called nuclear scanning, radionuclide imaging, and nuclear medicine scan. (See Figure 2-12C.) *Nuclear scan uses a very small amount of radioactivity and is not known to cause harm.*
tomography tō-MŎG-ră-fē *tom/o:* to cut, slice *-graphy:* process of recording	Any of several radiographic procedures in which specialized machines produce a film representing a detailed cross section, or slice (cut), of an area, tissue, or organ *Tomography is a valuable diagnostic tool for identifying space-occupying lesions, such as those found in the liver, brain, pancreas, and gallbladder. Types of tomography include PET (see Figure 2-12F), CT, and SPECT.*
computed tomography (CT) cŏm-PŪ-tĕd tō-MŎG-ră-fē	Tomography in which a narrow beam of x-rays rotates in a full arc around the patient to acquire multiple views of the body, which a computer interprets to produce cross-sectional images of an internal organ or tissue; previously called computerized axial tomography (CAT) *CT scans help detect tumor masses, accumulations of fluid, and bone displacements. CT may be performed with or without a contrast medium. (See Figures 2-12D and 2-13.)*
ultrasonography (US) ŭl-tră-sŏn-ŎG-ră-fē *ultra-:* excess, beyond *son/o:* sound *-graphy:* process of recording	Radiographic procedure in which a small transducer passed over the skin transmits high-frequency sound waves (ultrasound) that bounce off body tissues and are then recorded to produce an image of an internal organ or tissue; also called ultrasound and echo. (See Figure 2-14.) *In contrast to other imaging techniques, US does not use ionizing radiation (x-ray). It is used to evaluate fetal development; examine internal structures of the abdomen, brain, and heart; diagnose musculoskeletal disorders; and evaluate blood flow. (See Figure 2-12B.) The record produced by US is called a sonogram or echogram.*
x-ray	High-energy electromagnetic waves (x-rays) pass through the body onto a photographic film to produce an image of internal structures of the body for diagnosis and therapeutic purposes; also called radiograph *Soft body tissues, such as the stomach or liver, appear black or gray on the x-ray; dense body tissues, such as bone, appear white, making it useful in diagnosing fractures. Figure 2-12A is a chest radiograph showing widening of the mediastinum.*

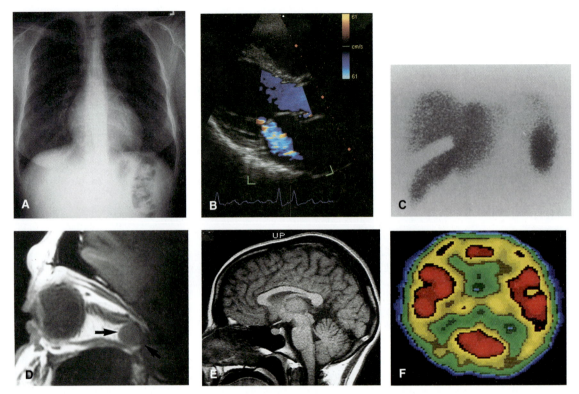

Figure 2-12 Medical imaging. (A) Chest radiograph. (B) Ultrasonogram of blood flow with color indicating direction. (C) Nuclear scan of the liver and spleen. (D) Computed tomography scan of eye showing a tumor below the optic nerve (arrow). (E) Magnetic resonance imaging scan of head. (F) Positron emission tomography scan of the brain. *(A) From McKinnis, L. Fundamentals of Orthopedic Radiology, page 149. F.A. Davis, 1997, with permission. (B) Courtesy of Suzanne Wambold, PhD, University of Toledo. (C) From Pittiglio, D.H. and Sacher, R.A. Clinical Hematology and Fundamentals of Hemostasis, page 302. F.A. Davis, 1987, with permission. (D, E, F) From Mazziotta, J.C., and Gilman, S. Clinical Brain Imaging: Principles and Applications, pages 27 and 298. Oxford University Press, 1992, with permission.*

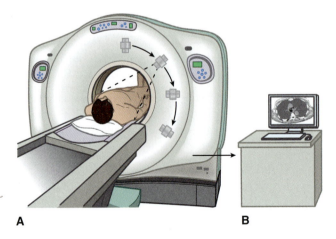

Figure 2-13 Computed tomography (CT) scan with motorized table (A) and computer (B).

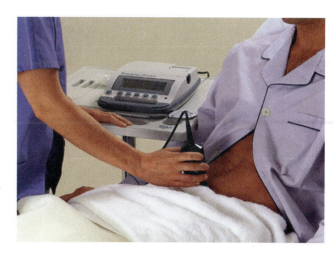

Figure 2-14 Ultrasonogram of the bladder. This bladder scan is performed at the bedside. It may be used instead of catheterization after the patient urinates to determine the amount of urine remaining in the bladder.

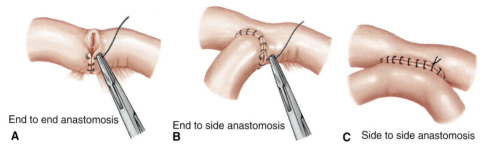

End to end anastomosis
A

End to side anastomosis
B

C   Side to side anastomosis

Figure 2-15 Anastomosis. (A) End-to-end anastomosis. (B) End-to-side anastomosis. (C) Side-to-side anastomosis.

Medical and Surgical Procedures

anastomosis ă-năs-tō-MŌ-sĭs	Connection between two vessels, such as the surgical joining of two ducts, blood vessels, or bowel segments, to allow flow from one to the other (See Figure 2-15.)
cauterize KAW-tĕr-īz	Destruction of abnormal tissue with an electrically heated instrument or chemicals (silver nitrate) *Cauterization is usually performed to destroy damaged or diseased tissues or coagulate blood vessels.*
incision and drainage (I&D)	Minor surgical procedure to release pus or pressure built up under the skin, such as from an abscess or boil

Pronunciation Help	*Long Sound*	ā in rāte	ē in rēbirth	ī in īsle	ō in ōver	ū in ūnite
	Short Sound	ă in ălone	ĕ in ĕver	ĭ in ĭt	ŏ in nŏt	ŭ in cŭt

WORD ELEMENTS REVIEW

This review provides a verification of your understanding of the word elements covered in this chapter. First, use a slash to break the term into its component parts and identify each element by labeling it P for prefix, WR for word root, CF for combining form, and S for suffix. Then, provide the meaning of the medical term. Remember to define the suffix first, define the beginning of the word second, and define the middle part of the term last. The first word is a sample completed for you.

Medical Term	Meaning
anter/ior *WR S*	*PT* to the front (of the body, organ, or structure)*
1. cephal/ad	
2. crani/o/meter	
3. epi/gastr/ic	
4. peri/umbilic/al	
5. poster/o/later/al	

*For adjective endings that mean pertaining to, use the abbreviation PT.

Match the medical terms that follow with definitions in the numbered list.

cauterize	endoscopy	septic
cephalad	hypogastric	superior
cytology	lateral	toxic
dorsal	radiology	transverse

6. _____ visual examination in or within (the body)

7. _____ PT under or below the stomach

8. _____ study of cells

9. _____ PT the side or to one side

10. _____ PT an infection

11. _____ PT poison

12. _____ toward the head

13. _____ study of radiation or an x-ray

14. _____ PT above or the upper part of a structure

15. _____ also called horizontal plane

Competency Verification: Check your answers in Appendix B: Answer Key, page 591. If you are not satisfied with your level of comprehension, review the vocabulary, and retake the review.

Correct Answers _____ × 6.67 = _____ % Score

Additional Medical Terms Review

Match the medical terms with the definitions in the numbered list.

adhesion   CT   inflammation   radiopharmaceutical
anastomosis   endoscope   MRI   septicemia
C&S   endoscopy   nuclear scan   tomography
cauterize   fluoroscopy   radiography   US

1. _____ uses a narrow beam of x-rays, which rotates in a full arc around the patient to obtain images of the body in cross-sectional slices.

2. _____ directs x-rays through the body to a fluorescent screen to view the motion of organs, such as the digestive tract and heart.

3. _____ employs high-frequency sound waves to produce images of internal structures of the body.

4. _____ employs magnetic energy (without ionizing x-rays) to produce cross-sectional images.

5. _____ is a laboratory test performed on a body fluid to identify the causative agent and its susceptibility to antibiotics.

6. _____ is a specialized lighted instrument to view the interior of organs and cavities.

7. _____ surgically joins two ducts, blood vessels, or bowel segments to allow flow from one to the other.

8. _____ is a protective response of body tissue that includes symptoms of redness, swelling, heat, and pain.

9. _____ is any of several radiographic techniques, such as CT, PET, or SPECT, that produce a film representing a detailed cross section of tissue structure.

10. _____ is a drug that contains a radioactive substance that travels to an area or a specific organ to be scanned.

11. _____ is a procedure to enable visualization of the interior of organs and cavities with a lighted instrument.

12. _____ is a procedure to burn abnormal tissue with electricity, heat, or chemicals.

13. _____ is a band of scar tissue that binds anatomical surfaces that normally are separate from each other.

14. _____ is a production of shadow images on photographic film.

15. _____ is a severe bacterial infection in the blood in which toxins circulating in blood cause severe systemic symptoms.

Competency Verification: Check your answers in Appendix B: Answer Key, page 591. If you are not satisfied with your level of comprehension, review the pathological, diagnostic, and therapeutic terms, and retake the review.

Correct Answers _____ × 6.67 = _____ % Score

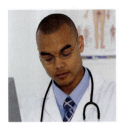

Medical Record Activities

The **medical record** is a chronological written account of a patient's examinations and treatments. It includes the patient's medical history and complaints, the physician's physical findings, the results of diagnostic tests and procedures, medication administration, and therapeutic procedures. Currently, the electronic medical record (**EMR**) is replacing the traditional paper-based medical record in doctor's offices, hospitals, clinics, and other health-care facilities. EMRs include general information, such as treatment and the medical history of a patient as it is collected by the individual medical practice. The EMR provides a platform to easily share medical documents among providers who are caring for the same patient so that there is continuity of treatment without duplication of effort.

In addition to ease of access, the EMR decreases errors associated with poor penmanship, lost pages, and misfiled records. It also provides instant documentation of health-care information that will be needed if legal issues arise. In addition, it is the basis for reimbursement of medical services. Therefore, it is important that all information entered into the medical record be complete, current, and correct, and that confidentiality be maintained.

Most hospitals, clinics, and other medical settings have converted some or all of their paper medical records to electronic versions. One significant difference between EMRs and paper medical records is that EMRs are universal—that is, instead of having different charts at different health-care facilities, a patient will have one electronic chart that can be accessed from numerous health-care facilities.

The medical record activities in subsequent chapters are designed to focus on the content and terminology of various types of medical records used in health-care facilities. In addition, the medical reports will help you develop the critical thinking skills necessary to interpret various reports you may encounter in a medical setting.

BODY STRUCTURE CHAPTER REVIEW

WORD ELEMENTS SUMMARY

The following table summarizes CFs, suffixes, and prefixes related to body structure.

Word Element	Meaning	Word Element	Meaning
Combining Forms			
abdomin/o	abdomen	**infer/o**	lower, below
anter/o	anterior, front	**inguin/o**	groin
caud/o	tail	**later/o**	side, to one side
cephal/o	head	**lumb/o**	loins (lower back)
cervic/o	neck; cervix uteri (neck of uterus)	**medi/o**	middle
chondr/o	cartilage	**nucle/o**	nucleus
crani/o	cranium (skull)	**pelv/o, pelv/i**	pelvis
cutane/o	skin	**poster/o**	back (of the body), behind, posterior
cyt/o	cell	**proxim/o**	near, nearest
dist/o	far, farthest	**radi/o**	radiation, x-ray; radius (lower arm bone on the thumb side)
dors/o	back (of the body)	**spin/o**	spine
fluor/o	luminous, fluorescence	**super/o**	upper, above
gastr/o	stomach	**thorac/o**	chest
hist/o	tissue	**umbilic/o**	umbilicus, navel
ili/o	ilium (lateral, flaring portion of the hip bone)	**ventr/o**	belly, belly side
Suffixes			
-ac, -al, -ar, -ary, -ous, -iac, -ic, -ior	pertaining to	**-meter**	instrument for measuring
-ad	toward	**-lysis**	separation; destruction; loosening
-graphy	process of recording	**-scopy**	visual examination
-logist	specialist in the study of	**-toxic**	poison
-logy	study of	**-verse**	turning
Prefixes			
endo-	in, within	**medi-**	middle
epi-	above, upon	**super-**	upper, above
hypo-	under, below; deficient	**trans-**	through, across

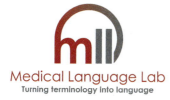

Medical Language Lab
Turning terminology into language

Visit the *Medical Language Lab* at medicallanguagelab.com. Use the flash-card word elements exercise to reinforce your study of word elements. We recommend you complete the flash-card activity before starting the Word Elements Review that follows.

Quadrants and Regions Review

In Figure A, label the four abdominopelvic quadrants; in Figure B, label the nine abdominopelvic regions.

Right upper quadrant (RUQ)
Left upper quadrant (LUQ)
Right lower quadrant (RLQ)
Left lower quadrant (LLQ)

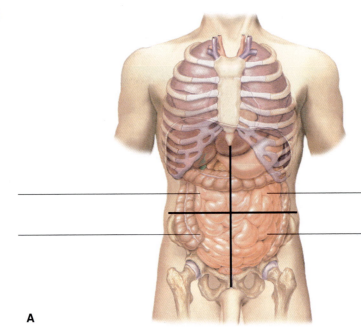

A

Right hypochondriac
Epigastric
Right lumbar
Right inguinal
Left hypochondriac
Umbilical
Left lumbar
Left inguinal
Hypogastric

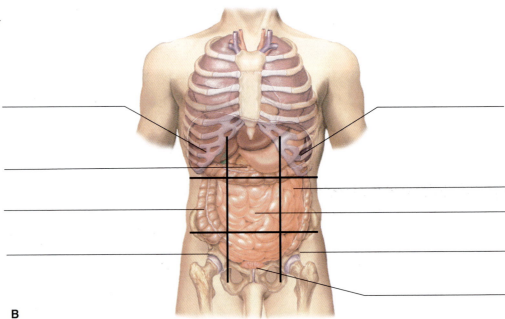

B

Competency Verification: Check your answers by referring to Figure 2-7, page 50.

Integumentary System

OBJECTIVES

Upon completion of this chapter, you will be able to:

• Describe the type of medical treatment the dermatologist provides.

• Identify the integumentary system structures by labeling the anatomical illustrations.

• Describe the primary functions of the integumentary system.

• Describe the diseases, conditions, and procedures related to the integumentary system.

• Apply your word-building skills by constructing various medical terms related to the integumentary system.

• Describe the common abbreviations and symbols related to the integumentary system.

• Recognize, define, pronounce, and spell terms correctly.

• Demonstrate your knowledge of this chapter by successfully completing the frames, reviews, and activities.

MEDICAL SPECIALTY: DERMATOLOGY

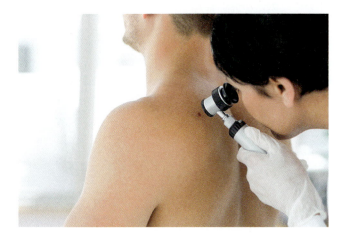

Dermatology is the medical specialty concerned with the diagnosis and treatment of diseases involving the skin and the relationship of skin lesions to systemic diseases. The physician who specializes in the diagnosis and treatment of skin diseases is called a *dermatologist*. The dermatologist's scope of practice includes management of skin cancers, moles, and other integumentary conditions. This specialist also uses various techniques for the enhancement and correction of cosmetic skin defects and prescribes measures to maintain the skin in a state of health.

Anatomy and Physiology Overview

The integumentary system consists of the skin and its accessory organs: hair, nails, sebaceous glands, and sweat glands. The skin is the largest organ in the body and protects the body from the external environment. It shields the body against injuries, infection, dehydration, harmful ultraviolet (UV) rays, and toxic compounds. Beneath the skin's surface is an intricate network of sensory receptors that register sensations of temperature, pain, and pressure. The millions of sensory receptors and a vascular network aid the functions of the entire body in maintaining homeostasis, which is the stable internal environment of the body. (See Figure 3-1.)

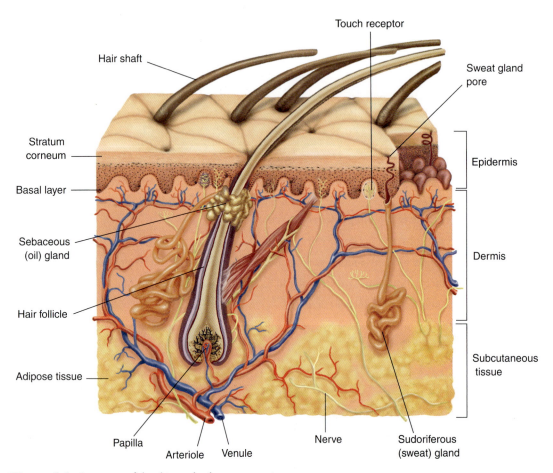

Figure 3-1 Structure of the skin and subcutaneous tissue.

WORD ELEMENTS

This section introduces word elements related to the integumentary system. Review the word elements and their meanings in the following table. Then, pronounce each term in the word analysis column, and place a √ in the box after you do so.

Word Element	Meaning	Word Analysis
Combining Forms		
adip/o	fat	**adip/o/cele** (ĂD-ĭ-pō-sēl ☐): hernia containing fat or fatty tissue *-cele:* hernia, swelling
lip/o		**lip/o/cyte** (LĬP-ō-sīt ☐): fat cell *-cyte:* cell
steat/o		**steat/itis** (stē-ă-TĪ-tĭs ☐): inflammation of fatty tissue *-itis:* inflammation
cutane/o	skin	**cutane/ous** (kū-TĀ-nē-ŭs ☐): pertaining to the skin *-ous:* pertaining to
dermat/o		**dermat/o/logist** (dĕr-mă-TŎL-ō-jĭst ☐): physician specializing in treating skin disorders *-logist:* specialist in the study of

derm/o		**hypo/derm/ic** (hī-pō-DĔR-mĭk ☐): pertaining to under or inserted under the skin, as in a hypodermic injection
		  hypo-: under, below, deficient
		  -ic: pertaining to

hidr/o	sweat	**hidr/aden/itis** (hī-drăd-ĕ-NĪ-tĭs ☐): inflammation of a sweat gland
		  aden: gland
		  -itis: inflammation
		
		Do not confuse hidr/o *(sweat) with* hydr/o *(water).*

sudor/o		**sudor/esis** (sū-dō-RĒ-sĭs ☐): condition of profuse sweating *-esis:* condition *Sudoresis is also referred to as* diaphoresis *and* hyperhidrosis.
ichthy/o	dry, scaly	**ichthy/osis** (ĭk-thē-Ō-sĭs ☐): abnormal condition of dryness and scaling of the skin *-osis:* abnormal condition; increase (used primarily with blood cells) *A mild form of ichthyosis, called winter itch, is common on the legs of older patients, especially during the dry winter months.*
kerat/o	horny tissue; hard; cornea	**kerat/osis** (kĕr-ă-TŌ-sĭs ☐): abnormal condition of overgrowth and thickening of the skin *-osis:* abnormal condition; increase (used primarily with blood cells)
melan/o	black	**melan/oma** (mĕl-ă-NŌ-mă ☐): malignant tumor of melanocytes that commonly begins in a darkly pigmented mole and can metastasize widely *-oma:* tumor *Melanomas are caused by intense exposure to sunlight and commonly metastasize throughout the body.*
myc/o	fungus (plural, *fungi*)	**dermat/o/myc/osis** (dĕr-mă-tō-mī-KŌ-sĭs ☐): fungal infection of the skin *dermat/o:* skin *-osis:* abnormal condition; increase (used primarily with blood cells)
onych/o	nail	**onych/o/malacia** (ŏn-ĭ-kō-mă-LĀ-shē-ă ☐): abnormal softening of the nails *-malacia:* softening

Continued

Word Element	Meaning	Word Analysis

pil/o	hair	**pil/o/nid/al** (pī-lō-NĪ-dăl ☐): pertaining to a growth of hair in a dermoid cyst or in a sinus opening on the skin
		  nid: nest
		  -al: pertaining to
		
		A pilonidal cyst commonly develops in the sacral region (fourth segment of the lower spinal column) of the skin. The cystic tumor contains elements derived from the ectoderm, such as hair, skin, sebum, or teeth.

trich/o		**trich/o/pathy** (trĭk-ŎP-ă-thē ☐): any disease of hair *-pathy:* disease
scler/o	hardening; sclera (white of eye)	**scler/o/derma** (sklĕr-ō-DĔR-mă ☐): chronic disease with abnormal hardening of the skin caused by formation of new collagen *-derma:* skin
seb/o	sebum, sebaceous	**seb/o/rrhea** (sĕb-or-Ē-ă ☐): discharge or flow of sebum; also called *seborrheic dermatitis* *-rrhea:* discharge, flow *Seborrhea is a common skin condition that mainly affects the scalp. It causes scaly patches, red skin, and stubborn dandruff. It can also affect oily areas of the body, such as the face, upper chest, and back.*
squam/o	scale	**squam/ous** (SKWĀ-mŭs ☐): covered with scales or scalelike *-ous:* pertaining to
xer/o	dry	**xer/o/derma** (zē-rō-DĔR-mă ☐): chronic skin condition characterized by excessive roughness and dryness *-derma:* skin *Xeroderma is a mild form of ichthyosis.*

<table>
<tr><td colspan="3">Suffixes</td></tr>
</table>

Word Element	Meaning	Word Analysis
-derma	skin	**py/o/derma** (pī-ō-DĔR-mă ☐): any pyogenic infection of the skin *py/o:* pus
-oid	resembling	**derm/oid** (DĔR-moyd ☐): resembling the skin *derm:* skin
-phoresis	carrying, transmission	**dia/phoresis** (dī-ă-fō-RĒ-sĭs ☐): condition of profuse sweating *dia-:* through, across *Diaphoresis is also referred to as* sudoresis *and* hyperhidrosis.
-plasty	surgical repair	**dermat/o/plasty** (DĔR-mă-tō-plăs-tē ☐): surgical repair of the skin *dermat/o:* skin
-therapy	treatment	**cry/o/therapy** (krī-ō-THĔR-ă-pē ☐): treatment using cold as a destructive medium *cry/o:* cold *Warts and actinic keratosis are some of the common skin disorders treated with cryotherapy.*

Pronunciation Help	*Long Sound*	ā in rāte	ē in rēbirth	ī in īsle	ō in ōver	ū in ūnite
	Short Sound	ă in ăpple	ĕ in ĕver	ĭ in ĭt	ŏ in nŏt	ŭ in cŭt

 Visit the *Medical Terminology Simplified* online resource center at FADavis.com for an audio exercise of the terms in this table to help master pronunciations and meanings of the selected medical terms.

SECTION REVIEW 3-1

For the following medical terms, first, write the suffix and its meaning. Then, translate the meaning of the remaining elements starting with the first part of the word. The first word is an example completed for you.

Term	Meaning
1. hypo/derm/ic	-ic: pertaining to; under, below, deficient; skin
2. melan/oma	_____
3. kerat/osis	_____
4. cutane/ous	_____
5. lip/o/cyte	_____
6. onych/o/malacia	_____
7. scler/o/derma	_____
8. dia/phoresis	_____
9. dermat/o/myc/osis	_____
10. cry/o/therapy	_____

Competency Verification: Check your answers in Appendix B: Answer Key, page 591. If you are not satisfied with your level of comprehension, review the vocabulary, and retake the review.

Correct Answers _____ x 10 = _____ % Score

Skin and Accessory Organs

The skin is a sensory organ that also provides protection for the body. The accessory organs of the skin include hair, nails, sebaceous glands, and sweat glands.

Skin

3-1   The skin is considered an organ and is composed of two layers of tissue: the outer epidermis, which is visible to the naked eye, and the inner layer, the dermis.

Identify and label the (1) **epidermis** and the (2) **dermis** in Figure 3-2.

---

epi/derm/is
ĕp-ĭ-DĔR-mĭs

derm/is
DĔR-mĭs

3-2   The epi/derm/is forms the protective covering of the body and does not have a blood or nerve supply. It is dependent on the dermis' network of capillaries for nourishment. As oxygen and nutrients flow out of the capillaries in the dermis, they pass through tissue fluid, supplying nourishment to the deeper layers of the epidermis.

When you talk about the outer layer of skin, you are referring to the

_____ / _____ / _____.

When you talk about the deeper layer of skin, consisting of nerve and blood vessels, you are talking about the _____ / _____.

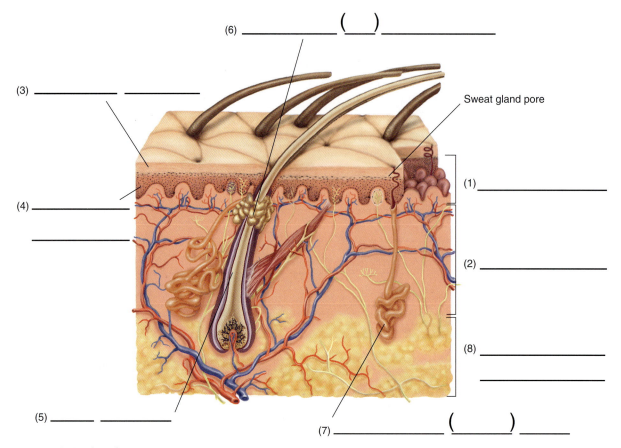

(6) _____ (__) _____

(3) _____ _____

Sweat gland pore

(4) _____

_____

(1) _____

(2) _____

(8) _____

_____

(5) _____ _____

(7) _____ (_____) _____

Figure 3-2 Identifying integumentary structures.

---

epi-

-is

3–3   The epi/derm/is is thick on the palms of the hands and the soles of the feet, but relatively thin over most other areas.

Identify the element in *epi/derm/is* that means

above or upon: _____.

a part of speech (noun): _____.

---

skin

3–4   The combining form (CF) *derm/o* refers to the skin. Derm/o/pathy is a

disease of the _____.

3–5   Although the epidermis is composed of several layers, the (3) **stratum corneum** and the (4) **basal layer** are of greatest importance.

The stratum corneum is composed of dead, flat cells. Its thickness is correlated with normal wear of the area it covers. Only the basal layer is composed of living cells. It is where new cells are continuously reproduced. Label these two structures in Figure 3-2.

3-6   As new cells form in the basal layer, they move toward the stratum corneum. Eventually, they die and become filled with a hard protein material called *keratin*. The relatively waterproof characteristic of keratin prevents body fluids from evaporating and moisture from entering the body. These keratinized cells gradually flake away and are replaced in a continuous cycle. The entire process by which a cell forms in the basal layers, rises to the surface, becomes keratinized, and sloughs off takes about 1 month.

Check the basal layer in Figure 3-1 to see the single row of newly formed cells in the deepest layer of the epi/derm/is.

---

skin

study, skin

3-7   In addition to ***derm/o,*** two other CFs for the skin are ***cutane/o*** and ***dermat/o.***

Cutane/ous means *pertaining to the* _____.

Dermat/o/logy is the _____ of the _____.

---

dermat/o/logist
dĕr-mă-TŎL-ō-jĭst

3-8   A physician who specializes in treating skin diseases is called a

_____ / _____ / _____.

---

skin

skin

3-9   The prefix *sub-* means *under* or *below;* the prefix *hypo-* means *under, below, deficient.*

A sub/cutane/ous injection occurs beneath the _____.

A hypo/derm/ic needle is inserted under the _____.

---

skin

3-10   *Sub/cutane/ous* literally means *pertaining to under the* _____.

---

skin

3-11   When you see the terms *derm/a, derm/is,* and *derm/oid,* you will know that

the roots refer to the _____.

---

skin

3-12   As discussed previously, suffixes *-al, -ic, -ior,* and *-ous* are adjective endings that mean *pertaining to.* Terms such as *derm/al* and *derm/ic* mean *pertaining to the*

_____.

---

melan/o/cyte
MĔL-ăn-ō-sīt

melan/oma
mĕl-ă-NŌ-mă

3-13   In the basal layer, specialized cells, called *melan/o/cytes,* produce a black pigment called *melanin.* Production of melanin increases with exposure to strong UV light. This exposure creates a suntan that provides a protective barrier from damaging effects of the sun.

The CF *melan/o* refers to the color black. Build a word that literally means

black cell: _____ / _____ / _____.

black tumor: _____ / _____.

3–14   Activity of melan/o/cytes is genetically regulated and inherited. Local accumulations of melanin are seen in pigmented moles and freckles. Environmental and physiological factors also play a role in skin color. Locate the basal layer in Figure 3-1.

---

albin/ism
ĂL-bĭn-ĭzm

3–15   Absence of pigment in the skin, eyes, and hair is most likely caused by an inherited inability to produce melanin. This lack of melanin results in the condition called *albin/ism*. A person with this condition is called an *albino*.

Deficiency or absence of pigment in the skin, hair, and eyes caused by an abnormality

in production of melanin is known as _____ / _____.

---

melanin
MĔL-ă-nĭn

3–16   The number of melan/o/cytes is about the same in all races. Differences in skin color are attributed to production of melanin. In people with dark skin, melan/o/cytes continuously produce large amounts of melanin. In people with light

skin, melan/o/cytes produce less _____.

When defining a medical word, first, define the suffix. Second, define the beginning of the word; finally, define the middle of the word. Following is an example of a term, which is translated as *abnormal condition of a skin fungus.*

dermat / o / myc / osis
(2)   (3)   (1)

3–17   Label Figure 3-2 as you learn about the parts of the dermis. The second layer of skin, the derm/is, contains the (5) **hair follicle,** (6) **sebaceous (oil) gland,** and (7) **sudoriferous (sweat) gland.**

---

inflammation, skin

3–18   Dermat/itis is an _____ of the _____ .

---

disease, skin

3–19   Derm/o/pathy is a disease of the skin; dermat/o/pathy is also a

_____ of the _____.

---

aden/oma
ăd-ĕ-NŌ-mă

3–20   An aden/oma is a benign (not malignant) neo/plasm in which the tumor cells form glands or glandlike structures. The tumor is usually well circumscribed, tending to compress, rather than infiltrate or invade, adjacent tissue.

Build a word that means *tumor composed of glandular tissue.*

_____ / _____

---

adip/ectomy
ăd-ĭ-PĔK-tō-mē

3–21   *Lip/o* and *adip/o* are CFs that mean *fat.* A lip/ectomy is excision of fat or adipose tissue.

Use *adip/o* to form another surgical term that means *excision of fat.*

_____ / _____

---

adip/o, lip/o **steat/o**	**3–22** *Adip/oma* and *lip/oma* are terms that mean *fatty tumor.* Both are benign tumors consisting of fat cells. The CFs in this frame that mean fat are _____ / _____ and _____ / _____. A third CF that refers to *fat* is _____ / _____.
	3–23 The dermis is attached to underlying structures of the skin by (8) **subcutaneous** tissue. Identify and label the layer of subcutaneous tissue in Figure 3-2.
sub/cutane/ous sŭb-kū-TĀ-nē-ŭs **lip/o/cytes** LĬP-ō-sītz	**3–24** Sub/cutane/ous tissue forms lip/o/cytes, also known as fat cells. Determine words in this frame that mean *pertaining to under or below the skin:* _____ / _____. *fat cells:* _____ / _____ / _____.
cell, tumor	**3–25** A lip/o/cyte is a fat _____, whereas an adip/oma is a fatty _____.

Competency Verification: Check your labeling of Figure 3-2 in Appendix B: Answer Key, page 592.

	3–26 Lip/o/suction is a form of plastic surgery in which sub/cutane/ous fat tissue is removed with a blunt-tipped cannula (tube) introduced into the fatty area through a small incision. Suction is then applied, and fat tissue is removed. Locate the sub/cutane/ous tissue in Figure 3-1.
fat	**3–27** Lip/o/suction is performed for cosmetic reasons. This surgical procedure removes localized areas of fat around the upper arms, breasts, abdomen, hips, legs, or buttocks, as shown in Figure 3-3. Lip/o/suction literally means *suction* *of* _____.
lip/ectomy lĭ-PĔK-tō-mē **ultra/son/ic** ŭl-tră-SŎN-ĭk	**3–28** Another type of lip/o/suction, ultra/son/ic-assisted lip/o/suction, uses ultra/son/ic waves to break up the fatty tissue before removal. This is also known as *suction-assisted lip/ectomy.* Identify the term that means *excision or removal of fat:* _____ / _____. *pertaining to excessive sound:* _____ / _____ / _____.
derm/o, dermat/o, **cutane/o**	**3–29** List three CFs that refer to the skin. _____ / _____, _____ / _____, and _____ / _____.

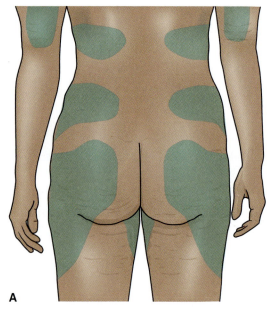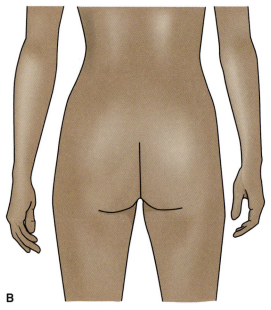

A　　　　　　　　　　　　　　　B

Figure 3-3 Liposuction. (A) Problem areas before liposuction. (B) Improved body contour after fluid retention and swelling diminishes.

dermat/o/plasty DĔR-mă-tō-plăs-tē **dermat/itis** dĕr-mă-TĪ-tĭs	**3–30**　Use *dermat/o* to form a word meaning *surgical repair (of the) skin:* _____ / _____ / _____. *inflammation (of the) skin:* _____ / _____.
dermat/o/plasty DĔR-mă-tō-plăs-tē	**3–31**　More specifically, *dermat/o/plasty* refers to any type of plastic surgery procedure of the skin, such as skin grafting, removal of a kel/oid, or a facelift. Build a word that means *surgical repair of the skin:* _____ / _____ / _____.
resembling	**3–32**　A **keloid** refers to a thickened scar that forms after an injury or surgical incision. (See Figure 3-4.) The suffix **-oid** means _____.
log **-ist** **-y**	**3–33**　The noun suffixes *-logy* and *-logist* contain the same root, *log/o,* which means *study of.* The *y* at the end of a term means *condition or process* and denotes a noun ending. The definitions of both suffixes are easier to remember if you analyze their components: *-logy* means study of; *-logist* means *specialist in the study of.* The root in each suffix that means *study of* is _____. The element in the suffix *-logist* that means specialist is _____. The element in the suffix *-logy* that means *condition or process* is _____.

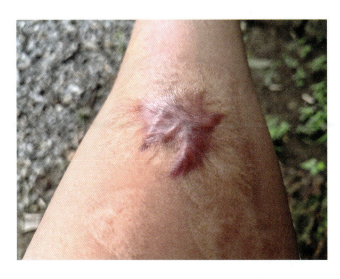

Figure 3-4 Close up of keloid scar on forearm following the healing of a wound resulting from an accident.

---

dermat/o/logy
dĕr-mă-TŎL-ō-jē

dermat/o/logist
dĕr-mă-TŎL-ō-jĭst

3-34 Refer to Frame 3–3 and use **dermat/o** to develop words that mean

study of the skin: _____ / _____ / _____ .

specialist who treats skin disorders: _____ / _____ /

_____ .

---

dermat/oma
dĕr-mă-TŌ-mă

dermat/o/pathy
dĕr-mă-TŎP-ă-thē

dermat/o/logy
dĕr-mă-TŎL-ō-jē

3-35 Use **dermat/o** to practice forming words that mean

tumor of the skin: _____ / _____ .

disease of the skin: _____ / _____ / _____ .

study of the skin: _____ / _____ / _____ .

---

hardening

3-36 Scler/osis is an abnormal condition of _____ .

---

skin

3-37 Scler/o/derma, a chronic hardening and thickening of the skin, is caused by new collagen formation. It is characterized by inflammation that ultimately develops into fibrosis (scarring), then sclerosis (hardening) of tissues.

Systemic scler/o/derma can be defined as hardening of the _____ .

---

system/ic scler/osis sĭs-TĔM-ĭk sklĕ-RŌ-sĭs **hardening**	**3–38** System/ic scler/osis, a form of scler/o/derma, is characterized by formation of thickened collagenous fibrous tissue, thickening of the skin, and adhesion to underlying tissues. The disease progresses to involve tissues of the heart, lungs, muscles, genit/o/urin/ary tract, and kidneys. A form of scler/o/derma that causes fibr/osis and scler/osis of multiple body systems is known as _____ / _____ _____ / _____. If you check **scler/o** in Appendix A: Glossary of Medical Word Elements, you will see that **scler/o** means *hardening; sclera (white of eye)*. In the integumentary system, however, **scler/o** specifically refers to _____.
horny tissue, hard **cornea**	**3–39** The CF **kerat/o** means *horny tissue; hard; cornea.* (The cornea of the eye is covered in Chapter 11.) When **kerat/o** is used in discussions of the skin, it refers to _____ _____ or _____. When **kerat/o** is used in discussions of the eye, it refers to the _____.
kerat/osis kĕr-ă-TŌ-sĭs	**3–40** Kerat/osis, a skin condition, is characterized by hard, horny tissue. A person with a skin lesion in which there is overgrowth and thickening of the epidermis most likely would be diagnosed with _____ / _____.
tumor	**3–41** A kerat/oma is a horny _____, also called *kerat/osis.*

Accessory Organs of the Skin

sebaceous sē-BĀ-shŭs **sudoriferous** sū-dŏr-ĬF-ĕr-ŭs	**3–42** Accessory organs of the skin include the sebaceous (oil) glands, sudoriferous (sweat) glands, hair, and nails. Refer to Figure 3-1 to complete this frame. Oil-secreting glands of the skin are called _____ glands. Sweat glands are called _____ glands.
comedos KŎM-ē-dōs **pustules** PŬS-tūlz	**3–43** Sebaceous glands are found in all areas of the body that have hair. The oily material, called sebum, is secreted by the sebaceous gland. It keeps hair and the skin soft and pliable and inhibits growth of bacteria on the skin. Increased activity of sebaceous glands at puberty may block the hair follicle and form blackheads (comedos). As bacteria feed on the sebum, they release irritating substances that produce inflammation. Large numbers of bacteria produce infection, forming whiteheads (pustules). Identify the medical term for *blackheads:* _____. *whiteheads:* _____.

Pink indicates a prefix. Blue indicates a suffix. Boldface indicates a word root or combining form.

sebaceous sē-BĀ-shŭs	**3–44** Comedos and pustules are the result of hypersecretion of sebum by the _____ (oil) glands.
sudoriferous sū-dŏr-ĬF-ĕr-ŭs	**3–45** Sweat glands that are not associated with hair follicles open to the surface of the skin through pores, as illustrated in Figure 3-1. These glands are stimulated by temperature increases or emotional stress and produce perspiration that evaporates on the surface of the skin and provides a cooling effect. Sweat, or perspiration, is produced by the _____ (sweat) glands.
hidr/osis hī-DRŌ-sĭs	**3–46** The CF for sweat is *hidr/o.* Use *-osis* to form a word that means: *abnormal condition of sweat:* _____ / _____.
sweat **gland** **inflammation**	**3–47** The term *dia/phoresis* denotes a *condition of profuse or excessive sweating.* The term *hidr/aden/itis* means: *hidr:* _____. *aden:* _____. *-itis:* _____.
excessive, above normal **sweat** **abnormal condition**	**3–48** The term *hyper/hidr/osis* also denotes a *condition of profuse or excessive sweating,* and it means *hyper-:* _____, _____ _____ *hidr:* _____ *-osis:* _____ _____
sweat, water	**3–49** Although *hidr/o* and *hydr/o* sound alike, they have different meanings. *Hidr/o* refers to _____. *Hydr/o* refers to _____.
an/hidr/osis ăn-hī-DRŌ-sĭs	**3–50** An/hidr/osis is an abnormal condition characterized by inadequate perspiration. When a person suffers from an absence of sweating, you would say the person has a condition called _____ / _____ / _____.
myc/osis mī-KŌ-sĭs	**3–51** The CF *myc/o* refers to a fungus (plural, *fungi*). Combine *myc/o* and *-osis* to form a word that means abnormal condition caused by fungi. _____ / _____
skin	**3–52** Dermat/o/myc/osis, a fungal infection of the skin, is caused by dermato-phytes, yeasts, and other fungi. When you see this term in a medical report, you will know it refers to a fungal infection of the _____.

fungus FŬN-gŭs	**3-53** Myc/o/dermat/itis, an inflammation of the skin, is caused by a _____.
derm/o/pathy dĕr-MŎP-ă-thē	**3-54** Use **derm/o** to form a medical term that means _disease of the skin._ _____ / _____ / _____
trich/o/pathy trĭk-ŎP-ă-thē **trich/osis** trĭ-KŌ-sĭs	**3-55** The CF **trich/o** refers to the hair. Construct medical terms that mean: _disease of the hair:_ _____ / _____ / _____. _abnormal condition of the hair:_ _____ / _____.
trich/o/myc/osis trĭk-ō-mī-KŌ-sĭs	**3-56** Combine **trich/o** + **myc** + **-osis** to form a medical term that means _abnormal condition of the hair caused by a fungus._ _____ / _____ / _____ / _____
hair	**3-57** Another CF for hair is **pil/o.** Whenever you see **pil/o** or **trich/o** in a word, you will know that it refers to the _____.
pil/o, -oid	**3-58** _Pil/o/cyst/ic_ refers to a _derm/oid cyst containing hair._ The element in this frame that means _hair_ is _____ / _____. The element in this frame that means _resembling_ is _____.

3-59   Label the structures of the fingernail in Figure 3-5 as you read the following material. Each nail is formed in the (1) **nail root** and is composed of keratin, a hard fibrous protein, which is also the main component of hair. As the nail grows from a (2) **matrix** of active cells beneath the (3) **cuticle**, it stays attached and slides forward over the epithelial layer, called the (4) **nailbed.** Most of the (5) **nail body** appears pink because of the underlying blood vessels. The (6) **lunula** is the crescent-shaped area at the base of the nail. It has a whitish appearance because the vascular tissue underneath does not show through.

Here is a review of the three basic rules of word building:
- **Rule 1:** The word root links a suffix that begins with a vowel.
- **Rule 2:** The combining form (root + **o**) links a suffix that begins with a consonant.
- **Rule 3:** The combining form (root + **o**) links a root to another root to form a compound word. (This rule holds true even if the next root begins with a vowel.)

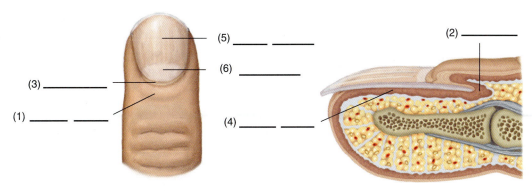

Figure 3-5 Structure of a fingernail.

onych/oma ŏn-ĭ-KŌ-mă **onych/o/pathy** ŏn-ĭ-KŎP-ăth-ē	**3–60**　The CF *onych/o* refers to the nail(s). Form medical words that mean *tumor of the nail (or nailbed):* _____ / _____ . *disease of the nail:* _____ / _____ / _____ .
onych/o/malacia ŏn-ĭ-kō-mă-LĀ-shē-ă	**3–61**　The term *malacia* means *abnormal softening of tissue.* This term is also used in words as a suffix. Build a word with *-malacia* that means *softening of the nail(s).* _____ / _____ / _____
onych/o **myc** **-osis**	**3–62**　Nails become white, opaque, thickened, and brittle when a person has a disease called *onych/o/myc/osis.* Identify elements in onych/o/myc/osis that mean nail: _____ / _____ . fungus: _____ . abnormal condition: _____ .
nail(s)	**3–63**　When you see the term *onych/o/myc/osis* in a medical chart, you will know that it means: an infection of the _____ caused by a fungus.
xer/o	**3–64**　The noun suffix *-derma* denotes *skin.* A person with excessive dryness of the skin has a condition called *xer/o/derma.* From xer/o/derma, identify the CF that means dry. _____ / _____
hernia, swelling	**3–65**　The suffix *-cele* refers to a _____ or _____ .
lip/o/cele LĬP-ō-sēl	**3–66**　A hernia containing fat or fatty tissue is called an *adip/o/cele* or _____ / _____ / _____ .

Competency Verification: Check your labeling of Figure 3-5 in Appendix B: Answer Key, page 592.

SECTION REVIEW 3-2

Using the following table, write the CF, suffix, or prefix that matches its definition in the space provided to the left of the definition. There may be more than one word element that matches a definition.

Combining Forms		Suffixes	Prefixes
adip/o	pil/o	-cele	epi-
cutane/o	scler/o	-derma	hypo-
derm/o	steat/o	-logist	
dermat/o	trich/o	-malacia	
hidr/o	xer/o	-osis	
lip/o		-pathy	
onych/o		-rrhea	

1. *nail* ___-Pathy___ disease
2. ___xer/o___ dry
3. ___steat/pil/o/ adip/o___ fat
4. ___-rr hea___ discharge, flow
5. ___cele___ hair
6. ___scler/o___ hardening; sclera (white of the eye)
7. ___-osis___ hernia; swelling
8. ___onyc/o___ nail
9. ___derma___ skin
10. ___malac'y___ softening
11. ___logist___ specialist in the study of
12. ___hypo___ above, upon
13. ___hyper___ abnormal condition; increase (used primarily with blood cells)
14. ___hidr/o___ sweat
15. ___epi___ under, below; deficient

Competency Verification: Check your answers in Appendix B: Answer Key, page 592. If you are not satisfied with your level of comprehension, go back to Frame 3–1, and rework the frames.

Correct Answers _____ x 6.67 = _____ % Score

When defining a medical word, first, define the suffix. Second, define the beginning of the word. Finally, define the middle of the word. Here is an example using the term:

sub / cutane / ous
(2)   (3)   (1)

Combining Forms Denoting Color

Skin

albin/ism
ĂL-bĭn-ĭzm

cyan/o/derma
sī-ă-nō-DĔR-mă

erythr/o/derma
ĕ-rĭth-rō-DĔR-mă

leuk/o/derma
loo-kō-DĔR-mă

melan/o/derma
mĕl-ăn-ō-DĔR-mă

xanth/oma
zăn-THŌ-mă

3-67 Examine the CFs that denote color and their meanings in the left-hand-side column of the table that follows. Examples of medical terms with their definitions are provided in the middle column. In the right-hand-side column, use a slash to break down each word into its basic elements.

Combining Form	Medical Term	Word Breakdown
albin/o: white	*albinism:* white condition	albinism
cyan/o: blue	*cyanoderma:* blue skin	cyanoderma
erythr/o: red	*erythroderma:* red skin	erythroderma
leuk/o: white	*leukoderma:* white skin	leukoderma
melan/o: black	*melanoderma:* black skin	melanoderma
xanth/o: yellow	*xanthoma:* yellow tumor	xanthoma

---

nouns

3-68 The *-a* ending in *cyan/o/derma, erythr/o/derma, leuk/o/derma,* and *melan/o/derma* designates that these words are (adjectives, nouns) _____.

---

erythr/o/derma
ĕ-rĭth-rō-DĔR-mă

melan/o/derma
mĕl-ăn-ō-DĔR-mă

xanth/o/derma
zăn-thō-DĔR-mă

xer/o/derma
zē-rō-DĔR-mă

3-69 Use *-derma* to build medical words that mean

skin that is red: __erythr__ / _o_ / __derma__.

skin that is black: __melan__ / _o_ / __derma__.

skin that is yellow: __xanth__ / _o_ / __derma__.

skin that is dry: __xer__ / _o_ / __derma__.

Cells

cells

cell

3-70 You already learned that a cell is the smallest basic unit of the human organism and that every tissue and organ in the human body is made up of cells.

Cyt/o/logy is the study of ___cells___.

The word elements **cyt/o** and **-cyte** are used to build words that refer to a

_____.

---

cells

3-71 *Cyt/o/logy* is the study of _____.

---

erythr/o/cyte
ĕ-RĬTH-rō-sīt

leuk/o/cyte
LOO-kō-sīt

melan/o/cyte
mĕl-ĂN-ō-sīt

xanth/o/cyte
ZĂN-thō-sīt

3–72   Use *-cyte* (cell) to form words that mean

cell that is red: _____ / _____ / _____.

cell that is white: _____ / _____ / _____.

cell that is black: _____ / _____ / _____.

cell that is yellow: _____ / _____ / _____.

-penia

leuk/o

cyt/o

3–73   Leuk/o/cyt/o/penia, an abnormal decrease in white blood cells (WBCs), may be caused by an adverse drug reaction, radiation poisoning, or a path/o/logic/al condition. The term *leuk/o/cyt/o/penia* is formed from the

suffix that means *decrease or deficiency:* _____.

CF that means *white:* _____ / _____.

CF that means *cell:* _____ / _____.

---

leuk/o/cyt/o/penia
loo-kō-sī-tō-PĒ-nē-ă

3–74   A deficiency in WBC production may be a sign of a path/o/logic/al

condition known as *leuk/o/penia* or _____ / _____ / _____ / _____ /

_____.

WBC

3–75   The abbreviation for *white blood cell* is _____.

---

blood

3–76   The suffix *-emia* is used in words to mean *blood condition*. Xanth/emia, an occurrence of yellow pigment in the blood, literally means *yellow*

_____.

---

xanth/omas
zăn-THŌ-măz

3–77   High cholesterol levels may cause small yellow tumors called

_____ / _____.

---

blood

white

3–78   Leuk/emia is a progressive malignant disease of the blood-forming organs. It is characterized by proliferation and development of immature leuk/o/cytes in blood and bone marrow.

Leuk/emia literally means *white* _____.

Leuk/o/cytes are _____ blood cells.

---

leuk/emia
loo-KĒ-mē-ă

3–79   A disease of unrestrained growth of immature WBCs is

called _____ / _____.

Pink indicates a prefix. Blue indicates a suffix. Boldface indicates a word root or combining form.

3-80   Melan/oma is a malignant neo/plasm (new growth) that originates in the skin and is composed of melan/o/cytes. The malignancy is attributed to a genetic predisposition and to exposure to ultraviolet light. (See Figure 3-6.)

melan/o/cyte
mĕl-ĂN-ō-sīt

melan/oma
mĕl-ă-NŌ-mă

Form medical words that literally mean:

black cell: _____ / _____ / _____.

black tumor: _____ / _____.

Boldface indicates a word root or combining form. **Boldface blue** indicates a suffix. **Boldface pink** indicates a prefix.

3-81   The lesion of melan/oma is characterized by its asymmetry, irregular border, and lack of uniform color. Malignant melan/oma is the most dangerous form of skin cancer because of its tendency to metastasize rapidly. Melanomas often metastasize to the lung(s), liver, bone, and brain.

melan/oma
mĕl-ă-NŌ-mă

The medical term that literally means *black tumor* is

_____ / _____.

3-82   Cyan/osis, also called *cyan/o/derma,* is caused by a deficiency of oxygen and an excess of carbon dioxide in the blood.

cyan/o/derma
sī-ă-nō-DĔR-mă

A person who is rescued from drowning exhibits a dark bluish or purplish discoloration of the skin. This condition is known as *cyan/osis* or

_____ / _____ / _____.

3-83   Use *-osis* to develop medical words that mean

cyan/osis
sī-ă-NŌ-sĭs

abnormal condition of blue (skin): _____ / _____.

erythr/osis
ĕr-ĭ-THRŌ-sĭs

abnormal condition of red (skin): _____ / _____.

melan/osis
mĕl-ăn-Ō-sĭs

abnormal condition of black (pigmentation): _____ / _____.

xanth/osis
zăn-THŌ-sĭs

abnormal condition of yellow (skin): _____ / _____.

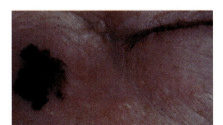

Cyanogri

Figure 3-6 Malignant melanoma. *From Goldsmith, LA, Lazarus, GS, and Tharp, MD: Adult and Pediatric Dermatology: A Color Guide to Diagnosis and Treatment. F.A. Davis, Philadelphia, 1997, p 146, with permission.*

increase

leuk/o/cyt/osis
loo-kō-sī-TŌ-sĭs

3–84   The suffix *-osis* is used in words to mean *abnormal condition*. However, when *-osis* is used in a word related to blood, it means *increase*. The complete meaning of *-osis* is *abnormal condition; increase (used primarily with blood cells)*.

The term *erythr/o/cyt/osis* is an _____ in red blood cells.

Use *leuk/o* (white) to build a term that means *increase in WBCs*:

_____ / _____ / _____ / _____ .

---

melan/oma
mĕl-ă-NŌ-mă

3–85   The most common skin cancers are basal cell carcinoma and squamous cell carcinoma.

Sun exposure, especially excessive tanning of the skin, can cause the lethal black

tumor called _____ / _____ .

---

carcin/oma
kăr-sĭ-NŌ-mă

3–86   Basal cell carcin/oma (BCC) is a skin cancer of the basal cell layer (deepest layer) of the epidermis. Metastasis is rare, but local invasion destroys underlying and adjacent tissue. This condition occurs most commonly on areas of the skin exposed to the sun. (See Figure 3-7.)

A type of skin cancer that affects the deepest layer of the epidermis is called basal cell

_____ / _____ .

---

carcin/oma
kăr-sĭ-NŌ-mă

in situ

3–87   There are two types of squamous cell carcinoma; those that are confined to the original site (in situ) and those that penetrate the surrounding tissue (invasive). Treatment includes surgical excision, cryotherapy, radiotherapy, or electrodesiccation and curettage.

A carcin/oma that affects the top layer of the epidermis is called squamous cell

_____ / _____ . (See Figure 3-8.)

When a squamous cell carcinoma is confined to the original site, it is known as

squamous cell carcinoma _____ _____ .

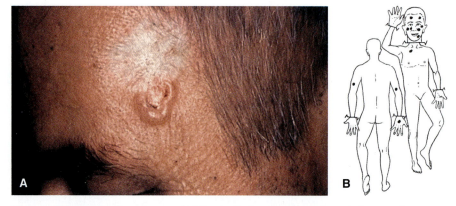

Figure 3-7 Basal cell carcinoma. (A) Pearly, flesh-colored papule with depressed center and rolled edge. (B) Common sites of basal cell carcinoma. *From Goldsmith, LA, Lazarus, GS, and Tharp, MD: Adult and Pediatric Dermatology: A Color Guide to Diagnosis and Treatment. F.A. Davis, Philadelphia, 1997, p 157, with permission.*

Pink indicates a prefix. Blue indicates a suffix. Boldface indicates a word root or combining form.

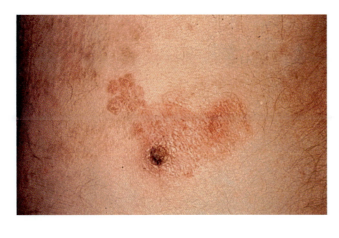

Figure 3-8 Squamous cell carcinoma, in which the surface is fragile and bleeds easily. *From Goldsmith, LA, Lazarus, GS, and Tharp, MD: Adult and Pediatric Dermatology: A Color Guide to Diagnosis and Treatment. F.A. Davis, Philadelphia, 1997, p 237, with permission.*

AIDS

Kaposi sarc/oma
KĂP-ō-sē săr-KŌ-mă

3-88   The CF *sarc/o* means *flesh (connective tissue).* Kaposi sarc/oma, a malignant skin tumor commonly associated with patients who are diagnosed with acquired immune deficiency syndrome (AIDS), is usually fatal. Initially, the tumor appears as a purplish brown lesion.

The abbreviation for *acquired immune deficiency syndrome* is _____.

The type of skin cancer associated with human immunodeficiency virus (HIV) is

_____ _____ / _____.

---

death

3-89   The CF *necr/o* is used in words to denote *death* or *necr/osis. Necr/o/tic* is a word that means *pertaining to necr/osis* or _____.

---

dead

3-90   The term *necr/osis* is used to denote the *death of areas of tissue or bone surrounded by healthy tissue.* Cellular necr/osis means that the cells are _____.

---

necr/osis
nĕ-KRŌ-sĭs

3-91   Bony necr/osis occurs when dead bone tissue results from the loss of blood supply (e.g., after a fracture). The term that means abnormal condition of death is

_____ / _____.

---

gangrene
GĂNG-grēn

3-92   Gangrene is a form of necr/osis associated with loss of blood supply. Before healing can take place, the dead matter must be removed.

When there is an injury to blood flow, a form of necr/osis may develop that is

known as _____.

---

self

self

self

3-93   In the English language, an *auto/graph* is a signature written by oneself. In medical words, *auto-* is used as a prefix and means *self, own.*

Auto/hypnosis is hypnosis of one's _____.

Auto/examination is an examination of one's _____.

An auto/graft is skin transplanted from one's _____.

---

auto/grafts
AW-tō-grăfts

3-94   A graft is tissue transplanted or implanted in a part of the body to repair a defect. Grafts done with tissue transplanted from the patient's own skin are called

_____ / _____.

SECTION REVIEW 3-3

Using the following table, write the CF, suffix, or prefix that matches its definition in the space provided to the left of the definition. There may be more than one word element that matches a definition.

Combining Forms		Suffixes		Prefixes
cyan/o	melan/o	-cyte	-osis	auto-
cyt/o	necr/o	-derma	-pathy	
erythr/o	xanth/o	-emia	-penia	
leuk/o		-oma	-rrhea	

1. _melan/o_ black
2. _cyan/o_ blue
3. _-emia_ blood condition
4. _cyte_ cell
5. _hpi_ decrease, deficiency
6. _pathy_ disease
7. _rrhea_ discharge, flow
8. _erythr/o_ red
9. _auto_ self, own
10. _derma_ skin
11. _-oma_ tumor
12. _leuk/o_ white
13. _xanth/o_ yellow
14. _necr/o_ death, necrosis
15. _-osis_ abnormal condition; increase (used primarily with blood cells)

Competency Verification: Check your answers in Appendix B: Answer Key, page 592. If you are not satisfied with your level of comprehension, go back to Frame 3–68, and rework the frames.

Correct Answers _____ × 6.67 = _____ % Score

Abbreviations

This section introduces abbreviations related to the integumentary system and their meanings.

Abbreviation	Meaning	Abbreviation	Meaning
AIDS	acquired immune deficiency syndrome	Dx	diagnosis
BCC	basal cell carcinoma	FH	family history
Bx, bx	biopsy	I&D	incision and drainage; irrigation and débridement
Derm	dermatology	PE	physical examination; pulmonary embolism; pressure-equalizing tube
HIV	human immunodeficiency virus	WBC, wbc	white blood cell

Additional Medical Terms

The following terms are additional terms related to the integumentary system. Recognizing and learning these terms will help you understand the connection between common signs, symptoms, and diseases and their diagnoses, as well as the rationale behind methods of treatment selected for a particular disorder.

Diseases and Conditions

abrasion
ă-BRĀ-zhŭn

Scraping, or rubbing away of a surface, such as skin, by friction

Abrasion may be the result of trauma, such as a skinned knee; therapy, as in dermabrasion of the skin to remove scar tissue; or normal function, such as the wearing down of a tooth by mastication.

---

abscess
ĂB-sĕs

Localized collection of pus at the site of an infection (characteristically, a staphylococcal infection)

An abscess can occur in any body part. Treatment includes oral antibiotics and incision and drainage (I&D) to drain the purulent material. (See Figure 3-9.)

furuncle
FŪ-rŭng-kl

Abscess that originates in a hair follicle; also called *boil*

carbuncle
KĂR-bŭng-kl

Cluster of furuncles in the subcutaneous tissue

Large furuncles with connecting channels to the skin surface form a carbuncle.

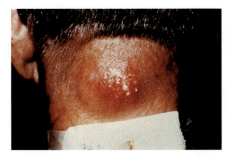

Figure 3-9 Abscess that has formed a furuncle in hair follicles of the neck. *From Goldsmith, LA, Lazarus, GS, and Tharp, MD. Adult and Pediatric Dermatology: A Color Guide to Diagnosis and Treatment. F.A. Davis, Philadelphia, 1997, p 364, with permission.*

acne
ĂK-nē

Inflammatory disease of sebaceous follicles of the skin, marked by comedos (blackheads), papules, and pustules

Acne is especially common in puberty and adolescence. It usually affects the face, chest, back, and shoulders. (See Figure 3-10.)

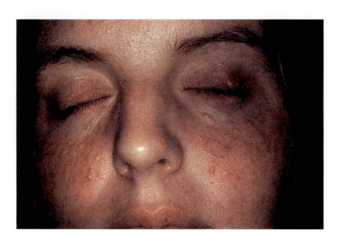

Figure 3-10 Acne. *From Goldsmith, LA, Lazarus, GS, and Tharp, MD: Adult and Pediatric Dermatology: A Color Guide to Diagnosis and Treatment. F.A. Davis, Philadelphia, 1997, p 227, with permission.*

alopecia
ăl-ō-PĒ-shē-ă

Absence or loss of hair, especially of the head; also known as *baldness*

burn

Tissue injury caused by contact with thermal, chemical, electrical, or radioactive agent

first-degree

Mild burn affecting the epidermis that causes redness (*erythema*), swelling, and pain without blisters or scar formation (See Figure 3-11A.)

second-degree

Burn affecting the epidermis and part of the dermis that causes erythema, blisters or large *bullae,* and pain with little or no scarring; also known as a *partial thickness burn* (See Figure 3-11B.)

third-degree

Severe burn that destroys the epidermis and dermis, and may involve the subcutaneous tissue and muscle layer beneath, that causes a white or charred appearance, with lack of sensation due to nerve ending destruction; also known as a *full thickness burn* (See Figure 3-11C.)

Due to the extensiveness of tissue destruction, skin grafting (dermatoplasty) is often required to promote skin closure and to protect the underlying tissue.

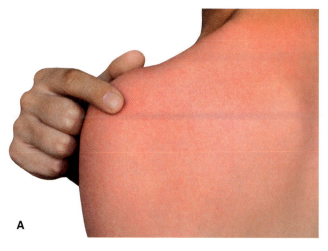

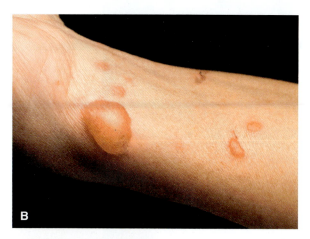

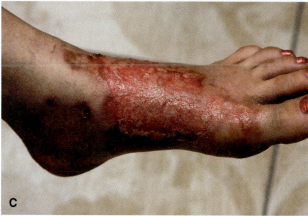

Figure 3-11 Burns. (A) Shoulder and upper back with first-degree burn from overexposure to the sun. (B) Forearm with second-degree burn from frying oil with small blisters and a large bulla. (C) Foot with third-degree burn from fire with destruction of the epidermis and damage to the subcutaneous tissue with charred and white borders.

cyst SĬST	Closed sac or pouch in or under the skin with a definite wall that contains fluid, semifluid, or solid material *The cyst may enlarge as sebum collects and may become infected.*
sebaceous sē-BĀ-shŭs	A cyst filled with sebum (fatty material) from a sebaceous gland

eczema ĔK-zĕ-mă	Redness of the skin caused by swelling of the capillaries *Eczematous rash may result from various causes, including allergies, irritating chemicals, drugs, scratching or rubbing of the skin, or sun exposure. It may be acute or chronic. (See Figure 3-12.)*

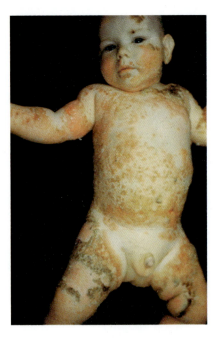

Figure 3-12 Scattered eczema of the trunk of an infant. *From Goldsmith, LA, Lazarus, GS, and Tharp, MD: Adult and Pediatric Dermatology: A Color Guide to Diagnosis and Treatment. F.A. Davis, Philadelphia, 1997, p 243, with permission.*

hemorrhage
HĔM-ĕ-rĭj
    hem/o: blood
    -rrhage: bursting
        forth (of)
	Loss of a large amount of blood in a short period, externally or internally
	
	Hemorrhage may be arterial, venous, or capillary.

contusion kŏn-TOO-zhŭn	Hemorrhage of any size under the skin in which the skin is not broken; also known as a *bruise*
ecchymosis ĕk-ĭ-MŌ-sĭs	Skin discoloration consisting of a large, irregularly formed hemorrhagic area with colors changing from blue-black to greenish brown or yellow; commonly called a *bruise* (See Figure 3-13.)
petechia pē-TĔ-kē-ă	Minute, pinpoint hemorrhagic spot on the skin *A petechia is a smaller version of an ecchymosis.*

hematoma
hēm-ă-TŌ-mă
    hemat: blood
    -oma: tumor
	Elevated, localized collection of blood trapped under the skin that usually results from trauma

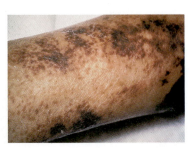

Figure 3-13 Ecchymosis. *From Harmening, DM. Clinical Hematology and Fundamentals of Hemostasis, 4th ed., F.A. Davis, Philadelphia, 2001, p 489, with permission.*

hirsutism HŬR-sūt-ĭzm	Condition characterized by excessive growth of hair or presence of hair in unusual places, especially in women *Hirsutism may be caused by hypersecretion of testosterone, or it may be caused by an adrenal neoplasm.*
impetigo ĭm-pě-TĪ-gō	Bacterial skin infection characterized by isolated pustules that become crusted and rupture
psoriasis sō-RĪ-ă-sĭs	Autoimmune disease characterized by itchy red patches covered with silvery scales (See Figure 3-14.) *Psoriasis seems to be genetically determined and is typically a lifelong condition. Various treatments help control symptoms, including topical treatments (lubricants, retinoids, corticosteroids, and saltwater immersions) and systemic treatments (UV light therapy and excimer light therapy).*

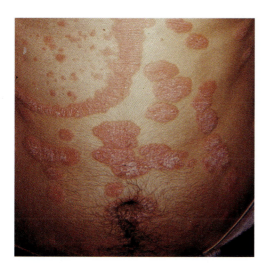

Figure 3-14 Psoriasis. *From Goldsmith, LA, Lazarus, GS, and Thar, MD. Adult and Pediatric Dermatology: A Color Guide to Diagnosis and Treatment. F.A. Davis, Philadelphia, 1997, p 258, with permission.*

scabies SKĀ-bēz	Contagious skin disease transmitted by the itch mite
skin lesion LĒ-zhŭn	Area of pathologically altered tissue caused by disease, injury, or a wound caused by external factors or internal disease *Evaluation of skin lesions, injuries, or changes to tissue helps establish the diagnosis of skin disorders. Lesions are described as primary or secondary. (See Figure 3-15.)*
primary lesion	Skin lesion caused directly by a disease process *A primary lesion is the initial reaction to pathologically altered tissue and may be flat or elevated.*
secondary lesion	Skin lesion that evolves from a primary lesion or that is caused by external forces, such as infection, scratching, trauma, or the healing process

PRIMARY LESIONS

FLAT LESIONS
Flat, discolored, circumscribed lesions of any size

Macule
Flat, pigmented, circumscribed area less than 1 cm in diameter.
Examples: freckle, flat mole, or rash that occurs in rubella.

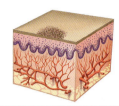

- -

ELEVATED LESIONS

Solid   *Fluid-filled*

Papule
Solid, elevated lesion less than 1 cm in diameter that may be the same color as the skin or pigmented.
Examples: nevus, wart, pimple, ringworm, psoriasis, eczema.

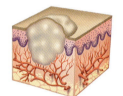

Vesicle
Elevated, circumscribed, fluid-filled lesion less than 0.5 cm in diameter.
Examples: poison ivy, shingles, chickenpox.

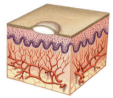

Nodule
Palpable, circumscribed lesion; larger and deeper than a papule (0.6 to 2 cm in diameter); extends into the dermal area.
Examples: intradermal nevus, benign or malignant tumor.

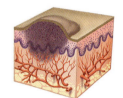

Pustule
Small, raised, circumscribed lesion that contains pus; usually less than 1 cm in diameter.
Examples: acne, furuncle, pustular psoriasis, scabies.

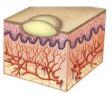

Tumor
Solid, elevated lesion larger than 2 cm in diameter that extends into the dermal and subcutaneous layers.
Examples: lipoma, steatoma.

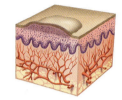

Bulla
A vesicle or blister larger than 1 cm in diameter.
Examples: second degree burns, severe poison oak, poison ivy.

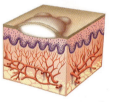

Wheal
Elevated, firm, rounded lesion with localized skin edema (swelling) that varies in size, shape, and color; paler in the center than its surrounding edges; accompanied by itching.
Examples: hives, insect bites, urticaria.

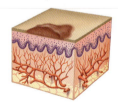

- -

SECONDARY LESIONS

DEPRESSED LESIONS
Depressed lesions caused by loss of skin surface

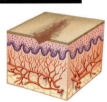

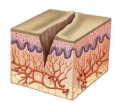

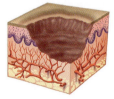

Excoriations
Linear scratch marks or traumatized abrasions of the epidermis.
Examples: scratches, abrasions, chemical or thermal burns.

Fissure
Small slit or cracklike sore that extends into the dermal layer; could be caused by continuous inflammation and drying.

Ulcer
An open sore or lesion that extends to the dermis and usually heals with scarring.
Examples: pressure sore, basal cell carcinoma.

Figure 3-15 Primary and secondary lesions.

tinea TĬN-ē-ă	Fungal infection whose name commonly indicates the body part affected; also called *ringworm* *Examples of tinea include tinea barbae (beard), tinea corporis (body), tinea pedis (athlete's foot), tinea versicolor (skin), and tinea cruris (jock itch).*
ulcer ŬL-sĕr	Lesion of the skin or mucous membranes marked by inflammation, necrosis, and sloughing of damaged tissues *Ulcers may be the result of trauma, caustic chemicals, intense heat or cold, arterial or venous stasis, cancers, drugs, and infectious agents.*
pressure ulcer	Skin ulceration caused by prolonged pressure, usually in a person who is bedridden; also known as decubitus ulcer or bedsore (See Figure 3-16.) *Pressure ulcers are most commonly found in skin overlying a bony projection, such as the hip, ankle, heel, shoulder, and elbow.*

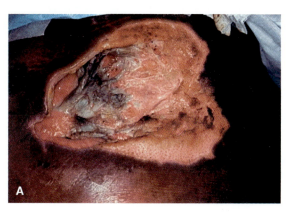
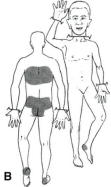

Figure 3-16 Pressure ulcer. (A) Deep pressure ulcer over a bony prominence in a bedridden patient. (B) Common sites of pressure ulcers. *From Goldsmith, LA, Lazarus, GS, and Tharp, MD: Adult and Pediatric Dermatology: A Color Guide to Diagnosis and Treatment. F.A. Davis, Philadelphia, 1997, p 445, with permission.*

urticaria ŭr-tĭ-KĀ-rē-ă	Allergic reaction of the skin characterized by eruption of pale red elevated patches that are intensely itchy; also called *wheals* or *hives*
verruca vě-ROO-kă	Rounded epidermal growths caused by a virus; also called *wart* *Types of warts include plantar warts, juvenile warts, and venereal warts. Warts may be removed by cryosurgery, electrocautery, or acids; however, they may regrow if the virus remains in the skin. (See Figure 3-17.)*

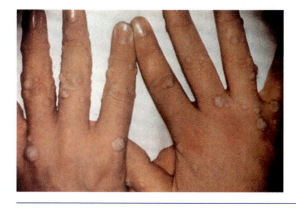

Figure 3-17 Verruca. *From Goldsmith, LA, Lazarus, GS, and Tharp, MD: Adult and Pediatric Dermatology: A Color Guide to Diagnosis and Treatment. F.A. Davis, Philadelphia, 1997, p 241, with permission.*

vitiligo vĭt-ĭl-Ī-gō	Localized loss of skin pigmentation characterized by milk-white patches; also called *leukoderma* (See Figure 3-18.)

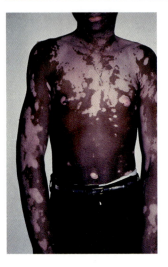

Figure 3-18 Vitiligo. *From Goldsmith, LA, Lazarus, GS, and Tharp, MD: Adult and Pediatric Dermatology: A Color Guide to Diagnosis and Treatment. F.A. Davis, Philadelphia, 1997, p 121, with permission.*

Diagnostic Procedures

biopsy (Bx, bx) BĪ-ŏp-sē	Removal of a small piece of living tissue from an organ or other part of the body for microscopic examination to confirm or establish a diagnosis, estimate prognosis, or follow the course of a disease *Types of biopsy include aspiration biopsy, needle biopsy, punch biopsy, shave biopsy, and frozen-section biopsy.*
skin test	Method for determining induced sensitivity (allergy) by applying or inoculating a suspected allergen or sensitizer into the skin and determining sensitivity (allergy) to the specific antigen by an inflammatory skin reaction to it *The most commonly used skin tests are the intradermal, patch, and scratch tests. (See Figure 3-19.)*

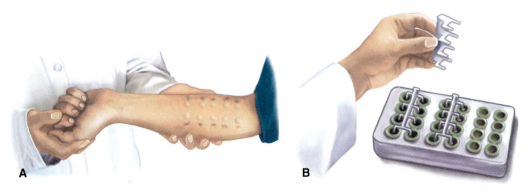

A   B

Figure 3-19 Skin tests. (A) Intradermal allergy test reactions. (B) Scratch (prick) skin test kit for allergy testing.

Medical and Surgical Procedures

cryosurgery krī-ō-SĔR-jĕr-ē	Use of subfreezing temperature, commonly with liquid nitrogen, to destroy abnormal tissue cells, such as unwanted, cancerous, or infected tissue
débridement dā-brēd-MŎN *or* dĭ-BRĒD-mĕnt	Treatment that involves removal of foreign material and dead or damaged tissue, especially in a wound, and is used to promote healing and prevent infection
excimer laser ĔK-sŭh-mĕr	Aims a high-intensity ultraviolet B (UVB) light dose of a very specific wavelength, and a handheld wand allows the energy to be delivered precisely to the affected areas without harming healthy skin around them; also called *exciplex laser* *Because the laser light never touches the surrounding skin, it reduces the risk of UV radiation exposure. Excimer lasers help treat mild to moderate psoriasis and require fewer and less vigorous treatments than other light therapies.*
fulguration fŭl-gū-RĀ-shŭn	Tissue destruction by means of a high-frequency electric current; also called *electrodesiccation* *Fulguration helps remove tumors and lesions within and on the body.*
incision and drainage (I&D)	Surgical procedure to release pus or pressure built up under the skin, such as in an abscess, and remove its contents
Mohs surgery MŌZ	Procedure in which layers of cancer-containing skin are progressively excised and examined until only cancer-free tissue remains; also called *micrographic surgery.*

skin graft	Surgical procedure to transplant healthy tissue to an injured site
	Human, animal, or artificial skin provides a temporary covering or permanent layer of skin over a wound or burn.
allograft ĂL-ō-grăft *allo-:* other, differing from the normal *-graft:* transplantation	Transplantation of healthy tissue from one person to another person; also called *homograft* *In an allograft, the skin donor is usually a cadaver. This type of skin graft is temporary and used to protect the patient against infection and fluid loss. The allograft is frozen and stored in a skin bank until needed.*
autograft AW-tō-grăft *auto-:* self, own *-graft:* transplantation	Transplantation of healthy tissue from one site to another site in the same individual
synthetic sĭn-THĔT-ĭk	Transplantation of artificial skin produced from collagen fibers arranged in a lattice pattern *With a synthetic skin graft, the recipient's body does not reject the synthetic skin (produced artificially), and healing skin grows into it as the graft gradually disintegrates.*
xenograft ZĔN-ō-grăft *xen/o:* foreign, strange *-graft:* transplantation	Transplantation (dermis only) from a foreign donor (usually a pig) and transferred to a human; also called *heterograft* *A xenograft is used as a temporary graft to protect the patient against infection and fluid loss.*
skin resurfacing	Repair of damaged skin, acne scars, fine or deep wrinkles, or tattoos, or improvement of skin tone irregularities by using topical chemicals, abrasion, or laser *In cosmetic surgery, skin resurfacing may involve dermabrasion, chemical peels, cutaneous lasers, and other techniques.*
chemical peel	Use of chemicals to remove outer layers of skin to treat acne scarring and general keratoses, as well as cosmetic purposes to remove fine wrinkles on the face; also called *chemabrasion*
cutaneous laser kū-TĀ-nē-ŭs *cutane:* skin *-ous:* pertaining to	Any of several laser treatments employed for cosmetic and plastic surgery *Cutaneous laser includes treatment of pigmented lesions, wrinkles, vascular malformations, and other cosmetic skin surface irregularities.*
dermabrasion DĔRM-ă-brā-zhŭn	Removal of acne scars, nevi, tattoos, or fine wrinkles on the skin through the use of sandpaper, wire brushes, or other abrasive materials on the epidermal layer

Pharmacology

Drug Category	Action
antibiotics ăn-tĭ-bī-ŎT-ĭks	Kill bacteria that cause skin infections
antifungals ăn-tĭ-FŬNG-găls	Kill fungi that infect the skin
antipruritics ăn-tĭ-proo-RĬT-ĭks	Reduce severe itching
corticosteroids kor-tĭ-kō-STĒR-oyds	Treat skin inflammation through anti-inflammatory action

Pronunciation Help	*Long Sound*	ā in rāte	ē in rēbirth	ī in īsle	ō in ōver	ū in ūnite
	Short Sound	ă in ăpple	ĕ in ĕver	ĭ in ĭt	ŏ in nŏt	ŭ in cŭt

Word Elements Review

This review provides a verification of your knowledge of the word elements covered in this chapter. First, use a slash to break the term into its component parts, and identify each element by labeling it P for prefix, WR for word root, CF for combining form, or S for suffix. Then, provide the meaning of the medical term. Remember to define the suffix first, define the beginning of the word second, and define the middle part of the term last. The first word is a sample completed for you.

Medical Term	Meaning
adip/oma *WR S*	tumor containing fat
1. anhidrosis	
2. dermatoplasty	
3. subcutaneous	
4. onychomalacia *onycho-nail malacia -nail.*	
5. lipectomy *fat remova*	

Match the medical terms that follow with the definitions in the numbered list.

carcinoma	lipocele	squamous
diaphoresis	lipocyte	trichopathy
keratoma	melanocyte	trichosis
leukocytopenia	melanoma	xeroderma

6. _____*lipocyte*_____ cell composed of fat
7. _____*melanoma*_____ black tumor
8. _____*tricopathy*_____ any disease of hair
9. _____*Squamous.*_____ covered with scales; scalelike
10. _____*Xeroderma.*_____ dry skin
11. _____*melanocyte*_____ black cell
12. _____ profuse sweating
13. _____ hernia containing fatty tissue
14. _____*Carcinoma*_____ cancerous tumor
15. _____*leukocytopenia.*_____ deficiency in white blood cell production

Competency Verification: Check your answers in Appendix B: Answer Key, page 592. If you are not satisfied with your level of comprehension, review the vocabulary, and retake the review.

Correct Answers _____ × 6.67 = _____ % Score

Additional Medical Terms Review

Match the medical terms that follow with the definitions in the numbered list.

alopecia	dermabrasion	scabies
comedo	eczema	tinea
corticosteroids	fulguration	urticaria
cryosurgery	furuncle	verruca
débridement	petechia	vitiligo

1. _Verruca_ is a rounded epidermal growth caused by a virus.

2. _Vitiligo_ is localized loss of skin pigmentation characterized by the appearance of milk-white patches.

3. _dermabrasion_ is a fungal skin disease, commonly called *ringworm,* whose name indicates the body part affected.

4. _____ is an abscess that originates in a hair follicle and is also called a *boil.*

5. _____ is a general term for an itchy red rash that may become crusted, thickened, or scaly.

6. _____ is an allergic reaction of the skin characterized by eruption of pale red elevated patches that are intensely itchy and is also called *hives.*

7. _____ are anti-inflammatory agents prescribed for skin inflammations.

8. _____ refers to use of revolving wire brushes or sandpaper to remove superficial scars on the skin.

9. _____ refers to the procedure in which diseased tissue is destroyed by a high-frequency electric current.

10. _____ refers to the use of liquid nitrogen to destroy or eliminate abnormal tissue cells.

11. _____ refers to removal of foreign material and dead or damaged tissue, especially in a wound.

12. _____ is a contagious skin disease transmitted by the itch mite.

13. _____ is the absence or loss of hair, especially of the head, and is also called *baldness.*

14. _____ is a blackhead.

15. _____ is a minute, hemorrhagic spot on the skin that is a smaller version of ecchymosis.

Competency Verification: Check your answers in Appendix B: Answer Key, page 593. If you are not satisfied with your level of comprehension, review the additional medical terms section, and retake the review.

Correct Answers _____ × 6.67 = _____ % Score

Primary and Secondary Lesions Review

Identify and label the following skin lesions using the terms in the following list.

bulla	*macule*	*pustule*	*vesicle*
excoriations	*nodule*	*tumor*	*wheal*
fissure	*papule*	*ulcer*	

PRIMARY LESIONS

FLAT LESIONS
Flat, discolored, circumscribed lesions of any size

Flat, pigmented, circumscribed area less than 1 cm in diameter.
Examples: freckle, flat mole, or rash that occurs in rubella.

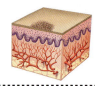

- -

ELEVATED LESIONS

Solid   *Fluid-filled*

Solid, elevated lesion less than 1 cm in diameter that may be the same color as the skin or pigmented.
Examples: nevus, wart, pimple, ringworm, psoriasis, eczema.

Elevated, circumscribed, fluid-filled lesion less than 0.5 cm in diameter.
Examples: poison ivy, shingles, chickenpox.

Palpable, circumscribed lesion; larger and deeper than a papule (0.6 to 2 cm in diameter); extends into the dermal area.
Examples: intradermal nevus, benign or malignant tumor.

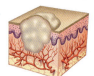

Small, raised, circumscribed lesion that contains pus; usually less than 1 cm in diameter.
Examples: acne, furuncle, pustular psoriasis, scabies.

Solid, elevated lesion larger than 2 cm in diameter that extends into the dermal and subcutaneous layers.
Examples: lipoma, steatoma.

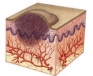

A vesicle or blister larger than 1 cm in diameter.
Examples: second degree burns, severe poison oak, poison ivy.

Elevated, firm, rounded lesion with localized skin edema (swelling) that varies in size, shape, and color; paler in the center than its surrounding edges; accompanied by itching.
Examples: hives, insect bites, urticaria.

- -

SECONDARY LESIONS

DEPRESSED LESIONS
Depressed lesions caused by loss of skin surface

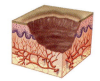

Linear scratch marks or traumatized abrasions of the epidermis.
Examples: scratches, abrasions, chemical or thermal burns.

Small slit or cracklike sore that extends into the dermal layer; could be caused by continuous inflammation and drying.

An open sore or lesion that extends to the dermis and usually heals with scarring.
Examples: pressure sore, basal cell carcinoma.

Competency Verification: Check your answers by referring to Figure 3-15, page 92. Review material that you did not answer correctly.

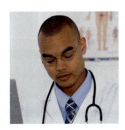

Medical Record Activities

To develop a working vocabulary of medical terms and to understand how those terms are used in the health-care industry, it is important that you complete the following activities.

MEDICAL RECORD ACTIVITY 3-1

CONSULTATION LETTER: SKIN CANCER CHECK

This activity contains a consultation letter for a skin cancer check. Read the consultation letter that follows and underline the medical terms. Then, complete the terminology and critical thinking exercises.

Consultation Letter

Dermatology and Cosmetic Surgery

1120 Park Shore Blvd.

Spring Garden, MI 12345

March 25, 20xx

Kim Lu, MD
786 Second Avenue
Spring Garden, MI 438112

Dear Doctor Lu:

RE: Joan Mears

Mrs. Mears, a 39-yr-old married woman, presented for a "skin cancer check." She readily volunteered information that she has spent a considerable amount of time out in the sun, although there is no family history of skin cancer.

I reassured the patient about typical changes of so-called idiopathic guttate hypomelanosis over her legs, plus a solitary seborrheic keratosis on her left wrist and a single cherry angioma over her left thigh.

Checking the sun-exposed sites, I did detect an early pigmented solar keratosis over her right zygoma. She also has numerous excoriated acne lesions on her face. After stressing the importance of photoprotection, I elected to freeze this precancer with liquid nitrogen on an applicator.

Mrs. Mears will return as required.

Kim Lu, M.D.
_____
Kim Lu, M.D.

KL:sr
D: 3/25/20xx; T: 3/25/20xx

Terminology 3-1

Terms listed in the following table come from the previous consultation letter. Use a medical dictionary, such as Taber's Cyclopedic Medical Dictionary; the appendices of this book; or other resources to define each term. Then pronounce the term and place a checkmark (✓) in the box after you do so.

Term	Definition
cherry angioma ăn-jē-Ō-mă ☐	
excoriated acne ĕks-KŌ-rē-ā-tĕd ĂK-nē ☐	
idiopathic guttate hypomelanosis ĭd-ē-ō-PĂTH-ĭk GOO-tāt hī-pō-mĕl-ă-NŌ-sĭs ☐	
photo-protection fō-tō-prō-TĔK-shŭn ☐	
pigmented solar keratosis PĬG-mĕnt-ĕd SŌ-lăr kĕr-ă-TŌ-sĭs ☐	
seborrheic keratosis sĕb-ō-RĔ-ĭk kĕr-ă-TŌ-sĭs ☐	

 Visit the *Medical Terminology Simplified* online resource center at FADavis.com to hear pronunciation and meanings of terms in this medical report.

Critical Thinking 3-1

Review the previous consultation letter to answer the following questions. Use a medical dictionary, such as Taber's Cyclopedic Medical Dictionary, *and other resources, if needed.*

1. What was the predisposing factor causing the patient's present condition?

   _____

   _____

2. What did the physician recommend to the patient to prevent future problems with solar keratosis?

   _____

   _____

3. What treatment did the physician perform on the precancerous lesions?

   _____

   _____

4. When does the physician want to see the patient again?

   _____

   _____

MEDICAL RECORD ACTIVITY 3-2

PROGRESS NOTE: PSORIASIS VULGARIS

This activity contains an office visit in which a patient is diagnosed with psoriasis vulgaris in various stages of severity. Read the progress note that follows and underline the medical terms. Then, complete the terminology and critical thinking exercises.

PROGRESS NOTE

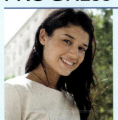

PATIENT NAME: Souza, Amanda
MEDICAL RECORD ID: 39-55659
DATE: November 19, 20xx

HISTORY: This 23-year-old white woman has experienced intermittent psoriasis in various stages of severity since her early teens. Since May, her condition has become more troublesome because of an increase in symptoms after being exposed to the sun. Her past history indicates she had chronic sinusitis of 3 years' duration. Her Bartholin gland was excised in 20xx. She has had pruritus of the scalp and abdominal regions. There is no family history of psoriasis. An uncle has had diabetes mellitus since age 43. Patient has occasional abdominal pains accompanied by diaphoresis and/or syncope.

PHYSICAL EXAMINATION: Psoriatic involvement of the scalp, external ears, trunk and, to a lesser degree, legs. There are many scattered erythematous (light ruby), thickened plaques covered by thick, yellowish white scales. A few areas on the legs and arms show multiple, sclerosed, brown macules and papules.

DIAGNOSES:
1. Psoriasis vulgaris
2. Multiple histiocytomas
3. Abdominal pain, by history
4. Rule out colitis, regional enteritis

PLAN: The patient has been referred to Dr. Henricks

Robert S. Dukota, M.D.

Robert S. Dukota, M.D.

RD:ks
D: 11/19/ T: 11/19/20xx

Terminology 3-2

Terms listed in the following table come from the previous progress note. Use a medical dictionary, such as Taber's Cyclopedic Medical Dictionary; *the appendices of this book; or other resources to define each term. Then pronounce the term, and place a checkmark (✓) in the box after you do so.*

Term	Definition
Bartholin gland BĂR-tō-lĭn ☐	
diabetes mellitus dī-ă-BĒ-tēz MĚ-lĭ-tŭs ☐	
diaphoresis dī-ă-fō-RĒ-sĭs ☐	
Dx	
enteritis ĕn-tĕr-Ī-tĭs ☐	
erythematous ĕr-ĭ-THĔM-ă-tŭs ☐	
FH	
histiocytoma hĭs-tē-ō-sī-TŌ-mă ☐	
macules MĂK-ūlz ☐	
papules PĂP-ūlz ☐	
PE	

Term	Definition
pruritus proo-RĪ-tŭs ☐	
psoriasis sō-RĪ-ă-sĭs ☐	
sclerosed sklĕ-RŌST ☐	
sinusitis sī-nŭs-Ī-tĭs ☐	
syncope SĬN-kō-pē ☐	
vulgaris vŭl-GĀ-rĭs ☐	

Visit the *Medical Terminology Simplified* online resource center at FADavis.com to hear pronunciation and meanings of terms in this medical report.

Critical Thinking 3-2

Review the previous progress note to answer the following questions. Use a medical dictionary, such as Taber's Cyclopedic Medical Dictionary, *and other resources, if needed.*

1. What causes psoriasis?

    _____

    _____

2. On what parts of the body does psoriasis typically occur?

    _____

    _____

3. How is psoriasis treated?

    _____

    _____

4. What is a histiocytoma?

    _____

    _____

MEDICAL RECORD ACTIVITY 3-3

CLINICAL APPLICATION

This activity is a clinical application that will help you integrate and reinforce your understanding of how the following medical terms are used in the clinical environment. Complete the clinically related sentences that follow by selecting an appropriate term from the list.

abscess	*biopsy*	*I&D*	*scabies*
alopecia	*débridement*	*petechia*	*ulcer*
antipruritics	*hirsutism*	*psoriasis*	*vitiligo*

1. A 16-year-old boy has an "extremely itchy rash" that began last week while camping. Following examination, he is diagnosed with poison ivy. To control the itching, the physician prescribes _____.

2. A 36-year-old female complains of hair growing on her face and upper lip. The physician explains that excessive growth of hair in unusual places, especially in females, is a condition known as _____.

3. A 38-year-old male is concerned that a mole could be cancerous because he has a family history of melanoma. The physician removes a small piece of tissue from the mole and sends it to the laboratory for microscopic examination, a procedure known as a(n) _____.

4. An 85-year-old male resident at a local nursing home presents for a follow-up visit with a deep pressure ulcer on his left hip. The wound is healing but requires removal of foreign material to prevent infection and promote healing, a procedure known as _____.

5. A 65-year-old obese patient complains of a large, painful sore, at the base of his spine, and the sore is oozing pus. He is diagnosed with a pilonidal cyst, and the physician informs him that he will remove the pus from the cyst. His nurse sets up the surgical tray for a procedure known as a(n) _____.

6. The mother of Lily, a 7-year-old girl, tells the physician that her daughter recently developed a rash on her hands and arms and itching of the scalp. She says the rash started several days after Lily spent the night at a friend's house. Upon close examination, the physician diagnoses Lily with a contagious skin disease transmitted by the itch mite. The physician charts a diagnosis of _____.

7. A 40-year-old woman with breast cancer is informed about the adverse effects of chemotherapy. She is concerned about the hair loss, also called _____, that commonly occurs with chemotherapy.

8. A 14-year-old boy accompanied by his mother complains of milk-white patches on his arms that have become more numerous. The mother states that there is a history of this condition on her side of the family. The physician explains that the boy most likely has _____, a hereditary condition characterized by localized loss of skin pigmentation.

9. A 50-year-old female complains of a sore on her buttocks. She states that the sore is very painful when she is sitting or having a bowel movement. The physician explains that she has _____, a localized collection of pus that is most likely the result of a bacterial infection.

10. A 25-year-old woman presents to the clinic with complaints of a rash on her lower legs. Upon examination, the physician notes small, red-purple spots on the skin, which he determines are caused by broken capillaries underneath the skin, which are hemorrhages known as _____.

Competency Verification: Check your answers in Appendix B: Answer Key, page 593. If you are not satisfied with your level of comprehension, review the material in this chapter, and retake the review.

Correct Answers _____ × 10 = _____ % Score

INTEGUMENTARY SYSTEM CHAPTER REVIEW

WORD ELEMENTS SUMMARY

The following table summarizes CFs, suffixes, and prefixes related to the integumentary system. Study the word elements and their meanings before completing the Vocabulary Review that follows.

Word Element	Meaning	Word Element	Meaning
Combining Forms			
adip/o, lip/o, steat/o	fat	melan/o	black
cutane/o, derm/o, dermat/o	skin	myc/o	fungus
cyt/o	cell	necr/o	death, necrosis
cyan/o	blue	onych/o	nail
erythr/o, erythemat/o	red	pil/o, trich/o	hair
hidr/o, sudor/o	sweat	scler/o	hardening; sclera (white of the eye)
hydr/o	water	squam/o	scale
ichthy/o	dry, scaly	xanth/o	yellow
kerat/o	horny tissue; hard; cornea	xer/o	dry
leuk/o	white		
Suffixes			
-al, -ous	pertaining to	-oma	tumor
-cele	hernia, swelling	-osis	abnormal condition; increase (used primarily with blood cells)
-cyte	cell	-pathy	disease
-derma	skin	-penia	decrease; deficiency
-emia	blood condition	-phagia	swallowing, eating
-esis	condition	-phoresis	carrying, transmission
-itis	inflammation	-plasty	surgical repair
-logist	specialist in the study of	-rrhea	discharge, flow
-logy	study of	-therapy	treatment
-malacia	softening	-tome	instrument to cut
Prefixes			
auto-	self, own	hypo-	under, below; deficient
epi-	above, on	sub-	under, below

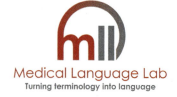

Medical Language Lab
Turning terminology into language

Visit the *Medical Language Lab* at medicallanguagelab.com. Use the flash-card word elements exercise to reinforce your study of word elements. We recommend you complete the flash-card activity before starting the Word Elements Review that follows.

Vocabulary Review

Match the medical term(s) that follow with the definitions in the numbered list.

autograft	*Kaposi sarcoma*	*onychomalacia*	*subcutaneous*
diaphoresis	*leukemia*	*onychomycosis*	*suction lipectomy*
ecchymosis	*lipocele*	*papules*	*trichopathy*
erythrocyte	*melanoma*	*pressure ulcer*	*xanthoma*
hirsutism	*onychoma*	*pustule*	*xeroderma*

1. _____ means beneath the skin.

2. _____ is a condition in which a person sweats excessively and is also called *sudoresis*.

3. _____ refers to any disease of hair.

4. _____ is a transplantation of healthy tissue from one site to another site in the same individual.

5. _____ is a type of malignant skin tumor associated with AIDS.

6. _____ refers to excision of subcutaneous fat tissue by use of a blunt-tipped cannula (tube) and is done for cosmetic reasons.

7. _____ is a fungal infection of the nails.

8. _____ is caused by prolonged pressure against an area of skin from a bed or chair.

9. _____ refers to excessive production of WBCs and literally means white blood.

10. _____ is a black-and-blue mark on the skin, also called a *bruise*.

11. _____ is a benign tumor of the nailbed.

12. _____ means excessive body hair, especially in women.

13. _____ is an elevated lesion containing pus, as seen in acne, furuncles, and psoriasis.

14. _____ is a medical term for warts, moles, and pimples.

15. _____ is a red blood cell.

16. _____ means excessive dryness of the skin.

17. _____ is a black tumor.

18. _____ refers to a hernia that contains fat or fatty cells.

19. _____ refers to a tumor containing yellow material.

20. _____ is an abnormal softening of the nail or nailbed.

Competency Verification: Check your answers in Appendix B: Answer Key, page 593. If you are not satisfied with your level of comprehension, review the chapter vocabulary, and retake the review.

Correct Answers: _____ × 5 = _____ % Score

Respiratory System

OBJECTIVES

Upon completion of this chapter, you will be able to:

• Describe the type of medical treatment the pulmonologist provides.

• Identify respiratory structures by labeling them on anatomical illustrations.

• Describe the primary functions of the respiratory system.

• Describe diseases, conditions, and procedures related to the respiratory system.

• Apply your word-building skills by constructing medical terms related to the respiratory system.

• Describe common abbreviations and symbols related to the respiratory system.

• Recognize, define, pronounce, and spell terms correctly.

• Demonstrate your knowledge of this chapter by successfully completing the frames, reviews, and activities.

MEDICAL SPECIALTY: PULMONOLOGY

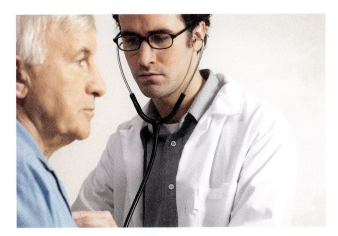

The medical specialty of **pulmonology,** also called **pulmonary medicine,** is the branch of medicine concerned with the diagnosis and treatment of diseases involving the structures of the lower respiratory tract, including the lungs, their airways and blood vessels, and the chest wall (thoracic cage). Medical doctors who treat respiratory disorders are called **pulmonologists.** Respiratory disorders include, but are not limited to, asthma, emphysema, chronic bronchitis, lung disease, and pulmonary vascular disease. Pulmonologists also care for patients requiring specialized ventilator support and lung transplantation. In general, pulmonologists are specialized to diagnose and manage pulmonary disorders, and chronic and acute respiratory failure, including those with COVID-19. Diagnosis and management of pulmonary disorders may include pulmonary function tests, arterial blood gas analysis, chest radiography, and chemical or microbiological tests.

Anatomy and Physiology Overview

The respiratory system consists of the upper and lower respiratory tracts. The upper tract includes the nose, pharynx, larynx, and trachea. The lower tract includes the left and right bronchi, bronchioles, alveoli, and lungs. (See Figure 4-1.) All of these organs work together to perform the mechanical and unconscious mechanisms of **respiration**. Respiration, or breathing, consists of external and internal processes:

- In **external respiration,** oxygen (O_2) is inhaled into the lungs and absorbed into the bloodstream. Carbon dioxide (CO_2) leaves the bloodstream and enters the lungs where it is expelled during exhalation.
- In **internal respiration**, O_2 and CO_2 are exchanged at the cellular level. O_2 leaves the bloodstream and is delivered to the tissue cells where it is used for energy. In exchange, CO_2 enters the bloodstream from the tissues and is transported back to the lungs for removal. Secondary functions of the respiratory system include warming air as it passes into the body and assisting in speech function by providing air for the larynx and vocal cords.

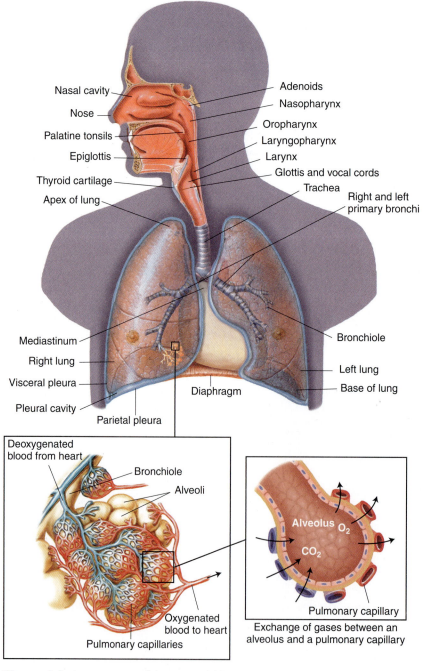

Figure 4-1 Anterior view of the upper and lower respiratory tracts.

WORD ELEMENTS

This section introduces word elements related to the respiratory system. Review the word elements and their meanings in the following table. Then, pronounce each term in the word analysis column, and place a ✓ in the box after you do so.

Word Element	Meaning	Word Analysis
Combining Forms Upper Respiratory Tract		
adenoid/o	adenoid	**adenoid**/ectomy (ăd-ĕ-noyd-ĔK-tō-mē ☐): excision of the adenoids *-ectomy:* excision, removal
laryng/o	larynx (voice box)	**laryng/o**/scope (lăr-ĬN-gō-skōp ☐): instrument for examining the larynx *-scope:* instrument for examining
nas/o	nose	**nas**/al (NĀ-zl ☐): pertaining to the nose *-al:* pertaining to
rhin/o		**rhin/o**/rrhea (rī-nō-RĒ-ă ☐): watery discharge from the nose *-rrhea:* discharge, flow *Allergies and a cold commonly cause rhinorrhea. The flow of cerebrospinal fluid from the nose after an injury to the head may also cause rhinorrhea.*
pharyng/o	pharynx (throat)	**pharyng**/itis (făr-ĭn-JĪ-tĭs ☐): inflammation of the pharynx, usually as a result of infection *-itis:* inflammation

tonsill/o	tonsils	peri/**tonsill**/ar (pĕr-ĭ-TŎN-sĭ-lăr ☐): pertaining to the area surrounding the tonsils
		   peri-: around
		   -ar: pertaining to

trache/o	trachea (windpipe)	**trache/o**/stomy (trā-kē-ŎS-tō-mē ☐): creation of an opening into the trachea *-stomy:* forming an opening (mouth) *Tracheostomy provides and secures an open airway.*
Lower Respiratory Tract		
alveol/o	alveolus (plural, *alveoli*)	**alveol**/ar (ăl-VĒ-ō-lăr ☐): pertaining to the alveoli *-ar:* pertaining to
bronchi/o	bronchus (plural, bronchi)	**bronchi**/ectasis (brŏng-kē-ĔK-tă-sĭs ☐): dilation of a bronchus or bronchi *-ectasis:* dilation, expansion *Bronchiectasis can be caused by the damaging effects of a long-standing infection.*
bronch/o		**bronch/o**/scope (BRŎNG-kō-skōp ☐): curved, flexible tube with a light for visual examination of the bronchi *-scope:* instrument for examining *A bronchoscope helps examine the bronchi or secure a specimen for biopsy or culture. It also can aspirate secretions or a foreign body from the respiratory tract.*
bronchiol/o	bronchiole	**bronchiol**/itis (brŏng-kē-ō-LĪ-tĭs ☐): inflammation of the bronchioles *-itis:* inflammation
pleur/o	pleura	**pleur**/itic (ploo-RĬT-ĭk ☐): pertaining to pleurisy *-itic:* pertaining to
pneum/o	air; lung	**pneum**/ectomy (nū-MĔK-tō-mē ☐): excision of all or part of a lung *-ectomy:* excision, removal
pneumon/o		**pneumon**/ia (nū-MŌ-nē-ă ☐): inflammation of one or both lungs, usually as a result of infection *-ia:* condition *Pneumonia is caused primarily by bacteria, viruses, and chemical irritants. Fluid, microorganisms, and white blood cells fill the alveoli and air passages, making breathing difficult.*

Continued

Word Element	Meaning	Word Analysis
pulmon/o	lung	**pulmon/o/logist** (pŭl-mō-NŎL-ō-jĭst ☐): physician who specializes in treating pathological conditions of the lungs *-logist:* specialist in the study of
thorac/o	chest	**thorac/o/pathy** (thō-răk-ŎP-ă-thē ☐): disease of the thorax or the organs it contains *-pathy:* disease
Suffixes		
-algia	pain	**pleur/algia** (ploo-RĂL-jē-ă ☐): pain in the pleura *pleur:* pleura
-dynia		**thorac/o/dynia** (thō-răk-ō-DĬN-ē-ă ☐): pain in the chest *thorac/o:* chest
-ectasis	dilation, expansion	**atel/ectasis** (ăt-ĕ-LĔK-tă-sĭs ☐): abnormal condition characterized by the collapse of the alveoli *atel:* incomplete; imperfect *Atelectasis is characterized by the collapse of the alveoli, preventing respiratory exchange of CO_2 and O_2 in parts of the lungs.*
-osis	abnormal condition; increase (used primarily with blood cells)	**cyan/osis** (sī-ă-NŌ-sĭs ☐): bluish discoloration of the skin and mucous membranes *cyan:* blue *Cyanosis is caused by deficiency of O_2 in blood.*
-osmia	smell	**an/osmia** (ăn-ŎZ-mē-ă ☐): loss or impairment of the sense of smell, which usually occurs as a temporary condition *an-:* without, not
-oxia	O_2	**hyp/oxia** (hī-PŎKS-ē-ă ☐): abnormally low level of O_2 at the cellular level *hyp-:* under, below, deficient *In hypoxia, tissues have a decreased amount of oxygen and cyanosis can result.*
-phagia	swallowing, eating	**aer/o/phagia** (ĕr-ō-FĂ-jē-ă ☐): swallowing air *aer/o:* air
-pnea	breathing	**a/pnea** (ăp-NĒ-ă ☐): temporary cessation of breathing *a-:* without, not *Apnea may be a serious symptom, especially in patients with other potentially life-threatening conditions. Some types of apnea include newborn, cardiac, and sleep apnea.*
-spasm	involuntary contraction, twitching	**pharyng/o/spasm** (făr-ĬN-gō-spăzm ☐): spasm of muscles in the pharynx *pharyng/o:* pharynx (throat)
-thorax	chest	**py/o/thorax** (pī-ō-THŌ-răks ☐): accumulation of pus in the thorax *py/o:* pus

Pronunciation Help	*Long Sound* *Short Sound*	ā in rāte ă in ăpple	ē in rēbirth ĕ in ĕver	ī in īsle ĭ in ĭt	ō in ōver ŏ in nŏt	ū in ūnite ŭ in cŭt

 Visit the *Medical Terminology Simplified* online resource center at FADavis.com for an audio exercise of the terms in this table. It will help you master pronunciations and meanings of the selected medical terms.

SECTION REVIEW 4-1

For the following medical terms, first, write the suffix and its meaning. Then, translate the meaning of the remaining elements starting with the first part of the word. The first word is an example completed for you.

Term	Meaning
1. laryng/o/scope	–scope: instrument for examining; larynx (voice box)
2. py/o/thorax	
3. hyp/oxia	
4. trache/o/stomy	
5. a/pnea	temporary cessation of breathing.
6. pulmon/o/logist	long
7. pneumon/ia	air/lung.
8. rhin/o/rrhea	nose discharge
9. an/osmia	smell
10. pneum/ectomy	excision of the part of the lung.

Competency Verification: Check your answers in Appendix B: Answer Key, page 594. If you are not satisfied with your level of comprehension, review the vocabulary, and retake the review.

Correct Answers _____ x 10 = _____ % Score

Respiratory System

Upper Respiratory Tract

nose, stomach	**4–1**　External openings of the nose are referred to as *nostrils* or *nares* (singular, naris). *Nas/o/gastr/ic* (NG) refers to the nose and stomach. This term describes procedures and devices associated with the nose and the stomach, such as *nas/o/gastr/ic* feeding and *nas/o/gastr/ic* suction.
	When you see the term *nas/o/gastr/ic tube,* you will know it refers to a tube inserted into the _____ and the _____.
pharynx (throat) FĂR-ĭnks	**4–2**　The term *tube* used in association with a medical procedure usually refers to a catheter. A catheter is a hollow, flexible tube inserted into a vessel or body cavity. Its purpose is to withdraw or instill fluids into a body cavity or vessel. A pharyng/eal suction catheter is a rigid tube that suctions mucous secretions to clear the airway for breathing.
	The combining form (CF) *pharyng/o* means _____ (_____).

nas/o, rhin/o	**4-3** The CFs for *nose* are _____ / _____ and _____ / _____.

para/nas/al păr-ă-NĀ-săl	**4-4** The prefix *para-* is a directional element that means *near, beside; beyond.* The para/nas/al sinuses are hollow spaces within the skull that open into the nasal cavities. They are lined with ciliated epithelium, which is continuous with the mucosa of the nasal cavities. (See Figure 4-2.) The term in this frame that means *near or beside the nose* is _____ /_____ / _____.

rhin/o/plasty RĪ-nō-plăs-tē **rhin/o/tomy** rī-NŎT-ō-mē	**4-5** The CFs *rhin/o* and *nas/o* refer to the nose. As a general rule, *nas/o* is not used to build surgical terms. However, if you are in doubt about which element to use, consult a medical dictionary. Form operative terms that mean *surgical repair of the nose:* _____ / _____ / _____. *incision of the nose:* _____ / _____ / _____.

rhin/o/rrhea rī-nō-RĒ-ă	**4-6** Rhin/o/rrhea is a *discharge from the nose.* Sneezing, tearing, and a runny nose are common symptoms of a cold. Build a term that means *discharge from the nose:* _____ / _____ / _____.

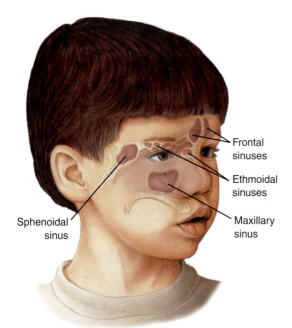

Figure 4-2 Paranasal sinuses.

Frontal
sinuses

Ethmoidal
sinuses

Maxillary
sinus

Sphenoidal
sinus

rhin/o/rrhagia rī-nō-RĂ-jē-ă **rhin/o/rrhea** rī-nō-RĒ-ă	**4-7** Whereas *rhin/o/rrhea* refers to a runny nose, *rhin/o/rrhagia* refers to a nosebleed. Profuse bleeding from the nose is charted with the Dx _____ /_____ /_____. A runny discharge from the nose is charted with the Dx _____ /_____ /_____.

> **!** When in doubt about the meaning of a word element, refer to Appendix A: Glossary of Medical Word Elements, page 575.

air, lung	**4-8** Air enters the nose and passes through the (1) **nasal cavity,** which contains a mucosal lining where inhaled air is moistened. Mucus and fine hairs trap inhaled dust particles, smoke, pollen, and bacteria to keep them from entering the lungs. Label the nasal cavity in Figure 4-3. The CFs *pneum/o* and *pneumon/o* mean _____; _____.
aer/o/phagia ĕr-ō-FĂ-jē-ă	**4-9** Swallowing air is not unusual in infants. It can occur as they suck on a nipple to obtain milk, water, or any liquid substance. Doing so commonly causes gaseous discomfort, which is relieved when the infant is burped. Combine *aer/o* + *-phagia* to form a medical term that means *swallowing air:* _____ / _____ / _____.
	4-10 After passing through the nasal cavity, air reaches the (2) **pharynx** (throat). Label the pharynx in Figure 4-3.
pharyng/o **myc** **-osis**	**4-11** From the term *pharyng/o/myc/osis,* determine the elements that mean *pharynx (throat):* _____ /_____. *fungus:* _____. *abnormal condition:* _____.
pharynx or throat FĂR-ĭnks	**4-12** Pharyng/o/myc/osis is a fungal disease of the _____.
pharynx FĂR-ĭnks	**4-13** The suffix *-plegia* means *paralysis. Pharyng/o/plegia* and *pharyng/o/paralysis* are terms used to describe muscle paralysis of the _____.
cancer KĂN-sĕr	**4-14** Smoking, drinking alcohol, and chewing tobacco can cause cancer (CA) of the pharynx. Patients with pharyng/eal CA may require some type of plastic surgery. When you see CA in a medical chart, you will know it is an abbreviation for _____.

A

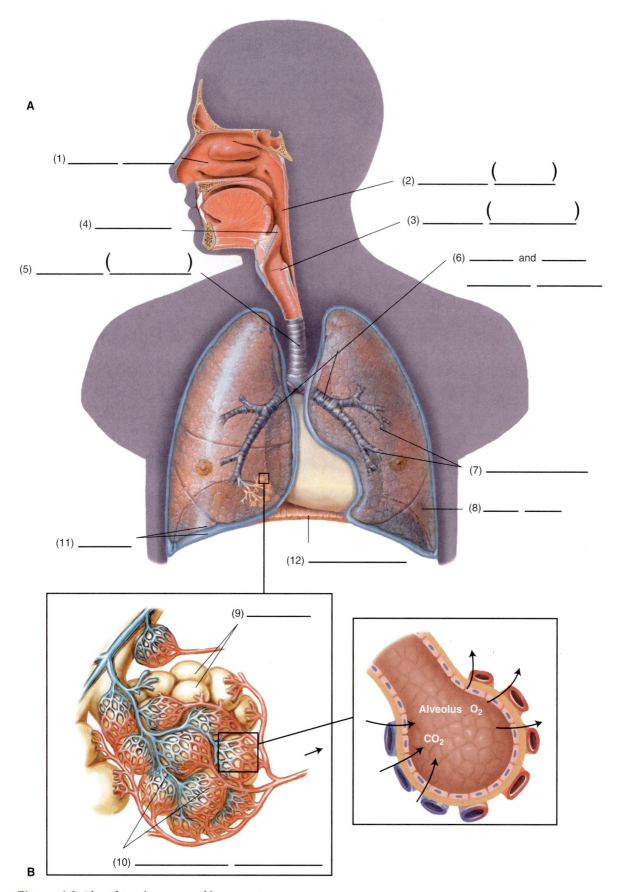

(1) _____ _____

(2) _____ _ (_____)

(3) _____ (_____)

(4) _____ _____

(5) _____ (_____)

(6) _____ and _____

_____ _____

(7) _____

(8) _____ _____

(11) _____

(12) _____

(9) _____

(10) _____ _____

Alveolus O_2

CO_2

B

Figure 4-3 Identifying the upper and lower respiratory tracts.

Pink indicates a prefix. Blue indicates a suffix. Boldface indicates a word root or combining form.

pharyng/itis făr-ĭn-JĪ-tĭs **pharyng/o/plasty** făr-ĬN-gō-plăs-tē **pharyng/o/tomy** făr-ĭn-GŎT-ō-mē **pharyng/o/tome** făr-ĬN-gō-tōm **pharyng/o/spasm** făr-ĬN-gō-spăzm	**4–15** Use *pharyng/o* to form medical words that mean *inflammation of the pharynx (throat):* _____ / _____. *surgical repair of the pharynx (throat):* _____ / ____ / _____. *incision of the pharynx (throat):* _____ / ____ / _____. *instrument to incise the pharynx (throat):* _____ / ____ / _____. *involuntary contraction or twitching of the pharynx (throat):* _____ / ____ / _____.
pharyng/o/cele făr-ĬN-gō-sēl	**4–16** Use *-cele* to build a word that literally means *hernia or swelling of the pharynx:* _____ / ____ / _____.
stricture, pharynx STRĬK-chūr, FĂR-ĭnks	**4–17** Pharyng/o/stenosis is a narrowing, or _____, of the _____.
	4–18 The (3) **larynx** (voice box) is responsible for sound production and makes speech possible. Label the larynx in Figure 4-3.
laryng/ectomy lăr-ĭn-JĔK-tō-mē	**4–19** When laryng/eal CA is detected in its early stages, a partial laryng/ectomy may be recommended. For extensive CA of the larynx, the entire larynx is removed. In either case, when excision of the larynx is performed, the surgery is called _____ / _____.
-stenosis laryng/o	**4–20** Laryng/o/stenosis is a narrowing or stricture of the larynx. Determine the elements that mean *narrowing, stricture:* _____. *larynx:* _____ / _____.

laryng/itis
lăr-ĭn-JĪ-tĭs

laryng/o/scope
lăr-ĬN-gō-skōp

laryng/o/scopy
lăr-ĭn-GŎS-kō-pē

laryng/o/stenosis
lăr-ĭn-gō-stĕ-NŌ-sĭs

4-21   Form medical words that mean

inflammation of the larynx:

_____ / _____.

instrument to view or examine the larynx:

_____ / _____ / _____.

visual examination of the larynx:

_____ / _____ / _____.

narrowing or stricture of the larynx:

_____ / _____ / _____.

4-22   A small leaf-shaped cartilage, called the (4) **epiglottis**, is located in the super/ior portion of the larynx. During swallowing, it closes off the larynx so that foods and liquids are directed into the esophagus. If anything except air passes into the larynx, a cough reflex attempts to expel the material to avoid a serious blockage of breathing. Label the epiglottis in Figure 4-3.

When defining a medical word, first define the suffix. Second, define the beginning of the word; finally, define the middle of the word. Here is an example of the term

bronch / o / pneumon / itis
(2)   (3)   (1)

SECTION REVIEW 4-2

Using the following table, write the CF, suffix, or prefix that matches its definition in the space provided to the left of the definition. There may be more than one word element that matches a definition.

Combining Forms		Suffixes		Prefixes
aer/o	*pharyng/o*	*-cele*	*-stenosis*	*a-*
hydr/o	*rhin/o*	*-ectasis*	*-stomy*	*an-*
laryng/o	*trache/o*	*-phagia*	*-therapy*	*neo-*
myc/o		*-plegia*	*-tome*	*para-*
nas/o		*-scopy*	*-tomy*	

1. _____ air

2. _____ near, beside; beyond

3. _____ fungus

4. _____ dilation, expansion

5. _____ forming an opening (mouth)

6. _____ incision

7. _____ instrument to cut

8. _____ larynx (voice box)

9. _____ hernia; swelling

10. _____ new

11. _____ nose

12. _____ paralysis

13. _____ pharynx (throat)

14. _____ narrowing, stricture

15. _____ swallowing, eating

16. _____ trachea (windpipe)

17. _____ treatment

18. _____ without, not

19. _____ visual examination

20. _____ water

Competency Verification: Check your answers in Appendix B: Answer Key, page 594. If you are not satisfied with your level of comprehension, go back to Frame 4–1, and rework the frames.

Correct Answers _____ x 5 = _____ % Score

Lower Respiratory Tract

bronchi/oles
BRŎNG-kē-ōlz

4-23   Continue to label structures in Figure 4-3, page 120, as you read the following material.

The (5) **trachea** (windpipe) is a cylindrical tube composed of smooth muscle embedded with a series of 16 to 20 C-shaped rings of cartilage. The trachea extends downward into the thoracic cavity, where it divides to form the (6) **right and left primary bronchi** (singular, *bronchus*). Each bronchus enters a lung and continues to subdivide into increasingly finer, smaller branches known as the (7) **bronchioles**.

The diminutive suffix *-ole* means *small, minute.* Thus, smaller segments of the bronchus are called _____ / _____.

bronchus
BRŎNG-kŭs

4-24   The continuous branching of the bronchi and bronchi/oles from the trachea throughout the lungs resembles an inverted tree. This series of respiratory tubes that branch into progressively narrower tubes as they extend into the lungs is known as the *bronchi/al tree.* Refer to Figure 4-1 to identify the structures of the bronchi/al tree.

The singular form of *bronchi* is _____.

cartilage
KĂR-tĭ-lĭj

4-25   The trachea's cartilaginous rings provide necessary rigidity to keep air passage open at all times. The CF *chondr/o* refers to *cartilage.*

Chondr/itis is an inflammation of _____.

chondr/o/plasty
KŎN-drō-plăs-tē

chondr/o/pathy
kŏn-DRŎP-ă-thē

chondr/oma
kŏn-DRŌ-mă

4-26   Form medical words that mean

surgical repair of cartilage: _____ / _____ / _____.

disease of cartilage: _____ / _____ / _____.

tumor (or tumorlike growth) of cartilage: _____ / _____.

trache/o/stomy
trā-kē-ŎS-tō-mē

4-27   On its way to the lungs, air passes from the larynx to the trachea (windpipe). In a life-threatening situation, when trache/al obstruction causes cessation of breathing, a trache/o/stomy is performed through the neck into the trachea to gain access below the blockage. (See Figure 4-4.)

When an emergency situation warrants creation of an opening (mouth) into the trachea, the procedure performed is a _____ / _____ / _____.

trache/o/malacia
trā-kē-ō-mă-LĀ-shē-ă

4-28   Softening of trache/al cartilage may be caused by pressure of the left pulmonary artery on the trachea. Use *-malacia* to form a word that literally means

softening of the trachea: _____ / _____ / _____.

Pink indicates a prefix. Blue indicates a suffix. **Boldface** indicates a word root or combining form.

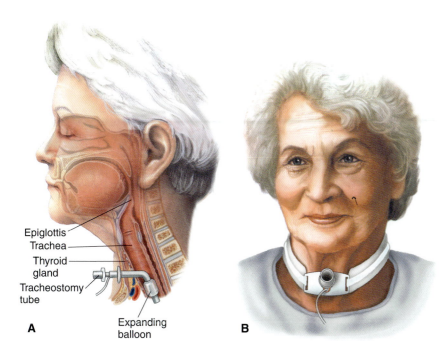

Epiglottis
Trachea
Thyroid gland
Tracheostomy tube
A
Expanding balloon
B

Figure 4-4 Tracheostomy. (A) Lateral view with tracheostomy tube in place. (B) Frontal view.

---

trache/o/pathy trā-kē-ŎP-ă-thē **trache/o/plasty** TRĀ-kē-ō-plăs-tē **trache/o/stenosis** trā-kē-ō-stĕn-Ō-sĭs **trache/o/tomy** trā-kē-ŎT-ō-mē	**4–29** Use **trache/o** to develop medical terms that mean *disease of the trachea:* _____ / _____ / _____ . *surgical repair of the trachea:* _____ / _____ / _____ . *narrowing or stricture of the trachea:* _____ / _____ / _____ . *incision of the trachea:* _____ / _____ / _____ .

4–30 Label the left lung in Figure 4-3 as you continue to read the material in this frame. Then, review the position of the trachea to see how it branches into right and left primary bronchi. Each primary bronchus (plural, *bronchi*) leads to a separate lung, the **right** and (8) **left lungs.** Structures of the bronchi and alveoli are part of the lungs, which are the organs of respiration (act of breathing).

---

bronchi BRŎNG-kē	**4–31** Change the singular form of *bronchus* to its plural form: _____ .

---

bronch/o/spasm BRŎNG-kō-spăzm	**4–32** Patients with asthma may experience wheezing caused by bronch/ial spasms. The medical term for this condition is *bronchi/o/spasm* or _____ / _____ / _____ .

---

bronchi/ectasis brŏng-kē-ĔK-tă-sĭs	**4-33** Chronic dilation of bronchi is called *bronchi/ectasis*. Chronic pneumon/ia or flu may result in dilation of bronchi. The medical term for this condition is _____ / _____ .
bronch/itis brŏng-KĪ-tĭs **bronch/o/spasm** BRŎNG-kō-spăzm **bronch/o/stenosis** brŏng-kō-stĕn-Ō-sĭs	**4-34** Use *bronch/o* to build medical words that mean *inflammation of bronchi:* _____ / _____ . *involuntary contraction or twitching of the bronchus:* _____ / _____ / _____ . *narrowing or stricture of bronchi:* _____ / _____ / _____ .
	4-35 Structurally, each primary bronchus is similar to that of the trachea, but as the bronchi subdivide into finer branches, the amount of cartilage in the walls decreases and finally disappears as it forms bronchi/oles. As cartilage diminishes, a layer of smooth muscle surrounding the tube becomes more prominent. Smooth muscles in the walls of bronchi/oles are designed to constrict or dilate the airways to maintain unobstructed air passages. Bronchi/oles eventually distribute air to the (9) **alveoli** (singular, *alveolus*), small clusters of grapelike air sacs of the lungs. Each alveolus is surrounded by a network of microscopic (10) **pulmonary capillaries**. Label the alveoli and pulmonary capillaries in Figure 4-3.
erythr/o/cytes ĕ-RĬTH-rō-sītz **oxygen** **carbon dioxide**	**4-36** The thin walls of the alveoli permit an exchange of gases between the alveolus and the surrounding capillaries. Blood flowing through the capillaries accepts oxygen (O_2) from the alveolus, while depositing carbon dioxide (CO_2) into the alveolus. Erythr/o/cytes in the blood carry O_2 to all parts of the body and CO_2 to the lungs for exhalation. The medical term for red blood cells is _____ / _____ / _____ . The abbreviation O_2 means _____ . The abbreviation CO_2 means _____ _____ .
alveoli ăl-VĒ-ō-lī	**4-37** If a lung disorder destroys or damages enough alveol/ar sacs, there is less surface area for gas exchange, and breathlessness results. Clusters of air sacs at the end of the bronchi/al tree are called _____ (plural).
O_2 CO_2	**4-38** The abbreviations O_2 and CO_2 are commonly seen in laboratory reports. Whenever you are in doubt about an abbreviation, refer to Appendix E, page 633, for a list of common abbreviations and symbols. The abbreviation for oxygen is _____ . The abbreviation for carbon dioxide is _____ .

Pink indicates a prefix. Blue indicates a suffix. Boldface indicates a word root or combining form.

4-39   Recall from the beginning of the chapter that the process of gas exchange between the atmosphere and body cells is called *respiration,* and it occurs in two phases. External respiration occurs each time we inhale (breathe in) air. This process results in a gas exchange (O_2 loading and CO_2 unloading) between air-filled chambers of the lungs and the blood in the pulmonary capillaries. Internal (cellular) respiration is the exchange of gases (O_2 unloading and CO_2 loading) between blood and body tissue cells. This process occurs in body tissues when O_2 (carried in blood from the lungs to nourish the body's cells) is exchanged for CO_2. The CO_2 travels in the bloodstream to the lungs and is exhaled through the mouth or nose. You may have to read this frame a few times to understand the process of respiration. See if you can differentiate between the two types of respiration and identify the symbols for oxygen and carbon dioxide.

Gas exchange between the body and the outside environment is called

_____ _____.

Gas exchange at the cellular level between blood and body tissue cells is called

_____ _____.

external respiration

internal respiration

---

inflammation, lung(s)
ĭn-flă-MĀ-shŭn

4-40   The CFs *pneum/o* and *pneumon/o* mean *air; lung.*
Pneumon/itis is an _____ of the _____.

---

air, lung

condition

4-41   Pneumon/ia, an acute inflammation and infection of the lungs in which alveoli fill with secretions, is a leading cause of death in the United States.

Analyze *pneumon/ia* by defining the word elements:

pneumon/o, which means _____ or _____

-ia, which means _____. (noun ending)

---

pneumon/ectomy
nū-mōn-ĔK-tō-mē

4-42   In patients with lung cancer, it may be necessary to remove part or all of the lung. (See Figure 4-5.)

Use *pneumon/o* to form a word that means *excision of a lung:*

_____ / _____.

---

pneumon/o/cele
nū-MŌN-ō-sēl

4-43   The suffix *-cele* means *hernia, swelling.* A hernial protrusion of lung tissue may be caused by a partial airway obstruction.

Use *pneumon/o* to form a word that means *herniation of the lung:*

_____ / _____ / _____.

---

pneumon/osis
nū-mōn-Ō-sĭs

pneumon/o/pathy
nū-mō-NŎP-ăth-ē

pneumon/ectomy
nū-mōn-ĔK-tō-mē

4-44   Use *pneumon/o* to build medical words that mean

abnormal condition of the lungs: _____ / _____.

disease of the lung: _____ / _____ / _____.

excision of a lung: _____ / _____.

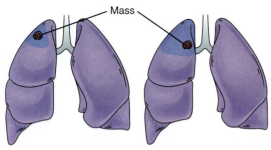

Wedge resection   Segmental resection

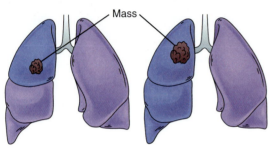

Lobectomy   Pneumonectomy

Figure 4-5 Types of pneumonectomy.

lung(s), air **black** **abnormal condition**	**4–45** Pneumon/o/melan/osis is an abnormal condition of black lung caused by inhalation of black dust (a disease common among coal miners), which is also called *pneumomelanosis* or *pneumoconiosis*. Analyze *pneumon/o/melan/osis* by defining the word elements *pneumon/o* means: _____ or _____. *melan/o* means: _____. *-osis* means: _____ _____.
excision *or* removal ĕk-SĬ-zhŭn	**4–46** Patients with lung CA may undergo a lob/ectomy, which is a(n) _____ of a lobe. (See Figure 4-5.)
lob/itis lō-BĬ-tĭs **lob/o/tomy** lō-BŎT-ō-mē **lob/ectomy** lō-BĔK-tō-mē	**4–47** Develop medical words that mean *inflammation of a lobe:* _____ / _____. *incision of a lobe:* _____ / _____ / _____. *excision of a lobe:* _____ / _____.
	4–48 Each lung is enclosed in a double-folded membrane called the (11) **pleura.** Label the pleura in Figure 4-3.
inflammation ĭn-flă-MĀ-shŭn	**4–49** Pleur/itis is an _____ of the pleura.

Pink indicates a prefix. Blue indicates a suffix. Boldface indicates a word root or combining form.

pleur/o	**4-50** From *pleur/o/dynia,* identify the CF for *pleura:* _____ / _____.
pleur/o/dynia, pleur/ algia ploo-rō-DĬN-ē-ă, ploo-RĂL-jē-ă	**4-51** Pain in the pleura is known as _____ / _____ / _____ or _____ / _____.
pneumon/o or pneum/o	**4-52** Pleur/o/pneumon/ia is pleurisy complicated with pneumonia. The CF for *air* or *lung* is _____ / _____.
pleur/itis ploo-RĪ-tĭs **pleur/o/cele** PLOO-rō-sēl	**4-53** Form medical words that mean *inflammation of the pleura:* _____ / _____. *hernia or swelling of the pleura:* _____ / ____ / _____.
inflammation, pleura PLOO-ră	**4-54** Pleurisy is an inflammation of the pleura. *Pleur/itis* is also an _____ of the _____.
inflammation, pleura PLOO-ră	**4-55** Whenever you see the word *pleur/isy* or *pleur/itis,* you will know it means _____ of the _____.
pleur/o/dynia ploo-rō-DĬN-ē-ă	**4-56** The suffixes *-algia* and *-dynia* refer to pain. The pleura commonly becomes inflamed when a person has pneumonia. This condition may cause pleur/algia, which is also called _____ / ____ / _____.
without, not **slow** **bad; painful; difficult** **good, normal** **rapid** **breathing**	**4-57** Prefixes *a-, brady-, dys-, eu-,* and *tachy-* are commonly attached to *-pnea* to describe various types of breathing conditions. Write the meanings of each of the following elements. *a-:* _____, _____. *brady-:* _____. *dys-:* _____ ; _____ ; _____. *eu-:* _____, _____. *tachy-:* _____. *-pnea:* _____.

a/pnea ĂP-nē-ă	**4-58** A/pnea is a temporary loss of breathing that results in brief or prolonged absence of spontaneous respiration. It is a serious symptom, especially in patients with other potentially life-threatening conditions. Causes include respiratory arrest or respiratory failure. A term that literally means *without breathing* is _____ / _____.
a/pnea ĂP-nē-ă	**4-59** When a/pnea occurs in premature infants, the immature central nervous system (CNS) fails to maintain a consistent respiratory rate. Thus, there are occasional long pauses between periods of regular breathing. An infant whose mother used cocaine during pregnancy is also likely to develop life-threatening a/pnea. When there is temporary cessation of breathing, the event is documented in the medical record as _____ / _____.
CPAP **OSA**	**4-60** Another type of a/pnea, obstructive sleep apnea (OSA), may be caused by enlarged tonsils that cause an airway obstruction. Treatment includes the use of a continuous positive airway pressure (CPAP) machine. (See Figure 4-6.) Provide the abbreviation that means *continuous positive airway pressure:* _____. *obstructive sleep apnea:* _____.
a/pnea ĂP-nē-ă **dys/pnea** dĭsp-NĒ-ă	**4-61** Because of airway obstruction, patients with OSA stop breathing multiple times each night. A/pnea is followed by a gasping breath that commonly awakens the patient and results in sleep deprivation, fatigue, and difficulty concentrating during the day. This condition occurs most commonly in middle-aged, obese men who snore excessively. Build a medical term that means *without or not breathing:* _____ / _____. *painful or difficult breathing:* _____ / _____.
dys/pnea dĭsp-NĒ-ă	**4-62** Dys/pnea is normal when caused by vigorous work or athletic activity. Dys/pnea can also occur as a result of various disorders of the respiratory system, such as pleurisy. A patient with pleurisy may experience _____ / _____.
eu- **-pnea**	**4-63** Eu/pnea is normal breathing, as distinguished from dys/pnea and a/pnea. From eu/pnea, determine word elements that mean *good, normal:* _____. *breathing:* _____.

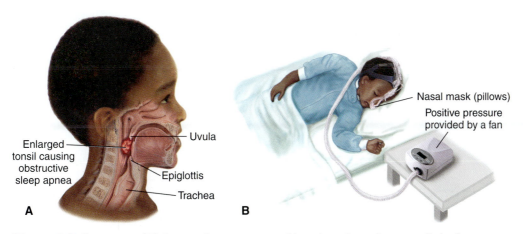

Figure 4-6 Sleep apnea. (A) Airway obstruction caused by enlarged tonsils, eventually leading to obstructive sleep apnea. (B) Continuous positive airway pressure (CPAP) machine.

-pnea **orth/o**	**4–64** Orth/o/pnea is a condition in which there is labored breathing in any posture except in the erect sitting or standing position. Identify word elements in this frame that mean *breathing:* _____. *straight:* _____ / _____.
thorac/o/tomy thō-răk-ŎT-ō-mē	**4–65** The CF *thorac/o* means chest. Form a word that means incision of the chest: _____ / _____ / _____.
thorac/o/centesis thō-răk-ō-sĕn-TĒ-sĭs	**4–66** To remove fluid from the thorac/ic cavity, a surgeon performs a surgical puncture of the chest. (See Figure 4-7.) This procedure is called *thoracentesis* or _____ / _____ / _____.
thoracentesis thō-ră-sĕn-TĒ-sĭs	**4–67** Fluid commonly builds up around the lung(s) in patients with CA or pneumonia. To remove fluid from the thorac/ic cavity, the physician performs the surgical procedure called *thorac/o/centesis,* also known as _____.
	4–68 The (12) **diaphragm** is a muscular partition that separates the lungs from the abdominal cavity and aids in the process of breathing. The CF *phren/o* refers to the diaphragm. Label the diaphragm in Figure 4-3.
phren/o	**4–69** The CF *phren/o* also refers to the mind. When you want to build words that refer to the diaphragm or mind, use the CF _____ / _____.
phren/o/spasm FRĔN-ō-spăzm	**4–70** Involuntary contraction or twitching of the diaphragm, also known as *hiccups,* is documented in the medical record as _____ / _____ / _____.

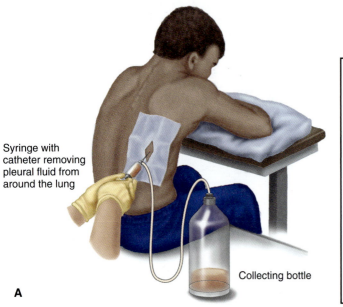

Syringe with catheter removing pleural fluid from around the lung

Collecting bottle

A

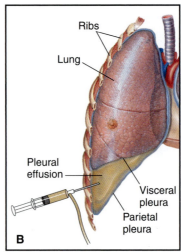

Ribs

Lung

Pleural effusion

Visceral pleura

Parietal pleura

B

Figure 4-7 Thoracentesis.

Competency Verification: Check your labeling of Figure 4-3 with Appendix B: Answer Key, page 594.

inspiration *or* **inhalation** ĭn-spĭ-RĀ-shŭn, ĭn-hă-LĀ-shŭn **expiration or exhalation** ĕks-pĭ-RĀ-shŭn, ĕks-hă-LĀ-shŭn	**4–71** Identify words in Figure 4-8 that mean *process of breathing air* *into the lungs:* _____. *out of the lungs:* _____.
inter/cost/al ĭn-tĕr-KŎS-tăl	**4–72** During inspiration, the diaphragm and the inter/cost/al muscles contract. As their name implies, the muscles between adjacent ribs are known as the _____ / _____ / _____ muscles.
descends **ascends**	**4–73** Examine Figure 4-8A and B and use the term *ascends* or *descends t*o complete this frame. During inspiration (or inhalation), the diaphragm _____. During expiration (or exhalation), the diaphragm _____.
muc/o **myc/o**	**4–74** Although the CFs *muc/o* and *myc/o* look similar, they have different meanings. Determine the CF that means *mucus:* _____ / _____. *fungus:* _____ / _____.

Pink indicates a prefix. Blue indicates a suffix. Boldface indicates a word root or combining form.

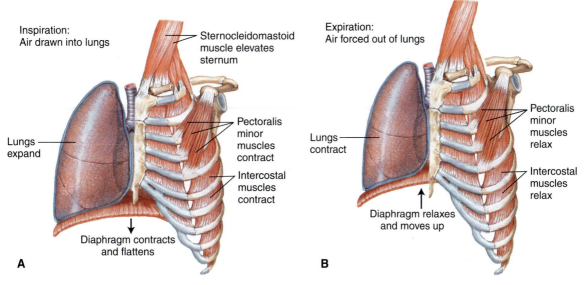

Inspiration:
Air drawn into lungs

Sternocleidomastoid muscle elevates sternum

Lungs expand

Pectoralis minor muscles contract

Intercostal muscles contract

Diaphragm contracts and flattens

A

Expiration:
Air forced out of lungs

Lungs contract

Pectoralis minor muscles relax

Intercostal muscles relax

Diaphragm relaxes and moves up

B

Figure 4-8 Position of the diaphragm during (A) inspiration and (B) expiration.

---

chronic bronch/itis brŏng-KĪ-tĭs	**4–75** Chronic bronch/itis is an inflammation of the bronchi that persists for a long time. This pulmon/ary disease is commonly caused by cigarette smoking and is characterized by increased production of mucus and obstruction of respiratory passages. Bronch/itis may be of short duration, but when it persists for a long time, it may be a more serious pulmon/ary disease called _____ _____ / _____.
bronchi/al BRŎNG-kē-ăl **bronch/itis** brŏng-KĪ-tĭs	**4–76** Chronic bronch/itis results in expectoration of mucus, sputum, or fluids by coughing or spitting. Use ***bronchi/o*** to build a term that means *pertaining to the bronchi*: _____ / _____. Use ***bronch/o*** to build a term that means inflammation of the bronchi: _____ / _____.
bronch/o **pneumon** **-ia**	**4–77** Pneumon/ia is lung inflammation caused by bacteria, viruses, fungi, or chemical irritants. Some pneumon/ias affect only one lobe of the lung (lobar pneumon/ia). Others, such as bronch/o/pneumon/ia, involve the surrounding areas of the bronchi, including the bronchioles, throughout the lung. Identify elements in *bronch/o/pneumon/ia* that mean *bronchus:* _____ / _____. *air; lung:* _____. *condition:* _____.

bronch/o/pneumon/ia brong-kō-nū-MŌ-nē-ă	**4–78** A type of pneumon/ia that involves the lungs and bronchi/oles is called _____ / _____ / _____.
-oles	**4–79** In Frame 4–78, the diminutive element that means *small or minute* is _____.
compromised, immunocompromised ĭm-ū-nō-KŎM-pră-mīzd	**4–80** *Pneumocystis* pneumon/ia (PCP) is closely associated with a compromised immune system, particularly in patients with acquired immune deficiency syndrome (AIDS). PCP is caused by a fungus that resides in or on the normal flora (potentially path/o/gen/ic organisms that reside in, but are harmless to, healthy individuals). The fungus becomes an aggressive path/o/gen in immunocompromised persons. Identify two terms in this frame that refer to an immune system incapable of resisting path/o/gen/ic organisms: _____ or _____.
PCP **AIDS**	**4–81** Identify the abbreviation for Pneumocystis *pneumon/ia:* _____. *Acquired immune deficiency syndrome:* _____.
***Pneumocystis* pneumonia** nū-mō-SĬS-tĭs nū-MŌ-nē-ă	**4–82** A type of pneumonia seen in patients with AIDS is _____ / _____.
COPD **asthma, emphys/ema** ĂZ-mă, ĕm-fĭ-SĒ-mă	**4–83** Chronic obstructive pulmonary disease (COPD), a group of respiratory disorders, is characterized by chronic, partial obstruction of the bronchi and lungs. Three major disorders included in COPD are asthma, chronic bronch/itis, and emphys/ema. (See Figure 4-9.) The abbreviation for *chronic obstructive pulmonary disease is* _____. Three major path/o/logic/al conditions associated with COPD are chronic bronch/itis, _____, and _____ / _____.
bronch/itis brong-KĪ-tĭs	**4–84** Chronic bronch/itis, an inflammation of the mucous membranes lining the bronchial airways, is characterized by increased mucus production resulting in a chronic productive cough. (See Figure 4-9A.) Cigarette smoking, environmental irritants, allergic response, and infectious agents cause this condition. The medical term that means *inflammation of bronchi* is _____ / _____.
emphys/ema ĕm-fĭ-SĒ-mă	**4–85** The CF *emphys/o* means *to inflate.* The suffix *-ema* means *state of; condition.* Emphys/ema is a chronic disease characterized by overexpansion and destruction of alveoli and is commonly associated with cigarette smoking. (See Figure 4-9B.) Destruction of alveoli occurs in the respiratory disease known as _____ / _____.

Pink indicates a prefix. Blue indicates a suffix. Boldface indicates a word root or combining form.

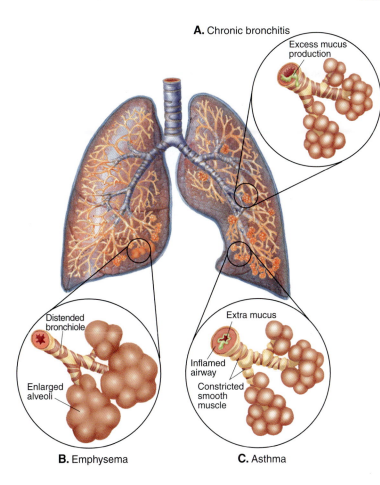

A. Chronic bronchitis

Excess mucus production

Distended bronchiole

Enlarged alveoli

B. Emphysema

Extra mucus

Inflamed airway

Constricted smooth muscle

C. Asthma

Figure 4-9 Chronic obstructive pulmonary disease (COPD). (A) Chronic bronchitis with inflamed airways and excessive mucus. (B) Emphysema with distended bronchioles and alveoli. (C) Asthma with narrowed bronchial tubes and swollen mucous membranes.

dys/pnea dĭsp-NĒ-ă	**4–86** Asthma is a respiratory condition characterized by recurrent attacks of labored or difficult breathing accompanied by wheezing. (See Figure 4-9C.) The medical term for painful or difficult breathing is _____ / _____.
metastasize *or* **metastasis** mĕ-TĂS-tă-sīz, mĕ-TĂS-tă-sĭs	**4–87** Lung CA, associated with smoking, is the leading cause of cancer-related deaths in men and women in the United States. It usually spreads rapidly and metastasizes to other parts of the body, making it difficult to diagnose and treat it in its early stages. When CA spreads to other parts of the body, the medical term used to describe that condition is _____.
tuberculosis tū-bĕr-kū-LŌ-sĭs **tubercles** TŪ-bĕr-klz	**4–88** Tuberculosis (TB), an infectious disease, produces small lesions, or tubercles, in the lungs. If left untreated, it infects the bones and organs of the entire body. An increase in TB is attributed to the increasing prevalence of AIDS. The abbreviation TB refers to _____. The name *tuberculosis* is derived from small lesions that appear in the lungs called _____.

SECTION REVIEW 4-3

Using the following table, write the CF, suffix, or prefix that matches its definition in the space provided to the left of the definition. There may be more than one word element that matches a definition.

Combining Forms		Suffixes		Prefixes	
bronch/o	orth/o	-cele	-scope	a-	tachy-
bronchi/o	pleur/o	-centesis	-spasm	brady-	
chondr/o	pneum/o	-ectasis	-stenosis	dys-	
hem/o	pneumon/o	-osis		eu-	
melan/o	thorac/o	-phobia		macro-	
myc/o		-pnea		micro-	

1. _____ abnormal condition; increase (used primarily with blood cells)

2. _____ slow

3. _____ bad; painful; difficult

4. _____ black

5. _____ breathing

6. _____ bronchus (plural, bronchi)

7. _____ blood

8. _____ chest

9. _____ dilation, expansion

10. _____ fear

11. _____ fungus

12. _____ good, normal

13. _____ hernia, swelling

14. _____ instrument for examining

15. _____ involuntary contraction, twitching

16. _____ large

17. _____ rapid

18. _____ air; lung

19. _____ pleura

20. _____ small

21. _____ straight

22. _____ narrowing, stricture

23. _____ surgical puncture

24. _____ without, not

25. _____ cartilage

Competency Verification: Check your Answers in Appendix B: Answer Key, page 594. If you are not satisfied with your level of comprehension, go back to Frame 4–23, and rework the frames.

Correct Answers _____ x 4 = _____ % Score

Abbreviations

This section introduces abbreviations related to the respiratory system and their meanings.

Abbreviation	Meaning	Abbreviation	Meaning
ABG	arterial blood gas	MRI	magnetic resonance imaging
AIDS	acquired immune deficiency syndrome	NMT	nebulized mist treatment
ARDS	acute respiratory distress syndrome	NG	nasogastric
CA	cancer; chronological age; cardiac arrest	O_2	oxygen
CF	cystic fibrosis	OSA	obstructive sleep apnea
CO_2	carbon dioxide	PCO_2, $PaCO_2$, PCO_2	partial pressure of carbon dioxide
COPD	chronic obstructive pulmonary disease	PCP	*Pneumocystis* pneumonia; primary care physician
COVID-19	coronavirus disease 2019	PE	pulmonary embolism
CPAP	continuous positive airway pressure	PFT	pulmonary function test
CT	computed tomography	pH	degree of acidity or alkalinity
DPT	diphtheria, pertussis, tetanus	PPD	purified protein derivative (substance used in a tuberculosis test)
Dx	diagnosis	PSG	polysomnography
EEG	electroencephalography, electroencephalogram	SARS	severe acute respiratory syndrome
ETT	endotracheal tube	SAT	saturation
FVC	forced vital capacity	SIDS	sudden infant death syndrome
HCO_3	bicarbonate	SOB	shortness of breath
HF	heart failure	TB	tuberculosis

Additional Medical Terms

The following terms are additional terms related to the respiratory system. Recognizing and learning these terms will help you understand the connections among common signs, symptoms, diseases, and their diagnoses as well as the rationale behind the methods of medical and surgical treatments selected for a particular disorder.

Diseases and Conditions

acidosis ăs-i-DŌ-sĭs	Excessive acidity of blood caused by an accumulation of acids or an excessive loss of bicarbonate *Respiratory acidosis is caused by abnormally high levels of CO_2 in the body.*
acute respiratory distress syndrome (ARDS) RĔS-pĭ-ră-tō-rē dĭs-TRĔS SĬN-drōm	Respiratory insufficiency marked by progressive hypoxia *ARDS is caused by severe inflammatory damage that causes abnormal permeability of the alveolar–capillary membrane. As a result, the alveoli fill with fluid, which interferes with gas exchange.*
adventitious breath sounds ăd-vĕn-TĬSH-ŭs	Abnormal breath sounds heard during respiration (breathing in and out) with the use of a stethoscope (auscultation) *Identifying the type of adventitious breath sound is important and assists the physician in determining a diagnosis.*
pleural rub PLOO-răl	Grating sound of the pleural linings rubbing against each other that is heard on auscultation; also called *friction rub* *A pleural rub helps diagnose pleurisy, pneumonia, and other conditions affecting the lungs. This condition occurs where the pleural layers are inflamed and have lost their lubrication.*
rales RĂLZ	Fine, crackling or bubbling sounds, commonly heard during inspiration when there is fluid in the alveoli; also called *crackles* *Rales are commonly associated with bronchitis, pneumonia, and heart failure (HF). Rales that do not clear after a cough may indicate pulmonary edema or fluid in the alveoli caused by HF or ARDS.*
rhonchi RONG-kē	Snoring, rumbling sounds heard upon auscultation of the chest during respiration *Rhonchi indicate inflammation and congestion of the bronchi caused by inflammation, mucus, or a foreign body that partially obstructs the bronchi.*
stridor STRĪ-dor	High-pitched, musical breathing sound made on inspiration and caused by obstruction in the pharynx or larynx, commonly heard without the use of a stethoscope *Stridor is characteristic of the upper respiratory disorder called croup. It is also caused by an allergic reaction, airway injury, throat abscess, or laryngitis.*
wheezes HWĒZ-ĕz	Continuous, high-pitched whistling sounds, usually heard during expiration and caused by narrowing of an airway *Wheezes occur in such conditions as asthma, croup, hay fever, and emphysema.*

anoxia
ăn-ŎK-sē-ă
   an: without, not
   -oxia: oxygen
	Total absence of O_2 in body tissues
	
	Anoxia is caused by a lack of O_2 in inhaled air or obstruction that prevents O_2 from reaching the lungs.

atelectasis ăt-ĕ-LĔK-tă-sĭs *atel:* -incomplete; imperfect *-ectasis:* dilation, expansion	Collapse of lung tissue, preventing respiratory exchange of O_2 and CO_2 *Atelectasis can be caused by obstruction of foreign bodies, excessive secretions, or pressure on the lung from a tumor. In fetal atelectasis, the lungs fail to expand normally at birth.*
coronavirus kŭh-RŌ-nŭh-vī-rŭs **COVID-19**	Group of viruses that can cause illnesses such as the common cold and severe acute respiratory syndrome (SARS) that is highly contagious and mainly spreads through respiratory droplets produced when an infected person breathes, talks, sneezes, or coughs Pandemic of new coronavirus that originated in China in 2019; common symptoms include loss of taste and smell, fever, cough, tiredness, and difficulty breathing with some experiencing worsened SOB and pneumonia after a week of onset *Those who are older, have existing chronic medical conditions, or immunosuppression are at an increased risk of severity. This pandemic has infected millions of Americans in the United States. Currently, several vaccines are available to prevent infections (See Figure 4.10).*
coryza kō-RĪ-ză	Acute inflammation of nasal passages accompanied by profuse nasal discharge; also called a *cold*
croup CROOP	Acute respiratory syndrome that occurs primarily in children and infants and is characterized by laryngeal obstruction and spasm, barking cough, and stridor

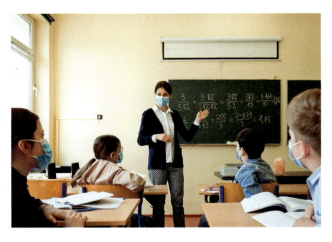

Figure 4-10 Teacher and students in the classroom wearing masks and social distancing 6 ft., the recommendation by medical experts to prevent the spread of COVID-19.

cystic fibrosis (CF)
SĬS-tĭk fĭ-BRŌ-sĭs
cyst: bladder
   -ic: pertaining to
fibr: fiber, fibrous
      tissue
-osis: abnormal
         condition;
         increase (used
         primarily with
         blood cells)
	Genetic disease of exocrine glands characterized by excessive secretions of thick mucus that does not drain normally, causing obstruction of passageways (including pancreatic and bile ducts and bronchi)
	
	CF leads to chronic airway obstruction, recurrent respiratory infection, bronchiectasis, and, eventually, respiratory failure.

empyema ĕm-pī-Ē-mă	Pus in a body cavity, especially in the pleural cavity (pyothorax) *Empyema is usually the result of a primary infection in the lungs.*
epiglottitis ĕp-ĭ-glŏt-Ī-tĭs *epiglott:* epiglottis *-itis:* inflammation	In the acute form, a severe, life-threatening infection of the epiglottis and surrounding area that occurs most commonly in children between ages 2 and 12 years with a sudden onset of fever, dysphagia, inspiratory stridor, and severe respiratory distress *Treatment of epiglottitis involves establishing an open airway for the person to breathe, including a breathing tube (intubation) and moistened (humidified) O_2. Also, intravenous (IV) therapy with antibiotics will be started immediately to help treat the infection by the bacteria.*
epistaxis ĕp-ĭ-STĂK-sĭs	Hemorrhage from the nose; also called *nosebleed*
hypoxemia hī-pŏks-Ē-mē-ă *hyp:* -under, below, deficient *ox:* oxygen *-emia:* blood	Deficiency of oxygen in blood, usually a sign of respiratory impairment; also called *low blood oxygen* *Blood oxygen can be measured by testing a sample of blood from an artery.*
hypoxia hī-PŎKS-ē-ă *hyp:* under, below, deficient *ox:* oxygen *-ia:* condition	Deficiency of O_2 in body tissues, usually a sign of respiratory impairment *Generalized hypoxia occurs in healthy people when they ascend to high altitudes, where it causes altitude sickness that may lead to potentially fatal complications.*

influenza
ĭn-floo-ĔN-ză

Acute, contagious respiratory infection characterized by sudden onset of fever, chills, headache, and muscle pain; also known as the *flu*

lung cancer
KĂN-sĕr

Pulmonary malignancy commonly attributed to cigarette smoking and inhalation of particles that lodge in the lung

Lung CA comprises various malignant neoplasms that may appear in the trachea, bronchi, or air sacs of the lungs. Survival rates are low in lung CA because of rapid metastasis and late detection.

pleural mesothelioma
PLOO-răl mĕz-ō-thē-lē-Ō-mă
   pleur/o: pleura
     -al: pertaining to
   meso: middle
   thel/i: nipple
   -oma: tumor

Aggressive, rare lung CA that develops in the pleura (mesothelium layer) caused primarily by the inhalation of microscopic asbestos fibers. (See Figure 4-11.)

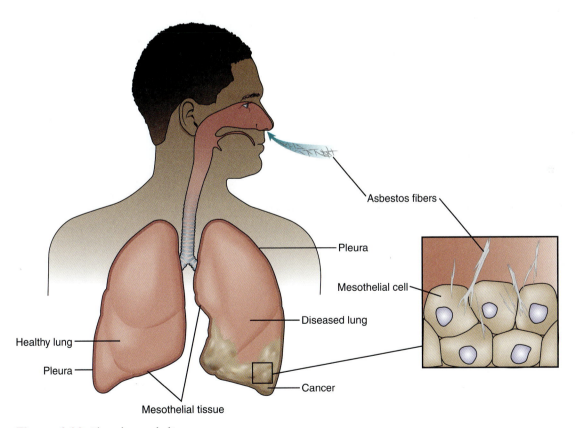

Asbestos fibers

Pleura

Mesothelial cell

Diseased lung

Cancer

Healthy lung

Pleura

Mesothelial tissue

Figure 4-11 Pleural mesothelioma.

pertussis pĕr-TŬS-ĭs	Acute infectious disease characterized by a cough with a sound like a "whoop"; also called *whooping cough* *Immunization of infants as part of the diphtheria, pertussis, tetanus (DPT) vaccine prevents the spread of pertussis.*
pleural effusion PLOO-răl ĕ-FŪ-zhŭn *pleur:* pleura *-al:* pertaining to	Abnormal presence of fluid in the pleural cavity *The fluid may contain blood (hemothorax), serum (hydrothorax), or pus (pyothorax). Treatment includes a surgical puncture of the chest using a hollow-bore needle (thoracentesis, thoracocentesis) to remove excess fluid.*
pneumothorax nū-mō-THŌ-răks *pneum/o:* air; lung *-thorax:* chest	Collection of air in the pleural cavity, causing the complete or partial collapse of a lung *Pneumothorax can occur with pulmonary disease (emphysema, lung CA, or TB) when pulmonary lesions rupture near the pleural surface, allowing communication between an alveolus or bronchus and the pleural cavity. It may also be the result of an open chest wound or a perforation of the chest wall that permits the entrance of air. (See Figure 4-12.)*
sudden infant death syndrome (SIDS)	Completely unexpected and unexplained death of an apparently healthy infant; also called *crib death* *SIDS is the most common cause of death occurring between the second week and first year of life.*

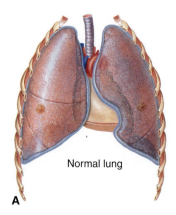
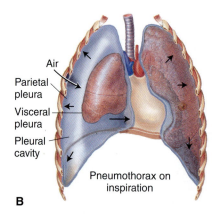
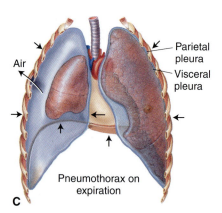

Figure 4-12 Pneumothorax. (A) Normal lung. (B) Pneumothorax on inspiration in which outside air rushes in due to disruption of chest wall and parietal pleura and the mediastinal contents shift to the side opposite the injury, compressing the uninjured lung. (C) Pneumothorax on expiration in which lung air rushes out as a result of disruption of visceral pleura and the mediastinal contents move toward the center.

Diagnostic Procedures

arterial blood gas (ABG) ăr-TĒ-rē-ăl *arteri:* artery *-al:* pertaining to	Measurement of the O_2 and CO_2 content of arterial blood by using various methods *ABG analysis is used to assess the adequacy of ventilation and oxygenation and the acid–base status of the body.*
bronchoscopy brŏng-KŎS-kō-pē *bronch/o:* bronchus (plural, bronchi) *-scopy:* visual examination	Visual examination of the interior bronchi using a bronchoscope, a flexible fiber-optic instrument with a light, which can be inserted through the nose or mouth (See Figure 4-13.) *Bronchoscopy may be performed to remove obstructions, obtain a biopsy specimen, or observe directly for pathological changes.*

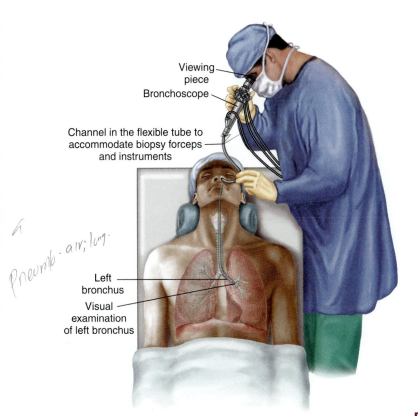

Figure 4-13 Bronchoscopy of the left bronchus.

computed tomography (CT) cŏm-PŪ-tĕd tō-MŎG-ră-fē *tom/o:* to cut, slice *-graphy:* process of recording	Radiographic study using a narrow beam of x-rays; the CT equipment rotates in a full arc around the patient to acquire multiple views of the body, and a computer interprets the images to produce a cross-sectional view of an internal organ or tissue; also called *computerized axial tomography (CAT) scanning* *In the respiratory system, CT detects lesions in the lungs and thorax, blood clots, and pulmonary embolism. CT may be performed with or without a contrast medium.*
COVID-19 tests	Laboratory tests performed to detect the presence of antibodies or the presence of the COVID-19 virus
antibody	Blood test to detect the presence of antibodies to determine past infection with the virus that causes COVID-19 *It can take 2 to 3 weeks to develop enough antibodies for detection and is important that testing not be done too soon.*
nose swab	Long swab is used to take a sample from the upper nasal cavity that is then sent to a laboratory for testing (See Figure 4-14.)

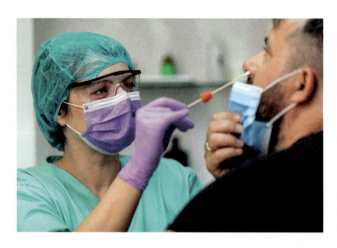

Figure 4-14 Doctor in protective workwear taking nose swab test from middle-aged man wearing face mask, during the COVID-19 pandemic outbreak.

magnetic resonance imaging (MRI) măg-NĔT-ĭc RĔZ-ĕn-ăns ĬM-ĭj-ĭng	Radiographic procedure that uses electromagnetic energy to produce multiplanar, cross-sectional images of the body *In the respiratory system, MRI produces a scan of the chest and lungs. MRI does not require a contrast medium, but it may be used to enhance visualization of internal structures.*
polysomnography (PSG) pŏl-ē-sŏm-NŎG-ră-fē *poly-:* many, much *somn/o:* sleep *-graphy:* process of recording	Test that diagnoses sleep disorders by recording various aspects of sleep, such as eye and muscle movements, respiration, and EEG patterns (See Figure 4-15.) *Electrodes on the head, face, and fingers as well as other monitors record the patient's brain waves, heart rate, and breathing, including eye and leg movements during the sleep study.*

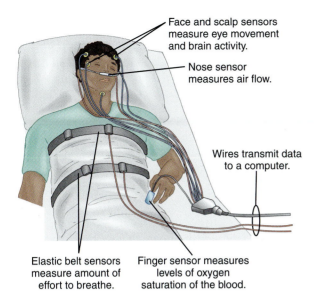

Face and scalp sensors measure eye movement and brain activity.

Nose sensor measures air flow.

Wires transmit data to a computer.

Elastic belt sensors measure amount of effort to breathe.

Finger sensor measures levels of oxygen saturation of the blood.

Figure 4-15 Polysomnography.

pulmonary function tests (PFTs) PŬL-mō-nĕ-rē	Group of tests that measure the capacity of the lungs and the volume of air during inhalation and exhalation *PFTs can diagnose lung diseases, measure the severity of lung impairments, and check to see how well treatment for a lung disease is working.*

spirometry
 spī-RŎM-ĕ-trē
    spir/o: to breathe
    -metry: act of
          measuring
	Common lung function test that measures and records the volume and rate of inhaled and exhaled air and is used to assess pulmonary function by means of a spirometer
	
	 Spirometry is most useful when assessing for obstructive lung diseases, especially asthma and COPD. (See Figure 4-16.)

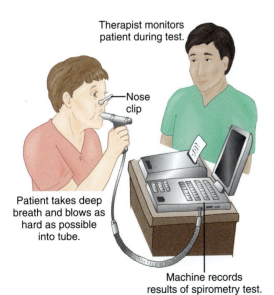

Therapist monitors patient during test.

Nose clip

Patient takes deep breath and blows as hard as possible into tube.

Machine records results of spirometry test.

Figure 4-16 Spirometry.

tuberculosis tests too-BĔRK-ū-lō-sĭs	Skin tests to determine whether a patient has been exposed to tuberculosis *A raised skin reaction after 48–72 hours indicates a prior exposure to tuberculosis with antibodies to the tuberculosis bacterium. A positive test is followed up with a chest x-ray to confirm whether or not the patient has active tuberculosis.*
Mantoux test	Screening test using an intradermal injection of purified protein derivative (PPD)
tine test	Screening test using a four-pronged device to puncture the skin and introduce PPD, part of the bacterium

Medical and Surgical Procedures

endotracheal intubation
ĕn-dŏ- TRĀ-kē-ăl ĭn-tū-BĀ-shŭn
  endo-: in, within
  trache-: trachea
    (windpipe)
  -al: pertaining to
	Insertion of an endotracheal tube (ETT) through the mouth or nose into the trachea (windpipe) just above the bronchi to provide air to patients who are unable to breathe on their own because of airway obstruction or respiratory failure, as well as to administer O$_2$, medication, or anesthesia. (See Figure 4-17.)
	
	A lighted laryngoscope is used to hold the airway open and helps visualize the vocal cords before insertion of the endotracheal tube.

postural drainage PŎS-chur-ăl	Use of body positioning to assist in removal of secretions from specific lobes of the lung, bronchi, or lung cavities

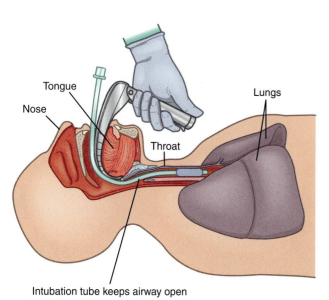

Figure 4-17 Endotracheal intubation.

Pharmacology

The following table lists common drug categories used to treat respiratory disorders, as well as their therapeutic actions.

Drug Category	Action
antituberculars ăn-tĭ-too- BĔR-kū-lărs	Used to treat tuberculosis, an infectious disease caused by *mycobacterium tuberculosis;* infection mainly affects the lungs but can also affect other organs *Several antituberculars are used in combination for effective treatment.*
bronchodilators brŏng-kō-DĬ-lă-tŏrz	Increase airflow by dilating constricted airways through relaxation of the smooth muscles that surround the bronchioles and bronchi *Bronchodilators are used to treat asthma, emphysema, COPD, and exercise-induced bronchospasm. Most bronchodilators provide metered dosages of the medication and may employ a spacer as a reservoir for the medication. (See Figure 4-18.)*
corticosteroids kor-tĭ-kō-STĔR-oyds	Decrease inflammation in the airways, reducing swelling and mucus production and making breathing easier *Corticosteroids are used to treat chronic lung conditions, such as COPD and asthma.*
mucolytics MŪ-kō-LĬT-ĭks	Liquefy sputum or reduce its viscosity so that it can be coughed up more easily
nebulized mist treatments (NMTs) NĔB-ū-līzd	Produce a fine spray (nebulizer) to deliver a medication directly into the lungs (See Figure 4-19.)

Pronunciation Help	*Long Sound*	ā in rāte	ē in rēbirth	ī in īsle	ō in ōver	ū in ūnite
	Short Sound	ă in ăpple	ĕ in ĕver	ĭ in ĭt	ŏ in nŏt	ŭ in cŭt

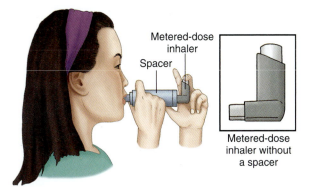

Figure 4-18 Inhaler with spacer.

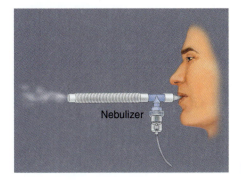

Figure 4-19 Nebulizer.

Word Elements Review

This review provides a verification of word elements covered in this chapter. First, use a slash to break the term into its component parts, and identify each element by labeling it P for prefix, WR for word root, CF for combining form, and S for suffix. Then, provide the meaning of the medical term. Remember to define the suffix first, define the beginning of the word second, and define the middle part of the term last. The first word is a sample completed for you.

Medical Term	Meaning
chondr/oma *WR S*	tumor containing cartilage
1. a/pnea	
2. pleur/o/dynia	
3. trache/o/stomy	
4. bronchi/ectasis	
5. pneumon/ectomy	

Match the medical following terms with the definitions in the numbered list.

anosmia   hemophobia   lobitis   rhinorrhea
emphysema   intercostal   pneumonia   thoracotomy
erythrocyte   laryngectomy   pneumonocentesis tracheostenosis

6. _____ red blood cell

7. _____ watery discharge from the nose

8. _____ incision into the chest

9. _____ surgical puncture of the lung

10. _____ chronic disease characterized by overexpansion and destruction of the alveoli

11. _____ narrowing or stricture of the trachea

12. _____ excision of the larynx

13. _____ loss or impairment of the sense of smell

14. _____ pertaining to the area between the ribs

15. _____ fear of blood

Competency Verification: Check your answers in Appendix B: Answer Key, page 595. If you are not satisfied with your level of comprehension, review the vocabulary, and retake the review.

Correct Answers _____ × 6.67 = _____ % Score

Additional Medical Terms Review

Match the following medical term(s) with the definitions in the numbered list.

acidosis	*coryza*	*epistaxis*	*lung cancer*	*rales*
ARDS	*COVID-19*	*hypoxemia*	*pertussis*	*rhonchi*
atelectasis	*cystic fibrosis*	*hypoxia*	*pleural effusion*	*SIDS*
bronchodilators	*epiglottitis*	*influenza*	*pneumothorax*	*stridor*

1. _____ is a high-pitched, musical breathing sound made on inspiration and caused by obstruction in the pharynx or larynx.

2. _____ refers to *nosebleed.*

3. _____ is a contagious respiratory infection characterized by the onset of fever, chills, headache, and muscle pain; also called *flu.*

4. _____ is excessive acidity of blood due to an accumulation of acids or excessive loss of bicarbonate.

5. _____ is acute inflammation of nasal passages accompanied by profuse nasal discharge; also called a *cold.*

6. _____ is a genetic disorder of exocrine glands characterized by excessive production of mucus, causing severe congestion within the lungs and pancreas.

7. _____ refers to a pulmonary malignancy commonly attributed to cigarette smoking.

8. _____ is an abnormal presence of fluid in the pleural cavity.

9. _____ refers to an accumulation of air in the pleural cavity.

10. _____ is fine, crackling or bubbling sounds, commonly heard during inspiration when there is fluid in the alveoli.

11. _____ are used to dilate bronchial walls to increase airflow.

12. _____ is a form of restrictive lung disease that follows severe infection or trauma in young, previously healthy individuals.

13. _____ is a recent virus in 2019 causing a public health emergency of international concern that is highly contagious and mainly spreads through respiratory droplets

14. _____ refers to a collapsed lung.

15. _____ is a severe, life-threatening infection of the epiglottis that occurs most commonly in children.

16. _____ is an acute infectious disease characterized by an explosive cough that is also called *whooping cough.*

17. _____ is a deficiency of O_2 in blood.

18. _____ refers to the unexpected, unexplained death of an apparently healthy infant.

19. _____ is a deficiency of O_2 in tissues.

20. _____ refers to abnormal chest sounds resembling snoring that is produced in obstructed airways.

Competency Verification: Check your answers in Appendix B: Answer Key, page 595. If you are not satisfied with your level of comprehension, review the pathological, diagnostic, and therapeutic terms, and retake the review.

Correct Answers _____ × 5 =_____ % Score

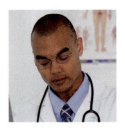

Medical Record Activities

To develop a working vocabulary of medical terms and to understand how those terms are used in the health-care industry, it is important that you complete the following activities.

MEDICAL RECORD ACTIVITY 4-1

REFERRAL LETTER: ALLERGIC RHINITIS

This activity contains a referral letter for a patient with an allergy. Read the consultation letter that follows, and underline the medical terms. Then, complete the terminology and critical thinking exercises.

REFERRAL LETTER

ENT Hospital Clinic

682 Lancaster

Dallas, TX 12345

April 5, 20xx

Elizabeth Gardner, MD
2728 Robert Blvd
Cleveland, OH 34569

Dear Dr. Gardner:

RE: Juanita Harding

I saw Ms. Harding today for complaints suggestive of allergic rhinitis. She has had a long history of nasal obstruction. Previously she was found to have mechanical destruction secondary to septal deformity and turbinate hypertrophy. She had a septoplasty and turbinate reduction the latter part of last year, and the procedure has significantly improved her airway compromise. She has noted some seasonal nasal symptoms of sneezing, watery rhinorrhea, a tickling of the palate, and burning of the eyes. This typically exacerbates in the spring and summer months. She is just beginning to experience the symptoms again at this time. She has nothing that would suggest recurrent sinusitis.

Her examination today revealed unremarkable otoscopic findings. Nasal examination revealed an essentially midline septum with improvement in the nasal airway after the septoplasty. The turbinates were lateralized inferiorly. The mucosa, however, throughout the nasal cavities appeared to be somewhat pale and edematous, with a serous discharge present. The sinuses were nontender. The nasopharynx was clear. The oral cavity and oropharynx were without mucosal lesion or induration. Neck was unremarkable to palpation.

My impression, based on her symptoms and findings, is allergic rhinitis. I have given her samples of Double Strength Vancenase AQ and Allegra for this. However, I think it would be best for her to see an allergist to undergo definitive allergy testing.

Sincerely yours,

Juan Perez, M.D.

_____

Juan Perez, M.D.

JP:rm

D: 4/5/20xx; T: 4/5/20xx

Terminology 4-1

Terms listed in the following table come from the referral letter Allergic Rhinitis. *Use a medical dictionary, such as Taber's Cyclopedic Medical Dictionary, the appendices of this book, or other resources to define each term. Then, pronounce the term, and place a ✓ in the box after you do so.*

Term	Definition
exacerbates ĕks-ĂS-ĕr-bātz ☐	
hypertrophy hī-PĔR-trŏ-fē ☐	
nasopharynx nā-zō-FĂR-ĭnks ☐	
otoscopic ō-tō-SKŎP-ĭc ☐	
rhinitis rī-NĪ-tĭs ☐	
rhinorrhea rī-nō-RĒ-ă ☐	
septoplasty SĔP-tō-plăs-tē ☐	
turbinate TŪR-bĭn-āt ☐	

Visit the *Medical Terminology Simplified* online resource center at FADavis.com to hear pronunciation and meanings of terms in this medical report.

Critical Thinking 4-1

Review the previous referral letter to answer the following questions. Use a medical dictionary, such as Taber's Cyclopedic Medical Dictionary, *and other resources, if needed.*

1. What surgeries did the patient have last year?

   _____

   _____

2. What was the outcome of last year's surgery?

   _____

   _____

3. What seasonal symptoms are currently noted by the patient?

   _____

   _____

4. How is the nasal mucosa described?

   _____

   _____

5. What was the recommendation of the physician?

   _____

   _____

MEDICAL RECORD ACTIVITY 4-2

PULMONARY FUNCTION REPORT

This activity contains the results of a pulmonary function test performed on a patient diagnosed with shortness of breath. Read the pulmonary function report note that follows, and underline the medical terms. Then, complete the terminology and critical thinking exercises.

PULMONARY FUNCTION REPORT

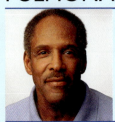

PATIENT NAME: Lewis, Malcolm
MEDICAL RECORD ID: 98-48178
DATE: August 6, 20xx

SMOKING HISTORY: 90 pack-years

DIAGNOSIS: Shortness of breath

COMMENTS: Ratio analysis: ABG—pH - 7.38, Pco_2 - 78, HCO_3 - 22, SAT - 94%

CALIBRATION: 3.00 L expected, 2.98 L measured

INTERPRETATION: A mild decrease in forced vital capacity. A moderate decrease in forced expiratory volume in 1 second. The timed vital capacity is mildly reduced. Maximum mid-flow is severely decreased. There is no significant improvement in airflow following inhalation of the bronchodilators.

IMPRESSION: Mild limitation to the airflow. Arterial blood gas analysis on room air on this patient reveals normoxemia with normal acid–base status.

John J. Spinella M.D
_____

John J. Spinella, M.D.

JJS:ba
D: 8/6/xx; T: 8/6/xx

Terminology 4-2

Terms listed in the following table come from Pulmonary Function Report. *Use a medical dictionary, such as* Taber's Cyclopedic Medical Dictionary, *the appendices of this book, or other resources to define each term. Then, pronounce the term, and place a checkmark (✓) in the box after you do so.*

Term	Definition
bronchodilators brŏng-kō-DĪ-lā-tŏrz ☐	
expiratory ĕks-PĪ-ră-tor-ē ☐	
pulmonary PŬL-mō-nĕ-rē ☐	
SOB	
vital capacity VĪ-tăl ☐	

Visit the *Medical Terminology Simplified* online resource center at FADavis.com to hear pronunciation and meanings of terms in this medical report.

Critical Thinking 4-2

Review the previous pulmonary function report to answer the following questions. Use a medical dictionary, such as Taber's Cyclopedic Medical Dictionary, *and other resources, if needed.*

1. Did this patient have any difficulty breathing?

   _____

   _____

2. What was the presenting diagnosis?

   _____

   _____

3. What was the hydrogen ion concentration?

   _____

   _____

4. What was the level of bicarbonate radical?

   _____

   _____

5. What was the partial pressure of carbon dioxide? (*Clue:* This patient is retaining carbon dioxide.)

   _____

   _____

MEDICAL RECORD ACTIVITY 4-3

CLINICAL APPLICATION

This activity is a clinical application that will help you integrate and reinforce your understanding of how the following medical terms are used in the clinical environment. Complete the following clinically related sentences by selecting an appropriate term from the list.

acidosis	*influenza*	*PFT*	*rales*
bronchodilator	*laryngoscope*	*pneumonia*	*thoracocentesis*
bronchorrhagia	*mucolytic*	*pneumothorax*	*tracheotomy*

1. A 25-year-old singer complains of hoarseness. Her physician prepares for a diagnostic test, explaining that he will use a _____ to view her vocal cords.

2. Joan S. presents to the emergency department (ED) complaining of fever, chills, headache, and generalized muscle pain. The physician diagnoses her with an acute respiratory viral infection and charts her condition as _____ .

3. A coal miner with a history of lung CA is admitted with bronchial hemorrhage. The physician documents this finding as _____, which is another term for bronchial hemorrhage.

4. Linda J., a 60-year-old patient, presents to the ED with fever, dehydration, and shortness of breath (SOB). Chest x-ray reveals a right lower lobe infiltrate. The physician diagnoses _____, an acute inflammation of the lungs caused by a bacterium, virus, or chemical irritant.

5. Xavier M. remains on chemotherapy with the major adverse effect of fluid accumulation in the right lung. The procedure to remove the fluid in the pleural space is known as _____ .

6. A 12-year-old boy with a recent diagnosis of asthma sees the nurse practitioner to learn about his new medication. The nurse informs him that an inhaler delivers the medication, which dilates constricted airways. She also tells him that the medication is called a _____ .

7. Upon arrival to a severe traffic accident, the emergency medical therapist (EMT) finds the driver unconscious, with his airway obstructed. The physician instructs the EMT over the emergency phone line to perform an incision into the trachea to open up the airway and restore breathing and oxygenation to the lungs. This surgical procedure is known as a(n) _____ .

8. Li W. presents to the pulmonology clinic with a chief complaint of SOB upon exertion. The physician orders a variety of tests to determine the capacity of the lungs to exchange O_2 and CO_2 efficiently, known as a _____ .

9. During Paul S.'s annual physical examination, the physician hears fine crackling and bubbling sounds during inspiration. He explains that he hears abnormal breath sounds caused by fluid in the lung. He further explains that these abnormal breath sounds may be caused by pneumonia and are called _____ .

10. Following her admission for emphysema, Vicky B. received her laboratory results that indicate excessively high levels of CO_2 in the body. The nurse explains that excessive CO_2 can cause high levels of acidity in the bloodstream, a condition called _____ .

Correct Answers _____ × 10 = _____ % Score

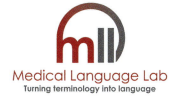
Medical Language Lab
Turning terminology into language

Visit the *Medical Language Lab* at *medicallanguagelab.com*. Use the flash-card activity to reinforce your study of word elements. We recommend you complete the flash-card activity before beginning the following Word Elements Chapter Review.

RESPIRATORY SYSTEM CHAPTER REVIEW

WORD ELEMENTS SUMMARY

The following table summarizes CFs, suffixes, and prefixes related to the respiratory system. Study the word elements and their meanings before completing the Vocabulary Review that follows.

Word Element	Meaning	Word Element	Meaning
Combining Forms			
acid/o	acid	my/o	muscle
adenoid/o	adenoids	myc/o	fungus
aer/o	air	nas/o, rhin/o	nose
alveol/o	alveolus (plural, *alveoli*)	or/o	mouth
arteri/o	artery	orth/o	straight
atel/o	incomplete, imperfect	ox/o	oxygen
bronch/o, bronchi/o	bronchus (plural, *bronchi*)	pharyng/o	pharynx (throat)
carcin/o	cancer	pleur/o	pleura
chondr/o	cartilage	pneum/o, pneumon/o	air; lung
epiglott/o	epiglottis	pulmon/o	lung
fibr/o	fiber, fibrous tissue	sinus/o	sinus, cavity
hem/o	blood	spir/o	to breathe
hydr/o	water	thorac/o	chest
laryng/o	larynx (voice box)	tom/o	to cut
melan/o	black	tonsill/o	tonsils
muc/o	mucus	trache/o	trachea (windpipe)
Suffixes			
-al, -ic, -ous	pertaining to	-phagia	swallowing, eating
-algia, -dynia	pain	-phobia	fear
-cele	hernia; swelling	-plasm	formation, growth
-centesis	surgical puncture	-plasty	surgical repair
-ectasis	dilation, expansion	-plegia	paralysis
-ectomy	excision, removal	-pnea	breathing
-emia	blood condition	-rrhagia	bursting forth (of)
-graphy	process of recording	-rrhaphy	suture
-ia	condition	-scope	instrument for examining
-ist	specialist	-scopy	visual examination
-logist	specialist in the study of	-spasm	involuntary contraction, twitching
-malacia	softening	-stenosis	narrowing, stricture

Word Element	Meaning	Word Element	Meaning
-metry	act of measuring	-therapy	treatment
-oma	tumor	-thorax	chest
-osis	abnormal condition; increase (used primarily with blood cells)	-tome	instrument to cut
-pathy	disease	-tomy	incision
Prefixes			
a-, an-	without; not	hyp-, hypo-	under, below; deficient
dys-	bad; painful; difficult	macro-	large
endo-	in, within	micro-	small
epi-	above, upon	neo-	new
eu-	good, normal	peri-	around

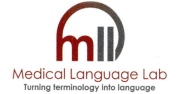

Medical Language Lab
Turning terminology into language

Visit the *Medical Language Lab* at the website *medicallanguagelab.com*. Use the flash-card exercise to reinforce your study of word elements. We recommend you complete the flash-card exercise before beginning the following Vocabulary Review.

Vocabulary Review

Match the medical terms with the definitions in the numbered list.

aerophagia	atelectasis	mucolytics	pyothorax
anosmia	catheter	pharyngoplegia	rhinoplasty
apnea	corticosteroids	pleurisy	TB
aspirate	COPD	pneumocystis	thoracentesis
asthma	croup	pneumothorax	tracheostomy

1. _____ refers to presence of pus in the chest.

2. _____ is a surgical puncture of the chest to remove fluid.

3. _____ is a respiratory condition marked by recurrent attacks of difficult or labored breathing accompanied by wheezing.

4. _____ is an acute respiratory syndrome of childhood characterized by laryngeal obstruction and spasm, barking cough, and stridor.

5. _____ is a surgical procedure that creates an opening through the neck into the trachea.

6. _____ decrease swelling, inflammation, and mucus production to promote easier breathing.

7. _____ is a temporary cessation of breathing.

8. _____ refers to swallowing air.

9. _____ refers to using suction to remove fluids from a body cavity.

10. _____ liquefy mucus to allow elimination through coughing more easily.

11. _____ is an abnormal condition characterized by collapse of alveoli.

12. _____ is the loss or impairment of the sense of smell.

13. _____ is paralysis of pharyngeal muscles.

14. _____ is inflammation of the pleura.

15. _____ is a type of pneumonia seen in patients with AIDS and in debilitated children.

16. _____ is a hollow, flexible tube that can be inserted into a vessel or cavity of the body to withdraw or instill fluids.

17. _____ refers to the surgical repair or plastic surgery of the nose.

18. _____ is an infectious disease that produces small lesions or tubercles in the lungs.

19. _____ refers to a group of respiratory disorders characterized by chronic bronchitis, asthma, and emphysema.

20. _____ is the presence of air in the pleural cavity.

Competency Verification: Check your answers in Appendix B: Answer Key, page 596. If you are not satisfied with your level of comprehension, review the chapter vocabulary and retake the review.

Correct Answers: _____ × 5 = _____ % Score

Cardiovascular and Lymphatic Systems

OBJECTIVES

Upon completion of this chapter, you will be able to:

- Describe the type of medical treatment the cardiologist, vascular surgeon, and immunologist provide.

- Identify the structures of the cardiovascular and lymphatic systems by labeling them on anatomical illustrations.

- Describe the primary functions of the cardiovascular and lymphatic systems.

- Describe diseases, conditions, and procedures related to the cardiovascular and lymphatic systems.

- Apply your word-building skills by constructing various medical terms related to the cardiovascular and lymphatic systems.

- Describe common abbreviations and symbols related to the cardiovascular and lymphatic systems.

- Recognize, define, pronounce, and spell terms correctly.

- Demonstrate your knowledge of this chapter by successfully completing the frames, reviews, and activities.

MEDICAL SPECIALTIES: CARDIOLOGY AND IMMUNOLOGY

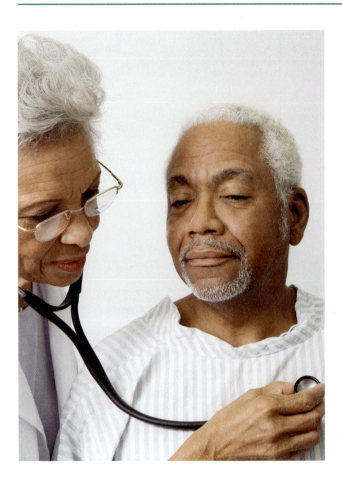

Cardiology

Cardiology is a branch of medicine associated with disorders of the heart as well as parts of the circulatory system. A **cardiologist** treats patients for heart disorders related to blood vessels and blockages. There are several subspecialties of cardiology which require additional training and board certification. A cardiologist who specializes in treating infants and children is known as a **pediatric cardiologist**. A cardiologist who performs surgeries is known as a **heart surgeon, cardiovascular surgeon**, or **cardiothoracic surgeon**.

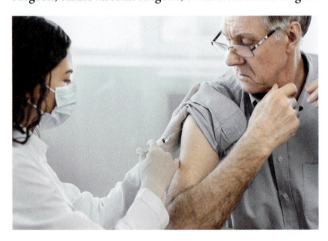

Immunology

Immunology is the medical specialty related to the lymphatic system and the immune response. The immune system is the body's defense against cancer cells and foreign invaders, such as bacteria and viruses. The ability to fight off disease and protect the body depends on an adequate functioning immune response. **Immunologists** are physicians who treat patients with autoimmune and immunodeficiency diseases, cancer, and patients who are undergoing bone marrow, organ, or stem cell transplantation.

Anatomy and Physiology Overview

The cardiovascular (CV) system includes the heart, which is essentially a muscular pump, and an extensive network of blood vessels. The main purpose of the CV system, also called the *circulatory system,* is to deliver oxygen, nutrients, and other essential substances to body cells and remove waste products of cellular metabolism. A complex network of blood vessels—including arteries, capillaries, and veins, all of which are connected to the heart—carries out this process. A healthy CV system is vital to a person's survival. A CV system that does not provide adequate circulation deprives tissues of oxygen and nutrients and fails to remove waste, and this results in irreversible changes to cells that could be life-threatening.

The lymphatic system is closely linked to the CV system and depends on the pumping action of the heart to circulate its substances throughout the body. The lymphatic system consists of a network of vessels and nodes, and a few specialized organs, including the tonsils, thymus, and spleen. Blood flows from the heart to blood capillaries and back to the heart. Lymph capillaries collect tissue fluid, which is returned to the blood. (See Figure 5-1.)

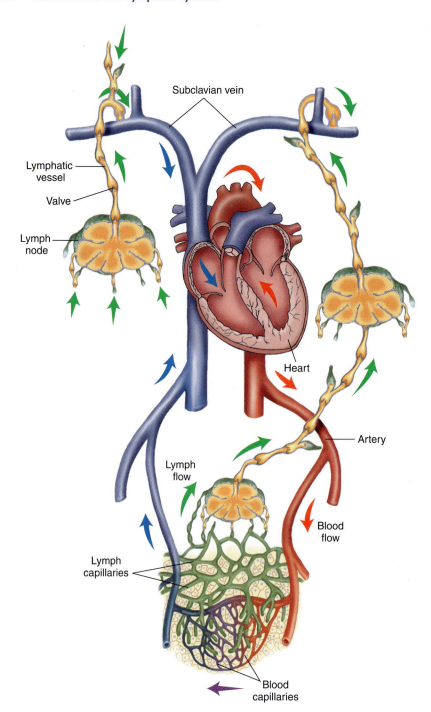

Figure 5-1 Interrelationship of the cardiovascular system with the lymphatic system, with blood flowing from the heart to blood capillaries and back to the heart and lymph capillaries collecting tissue fluid, which is returned to the blood (arrows indicating direction of blood and lymph flow).

WORD ELEMENTS

This section introduces word elements related to the cardiovascular system. Review the word elements and their meanings in the following table, then pronounce each term in the word analysis column, and place a ✓ in the box after you do so.

Word Element	Meaning	Word Analysis
Combining Forms		
angi/o	vessel (usually blood or lymph)	**angi/o/graphy** (ăn-jē-ŎG-ră-fē ☐): process of recording blood vessels *-graphy:* process of recording *Angiography is an x-ray visualization of the internal anatomy of the heart and blood vessels after the intravascular introduction of a contrast medium. It is used as a diagnostic aid to visualize blood vessel and heart abnormalities.*
aneurysm/o	widening, widened blood *vessel*	**aneurysm/o/rrhaphy** (ăn-ū-rĭz-MŎR-ă-fē ☐): suture of a blood vessel *-rrhaphy:* suture *Aneurysmorrhaphy closes the area of dilation and weakness in the wall of an artery. This condition may result from a congenital defect or a damaged vessel wall due to arteriosclerosis.*
aort/o	aorta	**aort/o/stenosis** (ăn-jē-ŎG-ră-fē ☐): narrowing of the aorta *-stenosis:* narrowing, stricture
arteri/o	artery	**arteri/o/scler/osis** (ăn-ū-rĭz-MŎR-ă-fē ☐): abnormal hardening of arterial walls *scler:* hardening; sclera (white of the eye) *-osis:* abnormal condition; increase (used primarily with blood cells) *Arteriosclerosis results in decreased blood supply, especially to the cerebrum and lower extremities.*
arteriol/o	arteriole	**arteriol/itis** (ăr-tēr-ē-ō-LĬ-tĭs ☐): inflammation of an arteriole *-itis:* inflammation
ather/o	fatty plaque	**ather/oma** (ăth-ĕr-Ō-mă ☐): fatty degeneration or thickening of the larger arterial walls, as in atherosclerosis *-oma:* tumor
atri/o	atrium	**atri/o/ventricul/ar** (ā-trē-ō-vĕn-TRĬK-ū-lăr ☐): pertaining to the atrium and the ventricle *ventricul:* ventricle (of heart or brain) *-ar:* pertaining to
cardi/o	heart	**cardi/o/megaly** (kăr-dē-ō-MĔG-ă-lē ☐): enlargement of the heart; also called *megalocardia* *-megaly:* enlargement
coron/o		**coron/ary** (KOR-ō-nă-rē ☐): pertaining to the heart *-ary:* pertaining to
phleb/o	vein	**phleb/itis** (flĕb-Ī-tĭs ☐): inflammation of a vein *-itis:* inflammation
ven/o		**ven/ous** (VĒ-nŭs ☐): pertaining to the veins or blood passing through them *-ous:* pertaining to
thromb/o	blood clot	**thromb/o/lysis** (thrŏm-BŎL-ĭ-sĭs ☐): breaking up of a thrombus *-lysis:* separation; destruction; loosening
varic/o	dilated vein	**varic/ose** (VĂR-ĭ-kōs ☐): pertaining to a dilated vein *-ose:* pertaining to; sugar
vas/o	vessel; vas deferens; duct	**vas/o/spasm** (VĂS-ō-spăzm ☐): spasm of a blood vessel *-spasm:* involuntary contraction, twitching

Continued

Word Element	Meaning	Word Analysis
vascul/o	vessel	**vascul**/ar (VĂS-kū-lăr ☐): pertaining to or composed of blood vessels *-ar:* pertaining to

ventricul/o	ventricle (of the heart or brain)	intra/**ventricul**/ar (ĭn-tră-věn-TRĬK-ū-lăr ☐): within a ventricle
		  intra: in, within
		    -ar: pertaining to

Suffixes		
-cardia	heart condition	tachy/**cardia** (tăk-ē-KĂR-dē-ă ☐): rapid heart rate *tachy-:* rapid

-gram	record, writing	electr/o/cardi/o/**gram** (ē-lěk-trō-KĂR-dē-ō-grăm ☐): record of electrical activity of the heart
		  electr/o: electricity
		  cardi/o: heart

-graph	instrument for recording	electr/o/cardi/o/**graph** (ē-lěk-trō-KĂR-dē-ŏ-grăf ☐): instrument for recording electrical activity of the heart
		  electr/o: electricity
		  cardi/o: heart

-graphy	process of recording	electr/o/cardi/o/**graphy** (ē-lěk-trō-kăr-dē-ŎG-ră-fē ☐): process of recording electrical activity of the heart
		  electr/o: electricity
		  cardi/o: heart
		
		Electrocardiography is a noninvasive test that records the electrical activity of the heart during contractions and rest. It helps diagnose abnormal cardiac rhythm and the presence of heart muscle (myocardial) damage.

-stenosis	narrowing, stricture	arteri/o/**stenosis** (ăr-tē-rē-ō-stě-NŌ-sĭs ☐): narrowing of an artery *arteri/o:* artery *Narrowing of an artery may be caused by fatty plaque buildup, scar tissue, or a blood clot.*

-um	structure, thing	endo/cardi/**um** (ěn-dō-KĂR-dē-ŭm ☐): structure within the heart
		  endo-: in, within
		  cardi: heart

Pronunciation Help	*Long Sound* *Short Sound*	ā in rāte ă in ăpple	ē in rēbirth ě in ěver	ī in īsle ĭ in ĭt	ō in ōver ŏ in nŏt	ū in ūnite ŭ in cŭt

 Visit the *Medical Terminology Simplified* online resource center at FADavis.com for an audio exercise of the terms in this table to help master pronunciations and meanings of the selected medical terms.

SECTION REVIEW 5-1

For the following medical terms, first, write the suffix and its meaning. Then, translate the meaning of the remaining elements, starting with the first part of the word. The first word is completed for you.

Term	Meaning
1. endo/cardi/um	–um: structure, thing; in, within; heart
2. cardi/o/megaly	Enlargement of heart
3. aort/o/stenosis	narrowing of aorta.
4. tachy/cardia	
5. phleb/it is	
6. thromb/o/lysis	breaking up of thrombus.
7. vas/o/spasm	twitching of blood vessels.
8. ather/oma	fatty plaque tumor
9. electr/o/cardi/o/graphy	electronic visual examination of heart.
10. atri/o/ventricul/ar	pertaining to atrium and ventricle.

Competency Verification: Check your answers in Appendix B: Answer Key, page 596. If you are not satisfied with your level of comprehension, review the vocabulary, and complete the review again.

Correct Answers _____ x 10 = _____ % Score

Cardiovascular System

Layers of the Heart Wall

5-1   The heart is a four-chambered muscular organ located in the mediastin/um, the area of the chest between the lungs. Its primary purpose is to pump blood through the arteries, veins, and capillaries. The walls of the heart are composed of three layers. Review the structures of the heart in Figure 5-2 and label the (1) **endocardium,** (2) **myocardium,** and (3) **pericardium.**

5-2   The endo/cardi/um, the inner membranous layer, lines the interior of the heart and the heart valves. The my/o/cardi/um, the middle muscular layer, is composed of a special type of muscle arranged in such a way that the contraction of muscle bundles results in squeezing or wringing of the heart chambers to eject blood from the chambers. The peri/cardi/um, a fibrous sac, surrounds and encloses the entire heart.

my/o/cardi/um
mī-ō-dē-ŭm

peri/cardi/um
pĕr-ĭ-KĂR-dē-ŭm

When we talk about the muscular layer of the heart, we are referring to the

_____ / _____ / _____ / _____.

When we talk about the fibrous sac that encloses the entire heart, we are referring to

the _____ / _____ / _____.

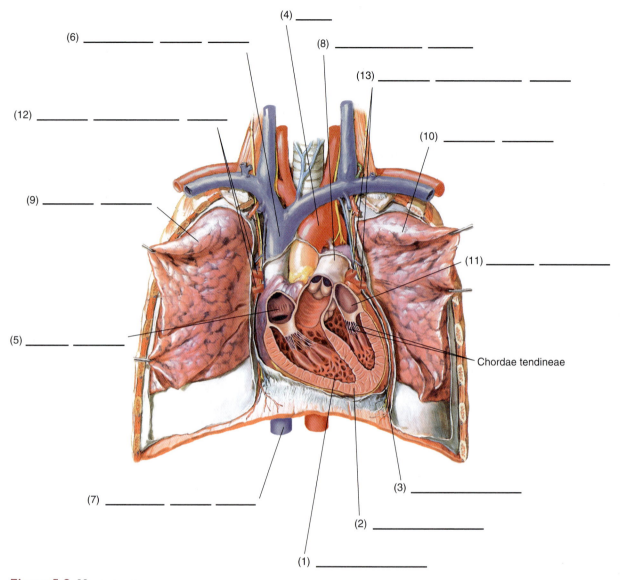

(4) _____

(6) _____ _____ _____

(8) _____ _____

(13) _____ _____ _____

(12) _____ _____ _____

(10) _____ _____

(9) _____ _____

(11) _____ _____

(5) _____ _____

Chordae tendineae

(7) _____ _____ _____

(3) _____

(2) _____

(1) _____

Figure 5-2 Heart structures.

---

peri/card/itis
pĕr-ĭ-kăr-DĪ-tĭs

peri/cardi/o/centesis
pĕr-ĭ-kăr-dē-ō-sĕn-TĒ-sĭs

5-3   The prefix *peri-* means *around.* Peri/card/itis is inflammation or infection of the pericardial sac and accumulation of pericardial fluid. When the fluid presses on the heart and prevents it from beating, the condition is known as *cardi/ac tamponade.* If necessary, peri/cardi/o/centesis may be performed.

Build medical terms that mean

inflammation around the heart: _____ / _____ / _____.

surgical puncture around the heart:

_____ / _____ / ____ / _____.

---

peri/cardi/ectomy
pĕr-ĭ-kăr-dē-ĔK-tō-mē

5-4   The surgical procedure that means excision of *all or part of the peri/cardi/um* is

_____ / _____ / _____.

Pink indicates a prefix. Blue indicates a suffix. Boldface indicates a word root or combining form.

peri/cardi/o/rrhaphy pĕr-ĭ-kăr-dē-OR-ă-fē	**5-5** Suturing a wound in the peri/cardi/um is called _____ / _____ / _____ / _____.
my/o/cardi/um mī-ō-KĂR-dē-ŭm	**5-6** Cross-striations of cardi/ac muscle provide the mechanics of squeezing blood out of the heart chambers to maintain the flow of blood in one direction. Identify the muscul/ar layer of the heart responsible for this function. _____ / _____ / _____ / _____
endo/cardi/um ĕn-dō-KĂR-dē-ŭm **peri/cardi/um** pĕr-ĭ-KĂR-dē-ŭm **my/o/cardi/um** mī-ō-KĂR-dē-ŭm	**5-7** Review the three layers of the heart by completing the following statements: The layer that lines the heart and the heart valves is known as the _____ / _____ / _____. The fibrous sac surrounding the entire heart and composed of two membranes separated by fluid is called the _____ / _____ / _____. The middle specialized muscular layer is called the _____ / _____ / _____ / _____.

Circulation and Heart Structures

5-8   The circulatory system is commonly divided into the cardiovascular system, which consists of the heart and blood vessels, and the lymphatic system, which consists of lymph vessels, lymph nodes, and lymphoid organs (spleen, thymus, and tonsils). Review Figure 5-1 to see the interrelationship of the cardiovascular system with the lymphatic system.

5-9   Some of the main vessels associated with circulation are illustrated in Figure 5-2. Observe the locations and label the structures as you read the following material. The (4) **aorta,** the largest blood vessel in the body, is the main trunk of systemic circulation. It starts and arches out at the left ventricle. Deoxygenated blood enters the (5) **right atrium** via two large veins, the **vena cavae** (*singular, vena cava*). The (6) **superior vena cava** conveys blood from the upper portion of the body (head, arms, and chest); the (7) **inferior vena cava** conveys blood from the lower portion of the body (abdomen, pelvis, and legs).

leuk/o/cytes LOO-kō-sīts **erythr/o/cytes** ĕ-RĬTH-rō-sīts **thromb/o/cytes** THRŎM-bō-sīts	**5-10** Blood is composed of a liquid solution, called plasma, in which solid components are suspended. The solid components of blood include red blood cells (erythr/o/cytes), white blood cells (leuk/o/cytes), and platelets (thromb/o/cytes). Blood makes up about 8% of the human body weight. (See Figure 5-3.) Identify the terms in this frame that mean *white blood cells:* _leuk_ / _o_ / _cytes_. *red blood cells:* _erythr_ / _o_ / _cytes_. *cell that clots:* _thromb_ / _o_ / _cytes_.

COMPOSITION OF BLOOD

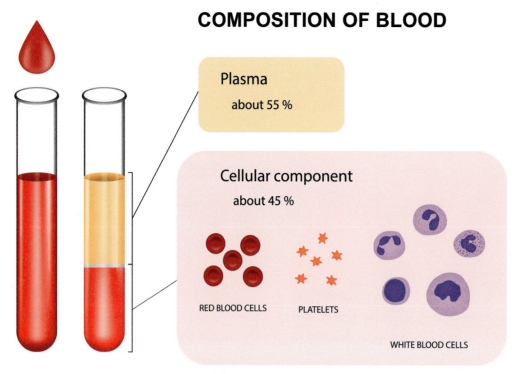

Figure 5-3 Composition of Blood.

erythr/o ĕ-RĬTH-rō **O₂**	**5-11** Erythr/o/cytes, are the most abundant cell type in the blood. The primary function of erythr/o/cytes is to transport oxygen (O_2) to body cells and deliver carbon dioxide to the lungs. The CF that means *red* is: _____/ _/ ___. Write the abbreviation for oxygen: _____*. *If you need help, refer to Appendix B, p. 585.
erythr/o/cytes ĕ-RĬTH-rō-sīts	**5-12** Red blood cells (RBCs) are important in identifying human blood type. Blood type is determined by the presence or absence of certain identifiers on the surface of RBCs. These identifiers, also called *antigens,* help the body's immune system to recognize its own RBC type. Table 5-1 lists blood types and their compatibility. Build a term that means *red blood cells:* _____

TABLE 5-I	BLOOD TYPES AND COMPATIBILITY			
Blood Type	**Antigen on RBC**	**Antigen on Plasma**	**Donate to**	**Receive From**
A	A	anti-B antibodies	A or AB	A or O
B	B	anti-A antibodies	B or AB	B or O
AB (universal recipient)	A and B	none	AB only	A, B, AB, O
O (universal donor)	none	anti-A and anti-B antibodies	A, B, AB, O	O

leuc/o/cytes or leuk/o/cytes LOO-kō-sīts	**5-13** White blood cells (WBCs), also called *leuk/o/cytes or leuc/o/cytes,* are the cells of the immune system that are involved in protecting the body against infectious disease and foreign invaders. All leuk/o/cytes are produced and derived from cells in bone marrow known as *hemat/o/poietic stem cells.* What cells protect the body from infection and foreign invaders? _____/ __/ _____
WBC **RBC** **O₂**	**5-14** Write the abbreviations that mean *white blood cell:* _____. *red blood cell:* _____. *oxygen:* _____.
thromb/o/cytes	**5-15** Platelets, also called thromb/o/cytes, are a component of blood, and their function (along with the coagulation factors) is to stop bleeding by clumping and clotting blood vessel injuries. Build a medical term that means cells that clot: _____ / _____ / _____.
deoxygenated dē-ŎK-sĭ-jĕn-ā-tĕd	**5-16** Blood in the veins, except for pulmonary veins, has a low oxygen content (deoxygenated) and a relatively high concentration of carbon dioxide. In contrast to the bright red color of the oxygenated blood in the arteries, deoxygenated blood has a dark blue to purplish color. The term in this frame that means low oxygen content is _____.
	5-17 Label Figure 5-2 as you continue to identify and learn about the structures and functions of the circulatory system. The (8) **pulmonary trunk** is the only artery that carries deoxygenated blood. As deoxygenated blood is pumped from the right ventricle, it enters the pulmonary trunk. The pulmonary trunk runs diagonally upward, then divides abruptly to form the branches of the right and left pulmonary arteries. Each branch conveys deoxygenated blood to the lungs. The (9) **right lung** has three lobes; the (10) **left lung** has two lobes. Oxygen-rich blood returns to the heart via four pulmonary veins, which deposit the blood into the (11) **left atrium.** There are two (12) **right pulmonary veins** and two (13) **left pulmonary veins.**

Competency Verification: Check your labeling of Figure 5-2 in Appendix B: Answer Key, page 597.

	5-18 Internally, the heart is composed of four chambers. (See Figure 5-4.) The upper chambers are the (1) **right atrium** (RA) and (2) **left atrium** (LA). The lower chambers are the (3) **right ventricle** (RV) and (4) **left ventricle** (LV). Locate and label the chambers of the heart in Figure 5-4.
atri/al Ā-trē-ăl	**5-19** The CF *atri/o* refers to the atrium. A term that means pertaining to the atrium is _____ / _____.
atrium, left Ā-trē-ŭm	**5-20** The heart consists of two upper chambers, the right _____ and the _____ atrium.

(17) _____ __ ___ _____

(16) _____

(6) _____ _____ _____ (   )

(10) Right _____
        _____

(11) Left _____
        _____

(13) Left _____
        _____

(12) Right _____
        _____

(2) Left _____ (   )

(15) _____ _____

(9) _____
        _____

(14) _____ _____

(1) Right _____ (   )

(8) _____
        _____

(4) _____
    _____ (   )

(7) _____ _____ _____ (   )

(5) _____
    _____ (   )

(3) _____ _____ (   )

(18) _____ _____

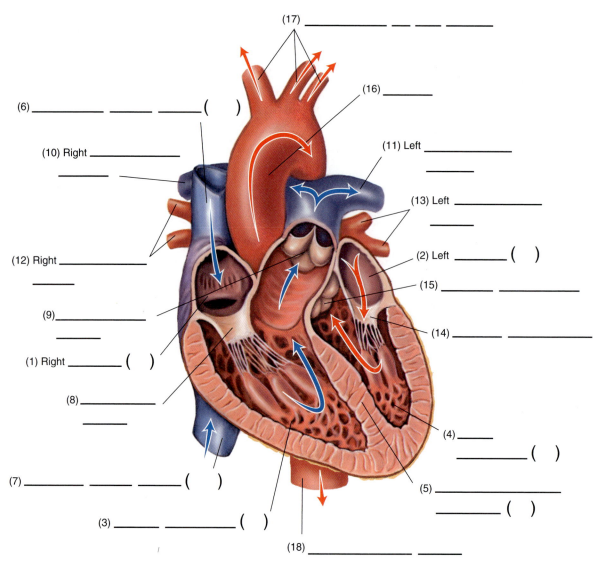

Figure 5-4 Internal structures of the heart (with *red arrows* designating oxygen-rich blood flow and *blue arrows* designating oxygen-poor blood flow).

ventricul/o/tomy věn-trĭk-ū-LŎT-ō-mē	**5-21** The CF **ventricul/o** means *ventricle (of the heart or brain).* A ventricle is a small cavity, such as the RV and LV of the heart or one of the cavities filled with cerebrospinal fluid in the brain. Incisions are sometimes performed into these cavities. An incision of a ventricle is known as a _____ / _____ / _____.
atrium, ventricle Ă-trē-ŭm, VĚN-trĭk-l	**5-22** The term *atri/o/ventricul/ar* (AV) refers to the atrium and the ventricle. It also pertains to a connecting conduction event between the atria and the ventricles. The singular form of atria is _____; the singular form of ventricles is _____.

ventricul/ar
věn-TRĬK-ū-lăr

5-23 *Flutter* is an a/rrhythm/ia in which there is very rapid but regular rhythm (250–300 beats per minute) of the atria or ventricles. The heart chambers do not have time to completely fill with blood before the next contraction. Flutter can progress to fibrillation.

When the flutter occurs in the atrium, it is called *atri/al flutter*. When the flutter occurs in the ventricle, it is called a _____ / _____ flutter.

a/rrhythm/ia
ă-RĬTH-mē-ă

my/o/cardi/um
mī-ō-KĂR-dē-ŭm

5-24 Flutter that progresses to fibrillation (a/rrhythm/ia in which there is a rapid, uncoordinated quivering of the my/o/cardi/um) can affect the atria or the ventricles.

Write the term that means

without rhythm: _____ / _____ / _____.

muscular layer of the heart: _____ / _____ / _____ /

_____.

atria
Ā-trē-ă

cardia
KĂR-dē-ă

septa
SĚP-tă

bacteria
băk-TĒ-rē-ă

5-25 The rule for forming plural words from singular words that end in *-um* is to drop *-um* and add *-a.* Practice modifying the following singular terms to their plural forms.

Singular	Plural
atrium	_____
cardium	_____
septum	_____
bacterium	_____

5-26 A wall or partition dividing a body space or cavity is known as a septum (plural, *septa*). Some septa are membranous; others are composed of bone or cartilage. Each is named according to its location in the body. In the heart, there are several septa, one of which is the interventricular septum (IVS), the partition that divides the LV from the RV. Label the (5) **interventricular septum** (IVS) in Figure 5-4.

IVS

IAS

5-27 The ventricles are separated by a thick muscular IVS, whereas the atria are separated by a thinner muscular **interatrial septum** (IAS).

The abbreviation of the septum situated between the

ventricles is: _____.

atria is: _____.

bacterium băk-TĒ-rē-ŭm **septum** SĔP-tŭm **atrium** Ā-trē-ŭm **cardium** KĂR-dē-ŭm	**5-28** Form singular words from the following plural words. Apply the rule that was covered in Frame 5–25. **Plural** **Singular** bacteria _____ septa _____ atria _____ cardia _____
rapid	**5-29** The prefix *tachy-* is used in words to mean *rapid*. *Tachy/cardia* is heart rate that is _____.
rapid eating	**5-30** *Tachy/pnea* refers to rapid breathing; *tachy/phagia* refers to rapid swallowing, or _____ _____.
brady/cardia brād-ē-KĂR-dē-ă	**5-31** The prefix *brady-* is used in words to mean slow. In people with symptoms of brady/cardia, the heart has difficulty pumping an adequate supply of blood to the tissues of the body. The medical term that literally means slow heart is _____ / _____.
brady/pnea brād-ĭp-NĒ-ă **brady/phagia** brād-ē-FĂ-jē-ă	**5-32** Form medical words that literally mean *slow breathing:* _____ / _____. *slow eating:* _____ / _____.
tachy/pnea tăk-ĭp-NĒ-ă. **tachy/phagia** tăk-ē-FĂ-jē-ă	**5-33** Construct medical words that mean *rapid breathing:* _____ / _____. *rapid eating:* _____ / _____.
RA **LA** **RV** **LV** **IVS**	**5-34** Review the chambers and structures of the heart by writing the abbreviation for the right atrium: _____. left atrium: _____. right ventricle: _____. left ventricle: _____. interventricular septum: _____.

Pink indicates a prefix. Blue indicates a suffix. Boldface indicates a word root or combining form.

Blood Flow Through the Heart

5-35   Although general information on the circulatory system was discussed previously, this section covers in greater detail the specific structures involved in the flow of blood through the heart. The heart's double pump serves two distinct circulations: pulmonary circulation, which is the short loop of blood vessels that runs from the heart to the lungs and back to the heart, and systemic circulation, which routes blood through a long loop to all parts of the body before returning it to the heart.

Continue to label Figure 5-4 as you read the following information. The RA receives oxygen-poor blood from all tissues except those of the lungs. The blood from the head and arms is delivered to the RA through the (6) **superior vena cava** (SVC). The blood from the legs and torso is delivered to the RA through the (7) **inferior vena cava** (IVC).

---

superior

inferior

5-36   Refer to Figure 5-4 and use the words superior or inferior to complete this frame.

The LA is _____ to the LV.

The RV is _____ to the RA.

5-37   Blood flows from the RA through the (8) **tricuspid valve** and into the RV. The leaflets (cusps) are shaped such that they form a one-way passage, which keeps the blood flowing in only one direction. Label the tricuspid valve in Figure 5-4.

---

tri/cuspid valve
trī-KŬS-pĭd

5-38   The prefix *tri-* means *three*. The valve that has three leaflets, or flaps, is the

_____ / _____ _____.

---

two

5-39   The prefix *bi-* refers to *two*. A bi/cuspid valve has _____ leaflets, or flaps.

5-40   The ventricles are the pumping chambers of the heart. As the RV contracts to pump oxygen-deficient blood through the (9) **pulmonary valve** into the pulmonary artery, the tri/cuspid valve remains closed, preventing a backflow of blood into the RA. When blood passes through the pulmonary trunk, also known as the main *pulmonary artery*, it branches into the (10) **right pulmonary artery** and the (11) **left pulmonary artery**. The pulmonary arteries carry the oxygen-deficient blood to the lungs. Label the structures introduced in this frame in Figure 5-4.

---

artery
ĂR-tĕr-ē

5-41   The CF *arteri/o* refers to an artery. Arteri/al bleeding is bleeding from an

_____.

---

arteries
ĂR-tĕr-ēs

5-42   Arteri/al circulation is movement of blood through the

_____.

---

arteri/o/rrhexis ăr-tē-rē-ō-RĔK-sĭs **arteri/o/rrhaphy** ăr-tē-rē-OR-ă-fē **arteri/o/pathy** ăr-tē-rē-ŎP-ă-thē **arteri/o/spasm** ăr-TĒ-rē-ō-spăzm	**5-43** Develop medical words that mean *rupture of an artery:* _____ / _____ / _____. *suture of an artery:* _____ / _____ / _____. *disease of an artery:* _____ / _____ / _____. *involuntary contraction or twitching of an artery:* _____ / _____ / _____.
stone, artery ĂR-tĕr-ē	**5-44** The suffix *-lith* refers to a *stone,* or *calculus.* An arteri/o/lith, also called an *arteri/al calculus,* is a calculus, or _____, in an _____.
11 **10**	**5-45** The right and left pulmonary arteries leading to the lungs branch and subdivide until they ultimately form capillaries around the alveoli. Carbon dioxide passes from blood into the alveoli and is expelled out of the lungs. Oxygen inhaled by the lungs is passed from the alveoli into blood. The left pulmonary artery is identified in Figure 5-4 as number _____. The right pulmonary artery is identified in Figure 5-4 as number _____.
	5-46 Oxygenated blood leaves the lungs and returns to the heart via the (12) **right pulmonary veins** and (13) **left pulmonary veins.** The four pulmonary veins empty into the LA. The LA contracts to force blood through the (14) **mitral valve** into the LV. Label the structures in Figure 5-4.
two	**5-47** The mitral valve, located between the LA and LV, is a bi/cuspid, or bi/leaflet, valve, which means that the number of leaflets or flaps that the mitral valve has is _____.
vein VĀN	**5-48** *Ven/o* is a combining form that means _____.
vein VĀN	**5-49** *Phleb/o* is another CF for *vein.* Phleb/o/tomy is a procedure used to draw blood from a _____.
phleb/o/rrhaphy flĕb-ŎR-ă-fē **phleb/o/rrhexis** flĕb-ō-RĔK-sĭs **phleb/o/stenosis** flĕb-ō-stĕ-NŌ-sĭs	**5-50** Use *phleb/o* to construct words that mean *suture of a vein:* _____ / _____ / _____. *rupture of a vein:* _____ / _____ / _____. *stricture or narrowing of a vein:* _____ / _____ / _____.

Pink indicates a prefix. Blue indicates a suffix. **Boldface** indicates a word root or combining form.

blood	**5-51** *Hemat/o* and *hem/o* mean _____.
hemat/o/logy hē-mă-TŎL-ō-jē **hemat/o/logist** hē-mă-TŎL-ō-jĭst	**5-52** Use *hemat/o* to form words that mean *study of blood:* _____ / _____ / _____. *specialist in the study of blood:* _____ / _____ / _____.
lymph vessels	**5-53** The CF *angi/o* means *vessel* (usually blood or lymph). An angioma is a tumor consisting primarily of blood or _____ _____.
hemangi/oma hē-măn-jē-Ō-mă	**5-54** *Hem/o* and *angi/o* can be combined into a new element that also means *blood vessel*. Use *hemangi/o* (blood vessel) to develop a word that means *tumor of blood vessels:* _____ / _____.
expansion	**5-55** Hemangi/ectasis is a dilation or _____ of a blood vessel.
	5-56 Label the structures in Figure 5-4 as you continue to learn about the heart. Contractions of the LV send oxygenated blood through the (15) **aortic valve** and into the (16) **aorta.** The three branches of the (17) **ascending aorta** transport blood to the head and arms. The (18) **descending aorta** transports the blood to the legs and the torso.
aort/o/pathy ā-ŏr-TŎP-ă-thē	**5-57** The aorta is the largest artery of the body and originates at the LV of the heart. The combining form *aort/o* refers to the aorta. Any disease of the aorta is called _____ / _____ / _____.
pulmon/ary PŬL-mō-nĕ-rē **vascul/ar** VĂS-kū-lăr **cardi/ac** KĂR-dē-ăk	**5-58** *Aortic stenosis,* a narrowing or stricture of the aortic valve, may be caused by congenital malformation or fusion of the cusps. The stenosis obstructs the flow of blood from the LV into the aorta, causing decreased cardi/ac output and pulmon/ary vascul/ar congestion. Treatment usually requires surgical repair. Identify the terms in this frame that mean *pertaining to the lungs:* _____ / _____. *pertaining to a vessel:* _____ / _____. *pertaining to the heart:* _____ / _____.

artery, small vein	**5-59** The suffixes *-ole* and *-ule* refer to *small, minute.* An arteri/ole is a small _____; a ven/ule is a _____ _____.
arteries ĂR-tĕr-ēz **arteri/oles** ăr-TĒ-rē-ōls	**5-60** Arteries are large vessels that convey blood away from the heart; they branch into smaller vessels called *arteri/oles.* The arteri/oles deliver blood to adjoining minute vessels called *capillaries.* Large vessels that transport blood away from the heart are called _____. Smaller vessels that are formed from arteries are called _____ / _____.
arteri/oles ăr-TĒ-rē-ōls	**5-61** Arteries convey blood to adjacent smaller vessels called _____ / _____.
capillaries KĂP-ĭ-lă-rēz	**5-62** Arteri/oles are thinner than arteries and carry blood to extending minute vessels called _____.
arteri/o/scler/osis ăr-tē-ō-sklĕ-RŌ-sĭs	**5-63** As a person ages, the arteries lose elasticity, thicken, become weakened, and deteriorate. Deterioration of arterial walls is also caused by constant high pressure needed to transport blood throughout the body. The medical term for an *abnormal condition of artery hardening* is _____ / _____ / _____ / _____.
superior vena cava VĒ-nă KĂ-vă **inferior vena cava** VĒ-nă KĂ-vă	**5-64** Capillaries carry blood from arteri/oles to ven/ules. Ven/ules form a collecting system to return oxygen-deficient blood to the heart through two large veins, the SVC and the IVC. Define the following abbreviations SVC: _____ _____ _____ IVC: _____ _____ _____
6, 7	**5-65** In Figure 5-4, the SVC is number _____; the IVC is number _____.
varic/ose VĂR-ĭ-kōs **competent**	**5-66** Normal veins have competent (healthy) valves and their ven/ous walls are strong enough to withstand the later/al pressure of blood that is exerted on them. Blood flows through competent valves in one direction, which is toward the heart. In varic/ose veins, also known as *varicosities,* dilation of veins from long periods of pressure prevents complete closure of the valves. (See Figure 5-5.) Identify the medical term in this frame that means *pertaining to a dilated vein:* _____ / _____. *healthy:* _____.

Pink indicates a prefix. Blue indicates a suffix. Boldface indicates a word root or combining form.

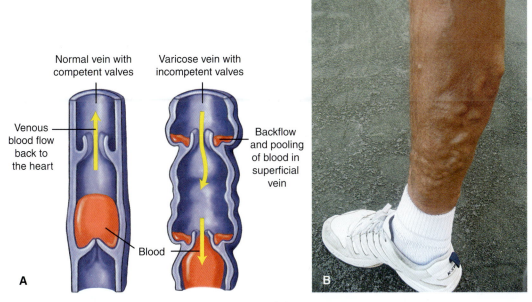

Figure 5-5 Healthy and unhealthy veins and valves. (A) Valve function in competent and incompetent valves. (B) Varicose veins.

varicosities văr-ĭ-KŎS-ĭ-tēz **incompetent**	**5-67** Incompetent (damaged) valves cause backflow of blood in the veins, causing enlarged, twisted superficial veins called *varicosities.* Identify the terms in this frame that mean *abnormally enlarged, twisted veins:* _____. *damaged:* _____ / _____.

Competency Verification: Check your labeling of Figure 5-4 in Appendix B: Answer Key, page 597.

Heart Valves

5-68 Label Figure 5-6 as you read the material about the heart valves and their cusps, also called *flaps.* Four heart valves maintain the flow of blood in one direction through the heart. The (1) **tricuspid valve** and the (2) **mitral valve** are situated between the upper and lower chambers and are attached to the heart walls by fibrous strands called (3) **chordae tendineae.** The (4) **pulmonary valve** and the (5) **aortic valve** are located at the exits of the ventricles.

Heart valves are composed of thin, fibrous cusps, covered by a smooth membrane called the *endocardium,* and reinforced by dense connective tissue. The aortic, pulmonary, and tricuspid valves contain (6) **three cusps;** the mitral valve contains (7) **two cusps.** The purpose of the cusps is to open and permit blood to flow through and seal shut to prevent backflow. The opening and closing of the cusps take place with each heartbeat.

mitral valve MĪ-trăl	**5-69** To classify a heart abnormality, it is important to identify the part of the organ in which the disorder occurs. A mitral valve murmur is caused by an incompetent, or faulty, valve. This type of murmur occurs in the valvular structure of the heart known as the _____ _____.

A

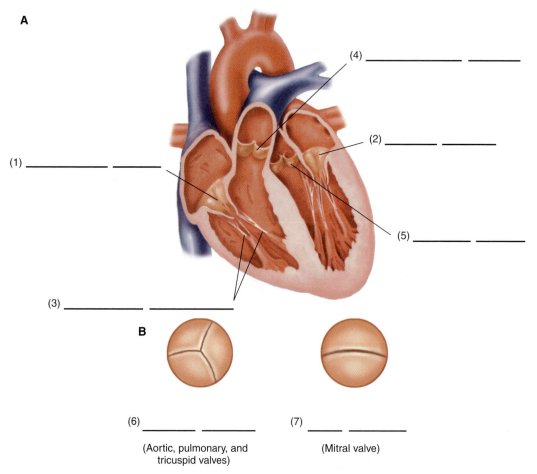

(4) _____ _____

(2) _____ _____

(1) _____ _____

(5) _____ _____

(3) _____ _____

B

(6) _____ _____
(Aortic, pulmonary, and
tricuspid valves)

(7) _____ _____
(Mitral valve)

Figure 5-6 Heart structures with valves and cusps. (A) Heart valves. (B) Valve cusps.

| valve | **5-70**   Replacement surgery can be performed to replace a damaged heart valve. When the tri/cuspid valve is damaged, it is replaced at the level of the tri/cuspid _____. |

Competency Verification: Check your labeling of Figure 5-6 in Appendix B: Answer Key, page 597.

SECTION REVIEW 5-2

Using the following table, write the CF, suffix, or prefix that matches its definition in the space provided to the left of the definition. There may be more than one word element that matches a definition.

Combining Forms		Suffixes		Prefixes
aort/o	my/o	-ectasis	-rrhaphy	bi-
arteri/o	phleb/o	-ole	-rrhexis	brady-
atri/o	scler/o	-osis	-spasm	epi-
cardi/o	ven/o	-pathy	-stenosis	peri-
hem/o	ventricul/o	-phagia	-ule	tachy-
hemat/o		-pnea		tri-

1. _____ abnormal condition; increase (used primarily with blood cells)

2. _____ above, on

3. _____ aorta

4. _____ around

5. _____ artery

6. _____ atrium

7. _____ blood

8. _____ breathing

9. _____ disease

10. _____ dilation, expansion

11. _____ hardening; sclera (white of the eye)

12. _____ heart

13. _____ involuntary contraction, twitching

14. _____ muscle

15. _____ rapid

16. _____ rupture

17. _____ slow

18. _____ small, minute

19. _____ suture

20. _____ narrowing, stricture

21. _____ swallowing, eating

22. _____ three

23. _____ two

24. _____ vein

25. _____ ventricle (of the heart or brain)

Competency Verification: Check your answers in Appendix B: Answer Key, page 597. If you are not satisfied with your level of comprehension, go back to Frame 5–1, and rework the frames.

Correct Answers _____ x 4 = _____ % Score

Conduction Pathway of the Heart

5-71   Label Figure 5-7 as you read the material about the conduction pathway of the heart. Primary responsibility for initiating the heartbeat rests with the (1) **sinoatrial (SA) node,** also known as the pacemaker of the heart. The SA node is a small region of specialized cardiac muscle tissue located on the posterior wall of the (2) **right atrium.**

---

electricity

5-72   The CF *electr/o* refers to electricity. *Electric/al* and electr/ic both mean pertaining to _____.

5-73   The electric/al current generated by the heart's pacemaker causes the atri/al walls to contract and forces the flow of blood into the ventricles. The wave of electricity moves to another region of the myo/cardi/um called the (3) **atrioventricular (AV) node.** Label the structure in Figure 5-7 to learn about the conduction pathway of the heart.

SA

RA

AV

5-74   Write the abbreviations for:

sinoatrial: _____.

right atrium: _____.

atri/o/ventricul/ar: _____.

---

atri/o/ventricul/ar
ā-trē-ō-věn-TRĬK-ū-lăr

electric/al

atri/al
Ā-trē-ăl

5-75   Identify the words in Frame 5–74 that mean

pertaining to the atrium and ventricles:

_____ / _____ / _____ / _____.

pertaining to electricity: _____ / _____.

pertaining to the atrium: _____ / _____.

5-76   The AV node instantaneously transmits impulses to the (4) **bundle of His,** a bundle of specialized fibers that transmits those impulses to the right and left (5) **bundle branches.** Label the structures in Figure 5-7.

5-77   From the right and left bundle branches, impulses travel through the (6) **Purkinje fibers** to the rest of the ventricul/ar my/o/cardi/um and bring about ventricul/ar contraction. Label the Purkinje (pŭr-KĬN-jē) fibers in Figure 5-7.

Competency Verification: Check your labeling of Figure 5-7 in Appendix B: Answer Key, page 597.

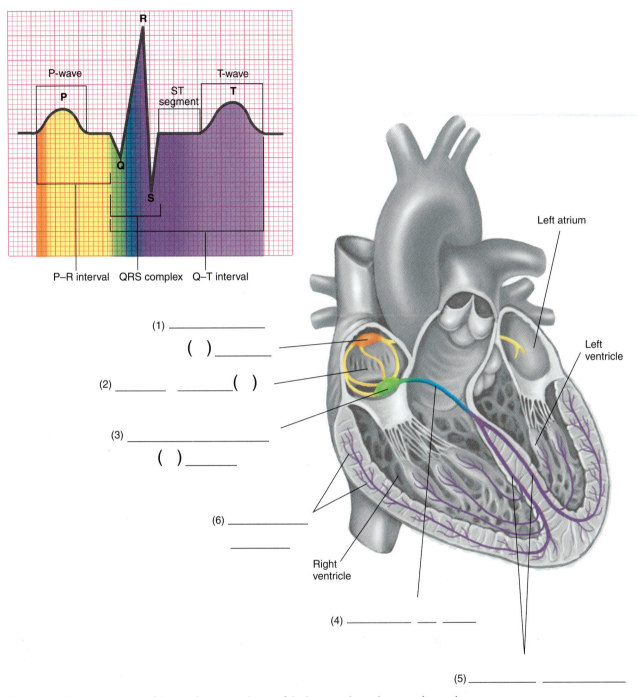

Figure 5-7 Anterior view of the conduction pathway of the heart with an electrocardiographic tracing of one normal heartbeat.

Cardiac Cycle and Heart Sounds

diastole
dī-ĂS-tō-lē

5-78 *The cardi/ac cycle* refers to the events of one complete heartbeat. Each contraction, or systole, of the heart is followed by a period of relaxation, or diastole. This cycle occurs 60 to 100 times per minute in the normal functioning heart.

The normal period of heart contraction is called *systole;* the normal period of heart relaxation is called _____.

systole SĬS-tō-lē **diastole** dī-ĂS-tō-lē **systole** SĬS-tō-lē	**5-79** When the heart is in the phase of relaxation, it is in diastole. When the heart is in the contraction phase, it is in _____. The pumping action of the heart consists of contraction and relaxation of the myocardial layer of the heart wall. During relaxation (diastole), blood fills the ventricles. The contraction that follows (systole) propels blood out of the ventricles and into the circulation. Write the medical term relating to the cardi/ac cycle that is in the phase of relaxation: _____. contraction: _____.
systole SĬS-tō-lē **diastole** dī-ĂS-tō-lē	**5-80** Blood pressure is recorded as systole/diastole. When a patient's blood pressure (BP) reading is 120/60, The 120 is known as _____ and 60 as _____.
-graphy **-gram**	**5-81** Recall the suffixes that mean *process of recording:* _____. *record, writing:* _____.
heart	**5-82** Electr/o/cardi/o/graphy is the process of recording electric/al activity generated by the _____.
record, heart	**5-83** An electr/o/cardi/o/gram is a _____ of electric/al activity generated by the _____.
electr/o/cardi/o/gram ē-lĕk-trō-KĂR-dē-ō-grăm	**5-84** *ECG* and *EKG* are abbreviations for *electr/o/cardi/o/gram.* To evaluate an abnormal cardi/ac rhythm, such as tachy/cardia, an ECG may be helpful. The abbreviations *ECG* and *EKG* refer to an _____ / _____ / _____ / _____ / _____.

 The following summary provides a brief, general interpretation of an ECG. A more comprehensive explanation of ECG abnormalities is beyond the scope of this book. Refer to Figure 5-7 as you read the text that follows.

A normal heart rhythm, or **sinus rhythm,** shows five waves on the ECG strip, which represent electrical changes as they spread through the heart. The waves are known as the **P waves, QRS waves,** and **T waves.**

The **P wave** represents atrial depolarization, conduction of an electrical impulse through the atria. These electrical changes cause atrial contraction. The **QRS waves,** commonly referred to as the *QRS complex,* represent ventricular depolarization, conduction of electrical impulses through the ventricle by way of the bundle of His and the Purkinje fibers. These electrical changes cause ventricular contraction. The T wave represents the electrical recovery and relaxation of the ventricles (during diastole).

electr/o/cardi/o/gram ē-lĕk-trō-KĂR-dē-ō-grăm	**5-85** Although the heart itself generates the heartbeat, such factors as hormones, drugs, and nervous system stimulation can also influence the heart rate. To evaluate a patient's heart rate, a physician may order an ECG, an abbreviation for _____ / _____ / _____ / _____ / _____.
micro/cardia mī-krō-KĂR-dē-ă	**5-86** Micro/cardia, an abnormal smallness of the heart, is a condition that is not usually compatible with a normal life. A person diagnosed with an underdeveloped heart suffers from the condition called _____ / _____.
enlargement, heart	**5-87** Megal/o/cardia is an enlargement of the heart. Cardi/o/megaly also means _____ of the _____.
cardi/o/megaly, **megal/o/cardia** kăr-dē-ō-MĔG-ă-lē, mĕg-ă-lō-KĂR-dē-ă	**5-88** In patients with high blood pressure, the heart must work extremely hard. As a result, it enlarges, similar to any other muscle in response to excessive activity or exercise. A patient who develops an enlarged heart has a condition called _____ / _____ / _____ or _____ / _____ / _____.
	5-89 Use your medical dictionary to define *angina pectoris* and *lumen*. _____ _____ _____ _____
-osis **scler** **ather/o**	**5-90** Coronary artery disease (CAD) affects the arteries and may cause various pathological conditions, including a reduced flow of oxygen and nutrients to the myocardium. (See Figure 5-8.) The most common type of CAD is coronary ather/o/scler/osis. It is now the leading cause of death in the Western world. Identify the word elements in this frame that mean *abnormal condition:* _____. *hardening:* _____. *fatty plaque:* _____ / _____.
arteri/o/scler/osis ăr-tē-rē-ō-sklĕ-RŌ-sĭs	**5-91** Arteri/o/scler/osis is a thickening, hardening, and loss of elasticity of arteri/al walls, which results in decreased blood supply. Thus, arteri/o/scler/osis is commonly referred to as *hardening of the arteries.* When the physician diagnoses a hardening of the arteries, the condition is recorded in the medical chart as _____ / _____ / _____ / _____.

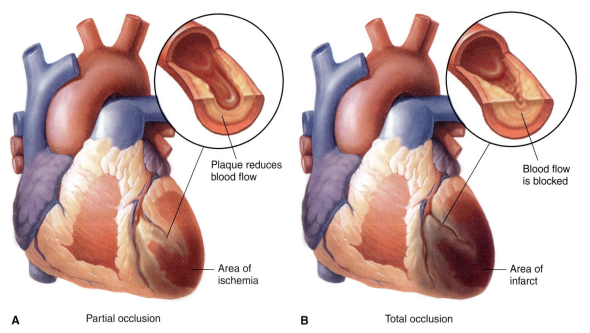

Figure 5-8 Coronary artery disease. (A) Partial occlusion. (B) Total occlusion.

| arteri/o/scler/osis
ăr-tē-rē-ō-sklĕ-RŌ-sĭs

ather/o/scler/osis
ăth-ĕr-ō-sklĕ-RŌ-sĭs | **5-92**   The carotid arteries are a common site of ather/o/scler/osis. When a piece of plaque breaks away from the site, it may travel to the brain, blocking blood flow and causing a stroke. (See Figure 5-9.)

Build medical words that mean

abnormal condition of arterial hardening:

_____ / _____ / _____ / _____.

abnormal condition of fatty plaque hardening:

_____ / _____ / _____ / _____. |

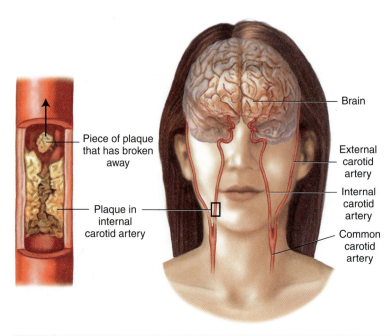

Figure 5-9 Atherosclerosis of the internal carotid artery.

Pink **indicates a prefix.** Blue **indicates a suffix. Boldface indicates a word root or combining form.**

ather/o **arteri/o** **scler/o** **my/o** **cardi**	**5-93** Ather/o/scler/osis, the most common form of arteri/o/scler/osis, is characterized by an accumulation of plaque within the arterial wall. This condition results in partial, and eventually total, occlusion. Both conditions develop over a long period and usually occur together. Indicate the word elements used to denote coronary artery disease that mean *fatty plaque:* _____ / _____. *artery:* _____ / _____. *hardening:* _____ / _____. *muscle:* _____ / _____. *heart:* _____.
excision or removal	**5-94** The CF *necr/o* refers to death or necrosis. *Necr/ectomy* is _____ of dead tissue.
cardi/ac KĂR-dē-ăk **necr/osis** nĕ-KRŌ-sĭs	**5-95** Necr/osis of the my/o/cardi/um occurs when there is insufficient blood supply to the heart. Eventually, such a condition may result in cardi/ac failure and death of the my/o/cardi/um. Identify the words in this frame that mean *pertaining to the heart:* _____ / _____. *abnormal condition of tissue death:* _____ / _____.
	5-96 A my/o/cardi/al infarction (MI), or *infarct,* is caused by occlusion of one or more coronary arteries. MI is a medical emergency requiring immediate attention. Using your medical dictionary, define *infarct.* _____ _____ _____
thromb/us THRŎM-bŭs	**5-97** The *CF* **thromb/o** is used in words to refer to a blood clot; the suffix *-us* means *condition,* structure. Combine **thromb/o** and *-us* to form a word that means *condition of a blood clot.* _____ / _____
thromb/ectomy thrŏm-BĔK-tō-mē	**5-98** Thromb/osis is a condition in which a stationary blood clot obstructs a blood vessel at the site of its formation. The surgical excision of a blood clot is called _____ / _____.

thrombi THRŎM-bī **anti-**	**5-99** Anti/coagulants are agents that prevent or delay blood coagulation; they are used in the prevention and treatment of a thrombus. The plural form of *thrombus* is _____. The element in this frame that means *against* is _____.
thromb/o/genesis thrŏm-bō-JĔN-ĕ-sĭs	**5-100** Use *-genesis* to form a word that means *producing or forming a blood clot.* _____ / _____ / _____
clot	**5-101** If the anti/coagulant does not dissolve the clot, it may be surgically removed. A thromb/ectomy is an excision of a blood _____.
anti/coagulant ăn-tī-kō-ĂG-ū-lănt	**5-102** To prevent blood coagulation, the physician uses an agent known as an _____ / _____.
thromb/o/lysis thrŏm-BŎL-ĭ-sĭs	**5-103** Use the surgical suffix *-lysis* to form a word that means *destruction or dissolving of a thrombus.* _____ / _____ / _____
thromb/o/lysis thrŏm-BŎL-ĭ-sĭs	**5-104** The surgical procedure to destroy or remove a clot is thromb/ectomy or _____ / _____ / _____.
aneurysm ĂN-ū-rĭzm	**5-105** An aneurysm is an abnormal dilation of the vessel wall caused by a weakness that causes the vessel to balloon and potentially rupture. There are three types of aneurysms: **fusiform,** with a dilation of the entire circumference of the artery; **saccular,** with bulging on only one side of the artery wall; and **dissecting,** with an inner layer tear (dissection) that causes a cavity to form and fill with blood with each heartbeat. (See Figure 5-10.) A ballooning out of the wall of the aorta is called an aort/ic _____.

Fusiform   Saccular   Dissecting

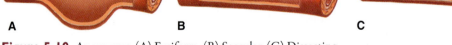

A   B   C

Figure 5-10 Aneurysms. (A) Fusiform. (B) Saccular. (C) Dissecting.

aorta ā-ŎR-tă	**5-106** If a cerebr/al aneurysm ruptures, the hem/o/rrhage occurs in the cerebrum or brain. If an aort/ic aneurysm ruptures, the hem/o/rrhage occurs in the _____.
aort/ic ā-ŎR-tĭk **hem/o/rrhage** HĔM-ĕ-rĭj **cerebr/al** SĔR-ĕ-brăl **aneurysm** ĂN-ū-rĭzm	**5-107** Identify the words in Frame 5-106 that mean *pertaining to the aorta:* _____ / _____. *bursting forth (of) blood:* _____ / _____ / _____. *pertaining to the cerebrum:* _____ / _____. *dilation of a vessel caused by weakness:* _____.

Lymphatic System

The lymphatic system consists of lymph, lymph vessels, lymph nodes, and three organs: the tonsils, thymus, and spleen. The lymphatic system has three main functions:

1. It drains excess interstitial fluid from tissue spaces and returns it to circulating blood.
2. It protects the body by defending against foreign or harmful agents, such as bacteria, viruses, and cancer (CA) cells.
3. It absorbs and transports digested fats to venous circulation. These fats are provided by aggregations of lymphatic tissue known as *Peyer patches* that are present in the lining of the ileum (small intestine).

The fluid (lymph) circulating through the lymphatic system comes from blood. It contains WBCs (leukocytes) responsible for immunity, as well as monocytes and lymphocytes. As certain constituents of blood plasma filtrate through tiny capillaries into the spaces between cells, they become interstitial fluid. Most interstitial fluid is absorbed from the interstitial (or intercellular) spaces by thin-walled vessels called *lymph capillaries.* At this point of absorption, interstitial fluid becomes lymph and is passed through lymphatic tissue called *lymph nodes.* The nodes are found in clusters in such areas as the neck (cervic/al lymph nodes), under the arm (axill/ary lymph nodes), the pelvis (ili/ac lymph nodes), and the groin (inguin/al lymph nodes). The nodes act as filters against foreign materials. Eventually, lymph reaches large lymph vessels in the upper chest and re-enters the bloodstream. (See Figure 5-1.)

WORD ELEMENTS

This section introduces word elements related to the lymphatic system. Review the word elements and their meanings in the following table. Then, pronounce each term in the word analysis column, and place a ✓ in the box after you do so.

Word Element	Meaning	Word Analysis
Combining Forms		
aden/o	gland	**aden/o**/pathy (ă-dĕ-NŎP-ă-thē ☐): disease of a gland *-pathy:* disease
agglutin/o	clumping, gluing	**agglutin**/ation (ă-dĕ-NŎP-ă-thē ☐): process of cells clumping together *-ation:* process (of)
immun/o	immune, immunity, safe	**immun/o**/gen (ĭ-MŪ-nō-jĕn ☐): producing immunity *-gen:* forming, producing, origin *An immunogen is a substance capable of producing an immune response.*
lymph/o	lymph	**lymph/o**/poiesis (lĭm-fō-poy-Ē-sĭs ☐): formation of lymphocytes or of lymphoid tissue *-poiesis:* formation, production
lymphaden/o	lymph gland (node)	**lymphaden**/itis (lĭm-făd-ĕn-Ī-tĭs ☐): inflammation of a lymph gland (node) *-itis:* inflammation
lymphangi/o	lymph vessel	**lymphangi**/oma (lĭm-făn-jē-Ō-mă ☐): tumor composed of lymphatic vessels *-oma:* tumor
phag/o	swallowing, eating	**phag/o**/cyte (FĂG-ō-sīt ☐): cell that swallows and eats (cellular debris) *-cyte:* cell *A phagocyte surrounds, engulfs, and digests microorganisms and cellular debris.*
splen/o	spleen	**splen/o**/megaly (splĕ-nō-MĔG-ă-lē ☐): enlargement of the spleen *-megaly:* enlargement
thym/o	thymus gland	**thym**/oma (thī-MŌ-mă ☐): tumor of the thymus gland, usually a benign tumor *-oma:* tumor
Suffix		
-phylaxis	protection	ana/**phylaxis** (ăn-ă-fĭ-LĂK-sĭs ☐): against protection *ana-:* against; up; back *Anaphylaxis is an extreme allergic reaction characterized by rapid decrease in blood pressure, as well as breathing difficulties, hives, and abdominal cramps.*

Pronunciation Help	*Long Sound*	ā in rāte	ē in rēbirth	ī in īsle	ō in ōver	ū in ūnite
	Short Sound	ă in ăpple	ĕ in ĕver	ĭ in ĭt	ŏ in nŏt	ŭ in cŭt

 Visit the *Medical Terminology Simplified* online resource center at FADavis.com for an audio exercise of the terms in this table to help master pronunciations and meanings of the selected medical terms.

SECTION REVIEW 5-3

For the following medical terms, first, write the suffix and its meaning. Then, translate the meaning of the remaining elements starting with the first part of the word. The first word is an example that is completed for you.

Term	Meaning
1. agglutin/ation	–ation: process (of); clumping, gluing
2. thym/oma	
3. phag/o/cyte	
4. lymphaden/itis	
5. splen/o/megaly	
6. aden/o/pathy	
7. ana/phylaxis	
8. lymphangi/oma	
9. lymph/o/poiesis	
10. immun/o/gen	

Competency Verification: Check your answers in Appendix B: Answer Key, page 598. If you are not satisfied with your level of comprehension, review the vocabulary, and retake the review.

Correct Answers _____ × 10 = _____ % Score

Lymphatic Structures

5-108   Similar to blood capillaries, (1) **lymph capillaries** are thin-walled tubes that carry lymph from the tissue spaces to larger (2) **lymph vessels.** Label these structures in Figure 5-11.

lymph/oma
lĭm-FŌ-mă

lymph/o/cyte
LĬM-fō-sīt

lymph/o/poiesis
lĭm-fō-poy-Ē-sĭs

5-109   Lymph/oma is a malignant tumor of lymph nodes and lymph tissue. Two main kinds of lymphomas are Hodgkin disease and non-Hodgkin lymphoma. These disorders are covered in the Diseases section of this chapter.

Use *lymph*/o to build terms that mean

tumor composed of lymph tissue: _____ / _____.

cell present in lymph tissue: _____ / _____ / _____.

formation or production of lymph:

_____ / _____ / _____.

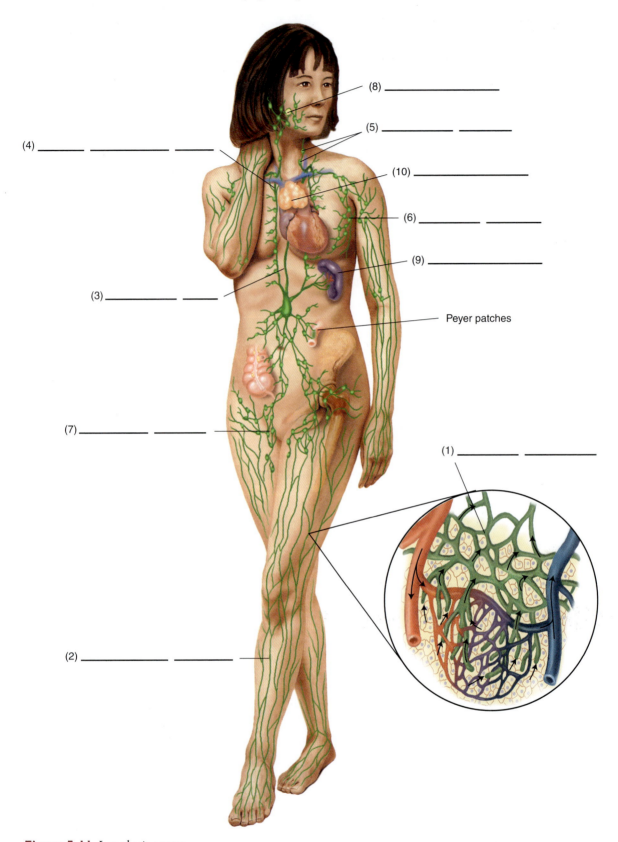

(8) _____

(5) _____ _____

(4) _____ _____ _____

(10) _____

(6) _____ _____

(9) _____

(3) _____ _____

Peyer patches

(7) _____ _____

(1) _____ _____

(2) _____ _____ _____

Figure 5-11 Lymphatic system.

vessels	**5-110** Recall that *angi/o* is used in words to denote a vessel (usually blood or lymph). Angio/card/itis is an inflammation of the heart and blood _____.
lymphangi/o	**5-111** Combine *lymph/o* and *angi/o* to form a new element that means *lymph vessel*. _____ / _____
lymphangi/oma lĭm-făn-jē-Ō-mă	**5-112** Use *lymphangi/o* to form a word that means tumor composed of *lymph vessels*. _____ / _____
angi/o/rrhaphy ăn-jē-OR-ă-fē **angi/o/plasty** ĂN-jē-ō-plăs-tē **angi/o/rrhexis** ăn-jē-ō-RĔK-sĭs	**5-113** Use *angi/o* to develop medical words that mean *suture of a vessel:* _____ / _____ / _____. *surgical repair of a vessel:* _____ / _____ / _____. *rupture of a vessel:* _____ / _____ / _____.
chest	**5-114** Similar to veins, lymph vessels contain valves that keep lymph flowing in one direction, toward the thorac/ic cavity. Thorac/ic means *pertaining to the* _____.
	5-115 The (3) **thoracic duct** and the (4) **right lymphatic duct** carry lymph into the veins in the upper thoracic region. Label these two ducts in Figure 5–11.
-edema **lymph**	**5-116** When a blockage prevents lymph fluid from flowing normally, the fluid builds up and leads to lymph/edema. Identify the word element in this frame that means: *swelling:* _____. *lymph:* _____.
lymph/edema lĭmf-ĕ-DĒ-mă	**5-117** Lymph/edema is most commonly caused by damage or removal of lymph nodes as part of cancer treatment. This results in a blockage which prevents lymph fluid from draining well and commonly occurs in the arms or legs. (See Figure 5-12.) Identify the term in this frame that means *swelling with lymph (fluid)*. _____ / _____

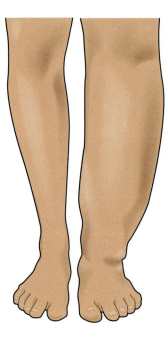

Figure 5-12 Lymphedema of the leg.

5-118   The major lymph node sites are the (5) **cervical nodes**, (6) **axillary nodes**, and (7) **inguinal nodes**. Label the three major lymph node sites in Figure 5-11.

cervic/al SĔR-vĭ-kăl **axill/ary** ĂK-sĭ-lăr-ē **inguin/al** ĬNG-gwĭ-năl	**5-119** Write the name of the lymph nodes located in the neck: _____ / _____. armpit: _____ / _____. groin (depression between the thigh and trunk): _____ / _____.

Tonsil, Spleen, and Thymus

5-120   The (8) **tonsil** is a small mass of lymphoid tissue in the mucous membranes of the pharynx and base of the tongue. Tonsils consist of several masses and are the first line of defense from the external environment. They act as a filter to protect against bacteria and other harmful substances that may enter the body through the nose or mouth. Label the tonsil in Figure 5-11.

5-121   The (9) **spleen** is located in the left upper quadrant (LUQ) of the abdomen and behind the stomach. It is the largest lymphatic organ in the body. Although the spleen is not essential to life, it plays an important role in the immune response by filtering blood in much the same way that lymph nodes filter lymph. Label the spleen in Figure 5-11.

Pink indicates a prefix. Blue indicates a suffix. Boldface indicates a word root or combining form.

path/o/gen
păth-ō-JĔN

hem/o/rrhage
HĔM-ĕ-rĭj

ven/ous
VĒ-nŭs

macro/phage
MĂK-rō-fāj

5-122   Path/o/gens of all types are filtered from circulating blood by the macro/phages of the spleen. The spleen also removes and destroys old RBCs from circulation. The spleen contains ven/ous sinuses that serve as a storage reservoir for blood. In emergencies, such as hem/o/rrhage, the spleen can release blood back into the general circulation.

Identify the term in this frame that refers to

micro/organ/ism capable of producing disease:

_____ / _____ / _____.

loss of large amounts of blood in a short period:

_____ / _____ / _____.

pertaining to a vein: _____ / _____.

phag/o/cyt/ic cell in the spleen:

_____ / _____.

5-123   The (10) **thymus,** also an endocrine gland, is a lymphatic organ. It is located near the middle of the chest (mediastinum) just beneath the sternum. Label the thymus in Figure 5-11.

immun/o

5-124   During fetal life and childhood, the thymus is quite large but becomes smaller with age as it completes most of its essential work during childhood. The thymus plays an important role in the body's ability to protect itself against disease (immunity), especially during the early years of growth.

What CF means *immune, immunity, safe*?

_____ / _____

T cells

5-125   The thymus secretes a hormone called *thymosin,* which stimulates the red bone marrow to produce T lymph/o/cytes, or T cells. T cells are important in the immune process. They originate in bone marrow but migrate and mature in the thymus. Upon maturation, T cells enter blood and circulate throughout the body, providing a mechanism of defense against disease because the cells attack and destroy foreign or abnormal cells.

Specific lymph/o/cytes that attack foreign agents, such as viruses, are known as

T lympho/cytes or _____.

cyt/o/tox/ic
sī-tō-TŎKS-ĭk

CA

5-126   Some T cells are called killer *T cells or cytotoxic T lymphocytes (CTLs)* because they secrete immun/o/logic/ally essential chemical compounds that destroy foreign cells. These killer cells are so named because they are capable of destroying specific cells. The killer cells also play a significant role in the body's resistance to proliferation of CA cells.

Specialized cells that provide surveillance against CA cells are called *killer*

T lymph/o/cytes or _____ / _____ / _____ / _____

T lymph/o/cytes.

The abbreviation for cancer is _____.

Competency Verification: Check your labeling of Figure 5-11 in Appendix B: Answer Key, page 598.

SECTION REVIEW 5-4

Using the following table, write the CF or suffix that matches its definition in the space provided to the left of the definition. There may be more than one word element that matches a definition.

Combining Forms

angi/o	lymph/o
aort/o	my/o
cardi/o	necr/o
cerebr/o	thromb/o
electr/o	
hem/o	

Suffixes

-al	-megaly
-cyte	-pathy
-gram	-plasty
-graphy	-rrhexis
-ic	-stenosis
-lysis	

1. _____ aorta

2. _____ blood

3. _____ blood clot

4. _____ cell

5. _____ cerebrum

6. _____ death, necrosis

7. _____ disease

8. _____ electricity

9. _____ enlargement

10. _____ heart

11. _____ lymph

12. _____ muscle

13. _____ process of recording

14. _____ record, writing

15. _____ pertaining to

16. _____ rupture

17. _____ separation; destruction; loosening

18. _____ narrowing, stricture

19. _____ surgical repair

20. _____ vessel (usually blood or lymph)

Competency Verification: Check your answers in Appendix B: Answer Key, page 598. If you are not satisfied with your level of comprehension, go back to Frame 5–108 and rework the frames.

Correct Answers _____ × 5 = _____ % Score

Abbreviations

This section introduces cardiovascular and lymphatic systems-related abbreviations and their meanings. Included are abbreviations contained in the medical record activities that follow.

Abbreviation	Meaning	Abbreviation	Meaning
ACE	angiotensin-converting enzyme (inhibitor)	HIV	human immunodeficiency virus
AED	automatic external defibrillator	HTN	hypertension
AICD	automatic implantable cardioverter–defibrillator	IAS	interatrial septum
AIDS	acquired immune deficiency syndrome	ICD	implantable cardioverter-defibrillator
AV	atrioventricular; arteriovenous	IVC	inferior vena cava
BMT	bone marrow transplant	IVS	interventricular septum
BP	blood pressure	LA	left atrium
CA	cancer; chronological age; cardiac arrest	LDL	low-density lipoprotein
CABG	coronary artery bypass graft	LUQ	left upper quadrant
CAD	coronary artery disease	LV	left ventricle
CBC	complete blood count	MI	myocardial infarction
CC	cardiac catheterization; chief complaint	MVP	mitral valve prolapse
CHB	complete heart block	PCI	percutaneous coronary intervention
CHF	congestive heart failure	PTCA	percutaneous transluminal coronary angioplasty
CTL	cytotoxic T lymphocyte	RA	right atrium
CV	cardiovascular	RBC	red blood cell
CVA	cerebrovascular accident; costovertebral angle	RV	right ventricle
DVT	deep vein thrombosis (also called deep venous thrombosis)	SA	sinoatrial (node)
EBV	Epstein-Barr virus	SLE	systemic lupus erythematosus; slit-lamp examination
ECG, EKG	electrocardiogram; electrocardiography	SVC	superior vena cava
ELISA	enzyme-linked immunosorbent assay (test to detect anti-HIV antibodies)	TIA	transient ischemic attack
HDL	high-density lipoprotein	US	ultrasound; ultrasonography
HF	heart failure	WBC	white blood cell

Additional Medical Terms

The following are additional terms related to the cardiovascular and lymphatic systems. Recognizing and learning these terms will help you understand the connection between common signs, symptoms, and diseases and their diagnoses, as well as the rationale behind methods of treatment selected for a particular disorder.

Diseases and Conditions

Cardiovascular System

anemia ă-NĒ-mē-ă *an:* without, not *-emia:* blood condition	Blood disorder characterized by a deficiency of red blood cell production and hemoglobin, increased red blood cell destruction, or blood loss
aplastic ā-PLĂS-tĭk	Failure of bone marrow to produce stem cells because it has been damaged by disease, cancer, radiation, or chemotherapy drugs; rare but serious form of anemia
pernicious pĕr-NĬSH-ŭs	Deficiency of erythrocytes resulting from inability to absorb vitamin B_{12} into the body, which plays a vital role in hematopoiesis
sickle cell	Inherited genetic disease of abnormal hemoglobin that produces sickle-shaped erythrocytes resulting in obstruction of normal blood flow *The incidence of sickle cell anemia is highest among African American and African ancestry. Figure 5-13 illustrates the effects of sickle cell anemia on the many body systems.*

thalassemia
thăl-ă-SĒ-mē-ă
 	
thalass/o: sea
  -emia: blood
        condition
	Group of hereditary anemias characterized by less hemoglobin and fewer red blood cells in the body than normal; usually seen in people of Mediterranean origin

angina pectoris ăn-JĪ-nă pĕk-TŌ-rĭs	Mild to severe pain or pressure in the chest caused by ischemia; also called *angina* *Angina pectoris usually results from atherosclerosis of the coronary arteries. It can occur while resting or during exercise and is a warning sign of an impending myocardial infarction (MI).*
bruit BRWĒ	Abnormal blowing sound heard on auscultation and caused by turbulent blood flow through an artery

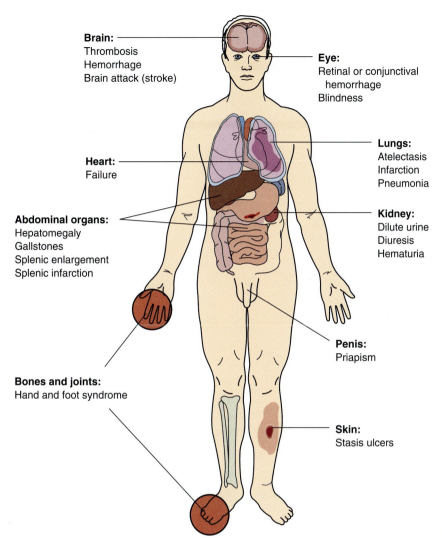

Brain:
Thrombosis
Hemorrhage
Brain attack (stroke)

Eye:
Retinal or conjunctival
hemorrhage
Blindness

Lungs:
Atelectasis
Infarction
Pneumonia

Heart:
Failure

Abdominal organs:
Hepatomegaly
Gallstones
Splenic enlargement
Splenic infarction

Kidney:
Dilute urine
Diuresis
Hematuria

Penis:
Priapism

Bones and joints:
Hand and foot syndrome

Skin:
Stasis ulcers

Figure 5-13 Clinical manifestations of sickle cell anemia/ From Williams & Hopper: Understanding Med/Surg, ed 2, p. 381.

deep vein thrombosis (DVT)
 VĀN thrŏm-BŌ-sĭs
  thromb: blood clot
  -osis: abnormal condition; increase (used primarily with blood cells)
	Formation of a blood clot in a deep vein of the body, occurring most commonly in the legs or thighs
	
	 Anticoagulants help dissolve clot formations and prevent further clotting. (See Figure 5-14.)

embolus
 ĔM-bŏ-lŭs
  embol: embolus (plug)
  -us: condition; structure
	Mass of undissolved matter—commonly a blood clot, fatty plaque, or air bubble—that travels through the bloodstream and becomes lodged in a blood vessel
	
	 Emboli may be solid, liquid, or gaseous. Occlusion of vessels from an embolus usually results in the development of an infarct.

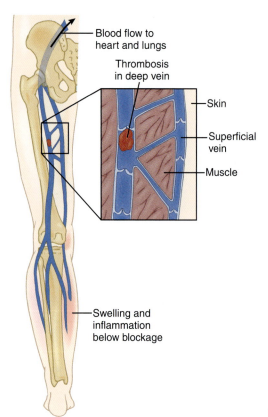

Blood flow to heart and lungs

Thrombosis in deep vein

Skin

Superficial vein

Muscle

Swelling and inflammation below blockage

Figure 5-14 Deep vein thrombosis.

heart block	Interference with normal conduction of electrical impulses that control activity of the heart muscle
	Heart block is usually specified by the location of the block and the type.
first-degree	Atrioventricular (AV) block in which the atrial electrical impulses are delayed by a fraction of a second before being conducted to the ventricles
	First-degree AV block is recognized on ECG by a prolonged PR interval. There is no specific treatment for first-degree AV block, but the condition is monitored because it may precede higher degrees of block.
second-degree	AV block in which occasional electrical impulses from the SA node fail to be conducted to the ventricles
	Because of the dropped beats in second-degree AV block, the QRS complexes are dropped periodically, usually every second, third, or fourth beat.
third-degree	AV block in which electrical impulses from the atria fail to reach the ventricles; also called *complete heart block (CHB)*
	In right- or left-bundle branch block, electrical impulses are unable to travel down the right or left bundle of His. Treatment for second- or third-degree heart block consists of atropine (a drug used to increase heart rate) or pacemaker insertion.

heart failure (HF)	Inability of the heart to pump sufficient blood to meet the metabolic needs of the body
congestive heart failure (CHF)	HF that occurs when blood returning to the heart backs up into the lungs or other parts of the body, causing congestion
	Symptoms of CHF include fluid retention of the lower extremities with pulmonary edema, shortness of breath, and activity intolerance.
hypertension hī-pĕr-TĔN-shŭn *hyper:* excessive, above normal *-tension:* to stretch	Consistently elevated blood pressure (BP) that is higher than 140/90 mm Hg, causing damage to the blood vessels and, ultimately the heart
ischemia ĭs-KĒ-mē-ă *isch:* to hold back; block *-emia:* blood	Deficiency of blood flow to an organ or tissue as a result of circulatory obstruction *In the cardiovascular system, causes of ischemia include arterial embolism, atherosclerosis, thrombosis, and vasoconstriction. (See the ischemic area of the myocardium in Figure 5-8.)*
mitral valve prolapse (MVP) MĪ-trăl VĂLV PRŌ-lăps	Condition in which the leaflets of the mitral valve prolapse into the LA during systole, resulting in incomplete closure and regurgitation (backflow) of blood (See Figure 5-15.)

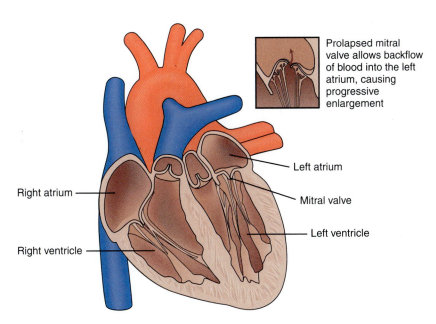

Prolapsed mitral valve allows backflow of blood into the left atrium, causing progressive enlargement

Right atrium

Right ventricle

Left atrium

Mitral valve

Left ventricle

Figure 5-15 Mitral valve prolapse.

myocardial infarction (MI)
mī-ō-KĂR-dē-ăl ĭn-FĂRK-shŭn
  my/o: muscle
  cardi: heart
    -al: pertaining to
	Necrosis of a portion of cardiac muscle caused by partial or complete occlusion of one or more coronary arteries; also called *heart attack*

patent ductus arteriosus PĂT-ĕnt DŬK-tŭs ăr-tē-rē-Ō-sŭs	Failure of the ductus arteriosus to close after birth, resulting in an abnormal opening between the pulmonary artery and the aorta
Raynaud disease rā-NŌ	Vascular disorder in which the fingers and toes become cold, numb, and painful as a result of temporary constriction of blood vessels in the skin *Episodes may be triggered by cold temperatures or emotional stress. It may also be an indicator of some other, more serious, problem.*
rheumatic heart disease rū-MĂT-ĭk	Streptococcal infection that causes damage to the heart valves and heart muscle, most commonly in children and young adults

Lymphatic System

acquired immune deficiency syndrome (AIDS) ă-KWĪRD ĭm-ŪN dē-FĬSH-ĕn-sē	Deficiency of cellular immunity induced by infection with HIV, characterized by increasing susceptibility to infections, malignancies, and neurological diseases *HIV is transmitted from person to person in cell-rich body fluids (notably blood and semen) through sexual contact, sharing of contaminated needles (as by intravenous drug abusers), or other contact with contaminated blood (as in accidental needlesticks among health-care workers).*
lymphoma lĭm-FŌ-mă	Any malignant tumor of lymph nodes or other lymph tissue
Hodgkin HŎJ-kĭn	Lymphoma characterized by painless, progressive enlargement of lymphoid tissue (usually first evident in cervical lymph nodes), splenomegaly, and the presence of unique Reed-Sternberg cells in the lymph nodes; also called *classic Hodgkin lymphoma*

non-Hodgkin
  non-HŎJ-kĭn
    lymph: lymph
    -oma: tumor
	Lymphoma that originates in the lymphatic system and develops from lymphocytes
	
	These lymphomas include a group of more than 20 different types of lymphomas that occur in older adults and do not show Reed-Sternberg cells.

Kaposi sarcoma
KĂP-ō-sē săr-KŌ-mă

   sarc: flesh (connective tissue)

   -oma: tumor

Malignancy of connective tissue, including bone, fat, muscle, and fibrous tissue; also called *malignant neoplasm of soft tissue*

Kaposi sarcoma is closely associated with AIDS and is commonly fatal because the tumors readily metastasize to various organs.

---

mononucleosis
mŏn-ō-nū-klē-Ō-sĭs

   mono-: on e

   nucle: nucleus

   -osis: abnormal condition; increase (used primarily with blood cells)

Acute infection caused by the Epstein-Barr virus (EBV) and characterized by a sore throat, fever, fatigue, and enlarged lymph nodes

---

systemic lupus erythematosus (SLE)
LŪ-pŭs ĕr-ĭ-thē-mă-TŌ-sĭs

Chronic inflammatory autoimmune disease characterized by unusual antibodies in the blood that target tissues of the body with a butterfly-shaped rash that appears on the face (See Figure 5-16.)

There is a sensitivity to sunlight, fatigue, and joint pain. Treatment includes anti-inflammatories, immunosuppressives, and corticosteroids. The rash tends to get worse when exposed to direct sunlight.

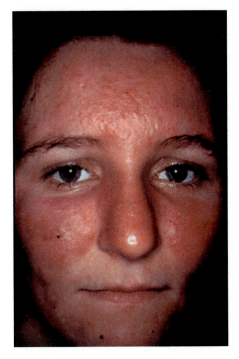

Figure 5-16 Butterfly rash of systemic lupus erythematosus. From Goldsmith, L.A. and Tharp, M.D.: Adult and Pediatric Dermatology, page 230. FA Davis, 1997, with permission.

Diagnostic Procedures

Cardiovascular System

cardiac catheterization (CC) KĂR-dē-ăk kăth-ĕ-tĕr-ĭ-ZĀ-shŭn *cardi:* heart *-ac:* pertaining to	Insertion of a catheter into the heart through a vein or artery, usually of an arm (brachial approach) or leg (femoral approach) to provide evaluation of the heart (See Figure 5-17.) *During CC, the cardiologist may also inject a contrast medium and take radiographs (angiography). Cardiac catheterization is used mainly in diagnosing and evaluating congenital, rheumatic, and coronary arterial lesions, including MI.*
cardiac enzyme studies KĂR-dē-ăk ĔN-zīm	Tests that measure levels of enzymes and proteins in blood; the levels increase with an injury to the heart muscle, such as from a heart attack *Cardiac enzyme studies help determine whether angina, shortness of breath, or abnormal electrocardiography results indicate a heart attack or imminent heart attack.*
echocardiography ĕk-ō-kăr-dē-ŎG-ră-fē *echo-:* a repeated sound *cardi/o:* heart *-graphy:* process of recording	Use of ultrasound to evaluate the heart and great vessels and diagnose cardiovascular lesions
electrocardiography (ECG, EKG) ē-lĕk-trō-kăr-dē-ŎG-ră-fē *electr/o:* electricity *cardi/o:* heart *-graphy:* process of recording	Creation and study of graphic records (electrocardiograms) produced by electric activity generated by the heart muscle; also called cardiography *A cardiologist analyzes an ECG, which is valuable in diagnosing cases of abnormal heart rhythm and myocardial damage.*

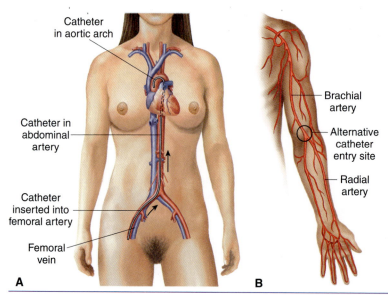

Figure 5-17 Cardiac catheterization. (A) Catheter insertion in the femoral vein or artery. (B) Catheter insertion in the brachial or radial artery.

Holter monitor
HŌL-ter MŎN-ĭ-tor

Device worn by a patient that records prolonged electrocardiograph readings (usually 24 hours) on a portable tape recorder while the patient conducts normal daily activities

Holter monitoring provides a record of cardiac arrhythmia that would not be discovered by means of an ECG of only a few minutes' duration. The patient keeps an activity diary to compare daily events with electrocardiographic tracings. (See Figure 5-18.)

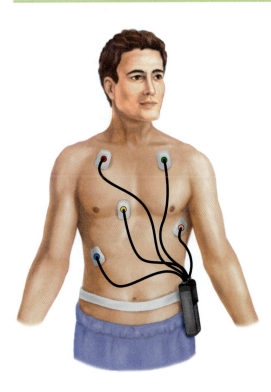

Figure 5-18 Holter monitor.

lipid panel
LĬP-ĭd

Panel of blood tests measuring cholesterol components to assess the risk of heart disease

A lipid panel consists of total cholesterol, high-density lipoprotein (HDL), low-density lipoprotein (LDL), and triglycerides.

stress test

Test in which an ECG is recorded under controlled exercise conditions (typically using a treadmill) to determine the heart's response to physical exertion (stress)

A stress test may show abnormal ECG tracings that do not appear during an ECG taken when the patient is resting. (See Figure 5-19.)

nuclear

Stress test that uses a radioisotope to evaluate coronary blood flow

In a nuclear stress test, the radioisotope is injected at the height of exercise. The area not receiving sufficient oxygen is visualized by decreased uptake of the isotope.

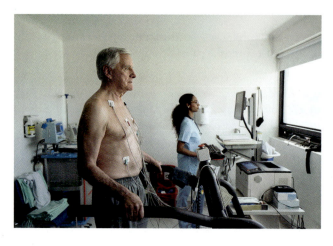

Figure 5-19 Patient performing stress test on a treadmill while the nurse views the cardiac monitor.

troponin I TRŌ-pō-nĭn	Blood test that measures protein released into the blood by damaged heart muscle (not skeletal muscle) *The troponin I test is a highly sensitive and specific indicator of recent MI.*

ultrasonography (US)
ŭl-tră-sŏn-ŎG-răf-ē
   ultra-: excess, beyond
   son/o: sound
  -graphy: process of
          recording
	Radiographic procedure in which a small transducer passed over the skin transmits high-frequency sound waves (ultrasound) that bounce off body tissues and are then recorded to produce an image of an internal organ or tissue; also called *ultrasound* and *echo*

Doppler DŎP-lĕr	Ultrasonography used to assess blood flow through blood vessels and the heart; also called *ultrasonography using sound pitch* *Doppler US detects alterations in blood flow caused by plaque or blood clots in arteries and veins. It is used to diagnose deep vein thrombosis (DVT), varicose veins, aneurysms, carotid artery occlusion, and other vessel abnormalities. (See Figure 5-20.)*

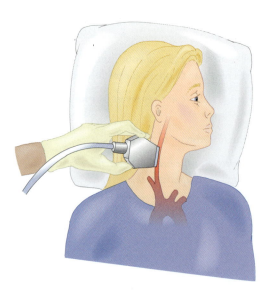

Figure 5-20 Doppler ultrasonography of the carotid artery.

Lymphatic System

bone marrow aspiration biopsy ăs-pĭ-RĀ-shŭn BĪ-ŏp-sē	Removal of living bone marrow tissue, usually taken from the sternum or iliac crest, for microscopic examination (See Figure 5-21.) *Bone marrow aspiration biopsy evaluates hematopoiesis by revealing the number, shape, and size of RBCs, WBCs, and platelet precursors.*
enzyme-linked immunosorbent assay (ELISA)	Blood test that detects antibodies in the blood, including screening for antibody to HIV *A positive result on the ELISA test indicates probable virus exposure and is confirmed with the Western blot test, which is more specific.*

lymphangiography
lĭm-făn-jē-ŎG-ră-fē
  lymph: ymph
  angi/o: vessel (usually blood or lymph)
  -graphy: process of recording
	Radiographic examination of lymph glands and lymphatic vessels after an injection of a contrast medium; used to identify enlarged lymph nodes, lymphomas, and areas of blocked lymphatic drainage
	
	Because lymph nodes filter and trap CA cells, this test is commonly used to determine lymph flow in areas that contain malignancy.

tissue typing	Technique that determines the histocompatibility of tissues used in grafts and transplants with the recipient's tissues and cells; also known as histocompatibility testing

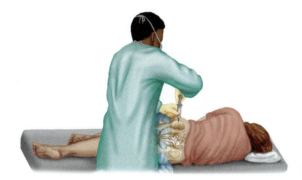

Figure 5-21 Bone marrow aspiration.

Medical and Surgical Procedures

Cardiovascular System

angioplasty
ĂN-jē-ō-plăs-tē

Endovascular procedure (under x-ray visualization) that widens or opens blocked coronary arteries to restore blood flow to the heart muscle; also called *coronary angioplasty*

Angioplasty relieves chest pain caused by reduced blood flow to the heart and minimizes damage to heart muscle caused by a heart attack. A coronary artery stent may also be placed during angioplasty to prevent closure of a coronary artery from an atherosclerotic lesion.

percutaneous transluminal coronary angioplasty (PTCA)
pĕr-kū-TĀ-nē-ŭs
trăns-LŪ-mĭ-năl
KOR-ō-nă-rē
ĂN-jē-ō-plăs-tē

Angioplasty in which a balloon catheter is inserted and threaded through the femoral or radial artery into the blocked coronary artery that is narrowed because of atherosclerosis (See Figure 5-22.)

Once the catheter is in place, the balloon is inflated and compresses the plaque outward against the wall of the artery. This widens the artery and restores blood flow. This procedure is also called percutaneous coronary intervention (PCI).

catheter ablation
KĂTH-ĕ-tĕr ăb-LĀ-shŭn

Uses of radiofrequency energy to destroy a small area of heart tissue that is causing arrhythmias; also called *radiofrequency ablation*

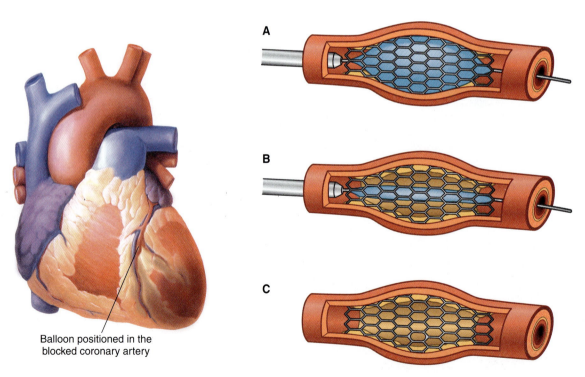

Balloon positioned in the blocked coronary artery

Figure 5-22 PTCA with stent placement. (A) Balloon inflated to widen the artery. (B) Deflated balloon. (C) Stent remains to hold artery open when catheter is removed.

cardioversion căr-dē-ō-VĔR-zhŭn *cardi/o:* heart *-version:* turning	Delivery of brief discharges of electricity that pass across the chest to stop a cardiac arrhythmia and restore normal sinus rhythm; also called *defibrillation* (See Figure 5-23.) *A defibrillator is the electrical device used for cardioversion.*

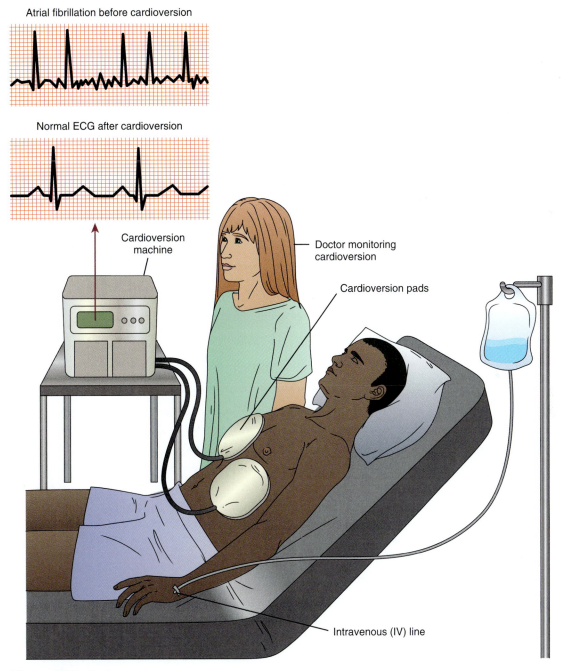

Atrial fibrillation before cardioversion

Normal ECG after cardioversion

Cardioversion machine

Doctor monitoring cardioversion

Cardioversion pads

Intravenous (IV) line

Figure 5-23 Cardioversion.

coronary artery bypass graft (CABG)

Bypass surgery that creates new routes around narrowed or blocked arteries to allow sufficient blood flow to deliver oxygen and nutrients to the heart muscle; also called *coronary artery bypass surgery* (See Figure 5-24.)

CABG is performed to relieve angina and reduce the risk of death caused by coronary artery disease. Arteries or veins from elsewhere in the patient's body are grafted to the coronary arteries to bypass atherosclerotic narrowings and improve blood supply to the coronary circulation supplying the myocardium.

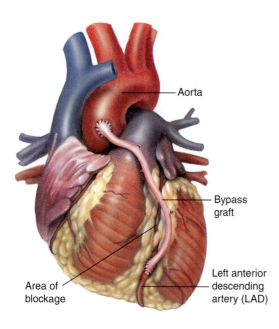

Aorta

Bypass graft

Left anterior descending artery (LAD)

Area of blockage

Figure 5-24 Coronary artery bypass graft (CABG).

defibrillator
dē-FĬB-rĭ-lā-tor

Device designed to administer a defibrillating electric shock to restore normal SA

There are two types of defibrillators: automatic implantable cardioverter-defibrillators (AICDs) and automatic external defibrillators (AEDs).

automatic implantable cardioverter-defibrillator (AICD)
căr-dē-ō-VĔR-tĕr
dē-FĬB-rĭ-lā-tor

Surgically implanted defibrillator that automatically detects and corrects potentially fatal arrhythmias, such as ventricular fibrillations; also called *implantable cardioverter-defibrillator (ICD)* (See Figure 5-25.)

An AICD is implanted, usually in the chest, in a patient who is at high risk for developing a serious arrhythmia. It has leads (wires) that go to the heart, sense its rhythm, and deliver an electrical shock, if needed.

automatic external defibrillator (AED)
dē-FĬB-rĭ-lā-tor

Portable computerized defibrillator that analyzes the patient's heart rhythm and delivers an electrical shock to stimulate a heart in cardiac arrest (CA)

An AED is kept on emergency response vehicles and in public places, such as recreation facilities, and is designed to be used by trained first-responder personnel or lay people.

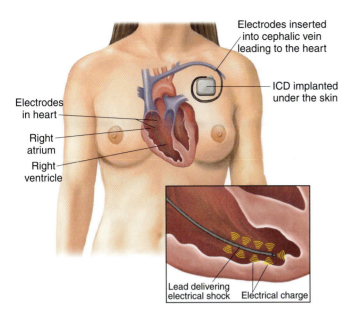

Electrodes inserted into cephalic vein leading to the heart

ICD implanted under the skin

Electrodes in heart

Right atrium

Right ventricle

Lead delivering electrical shock   Electrical charge

Figure 5-25 Automatic implantable cardioverter-defibrillator (AICD).

---

endarterectomy
ĕnd-ăr-tĕr-ĔK-tō-mē
   end-: in, within
   arter: artery
   -ectomy: excision, removal

carotid
kă-RŎT-ĭd

Surgical removal of the lining of an artery

Endarterectomy is performed on almost any major artery, such as the carotid or femoral artery, when it is diseased or blocked.

Endarterectomy of an occluded carotid artery

Carotid endarterectomy reduces the risk of stroke when it is performed on a patient with moderate or severe stenosis of the artery, with or without a history of transient ischemic attacks (TIAs). (See Figure 5-26.)

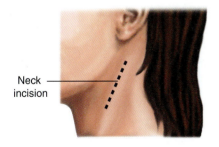

Neck incision

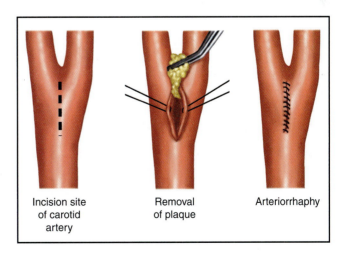

Incision site of carotid artery

Removal of plaque

Arteriorrhaphy

Figure 5-26 Carotid endarterectomy.

sclerotherapy
sklĕr-ō-THĔR-ă-pē
　　scler/o: hardening;
　　　　sclera (white
　　　　of the eye)
　　-therapy: treatment

Chemical injection into a varicose vein that causes inflammation and formation of fibrous tissue, which closes the vein

When a vein closes, it can no longer fill with blood. In a few weeks, the treated varicose vein fades.

valvuloplasty
VĂL-vū-lō-plăs-tē
　　valvul/o: valve
　　-plasty: surgical repair

Plastic or restorative surgery on a heart valve to correct a prolapse or stenosis

A special type of valvuloplasty, called balloon valvuloplasty, involves insertion of a balloon catheter to open a stenotic heart valve. Inflation of the balloon decreases the constriction.

Lymphatic System

lymphangiectomy
lĭm-făn-jē-ĔK-tō-mē
　　lymph: lymph
　　angi: vessel (usually
　　　　blood or
　　　　lymph)
　　-ectomy: excision,
　　　　removal

Removal of a lymph vessel

**bone marrow transplant
(BMT)**

Infusion (transplantation) of healthy bone marrow stem cells to stimulate blood cell production once diseased bone marrow is destroyed by radiation or chemotherapy drugs

BMT is used to treat patients with leukemia and lymphoma. It can be autologous (from the patient's own bone marrow) or allogenic (from a compatible donor).

Pharmacology

The following table lists some common drug categories used to treat cardiovascular and lymph disorders, as well as their therapeutic actions.

Drug Category	Action
Cardiovascular System	
anticoagulants ăn-tĭ-kō-ĂG-ū-lănts	Prevent blood clot formation *Anticoagulants decrease the risk of stroke and DVT and are also used postoperatively to prevent clot formation.*
antiarrhythmics ăn-tē-ă-RĬTH-mĭks	Counteract cardiac arrhythmias (dysrhythmias) by stabilizing the electrical conduction system of the heart
antihypertensives ăn-tē-hī-pĕr-TĔN-sĭvs	Treat hypertension (high blood pressure) *Antihypertensives prevent complications of high blood pressure, such as stroke and MI. There are many classes of antihypertensives that lower blood pressure by different means. Some of the most widely used include beta blockers, diuretics, and angiotensin-converting enzyme (ACE) inhibitors.*
beta blockers	Decrease heart rate and dilate arteries by blocking beta receptors *Beta blockers are used to treat angina, arrhythmias, and hypertension.*
diuretics dī-ū-RĔT-ĭks	Block sodium from being absorbed back into blood *Diuretics reduce fluid buildup in the body, including fluid in the lungs, a common symptom of heart failure, by increasing the secretion of urine. They are commonly prescribed in treating hypertension and heart failure.*
statins STĂ-tĭnz	Lower cholesterol levels in blood and reduce production of cholesterol in the liver by blocking the enzyme that produces it
thrombolytics thrŏm-bō-LĬT-ĭks	Dissolve blood clots and help prevent damage to the heart muscle; commonly called *clot busters* *Thrombolytics help manage stroke and may also stop a heart attack that would otherwise be deadly.*
Lymphatic System	
antivirals an-tĭ-VĪ-rălz	Inhibit development of specific viruses *Antivirals are used to treat HIV infection and AIDS.*
immunosuppressants ĭm-ū-nō-sū-PRĔSS-ănts	Suppress the immune response to prevent organ rejection after transplantation or to slow the progression of autoimmune disease

Pronunciation Help	*Long Sound*	ā in rāte	ē in rēbirth	ī in īsle	ō in ōver	ū in ūnite
	Short Sound	ă in ăpple	ĕ in ĕver	ĭ in ĭt	ŏ in nŏt	ŭ in cŭt

Word Elements Review

This review provides a verification of word elements covered in this chapter. First, use a slash to break the term into its component parts, and identify each element by labeling it P for prefix, WR for word root, CF for combining form, and S for suffix. Then, provide the meaning of the medical term. Remember to define the suffix first; second, define the beginning of the word; and last, define the middle part of the term. The first word is a sample completed for you.

Medical Term	Meaning
splen/o/megaly 　　CF　　S	enlargement of the spleen
1. lymphangi/oma	
2. hemat/o/poiesis	
3. phleb/o/stenosis	
4. thromb/ectomy	
5. peri/cardi/o/centesis	

Match the following medical terms with the definitions in the numbered list.

agglutination	arrhythmia	electrocardiograph	lymphopoiesis
aneurysmorrhaphy	arteriosclerosis	immunogen	tachycardia
angioplasty	atherectomy	intraventricular	vasospasm

6. _____ process of cells clumping together

7. _____ heart rate that is rapid

8. _____ condition of hardening of an artery

9. _____ suture of a widened blood vessel

10. _____ involuntary contraction or twitching of a blood vessel

11. _____ instrument for recording the electrical activity of the heart

12. _____ within a ventricle

13. _____ excision of fatty plaque

14. _____ without rhythm

15. _____ producing immunity

Competency Verification: Check your answers in Appendix B: Answer Key, pages 598 and 599. If you are not satisfied with your level of comprehension, review the vocabulary, and retake the review.

Correct Answers _____ × 6.67 = _____ % Score

Additional Medical Terms Review

Match the following medical term(s) with the definitions in the numbered list.

AIDS	*embolus*	*ischemia*	*statins*
bruit	*fibrillation*	*lymphangiography*	*thrombolytics*
CABG	*HF*	*mononucleosis*	*tissue typing*
Doppler US	*Hodgkin lymphoma*	*Raynaud disease*	*troponin I*
DVT	*Holter monitor*	*rheumatic heart disease*	*valvuloplasty*

1. _____ is an acute infection caused by EBV and characterized by a sore throat, fever, fatigue, and enlarged lymph nodes.

2. _____ are drugs that dissolve a blood clot.

3. _____ is a mass of undissolved matter present in a blood vessel.

4. _____ refers to formation of a blood clot in a deep vein of the body.

5. _____ are drugs used to lower blood cholesterol levels.

6. _____ is an abnormal blowing sound caused by turbulent blood flow.

7. _____ is ultrasonography used to assess blood flow through the blood vessels and the heart.

8. _____ is a streptococcal infection that causes damage to heart valves and heart muscle.

9. _____ is a small portable device worn on a patient during normal activity to obtain a record of cardiac arrhythmia.

10. _____ is a vascular disorder in which fingers and toes become cold, numb, and painful.

11. _____ is a deficiency of blood flow leading to necrosis of the myocardium.

12. _____ refers to malignant tumors of the lymphatic system.

13. _____ is a transmissible infection caused by HIV.

14. _____ is a condition in which the ability of the heart to pump blood is impaired.

15. _____ is an arrhythmia of heart fibers.

16. _____ refers to restorative surgery on a valve, especially a cardiac valve.

17. _____ is a radiographic examination of lymph glands and lymphatic vessels after an injection of a contrast medium; used to identify pathological conditions of the lymphatic system.

18. _____ is also known as histocompatibility testing.

19. _____ refers to a blood test that measures protein released into the blood by damaged heart muscle.

20. _____ refers to bypassing one or more blocked coronary arteries to restore blood flow.

Competency Verification: Check your answers in Appendix B: Answer Key, page 599. If you are not satisfied with your level of comprehension, review the additional medical terms, and retake the review.

Correct Answers _____ × 4 = _____ % Score

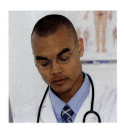

Medical Record Activities

To develop a working vocabulary of medical terms and to understand how those terms are used in the health-care industry, it is important that you complete the following activities.

MEDICAL RECORD ACTIVITY 5-1

EMERGENCY DEPARTMENT REPORT: RULE OUT MYOCARDIAL INFARCTION

This activity contains an emergency department report on a patient who presents with chest pain. Read the emergency department report that follows, and underline the medical terms. Then complete the terminology and critical thinking exercises.

EMERGENCY DEPARTMENT REPORT

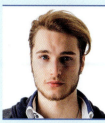

PATIENT NAME: Nichols, James
MEDICAL RECORD ID: 68-19347
DATE: May 1, 20xx

CHIEF COMPLAINT: Patient complains of chest pain.

PRESENT ILLNESS: Patient is a 22-year-old male, who states that he has had two previous myocardial infarctions related to his use of cocaine. The patient states he has not used cocaine for the last 3 months. He describes the pain as midsternal pain, a burning type sensation that lasted several seconds. The patient took one of his own nitroglycerin tablets without any relief. The patient became concerned and came into the emergency department. In the emergency department, the patient states that his pain is a 3 on a scale of 1 to 10. He feels much more comfortable. He denies any shortness of breath or dizziness and states that the pain feels unlike the pain of his myocardial infarction. The patient has no other complaints at this time.

PAST HISTORY: The patient's past medical history is significant for status post myocardial infarction in January of 19xx and again in April of 19xx. Both were related to illegal use of cocaine.

ALLERGIES: None

MEDICATIONS: Nitroglycerin p.r.n.

PHYSICAL EXAMINATION

GENERAL: A well-developed, well-nourished, white male in no acute distress. He is alert, oriented x3, and lying comfortably on the bed. **VITAL SIGNS:** Temperature 98.2, blood pressure 138/80 mm Hg, pulse 100 beats/min, respirations 18 breaths/min. **HEENT:** Normocephalic. The pupils are equal, round, and reactive. Extraocular movements are intact. **NECK:** Supple with full range of motion. No rigidity. **CHEST:** Nontender. **LUNGS:** Clear to auscultation. **HEART:** Regular rate and rhythm. No murmurs present. **ABDOMEN:** Soft, nondistended, nontender with active bowel sounds. **EXTREMITIES:** Unremarkable. **NEUROLOGIC:** Unremarkable.

LABORATORY DATA: Complete blood count (CBC), chemistry profile, and cardiac enzymes, all within normal limits. Chest x-ray was normal. Electrocardiogram showed normal sinus rhythm with no acute ST or T-wave segment changes. There were no acute changes seen on the electrocardiogram. O2 saturation was 98%.

HOSPITAL COURSE: The patient had a stable, uncomplicated emergency department course. The patient received 45 cc of Mylanta and 10 cc of viscous lidocaine with complete relief of his chest pain. The patient had no further complaints and stated that he felt much better shortly thereafter.

DIAGNOSIS: 1. Angina pectoris. 2. Possible esophageal reflux.

PLAN: Patient discharged from the emergency department in stable, ambulatory, good condition, with instructions to use Mylanta for his abdominal pain and to follow up with his internist in the next 2 to 3 days.

Edward Tohme M.D.

Edward Tohme, M.D.

ET: bc
D: 5/1/xx; T: 5/1/xx

Terminology 5-1

Terms listed in the following table come from the consultation letter Emergency Department Report: Rule Out Myocardial Infarction. *Use a medical dictionary, such as* Taber's Cyclopedic Medical Dictionary; *the appendices of this book; or other resources to define each term. Then, pronounce the term, and place a checkmark (✓) in the box after you do so.*

Term	Definition
auscultation aws-kŭl-TĀ-shŭn ☐	
electrocardiogram ē-lĕk-trō-KĂR-dē-ō-grăm ☐	
esophageal reflux ē-sŏf-ă-JĒ-ăl RĒ-flŭks ☐	
extraocular ĕks-tră-ŎK-ū-lăr ☐	
lidocaine LĪ-dō-kān ☐	
midsternal mĭd-STĔR-năl ☐	
murmur MĔR-mĕr ☐	
Mylanta mī-LĂN-tă ☐	
myocardial infarction mī-ō-KĂR-dē-ăl ĭn-FĂRK-shŭn ☐	

Term	Definition
nitroglycerin nī-trō-GLĬS-ĕr-ĭn ☐	
normocephalic nor-mō-sĕ-FĂL-ĭk ☐	
ST	
T-wave	

 Visit the *Medical Terminology Simplified* online resource center at FADavis.com to hear pronunciation and meanings of the selected terms in this medical report listed in the previous table.

Critical Thinking 5-1

Review the Emergency Department Report: Rule Out Myocardial Infarction *from earlier to answer the following questions. Use a medical dictionary, such as* Taber's Cyclopedic Medical Dictionary, *and other resources, if needed.*

1. What symptoms did the patient experience before admission to the hospital?

_____

_____

2. What was found during the clinical examination?

_____

_____

3. What was the cause of the patient's prior myocardial infarctions?

_____

_____

4. Did the patient have a prior history of heart problems? If so, describe them.

_____

_____

5. How was the chest pain treated?

_____

_____

MEDICAL RECORD ACTIVITY 5-2

OPERATIVE REPORT: CARDIAC CATHETERIZATION

This activity contains an operative report of a cardiac catheterization. Read the operative report that follows, and underline the medical terms. Then, complete the terminology and critical thinking exercises.

OPERATIVE REPORT

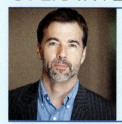

PATIENT NAME: Mathis, Emory
MEDICAL RECORD ID: 18-1239747192
DATE: June 23, 20xx

SURGEON: George A. Smale, M.D.   **ANESTHESIOLOGIST:** Jeffrey Myerson, M.D.

ANESTHESIA: IV sedation per cardiac catheterization protocol.

PRIMARY INDICATION: Chest pain.

ESTIMATED BLOOD LOSS: Less than 10 mL.

ESTIMATED CONTRAST: Less than 150 mL.

PROCEDURE:

Patient was prepared and draped in a sterile fashion, and 20 mL of 1% lidocaine was infiltrated into the right groin. A No. 6 French Cordis right femoral arterial sheath was placed, and a No. 6 French JL-5 and JR-4 catheter was used to engage the left and right coronary. A No. 6 French pigtail was used for left ventricular angiography. Angioplasty was performed, and further dictation is under the angioplasty report. There were minor irregularities, with a maximal 25% stenosis just after the first diagonal. The remainder of the vessel was free of significant disease.

A 0.014, high-torque, floppy, extra support, exchange-length wire was used to cross the stenosis in the distal right coronary artery. A 3.5 × 20-mm Track Star balloon was inflated in the right coronary artery in the distal portion. The initial stenosis was 50% to 75% with an ulcerated plaque, and the final stenosis was 20% with no significant clot seen in the region. The patient had significant ST elevations in the inferior leads and severe throat tightness and shortness of breath. This would resolve immediately with the inflation of the balloon. The catheters were removed, and the sheath was changed to a No. 8 French Arrow sheath. The patient will be on heparin over the next 12 hours.

IMPRESSION:

1. Two-vessel coronary artery disease with a 75% obtuse marginal and a 75% right coronary arterial lesion.
2. Normal left ventricular function.
3. Successful angioplasty to right coronary artery, with initial stenosis of 75% and a final stenosis of 20%.

RECOMMENDATIONS:

1. Routine postcardiac catheterization care.
2. Refer to cardiac rehab.
3. Aspirin 81 mg daily; Plavix 75 mg p.o. daily.

George A. Smale M.D.

George A. Smale, M.D.

GAS: rm
D: 6/23/20xx; T: 6/23/20xx

Terminology 5-2

Terms listed in the following table come from the Operative Report: Cardiac Catheterization. *Use a medical dictionary, such as* Taber's Cyclopedic Medical Dictionary; *the appendices of this book; or other resources to define each term. Then, pronounce the term, and place a checkmark (✓) in the box after you do so.*

Term	Definition
angiography ăn-jē-ŎG-ră-fē ☐	
angioplasty ĂN-jē-ō-plăs-tē ☐	
catheter KĂTH-ĕ-tĕr ☐	
heparin HĔP-ă-rĭn ☐	
lidocaine LĬ-dō-kān ☐	
Plavix PLĂ-vĭx ☐	
sheath SHĒTH ☐	
ST elevations	
stenosis stĕ-NŌ-sĭs ☐	

 Visit the *Medical Terminology Simplified* online resource center at FADavis.com to hear pronunciation and meanings of the selected terms in this medical report listed in the previous table.

Critical Thinking 5-2

Review the medical record Operative Report: Cardiac Catheterization *to answer the following questions. Use a medical dictionary, such as* Taber's Cyclopedic Medical Dictionary, *and other resources, if needed.*

1. Which coronary arteries were under examination?

   _____

   _____

2. Which surgical procedure was used to clear the stenosis?

   _____

   _____

3. What symptoms did the patient exhibit before balloon inflation?

   _____

   _____

4. Why was the patient put on heparin?

   _____

   _____

MEDICAL RECORD ACTIVITY 5-3

CLINICAL APPLICATION

This clinical application activity will help you integrate and reinforce your understanding of how the following medical terms are used in the clinical environment.

AIDS	cardiac catheterization	Holter monitor	mononucleosis
angina pectoris	heart failure	Kaposi sarcoma	statin
beta blocker	Hodgkin disease	lymphangiography	thrombolytics

1. A 49-year-old male presents to the emergency department with complaints of shortness of breath and a feeling of pressure in the center of his chest. An ECG is performed. No abnormalities are present. The physician assesses the patient with pain in the chest caused by ischemia. He charts the diagnosis as _____.

2. A 22-year-old male with HIV presents with a rash. His physician examines the lesions and determines a malignancy of connective tissue closely associated with AIDS, known as _____.

3. A 16-year-old girl presents to the physician with her mother. The girl has a sore throat, temperature of 101.4°F, and extreme fatigue. The physician also finds that she has enlarged cervical lymph nodes. He diagnoses her with an infection caused by EBV, called _____.

4. A 24-year-old male with a history of intravenous drug abuse complains of fever, night sweats, and weight loss. The physician suspects an infectious disease caused by HIV and charts his diagnosis as _____.

5. This 48-year-old male is seen during a follow-up visit for hypertension. The physician determines that treatment is required. She prescribes a medication to slow the patient's heart rate and lower his blood pressure. This type of medication is called a _____.

6. Jason reviews the results of blood tests with his physician, who tells him that he has hypercholesterolemia, a condition of elevated cholesterol in the blood. To reduce his cholesterol level and block production of a liver enzyme that produces it, the physician prescribes the medication known as a(n) _____.

7. Mr. Feller tells the cardiologist that he is experiencing occasional irregularities of heartbeat. To help assess the patient's condition, he will wear an instrument that records electrocardiographic readings over a 24-hour period. This instrument is known as a(n) _____.

8. A 21-year-old male is seen for a routine physical examination. The physician finds an enlarged cervical lymph node and splenomegaly. She orders a biopsy of the lymph node to look for the presence of Reed-Sternberg cells and determine whether the patient has _____.

9. The nurse prepares a 53-year-old female diagnosed with coronary artery disease for a procedure to evaluate the extent of the disease. The surgical procedure involves a catheter inserted into the heart, usually through a vein (femoral approach) or artery (brachial approach), and is called _____.

10. Mrs. T. presents with a complaint of swollen feet and legs. The physician confirms a diagnosis of edema on the face, neck, and chest. She orders a radiographic examination of the lymph glands and lymphatic vessels to view the path of lymph flow. This procedure is called a(n) _____.

Competency Verification: Check your answers in Appendix B: Answer Key, page 599. If you are not satisfied with your level of comprehension, review the material in this chapter, and retake the review.

Correct Answers _____ × 10 = _____ % Score

CARDIOVASCULAR AND LYMPHATIC SYSTEMS CHAPTER REVIEW

WORD ELEMENTS SUMMARY

The following table summarizes CFs, suffixes, and prefixes related to the cardiovascular and lymphatic systems. Study the word elements and their meanings before completing the Vocabulary Review that follows.

Word Element	Meaning	Word Element	Meaning
Combining Forms			
aden/o	gland	**lymph/o**	lymph
aneurysm/o	a widening, a widened blood vessel	**my/o**	muscle
angi/o	vessel (usually blood or lymph)	**necr/o**	death, necrosis
aort/o	aorta	**phleb/o, ven/o**	vein
arteri/o	artery	**rrhythm/o**	rhythm
ather/o	fatty plaque	**sarc/o**	flesh (connective tissue)
atri/o	atrium	**scler/o**	hardening; sclera (white of the eye)
cardi/o, coron/o	heart	**thromb/o**	blood clot
cerebr/o	cerebrum	**varic/o**	dilated vein
embol/o	embolus (plug)	**vas/o**	vessel; vas deferens; duct
hem/o	blood	**vascul/o**	vessel
isch/o	to hold back; block	**ventricul/o**	ventricle (of the heart or brain)
Suffixes			
-al, -ic, -ary	pertaining to, relating to	**-pathy**	disease
-cardia	heart condition	**-phagia**	swallowing, eating
-cyte	cell	**-phobia**	fear
-ectasis	dilation, expansion	**-phylaxis**	protection
-ectomy	excision, removal	**-plasty**	surgical repair
-emia	blood	**-pnea**	breathing
-genesis	forming, producing, origin	**-poiesis**	formation, production
-gram	record, writing	**-rrhaphy**	suture
-graphy	process of recording	**-rrhexis**	rupture
-ia	condition	**-spasm**	involuntary contraction, twitching
-lith	stone, calculus	**-stenosis**	narrowing, stricture
-lysis	separation; destruction; loosening	**-tension**	to stretch
-malacia	softening	**-therapy**	treatment
-megaly	enlargement	**-tomy**	incision
-oid	resembling	**-um**	structure, thing

Continued

Word Element	Meaning	Word Element	Meaning
-ole, -ule	small, minute	-us	condition, structure
-oma	tumor	-version	turning
-osis	abnormal condition; increase (used primarily with blood cells)		
Prefixes			
a-	without, not	epi-	above, upon
anti-	against	micro-	small
bi-	two	peri-	around
brady-	slow	tachy-	rapid
echo-	a repeated sound	trans-	across, through
endo-	in, within	tri-	three

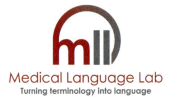

Medical Language Lab
Turning terminology into language

Visit the *Medical Language Lab* at *medicallanguagelab.com*. Use the flash-card activity to reinforce your study of word elements. We recommend you complete the flash-card activity before starting the following Vocabulary Review

Vocabulary Review

Match the medical term(s) with the definitions in the numbered list.

agglutination	*arteriosclerosis*	*ECG*	*pacemaker*
anaphylaxis	*capillaries*	*hemangioma*	*phagocyte*
aneurysm	*cardiomegaly*	*malaise*	*statins*
angina pectoris	*desiccated*	*MI*	*systole*
arterioles	*diastole*	*myocardium*	*tachypnea*

1. _____ refers to the muscular layer of the heart.

2. _____ means rapid breathing.

3. _____ is a disease characterized by an abnormal hardening of the arteries.

4. _____ is a cell that engulfs and digests cellular debris.

5. _____ refers to the contraction phase of the heart.

6. _____ refers to the relaxation phase of the heart.

7. _____ is a record of the electrical impulses of the heart.

8. _____ means a vague feeling of bodily discomfort, which may be the first indication of an infection or disease.

9. _____ means dried thoroughly; rendered free from moisture.

10. _____ means enlarged heart.

11. _____ refers to weakness in the vessel wall that balloons and eventually bursts.

12. _____ is severe pain and constriction about the heart caused by an insufficient supply of oxygenated blood to the heart.

13. _____ is necrosis of an area of muscular heart tissue after cessation of blood supply.

14. _____ is a process of cells clumping together.

15. _____ are used to lower cholesterol levels in blood.

16. _____ is an allergic reaction characterized by a rapid decrease in blood pressure.

17. _____ are the smallest vessels of the circulatory system.

18. _____ is a tumor composed of blood vessels.

19. _____ are small arteries.

20. _____ maintains primary responsibility for initiating the heartbeat.

Competency Verification: Check your answers in Appendix B: Answer Key, page 597. If you are not satisfied with your level of comprehension, review the chapter vocabulary, and retake the review.

Correct Answers: _____ × 5 = _____ % Score

Digestive System

OBJECTIVES

Upon completion of this chapter, you will be able to:

• Describe the type of medical treatment the gastroenterologist provides.

• Identify digestive system structures by labeling them on anatomical illustrations.

• Describe the primary functions of the digestive system.

• Describe diseases, conditions, and procedures related to the digestive system.

• Apply your word-building skills by constructing various medical terms related to the digestive system.

• Describe common abbreviations and symbols related to the digestive system.

• Recognize, define, pronounce, and spell terms correctly.

• Demonstrate your knowledge of this chapter by successfully completing the frames, reviews, and activities.

MEDICAL SPECIALTY: GASTROENTEROLOGY

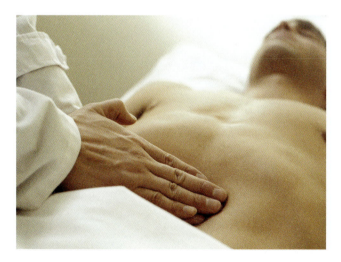

Medical doctors who treat diseases and disorders of the **digestive system,** also called the *gastrointestinal (GI) system,* are known as **gastroenterologists.** They employ various diagnostic procedures to evaluate and treat disorders of the GI system. One of the commonly used diagnostic procedures is known as **endoscopy.** This procedure involves the use of a flexible lighted instrument to examine the organs of the digestive system and is effectively used to inspect the esophagus, stomach, intestines, and bile ducts. Endoscopy has made it possible to identify various pathological conditions, including cancers, at an early stage. In addition to endoscopy, imaging procedures, blood tests, and tissue biopsies help establish or verify the initial diagnosis.

Anatomy and Physiology Overview

The primary function of the digestive system is to break down food, prepare it for absorption, and eliminate waste substances. The digestive system consists of a digestive tube, called the **GI tract** or *alimentary canal.* It includes the esophagus, stomach, intestines, and accessory organs: the liver, gallbladder, and pancreas. The GI tract, extending from the oral cavity (mouth) to the anus, varies in size and structure in several distinct regions. It terminates at the anus, where solid wastes are eliminated from the body by means of defecation. (See Figure 6-1.)

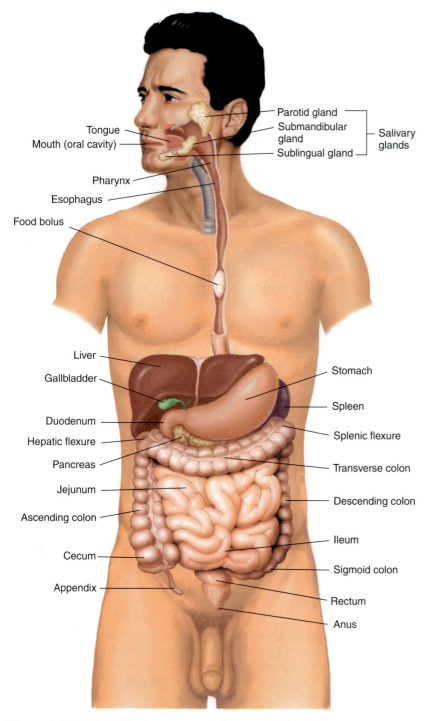

Figure 6-1 Organs of the digestive system (anterior view).

WORD ELEMENTS

This section introduces word elements related to the digestive system. Review the word elements and their meaning in the following table. Then, pronounce each term in the word analysis column, and place a ✓ in the box after you do so.

Word Element	Meaning	Word Analysis
Combining Forms		
Oral Cavity		
dent/o	teeth	**dent**/ist (DĔN-tĭst ☐): specialist who diagnoses and treats diseases and disorders of the oral cavity (teeth and gums) *-ist:* specialist

odont/o		**orth**/**odont**/ist (ŏr-thō-DŎN-tĭst ☐): dental specialist in prevention and correction of abnormally positioned or misaligned teeth
		  orth: straight
		    -ist: specialist

gingiv/o	gum(s)	**gingiv**/itis (jĭn-jĭ-VĪ-tĭs ☐): inflammation of the gums *-itis:* inflammation

gloss/o	tongue	hypo/**gloss**/al (hī-pō-GLŎS-ăl ☐): pertaining to under the tongue
		  hypo-: under, below; deficient
		    -al: pertaining to

lingu/o		sub/**lingu**/al (sŭb-LĬNG-gwăl ☐): pertaining to under the tongue
		  sub-: under, below
		    -al: pertaining to

or/o	mouth	**or**/al (OR-ăl ☐): pertaining to the mouth *-al:* pertaining to
stomat/o		**stomat**/o/pathy (stō-mă-TŎP-ă-thē ☐): disease of the mouth *-pathy:* disease
ptyal/o	saliva	**ptyal**/ism (TĪ-ă-lĭzm ☐): condition of excessive salivation *-ism:* condition
sial/o	saliva, salivary gland	**sial**/o/rrhea (sī-ă-lō-RĒ-ă ☐): excessive flow of saliva; also called *hypersalivation* or *ptyalism* *-rrhea:* discharge, flow
Esophagus, Pharynx, and Stomach		
esophag/o	esophagus	**esophag**/o/scope (ē-SŎF-ă-gō-skōp ☐): instrument for examining the esophagus *-scope:* instrument for examining

pharyng/o	pharynx (throat)	**pharyng**/o/tonsill/itis (fă-rĭng-gō-tŏn-sĭ-LĪ-tĭs ☐): inflammation of the pharynx and tonsils
		  tonsill: tonsils
		    -itis: inflammation

gastr/o	stomach	**gastr**/o/scopy (găs-TRŎS-kō-pē ☐): visual examination of the stomach *-scopy:* visual examination *A gastroscope is a flexible, fiberoptic instrument used to inspect the interior of the stomach.*

pylor/o	pylorus	**pylor**/o/my/o/tomy (pī-lor- ō-mī-ŎT-ō-mē ☐): incision of the pylorus muscle layer (sphincter in the lower portion of the stomach)
		  -tomy: incision
		  my/o: muscle
		
		Pyloromyotomy is performed on a newborn to correct a congenital defect that blocks the flow of food from the stomach into the small intestine.

Continued

Word Element	Meaning	Word Analysis
Suffixes		
-algia	pain	gastr/**algia** (găs-TRĂL-jē-ă ☐): pain in the stomach *gastr:* stomach
-dynia		gastr/o/**dynia** (găs-trō-DĬN-ē-ă ☐): pain in the stomach *gastr/o:* stomach
-emesis	vomiting	hyper/**emesis** (hī-pĕr-ĔM-ĕ-sĭs ☐): excessive vomiting *hyper-:* excessive, above normal
-megaly	enlargement	gastr/o/**megaly** (găs-trō-MĔG-ă-lē ☐): enlargement of the stomach *gastr/o:* stomach
-orexia	appetite	an/**orexia** (ăn-ō-RĔK-sē-ă ☐): loss of appetite *an-:* without, not *Anorexia can result from various conditions, such as adverse effects of medication, as well as other physical or psychological causes.*
-pepsia	digestion	dys/**pepsia** (dĭs-PĔP-sē-ă ☐): difficult or painful digestion; also called *indigestion* *dys-:* bad; painful; difficult *Dyspepsia is a feeling of epigastric discomfort after eating.*
-phagia	swallowing, eating	dys/**phagia** (dĭs-FĀ-jē-ă ☐): difficulty swallowing or eating *dys-:* bad; painful; difficult
-rrhea	discharge, flow	dia/**rrhea** (dī-ă-RĒ-ă ☐): discharge or flow of watery stools from the bowel *dia-:* through, across

Pronunciation Help	*Long Sound*	ā in rāte	ē in rēbirth	ī in īsle	ō in ōver	ū in ūnite
	Short Sound	ă in ăpple	ĕ in ĕver	ĭ in ĭt	ŏ in nŏt	ŭ in cŭt

Visit the *Medical Terminology Simplified* online resource center at FADavis.com for an audio exercise of the terms in this table to help master pronunciations and meanings of the selected medical terms.

SECTION REVIEW 6-1

For the following medical terms, first, write the suffix and its meaning. Then, translate the meaning of the remaining elements starting with the first part of the word. The first word is an example completed for you.

Term	Meaning
1. gingiv/itis	–itis: inflammation; gum(s)
2. dys/pepsia	
3. pylor/o/my/o/tomy	
4. dent/ist	
5. esophag/o/scope	
6. gastr/o/scopy	
7. dia/rrhea	
8. hyper/emesis	
9. an/orexia	
10. sub/lingu/al	

Competency Verification: Check your Answers in Appendix B: Answer Key, page 600. If you are not satisfied with your level of comprehension, review the vocabulary, and retake the review.

Correct Answers _____ x 10 = _____ % Score

Upper Gastrointestinal Tract

The upper GI tract consists of the oral cavity, esophagus, pharynx, and stomach.

Oral Cavity

6-1   Label the structures in Figure 6-2 as you read the material in the following frames. Chemical and mechanical processes of digestion begin in the (1) **oral cavity** (mouth) when food is chewed to make it easier to swallow.

stomat/o

or/o

6-2   The CFs for the mouth are *or/o* and *stomat/o*.

From *stomat/itis*, construct the CF for *mouth*:

_____/ _____.

From *or/al*, construct the CF for *mouth*: _____/ _____.

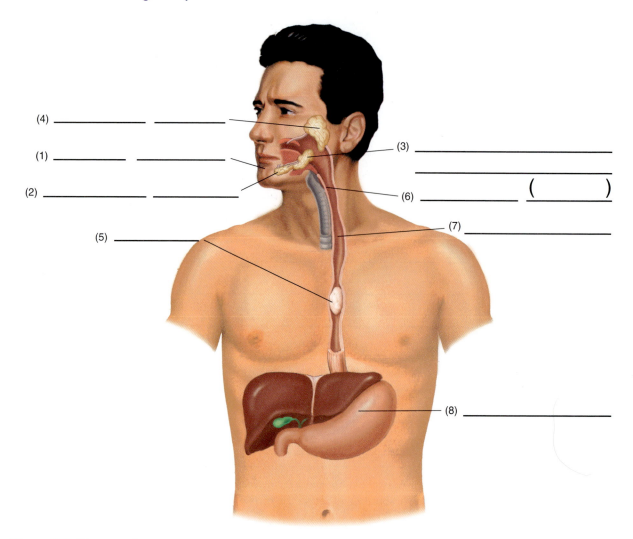

Figure 6-2 The upper GI tract.

stomat/itis stō-mă-TĪ-tĭs	**6–3** The suffix *-itis* refers to *inflammation*. It is used in all body systems to describe an inflammation of a particular organ. Use ***stomat/o*** to form a word that means *inflammation of the mouth*. _____ / _____
pain, mouth **pain, mouth**	**6–4** The suffixes *-dynia* and *-algia* refer to *pain*. *Stomat/o/dynia* is a(n) _____ in the _____. *Stomat/algia* is a(n) _____ in the _____.
combining form *or* combining vowel	**6–5** The suffixes *-dynia* and *-algia* are used interchangeably. Because *-algia* begins with a vowel, use a word root (WR) to link the suffix. Because *-dynia* begins with a consonant, use a _____ _____ to link the suffix.

Pink indicates a prefix. Blue indicates a suffix. Boldface indicates a word root or combining form.

	6-6 There are three pairs of salivary glands: the (2) **sublingual gland,** the (3) **sub-mandibular gland,** and the (4) **parotid gland.** The salivary glands, whose primary function is to secrete saliva into the oral cavity, are richly supplied with blood vessels and nerves. Label the salivary glands in Figure 6-2.
sial/o	**6-7** During the chewing process, salivary secretions begin the chemical breakdown of food. The CF **sial/o** means *saliva, salivary glands.* From *sial/ic,* which means *pertaining to saliva,* construct the CF for *saliva or salivary gland.* _____ / _____
sial/itis sī-ă-LĬ-tĭs	**6-8** Use **sial/o** + **-*itis*** to form a word that means *inflammation of a salivary gland.* _____ / _____
saliva **flow** **saliva** **condition**	**6-9** *Sial/o/rrhea,* more commonly called *ptyal/ism* or *hyper/salivation,* refers to *excessive secretion of saliva.* Analyze *sial/o/rrhea* by defining the elements: The CF **sial/o** refers to *salivary glands* or _____. The suffix *-rrhea* refers to *discharge* or _____. The CF **ptyal/o** refers to _____. The suffix *-ism* refers to _____.
tongue	**6-10** The CF **lingu/o** means *tongue.* The prefix *sub-* means *under.* *Sub/lingu/al* means *pertaining to under or below the* _____.
jaw	**6-11** The CF **maxill/o** means *jaw. Sub/maxill/ary* is a directional term that means *under the* _____.
below **below** **above**	**6-12** Refer to Figure 6-1, and use the directional terms "below" or "above" to complete this frame. The *sub/lingu/al* gland is located _____ the tongue. The *sub/mandibul/ar* gland is located _____ the parotid gland. The tongue is located _____ the esophagus.
abnormal condition, mouth	**6-13** The suffix *-osis* means *abnormal condition, increase (used primarily with blood cells). Stomat/osis* literally means _____ _____ of the _____.
myc	**6-14** *Stomat/o/myc/osis* is an *abnormal condition of a mouth fungus.* From *stomat/o/myc/osis,* identify the root that means *fungus.* _____

abnormal condition **fungus**	**6-15** Whenever you see *-osis* in a word, you will know it means _____ _____ *or increase (used primarily with blood cells).* Whenever you see *myc/o* in a word, you will know it refers to a _____.
myc/osis mī-KŌS-sĭs	**6-16** Two types of mycoses are athlete's foot and thrush. Change the plural form *mycoses* to its singular form. _____ / _____
-logist	**6-17** The CF *log/o* means *study of.* Combine *log/o* and *-ist* to form a new suffix that means *specialist in the study of.* _____
gastr/o/logist găs-TRŎL-ō-jĭst **enter/o/logist** ĕn-tĕr-ŎL-ō-jĭst **gastr/o/enter/o/logist** găs-trō-ĕn-tĕr-ŎL-ō-jĭst	**6-18** Recall that *-logist* means *specialist in the study of.* The gastr/o/logist, enter/o/logist, and gastr/o/enter/o/logist are medical specialists who diagnose and treat digestive disorders. Build medical words that mean *specialist who treats stomach disorders:* _____ / _____ / _____. *specialist who treats intestin/al disorders:* _____ / _____ / _____. *specialist who treats stomach and intestin/al disorders:* _____ / _____ / _____ / _____ / _____.
gastr/o/logy găs-TRŎL-ō-jē **gastr/o/enter/o/logist** găs-trō-ĕn-tĕr-ŎL-ō-jĭst	**6-19** Use *-logy* or *-logist* to form medical words that mean *study of the stomach:* _____ / _____ / _____. *specialist in the study of the stomach and intestines:* _____ / _____ / _____ / _____ / _____.
bowel movement **fasting blood sugar** **diagnosis** dī-ăg-NŌ-sĭs **gastr/o/intestin/al** găs-trō-ĭn-TĔS-tĭn-ăl	**6-20** Standardized abbreviations are commonly used in medical reports and insurance claims. Abbreviations are summarized at the end of each chapter and in Appendix E: Abbreviations, page 633. If needed, use one of those references to complete this frame. BM: _____ _____. FBS: _____ _____ _____. Dx: _____. GI: _____ / _____ / _____ / _____.
dent/o, odont/o	**6-21** Most of us take our teeth for granted. We do not think about the important mechanical function they perform in the first step of the digestive process—breaking food down into smaller pieces. The CFs for *teeth* are _____ / _____ and _____ / _____.

teeth, gums, diagnosis dī-ăg-NŌ-sĭs	**6–22** A dent/ist specializes in the prevention, Dx, and treatment of diseases of the teeth and gums. Dentistry is the branch of medicine dealing with the care of the _____ and _____. The abbreviation *Dx* means _____.
pain, tooth **odont/algia** ō-dŏn-TĂL-jē-ă	**6–23** *Odont/algia* literally means _____ in a _____. *Toothache* is another word for *odont/o/dynia* or _____ / _____.
specialist, teeth	**6–24** An orth/odont/ist is a dent/al specialist who corrects the abnormal position and misalignment of teeth. *Orth/o* means *straight*. *Orth/odont/ist* literally means _____ *in straight* _____.
odont **orth** **-ist**	**6–25** From *orth/odont/ist,* determine the root for *teeth:* _____. root for *straight:* _____. element that means *specialist:* _____.
orth/odont/ist ŏr-thō-DŎN-tĭst	**6–26** Being fitted for braces to straighten teeth requires a dent/al specialist known as an _____ / _____ / _____.
specialist **around** **teeth**	**6–27** Another dent/al specialist, the peri/odont/ist, treats abnormal conditions of tissues surrounding the teeth, including the gums and bones. (Use Appendix A: Glossary of Medical Word Elements on page 575 whenever you need help to work the frames.) The suffix *-ist* refers to _____. The prefix *peri-* refers to _____. The root *odont* refers to _____.
gingiv/o	**6–28** Gingiv/itis, a general term for *inflammation of the gums,* is usually caused by accumulation of food particles in crevices between the gums and teeth. From *gingiv/itis,* construct the CF for *gums.* _____ / _____
gingiv/itis jĭn-jĭ-VĪ-tĭs	**6–29** Form a word that means *inflammation of the gums.* _____ / _____
inflammation, teeth **inflammation, gums**	**6–30** Primary symptoms of gingiv/itis are bleeding gums. This condition can lead to a more serious disorder called *peri/odont/itis.* Gingiv/itis is best prevented by correct brushing of teeth and proper gum care. *Peri/odont/itis* means an _____ *around the* _____. *Gingiv/itis* means _____ *of the* _____.

Esophagus, Pharynx, and Stomach

6–31   Continue labeling Figure 6-2 as you read the material in this frame. After food is chewed, it is formed into a round, sticky mass called a (5) **bolus.** The bolus is pushed by the tongue into the (6) **pharynx** (throat), where it begins its descent down the (7) **esophagus** to the (8) **stomach.**

---

pharyng/itis

pharyng/o/dynia or **pharyng/algia**
fă-RĬNG-gō-dĭn-ē-ă,
făr-ĭn-GĂL-jē-ă

6–32   The funnel-shaped pharynx serves as a passageway to the respiratory and GI tracts and provides a resonating chamber for speech sounds. Use the CF **pharyng/o** (throat) to construct words that mean

inflammation of the throat: _____ / _____.

pain in the throat: _____ / _____ / _____ or

_____ / _____.

---

peristalsis
pĕr-ĭ-STĂL-sĭs

6–33   Food is propelled through the GI tract by coordinated, rhythmic muscle contractions called *peristalsis.* (See Figure 6-2.)

The bolus is transported to the stomach by involuntary muscle contractions known

as _____.

6–34   Gastr/ic juices in the stomach coupled with mechanical churning turn the bolus into a semiliquid mass called *chyme.* The chyme slowly leaves the stomach and continues the process of digestion as it enters the first part of the small intestine (duodenum). Review Figure 6-1 to follow the digestive path of the bolus as it enters the duodenum.

Competency Verification: Check your labeling of Figure 6-2 in Appendix B: Answer Key, page 600.

---

esophag/eal, gastr/ic
ē-sŏf-ă-JĒ-ăl, GĂS-trĭk

6–35   Peptic ulcer disease (PUD) is a condition in which the lining of the esophagus, stomach, or duodenum is eroded, usually from infection with *Helicobacter pylori.* (See Figure 6-3.) Ulcers are named by their location: *esophag/eal, gastr/ic,* or *duoden/al.* Peptic ulcers that occur in the small intestine are called *duoden/al ulcers;*

peptic ulcers that occur in the esophagus are called

_____ / _____ ulcers;

peptic ulcers that occur in the stomach are called

_____ / _____ ulcers.

---

muc/oid
MŪ-koyd

muc/ous
MŪ-kŭs

6–36   The erosion in the lining of the esophagus, stomach, and duodenum in PUD can also be caused by an increase in the concentration of hydrochloric acid and pepsin. As a result, the damaged mucosa is unable to secrete enough mucus to act as a barrier against the acid, which, combined with hypersecretion of acid, creates a large amount of acid moving into the duodenum. As a result, peptic ulcers occur more commonly in the duodenum. Use *muc/o* to build a term meaning

resembling mucus: _____ / _____.

pertaining to mucus: _____ / _____.

Pink indicates a prefix. Blue indicates a suffix. Boldface indicates a word root or combining form.

Peptic Ulcers

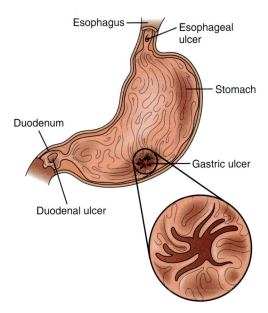

Figure 6-3 Peptic ulcer disease.

gastr/itis, peptic ulcer disease găs-TRĪ-tĭs	**6-37** Gastr/ic ulcers may cause severe pain and inflammation of the stomach. A medical term that means *inflammation of the stomach is* _____ / _____. PUD is the abbreviation for _____ _____ _____.
gastr/algia găs-TRĂL-jē-ă	**6-38** *Gastr/o/dynia* is the medical term for pain in the *stomach*. Another term that means *pain in the stomach is* _____ / _____.
stomach	**6-39** *Gastr/o/megaly* and *megal/o/gastr/ia* mean *enlargement of the* _____.
megal/o/gastr/ic mĕg-ă-lō-GĂS-trĭk	**6-40** In *megal/o/gastr/ia*, the suffix *-ia* is a noun ending that denotes a condition. Use *-ic* to change this word to an adjective. _____ / _____ / _____ / _____
endo/scopy ĕn-DŎS-kō-pē	**6-41** Endo/scopy is a *visual examination of a hollow organ or cavity using a rigid or flexible fiberoptic tube and lighted optical system.* The term in this frame that means *visual examination in or within (an organ)* is _____ / _____.

gastr/o/scopy
găs-TRŎS-kō-pē

endo/scope
ĔN-dō-skōp

6-42   An endo/scope is used to perform endo/scopy. The organ being examined dictates the name of the endo/scop/ic procedure. For example, visual examination of the esophagus is called *esophag/o/scopy,* and visual examination of the stomach is called *gastr/o/scopy.*

Endo/scopy is performed for bi/opsy, aspirating fluids, and coagulating bleeding areas. A surgeon can also pass a laser through the endo/scope for endo/scop/ic surgeries. A camera or video recorder is commonly used during endo/scop/ic procedures to provide a permanent record of the findings.

When the physician examines the stomach, the endoscopic procedure is called

_____ / _____ / _____.

The instrument used to examine within (a body cavity or organ) is an

_____ / _____ / _____.

---

esophag/o/gastr/o/
duoden/o/scopy
ĕ-SŎF-ă-gō-găs-trō-dū-ŏd-ĕ-NŎS-kō-pē

6-43   Upper GI endoscopy, also referred to as *esophag/o/gastr/o/duoden/o/scopy* (EGD), includes visualization of the esophagus, stomach, and duodenum.

Define the meaning of the abbreviation *EGD* by breaking the term down into its component parts.

_____ / _____ / _____ / _____ / _____ / _____ /

_____

---

esophag/o/plasty
ē-SŎF-ă-gō-plăs-tē

gastr/o/plasty
GĂS-trō-plăs-tē

6-44   Use *-plasty* to form medical words that mean

surgical repair of the esophagus: _____ / _____ / _____.

surgical repair of the stomach: _____ / _____ / _____.

6-45   Common surgical suffixes that refer to *cutting* are summarized below. Review and use them to complete subsequent frames related to operative procedures.

Surgical Suffix	Meaning
-ectomy	excision, removal
-tome	instrument to cut
-tomy	incision

---

esophagus
ē-SŎF-ă-gŭs

6-46   Whenever you see a word with the WR *tom* in it, relate it to an incision.
Esophag/o/tomy is an *incision through the wall of the* _____.

---

esophag/o/tome
ē-SŎF-ă-gō-tōm

6-47   When esophag/eal surgery necessitates an incision, the physician will ask for

an instrument called an _____ / _____ / _____.

---

gastr/ectomy
găs-TRĔK-tō-mē

6-48   A surgical procedure to remove all or, more commonly, part of the stomach

is called a _____ / _____.

Pink indicates a prefix. Blue indicates a suffix. Boldface indicates a word root or combining form.

gastr/o/tomy găs-TRŎT-ō-mē	**6-49** Develop a word that means *incision of the stomach*. _____ / _____ / _____
carcin/oma kăr-sĭ-NŌ-mă	**6-50** Cancer (CA) is a general term used to indicate various types of malignant neoplasms. Most cancers invade surrounding tissues and metastasize (spread) to other sites in the body. The combining form (CF) for *cancer* is **carcin/o.** Combine **carcin/o** + *-oma* to build a word that means *cancerous tumor.* _____ / _____
cancer	**6-51** CA, especially sarc/oma, can recur even though the tumor is excised. Ultimately, it may cause death. Whenever you see CA in a medical report, you will know it means _____.
cancerous *or* malignant	**6-52** A carcin/oma is a tumor that is _____.
cancer **tumor**	**6-53** The largest group of carcin/omas are solid tumors derived from epithelial tissue, which is the tissue that lines the surfaces of the body. It includes the skin and the tissues that line the internal organs, including the digestive organs. Analyze *carcin/oma* by defining the elements *carcin:* _____. *-oma:* _____.
gastr/itis găs-TRĪ-tĭs **epi/gastr/ic** ĕp-ĭ-GĂS-trĭk	**6-54** *Epi-* means *above, upon*. Epi/gastr/ic pain may result from an acute form of gastr/itis. Identify words in this frame that mean *inflammation of the stomach:* _____ / _____. *pertaining to above or upon the stomach:* _____ / _____ / _____.
hyper/emesis hī-pĕr-ĔM-ĕ-sĭs	**6-55** *Emesis* is a term that means *vomiting;* however, it may also be used as a suffix. A symptomatic term that means *excessive vomiting* is *hyper* / _____.
hyper- **-emesis**	**6-56** Hyper/emesis is characterized by excessive vomiting. Unless treated, it can lead to malnutrition. Determine elements in this frame that mean *excessive, above normal:* _____. *vomiting:* _____.

hemat/emesis hĕm-ăt-ĔM-ĕ-sĭs	**6-57** *Hemat/o* refers to *blood*. A patient with acute gastr/itis or a peptic ulcer may vomit blood. Build a word that means *vomiting blood*. _____ / _____
hemat/emesis hĕm-ăt-ĔM-ĕ-sĭs	**6-58** Bleeding in the stomach may be caused by a gastr/ic ulcer and may lead to vomiting of blood. A Dx of vomiting blood is entered in the medical record as _____ / _____ .
-pepsia **dys-**	**6-59** *Dys/pepsia* literally means *painful or difficult digestion* and is a form of gastric indigestion. It is not a disease in and of itself, but may be a symptom of disease. Determine word elements in this frame that mean *digestion:* _____ . *bad, painful, difficult:* _____ .
dys/pepsia dĭs-PĔP-sē-ă	**6-60** Over-the-counter antacids (agents that neutralize acidity) usually provide prompt relief of pain from _____ / _____ .
dys/phagia dĭs-FĀ-jē-ă **bad, painful, difficult** **swallowing, eating**	**6-61** The suffix *-phagia* means *swallowing, eating*. Use *dys-* and *-phagia* to form a word that means *difficult or painful swallowing*. _____ / _____ Analyze *dys/phagia* by defining its elements *dys-:* _____ , _____ , _____ . *-phagia:* _____ , _____ .
aer/o	**6-62** Swallowing air, usually followed by belching and gastric distention, is a condition known as aer/o/phagia. The CF for *air* is _____ / _____ .
aer/o/phagia ĕr-ō-FĀ-jē-ă	**6-63** Infants have a tendency to swallow air as they suck milk from a bottle, a condition charted as _____ / _____ / _____ .

Pink indicates a prefix. Blue indicates a suffix. Boldface indicates a word root or combining form.

SECTION REVIEW 6-2

Using the following table, write the CF, suffix, or prefix that matches its definition in the space provided to the left of the definition. There may be more than one word element that matches a definition.

Combining Forms		Suffixes		Prefixes
dent/o	*odont/o*	*-al*	*-orexia*	*an-*
gastr/o	*or/o*	*-ary*	*-pepsia*	*dia-*
gingiv/o	*orth/o*	*-algia*	*-phagia*	*dys-*
gloss/o	*pylor/o*	*-dynia*	*-rrhea*	*hyper-*
lingu/o	*sial/o*	*-ic*	*-scope*	*hypo-*
myc/o	*stomat/o*	*-ist*	*-tomy*	*peri-*
		-oma		

1. _____ tumor

2. _____ pertaining to

3. _____ around

4. _____ under, below; deficient

5. _____ discharge, flow

6. _____ fungus

7. _____ gum(s)

8. _____ pylorus

9. _____ bad; painful; difficult

10. _____ excessive; above normal

11. _____ saliva, salivary gland

12. _____ stomach

13. _____ specialist

14. _____ straight

15. _____ teeth

16. _____ through; across

17. _____ tongue

18. _____ instrument for examining

19. _____ incision

20. _____ appetite

21. _____ mouth

22. _____ pain

23. _____ swallowing, eating

24. _____ without, not

25. _____ digestion

Competency Verification: Check your answers in Appendix B: Answer Key, page 600. If you are not satisfied with your level of comprehension, go back to Frame 6–1, and rework the frames.

Correct Answers _____ x 4 = _____ % Score

WORD ELEMENTS

This section introduces word elements related to the digestive system. Review the word elements and their meanings in the following table. Then, pronounce each term in the word analysis column, and place a ✓ in the box after you do.

Word Element	Meaning	Word Analysis
Combining Forms		
Small Intestine		
duoden/o	duodenum (first part of the small intestine)	**duoden/o/scopy** (dū-ŏd-ĕ-NŎS-kō-pē ☐): visual examination of the duodenum -*scopy:* visual examination
enter/o	intestine (usually the small intestine)	**enter/o/pathy** (ĕn-tĕr-ŎP-ă-thē ☐): any intestinal disease -*pathy:* disease
jejun/o	jejunum (second part of the small intestine)	**jejun/o/rrhaphy** (jĕ-joo-NOR-ă-fē ☐): suture of the jejunum -*rrhaphy:* suture
ile/o	ileum (third part of the small intestine)	**ile/o/stomy** (ĭl-ē-ŎS-tō-mē ☐): incision of the ileum (ileostomy) and creation of a permanent opening -*stomy:* * forming an opening (mouth) *Ileostomy is performed after a total colectomy. The ileum is pulled out through the abdominal wall. The edges of the wall of the colon are rolled to make a mouth (stoma), which is then sutured to the abdominal wall. The patient wears a plastic pouch on the abdomen to collect feces.*
Large Intestine		

append/o
 	
appendic/o
	appendix	**append/ectomy** (ăp-ĕn-DĔK-tō-mē ☐): removal of the appendix
		    -*ectomy:* excision, removal
		
		Appendectomy is performed to remove a diseased appendix that is in danger of rupturing.
		appendic/itis (ă-pĕn-dĭ-SĪ-tĭs ☐): inflammation of the appendix
		    -*itis:* inflammation
		
		Surgical treatment of appendicitis is appendectomy within 48 hours of the first symptom.

col/o
 	
colon/o
	colon	**col/o/stomy** (kō-LŎS-tō-mē ☐): creation of an opening between the colon and the abdominal wall
		    -*stomy:* * forming an opening (mouth)
		
		A colostomy creates a place for fecal matter to exit the body other than through the anus. It may be temporary or permanent.
		colon/o/scopy (kō-lŏn-ŎS-kō-pē ☐): visual examination of the inner surface of the colon using a long, flexible endoscope
		    -*scopy:* visual examination

proct/o	anus, rectum	**proct/o/logist** (prŏk-TŎL-ō-jĭst ☐): physician who specializes in treating disorders of the colon, rectum, and anus -*logist:* specialist in the study of

Word Element	Meaning	Word Analysis
rect/o	rectum	**rect/o/cele** (RĔK-tō-sēl ☐): herniation or protrusion of the rectum; also called *proctocele* *-cele:* hernia, swelling
sigmoid/o	sigmoid colon	**sigmoid/o/tomy** (sĭg-moyd-ŎT-ō-mē ☐): incision of the sigmoid colon *-tomy:* incision

Pronunciation Help	*Long Sound*	ā in rāte	ē in rēbirth	ī in īsle	ō in ōver	ū in ūnite
	Short Sound	ă in ăpple	ĕ in ĕver	ĭ in ĭt	ŏ in nŏt	ŭ in cŭt

*When the suffix *-stomy* is used with a combining form that denotes an organ, it refers to a surgical opening to the outside of the body.

 Visit the *Medical Terminology Simplified* online resource center at FADavis.com for an audio exercise of the terms in this table to help master pronunciations and meanings of the selected medical terms.

SECTION REVIEW 6-3

For the following medical terms, first, write the suffix and its meaning. Then, translate the meaning of the remaining elements starting with the first part of the word. The first word is an example that is completed for you.

Term	Meaning
1. duoden/o/scopy	–scopy: visual examination; duodenum (first part of the small intestine)
2. appendic/itis	_____
3. enter/o/pathy	_____
4. col/o/stomy	_____
5. rect/o/cele	_____
6. sigmoid/o/tomy	_____
7. proct/o/logist	_____
8. jejun/o/rrhaphy	_____
9. append/ectomy	_____
10. ile/o/stomy	_____

Competency Verification: Check your answers in Appendix B: Answer Key, page 600. If you are not satisfied with your level of comprehension, review the vocabulary, and retake the review.

Correct Answers _____ x 10 = _____ % Score

Lower Gastrointestinal Tract

The lower GI tract consists of the small and large intestine as well as the anus and rectum.

Small and Large Intestines

6–64   The small intestine is a continuation of the GI tract. It is where digestion of food is completed as nutrients are absorbed into the bloodstream through tiny, fingerlike projections called *villi*. Any unabsorbed material is passed on to the large intestine to be excreted from the body. There are three parts of the small intestine: the (1) **duodenum**, the (2) **jejunum**, and the (3) **ileum.** Label these parts in Figure 6-4.

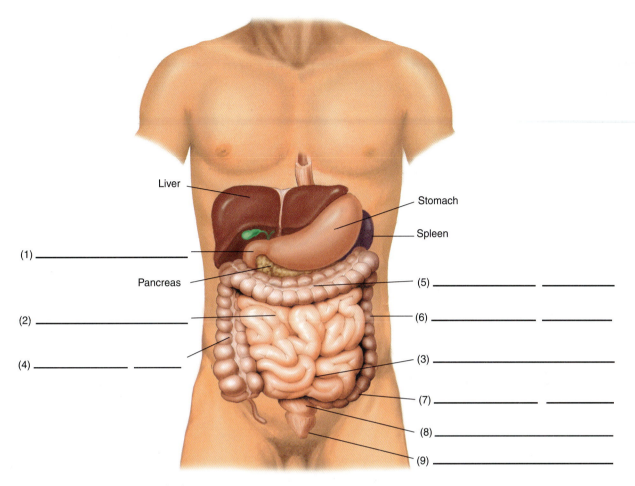

Figure 6-4 Small intestine and colon.

---

duodenum dū-ŎD-ĕ-nŭm **jejunum** jĕ-JŪ-nŭm **ileum** ĬL-ē-ŭm	**6-65** Here is a review of the small intestine. The CF *duoden/o* refers to the first part of the small intestine, called the _____. The CF *jejun/o* refers to the second part of the small intestine, called the _____. The CF *ile/o* refers to the third part of the small intestine, called the _____.
duoden/ectomy dū-ŏd-ĕ-NĔK-tō-mē **jejun/ectomy** jē-jū-NĔK-tō-mē **ile/ectomy** ĭl-ē-ĔK-tō-mē	**6-66** Duoden/ectomy, jejun/ectomy, and ile/ectomy are total or partial excisions of different sections of the small intestine. Build a word that means *excision of the duodenum:* _____ / _____. *excision of the jejunum:* _____ / _____. *excision of the ileum:* _____ / _____.

duodenum, duoden/o dū-ŎD-ĕ-nŭm **jejunum, jejun/o** jĕ-JŪ-nŭm **ileum, ile/o** ĬL-ē-ŭm	**6-67** Name the three parts of the small intestine and their CFs. **Part** **Combining Form** 1. _____ _____ / _____ 2. _____ _____ / _____ 3. _____ _____ / _____
duodenum dū-ŎD-ĕ-nŭm	**6-68** Duoden/o/stomy is performed to form an opening (mouth) into the _____.
opening, jejunum jē-JŪ-nŭm	**6-69** Jejun/o/stomy is a surgical procedure that means *forming an* _____ *into the* _____.
opening, ileum ĬL-ē-ŭm	**6-70** When the colon is removed because of colon CA, an ile/o/stomy is performed. The patient must wear an ile/o/stomy bag to collect fecal material from the ile/um. The surgical procedure *ile/o/stomy* means *forming an* _____ *into the* _____.
-stomy	**6-71** The medical term *stoma* refers to an *opening shaped like a mouth*. The suffix that means *forming an opening (mouth)* is _____.
-tomy **jejun/o/tomy** jĕ-jū-NŎT-ō-mē	**6-72** For patients who cannot eat by mouth, a jejun/al (pertaining to the jejunum) feeding tube is commonly placed through a jejun/o/tomy incision. The surgical suffix that means *incision* is _____. An *incision of the jejunum* is called _____ / _____ / _____.
ile/o/tomy ĭl-ē-ŎT-ō-mē	**6-73** *Incision of the ileum* is called _____ / _____ / _____.
ileum ĬL-ē-ŭm **suture**	**6-74** The suffix *-rrhaphy* refers to *suture (sew)*. Ile/o/rrhaphy is performed to surgically repair the ile/um. Analyze *ile/o/rrhaphy* by defining its elements. *ile/o:* _____ *-rrhaphy:* _____
duoden/ectomy dū-ŏd-ĕ-NĔK-tō-mē **duoden/o/rrhaphy** dū-ŏ-dĕ-NOR-ă-fē	**6-75** In a bleeding duoden/al ulcer, a suture over the bleeding portion can prevent the necessity of duoden/ectomy. Develop surgical words that mean *excision of the duodenum:* _____ / _____. *suture of the duodenum:* _____ / _____ / _____.

Pink indicates a prefix. Blue indicates a suffix. Boldface indicates a word root or combining form.

jejun/o/rrhaphy jĕ-joo-NOR-ă-fē **ile/o/rrhaphy** ĭl-ē-OR-ă-fē	**6-76** Form surgical words that mean *suture of the jejunum:* _____ / _____ / _____. *suture of the ileum:* _____ /_____ / _____.
stomach, duodenum dū-ŎD-ĕ-nŭm	**6-77** Gastr/o/duoden/o/stomy is the *formation of an opening between the* _____ *and* _____.
stomach, ileum ĬL-ē-ŭm	**6-78** *Gastr/o/ile/o/stomy* is the *formation of an opening between the* _____ *and* _____.
stomach, small intestine	**6-79** Anastomosis (connection between two vessels, bowel segments, or ducts) is performed to provide a connection from one structure to another. Gastr/o/enter/o/anastomosis is a *surgical connection between the* _____ *and* _____ _____.
gastr/o/enter/o/ anastomosis, gastr/o/ enter/o/stomy găs-trō-ĕn-tĕr-ō-ă-năs-tō-MŌ-sĭs, găs-trō-ĕn-tĕr-ŎS-tō-mē	**6-80** Gastr/o/enter/o/anastomosis, also called *gastr/o/enter/o/stomy,* may be performed when there is a malignant or benign gastr/o/duoden/al disease. Identify terms in this frame that mean *creation of a passage between the stomach and some part of the small intestine.* _____ / _____ / _____ / _____ / _____ *and* _____ / _____ / _____ / _____ / _____
-stomy	**6-81** Another type of anastomosis, gastr/o/duoden/o/stomy, is a procedure in which the lower part of the stomach is excised and the remainder is anastomosed to the duodenum. The element in this frame that means *forming an opening (mouth)* is _____.
ileum ĬL-ē-ŭm	**6-82** Most absorption of food takes place in the third part of the small intestine, which is the _____.
inflammation, ileum ĬL-ē-ŭm	**6-83** Crohn disease, a chronic inflammation of the ile/um, may affect any part of the intestinal tract. This disease is distinguished from closely related bowel disorders by its inflammatory pattern; it is also called *regional ile/itis.* *Ile/itis* means _____ *of the* _____.
enter/o	**6-84** *Enter/al means pertaining to the intestine (usually the small intestine).* From *enter/al,* construct the CF for *intestine.* _____ / _____

enter/ectomy
ĕn-tĕr-ĚK-tō-mē

enter/o/rrhaphy
ĕn-tĕr-OR-ă-fē

6-85   Build medical terms that mean

excision of intestine (usually small): _____ / _____.

suture of intestine (such as an intestinal wound): _____ / _____

/ _____.

6-86   Continue labeling Figure 6-4 as you read the following: The large intestine, also called the *colon,* extends from the ileum of the small intestine to the anus. The colon consists of four segments: (4) **ascending colon,** (5) **transverse colon,** (6) **descending colon,** and (7) **sigmoid colon.**

col/ectomy
kō-LĚK-tō-mē

col/itis
kō-LĪ-tĭs

col/o/tomy
kō-LŎT-ō-mē

6-87   The CF *col/o* refers to the colon.

Form medical words that mean

excision of the colon: _____ / _____.

inflammation of the colon: _____ / _____.

incision of the colon: _____ / _____ / _____.

col/o/stomy
kō-LŎS-tō-mē

col/o/rrhaphy
kō-LOR-ă-fē

6-88   Col/o/stomy is the surgical creation of an opening into the colon (through the surface of the abdomen). It may be temporary or permanent and may be performed as treatment for CA or diverticul/itis. Col/o/stomy allows elimination of feces into a bag attached to the skin. (See Figure 6-5.)

Build medical terms that mean

forming an opening (mouth) into the colon: _____ / _____ / _____.

suture of the colon: _____ / _____ / _____.

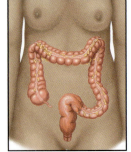
A

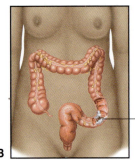
B — Intestinal obstruction

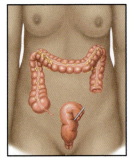
C — Excision of diseased colon

Healthy colon

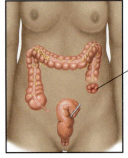
D — Stoma / Colostomy performed to attach healthy tissue to abdomen.

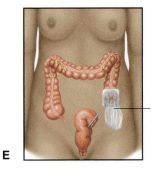
E — Colostomy bag attached to stoma.

Figure 6-5 Colostomy.

Pink indicates a prefix. Blue indicates a suffix. Boldface indicates a word root or combining form.

6-89   Absorption of water by the colon changes intestin/al contents from a fluid to a more solid consistency known as *feces* or *stool.* Use your medical dictionary to define *feces.*

---

peristalsis
pĕr-ĭ-STĂL-sĭs

6-90   Recall that the muscular contractions that propel a bolus through the digestive system are known as *peristalsis.* These muscular contractions also move feces through the colon during the process of defecation.

Elimination of waste products from the colon is possible because of the wavelike

contractions known as _____.

---

liver

spleen

6-91   The ascending colon is located superior to the cecum. (See Figure 6-1.) It curves horizontally at the hepatic flexure and descends at the splenic flexure.

Name the organ that is in close proximity to the

hepat/ic flexure: _____.

splen/ic flexure: _____.

6-92   The sigmoid colon is S-shaped and extends from the descending colon into the (8) **rectum.** The rectum terminates in the lower opening of the gastrointestinal tract, the (9) **anus.** Label Figure 6-4 to identify and locate the rectum and anus.

---

sigmoid/o

6-93   Sigmoid/ectomy, an excision of all or part of the sigmoid colon, is most commonly performed to remove a malignant tumor. A large percentage of lower bowel cancers occur in the sigmoid colon.

From sigmoid/ectomy, construct the CF for sigmoid colon.

_____ / _____

---

sigmoid/itis
sĭg-moyd-Ī-tĭs

6-94   Form a term that means *inflammation of the sigmoid colon.*

_____ / _____

Competency Verification: Check your labeling of Figure 6-4 in Appendix B: Answer Key, page 601.

Rectum and Anus

inflammation, rectum
RĔK-tŭm

6-95   The CF *rect/o* refers to the rectum. Rect/itis is a(n)

_____ of the _____.

---

pain

6-96   *Proct/algia* refers to a neur/o/logic/al *pain in or around the anus or lower rectum,* which is also called *rect/algia.* Whenever you see -*algia* in a term, you will

know it means _____.

---

surgical repair, rectum
RĔK-tŭm

6-97   Rect/o/plasty is a _____ _____ of

the _____.

through, across **discharge, flow**	**6-98** *Dia-* is a prefix that means *through, across.* Dia/rrhea refers to frequent passage of watery bowel movements. Analyze *dia/rrhea* by defining the elements. *dia-:* _____, _____ *-rrhea:* _____, _____
dia/rrhea dī-ă-RĒ-ă	**6-99** A patient with an irritable bowel may experience frequent passage of watery bowel movements or have symptoms of a condition called _____ / _____.
stenosis stě-NŌ-sĭs	**6-100** Stenosis is an abnormal narrowing or stricture of a body passage, especially a tube or canal. When the pylorus, a narrow opening between the stomach and duodenum, becomes strictured or narrowed, food cannot pass through the stomach to the intestine. This condition may result in an obstruction. A narrowing or stricture of the pylorus is called *pyloric* _____.
pylor/ic stenosis pī-LOR-ĭk stě-NŌ-sĭs **pylor/o/my/o/tomy** pī-lōr-ō-mī-ŎT-ō-mē	**6-101** Pylor/ic stenosis is a disorder in infants that blocks food from entering the small intestine. In pylor/ic stenosis, the muscular valve (pylorus) thickens and becomes abnormally large, blocking food from entering the small intestine. (See Figure 6-6.) The retained feedings cause the infant to vomit and to lose weight. Infants with pylor/ic stenosis seem to be hungry all the time. Pylor/o/my/o/tomy may be necessary to treat pylor/ic stenosis. The disorder in which food is blocked from entering the small intestine is called _____ / _____ _____. The surgical procedure in which an incision into the circular muscles of the pylorus is made to treat pyloric stenosis is called _____ / _____ / _____ / _____ / _____.

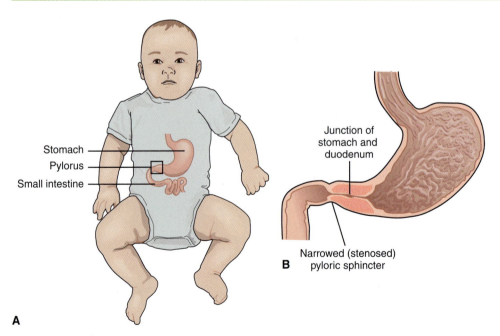

Stomach
Pylorus
Small intestine

Junction of stomach and duodenum

Narrowed (stenosed) pyloric sphincter

A   **B**

Figure 6-6 Pyloric stenosis.

proct/itis
prŏk-TĪ-tĭs

6-102 The CF *proct/o* refers to the *anus and rectum.* Locate the anus and rectum in Figure 6-1.

Inflammation of the anus and rectum is known as

_____ / _____.

---

rectum
RĔK-tŭm

rectum, anus
RĔK-tŭm, Ā-nŭs

6-103 The word *spasm* refers to an *involuntary contraction or twitching.* It is also used in medical words as a suffix.

Rect/o/spasm is an involuntary contraction of the _____.

Proct/o/spasm is an involuntary contraction of the _____ *and* _____.

---

path/o/log/ical
păth-ō-LŎJ-ĭ-kăl

6-104 Endo/scopy is an important tool in establishing or confirming a Dx or detecting a path/o/log/ical condition. A video recorder is commonly used during an endo/scop/ic procedure to guide the endo/scope and document abnormalities.

Determine the word in this frame that means *study of disease.*

_____ / _____ / _____ / _____

---

sigmoid/o/scopy
sĭg-moy-DŎS-kō-pē

colon/o/scopy
kō-lŏn-ŎS-kō-pē

6-105 Colon/o/scopy is a visual examination of the entire length of the colon; sigmoid/o/scopy is a visual examination of only the lower third of the colon. (See Figure 6-4.) Colon/o/scopy is used to screen for colon CA. The American Cancer Society recommends a first colon/o/scopy at age 45. It is recommended earlier if there is a family history (FH) of colon cancer. (See Figure 6-7.)

Visual examination of the sigmoid colon is called

_____ / _____ / _____.

Visual examination of the colon is called *col/o/scopy* or

_____ / _____ / _____.

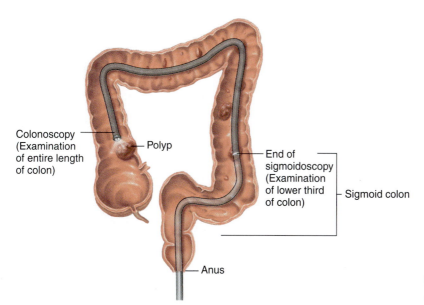

Colonoscopy
(Examination
of entire length
of colon)

Polyp

End of
sigmoidoscopy
(Examination
of lower third
of colon)

Sigmoid colon

Anus

Figure 6-7 Sigmoidoscopy and colonoscopy.

carcin/oma kăr-sĭ-NŌ-mă	**6–106** Examine Figure 6-8 to learn the symptoms related to the location of carcin/oma in the colon. Build a word that means a *cancerous tumor*. _____ / _____.
IV	**6–107** When the early stage of colon CA is undetected, metastasis, the spreading of CA cells, occurs. Figure 6-9 illustrates the progression of colon cancer and its stages. When cancer spreads from its original site to other organs, it is in stage _____.

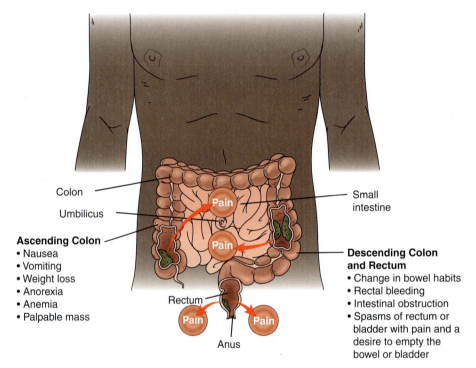

Figure 6-8 Symptoms of carcinoma of the colon, in which pain usually radiates toward the umbilicus or perianal area.

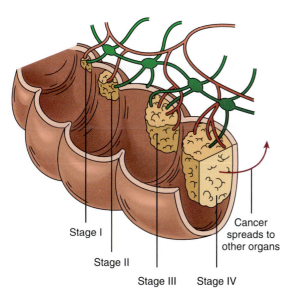

Stage I

Stage II

Stage III   Stage IV

Cancer
spreads to
other organs

Figure 6-9 *Stages of colon cancer.*

---

sigmoid/o/scope
sĭg-MOY-dō-skōp

6–108 A sigmoid/o/scope, a flexible fiberoptic tube that permits transmission of light to visualize images around curves and corners, is placed through the anus to assess the gastro/intestin/al tract.

To examine the colon, the physician uses a flexible fiberoptic instrument called a

_____ / _____ / _____.

---

sigmoid/ectomy
sĭg-moyd-ĔK-tō-mē

carcin/oma
kăr-sĭ-NŌ-mă

6–109 The sigmoid colon is S-shaped and is the last part of the colon. (See Figure 6-4.) Sigmoid/ectomy is most commonly performed for carcin/oma of the sigmoid colon.

Identify words in this frame that mean

excision of the sigmoid colon: _____ / _____.

cancerous tumor: _____ / _____.

SECTION REVIEW 6-4

Using the following table, write the CF or suffix that matches its definition in the space provided to the left of the definition. There may be more than one word element that matches a definition.

Combining Forms

col/o	jejun/o
colon/o	proct/o
duoden/o	rect/o
enter/o	sigmoid/o
ile/o	

Suffixes

-rrhaphy	-tome
-scopy	-tomy
-spasm	
-stenosis	
-stomy	

1. _____ intestine (usually small intestine)

2. _____ instrument to cut

3. _____ rectum

4. _____ involuntary contraction, twitching

5. _____ ileum (third part of the small intestine)

6. _____ visual examination

7. _____ jejunum (second part of the small intestine)

8. _____ colon

9. _____ duodenum (first part of the small intestine)

10. _____ forming an opening (mouth)

11. _____ anus, rectum

12. _____ narrowing, stricture

13. _____ suture

14. _____ incision

15. _____ sigmoid colon

Competency Verification: Check your answers in Appendix B: Answer Key, page 601. If you are not satisfied with your level of comprehension, go back to Frame 6–64, and rework the frames.

Correct Answers _____ × 6.67 = _____ % Score

Pink indicates a prefix. Blue indicates a suffix. Boldface indicates a word root or combining form.

WORD ELEMENTS

This section introduces word elements related to the accessory organs of digestion. Review the word elements and their meanings in the following table. Then, pronounce each term in the word analysis column, and place a ✓ in the box after you do so.

Word Element	Meaning	Word Analysis
Combining Forms		
cholangi/o	bile vessel	**cholangi**/ole (kō-LĂN-jē-ōl ☐): small terminal portion of the bile duct *-ole:* small, minute
chol/e*	bile, gall	**chol**/e/lith (kō-lē-LĬTH ☐): gallstone *-lith:* stone, calculus
cholecyst/o	gallbladder	**cholecyst**/ectomy (kō-lē-sĭs-TĚK-tō-mē ☐): removal of the gallbladder through laparoscopic or open surgery *-ectomy:* excision, removal *Cholecystectomy can be performed as open surgery or laparoscopically (placing a tube into the abdomen).*
choledoch/o	bile duct	**choledoch**/o/tomy (kō-lĕd-ō-KŎT-ō-mē ☐): incision of the common bile duct *-tomy:* incision
hepat/o	liver	**hepat**/itis (hĕp-ă-TĪ-tĭs ☐): inflammation of the liver *-itis:* inflammation
pancreat/o	pancreas	**pancreat**/itis (păn-krē-ă-TĪ-tĭs ☐): inflammation or infection of the pancreas *-itis:* inflammation
Suffixes		
-iasis	abnormal condition (produced by something specified)	chol/e/lith/**iasis** (kō-lē-lĭ-THĪ-ă-sĭs ☐): presence or formation of gallstones *chol/e:* bile, gall *lith/o:* stone, calculus
-megaly	enlargement	hepat/o/**megaly** (hĕp-ă-tō-MĚG-ă-lē ☐): enlargement of the liver *hepat/o:* liver *Hepatomegaly may be caused by infection; fatty infiltration, as in alcoholism; biliary obstruction; or malignancy.*
-prandial	Meal	post/**prandial** (pōst-PRĂN-dē-ăl ☐): following a meal *post-:* after, behind

Pronunciation Help	Long Sound	ā in rāte	ē in rēbirth	ī in īsle	ō in ōver	ū in ūnite
	Short Sound	ă in ăpple	ĕ in ĕver	ĭ in ĭt	ŏ in nŏt	ŭ in cŭt

*Using the combining vowel e instead of o is an exception to the rule.

 Visit the *Medical Terminology Simplified* online resource center at FADavis.com for an audio exercise of the terms in this table. It will help you master pronunciations and meanings of medical terms.

SECTION REVIEW 6-5

For the following medical terms, first, write the suffix and its meaning. Then, translate the meaning of the remaining elements starting with the first part of the word. The first word is completed for you.

Term	Meaning
1. hepat/itis	–itis: inflammation; liver
2. hepat/o/megaly	_____
3. chol/e/lith	_____
4. cholangi/ole	_____
5. cholecyst/ectomy	_____
6. post/prandial	_____
7. chol/e/lith/iasis	_____
8. choledoch/o/tomy	_____
9. pancreat/o/lith	_____
10. pancreat/itis	_____

Competency Verification: Check your answers in Appendix B: Answer Key, page 601. If you are not satisfied with your level of comprehension, go back to the word elements tables, and retake the review.

Correct Answers _____ x 10 = _____ % Score

Accessory Organs of Digestion

The accessory organs of digestion include the liver, gallbladder, and pancreas.

liver, gallbladder, pancreas	**6–110** Label Figure 6-10 as you learn about the accessory organs of digestion. Even though food does not pass through the (1) **liver,** (2) **gallbladder,** and (3) **pancreas,** these organs play a vital role in proper digestion and absorption of nutrients. The gallbladder serves as a storage site for bile, which is produced by the liver. When bile is needed for digestion, the gallbladder releases it through ducts into the (4) **duodenum** through the (5) **common bile duct.** The three accessory organs of digestion are the _____, _____, and _____.
hepat/o **cholecyst/o** **pancreat/o**	**6–111** Construct CFs for liver: _____ /_____. gallbladder: _____ /_____. pancreas: _____ /_____.

Pink indicates a prefix. Blue indicates a suffix. Boldface indicates a word root or combining form.

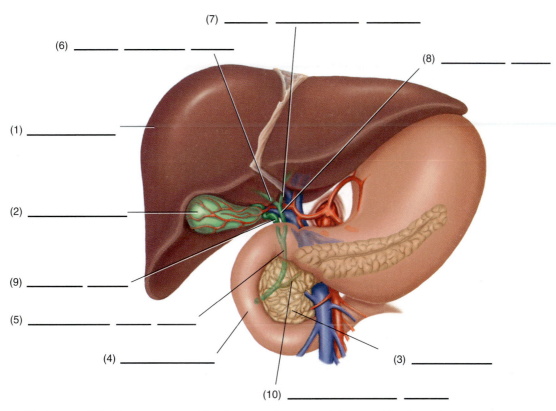

Figure 6-10 Liver, gallbladder, pancreas, and duodenum with associated ducts and blood vessels.

Liver

hepat/itis hĕp-ă-TĪ-tĭs	**6-112** Hepat/itis, an inflammatory condition of the liver, may be caused by bacteri/al or viral infection, parasitic infestation, alcohol, drugs, toxins, or transfusion of incompatible blood. It may be mild and brief or severe and life threatening. When a person has inflammation of the liver caused by a virus, the Dx is most likely _____ / _____.
hepat/o/megaly hĕp-ă-tō-MĔG-ă-lē	**6-113** Hepat/itis may be characterized by an enlarged liver. The medical term for an enlarged liver is _____ / _____ / _____.
hepat/oma hĕp-ă-TŌ-mă	**6-114** Hepat/o/megaly may be a symptom of a malignant tumor of the liver called *hepat/oma*. The tumor occurs most commonly in association with hepat/itis or liver cirrh/osis. The Dx of a liver tumor is charted as _____ / _____.
hepat/itis hĕp-ă-TĪ-tĭs	**6-115** Hepatitis B, the most common infectious hepatitis seen in hospitals, is transferred through blood and body secretions. As a preventive measure, hospital personnel are usually required to be vaccinated. The medical term for *inflammation of the liver* is _____ / _____.

hepat/o/dynia, hepat/algia hĕp-ă-tō-DĬN-ē-ă, hĕp-ă-TĂL-jē-ă **hepat/o/rrhaphy** hĕp-ă-TŎR-ă-fē **hepat/ectomy** hĕp-ă-TĔK-tō-mē	**6–116** Form medical words that mean *pain in the liver:* _____ / _____ / _____ *or* _____ / _____. *suture of the liver:* _____ / _____ / _____. *excision of (a portion of) the liver:* _____ / _____.
hepat/o/cyte HĔP-ă-tō-sīt	**6–117** Combine *hepat/o* and *-cyte* to form a word that means *liver cell.* _____ / _____ / _____
	6–118 Identify and label the following structures in Figure 6-10 as you read about the accessory organs of digestion. Bile is released from the gallbladder and also drained directly from the liver through the (6) **right hepatic duct** and the (7) **left hepatic duct.** These two ducts eventually form the (8) **hepatic duct.** The (9) **cystic duct** merges with the hepatic duct to form the common bile duct and the (10) **pancreatic duct.** These ducts carry their digestive juices into the duodenum.
hepat/ic hĕ-PĂT-ĭk **cyst/ic** SĬS-tĭk **pancreat/ic** păn-krē-ĂT-ĭk	**6–119** Use *-ic* to form medical words that mean *pertaining to the liver:* _____ / _____. *pertaining to the bladder:* _____ / _____. *pertaining to the pancreas:* _____ / _____.
hepat/ic, cyst/ic, pancreat/ic hĕ-PĂT-ĭk, SĬS-tĭk, păn-krē-ĂT-ĭk	**6–120** Refer to Frame 6–122 to write the names of the ducts responsible for transporting digestive juices. _____ / _____ duct, _____ / _____ duct, _____ / _____ duct, and common bile duct.

Competency Verification: Check your labeling of Figure 6-10 in Appendix B: Answer Key, page 601.

Gallbladder

vomiting	**6–121** The CF *chol/e* means *bile, gall. Chol/emesis* means _____ bile.
cholecyst/o	**6–122** Bile, also called *gall,* is a yellow-green bitter secretion produced by the liver and stored in the gallbladder. It receives its color from the presence of bile pigments, such as bilirubin. Bile passes from the gallbladder through the common bile duct into the small intestine. Bile emulsifies (breaks down) fats and prepares them for further digestion and absorption in the small intestine. Combine *chol/e* and *cyst/o* to develop the CF _____ / _____.

Pink indicates a prefix. Blue indicates a suffix. Boldface indicates a word root or combining form.

gallbladder	**6-123** Cholecyst/itis means *inflammation of the* _____.
o	**6-124** The vowel *e* in **chol/e** is an exception to the rule of using an _____ as a connecting vowel.
bile, gall **vomiting**	**6-125** When a patient vomits bile, the condition is called *chol/emesis.* Analyze *chol/emesis* by defining the elements. The CF **chol/e** refers to _____ *or* _____. The suffix *-emesis* refers to _____.
liver	**6-126** The suffix *-lith* is used in words to mean *stone,* or *calculus.* A hepat/o/lith is a stone, or calculus, in the _____.
pancreat/o/lith păn-krē-ĂT-ō-lĭth **cholecyst/o/lith** kō-lē-SĬS-tō-lĭth **hepat/o/lith** hĕp-Ă-tō-lĭth	**6-127** Form medical words that mean *stone, or calculus, in the pancreas:* _____ / _____ / _____. *stone, or calculus, in the gallbladder:* _____ / _____ / _____. *stone, or calculus, in the liver:* _____ / _____ / _____.
chol/e	**6-128** Chol/e/liths are gallstones; chol/e/lith/iasis is an abnormal condition of gallstones. Unless the gallstones obstruct a biliary duct, the condition may remain asymptomatic. Exact causes of gallstones are unknown; however, they occur more commonly in women, older people, and obese people. Figure 6-11 illustrates sites of gallstones. From chol/e/lith, determine the CF that means *bile, gall.* _____ / _____
chol/e/lith kō-lĕ-LĬTH	**6-129** The most common type of gallstone contains cholesterol. These calculi are formed in the gallbladder or bile ducts. The medical name for gallstone is _____ / _____ / _____.
jaund/o **hyper-** **-emia**	**6-130** Jaund/ice, a yellowish discoloration of the skin and whites of the eyes (sclerae), is due to abnormally high levels of bilirubin in blood (hyper/bilirubin/emia). This condition is usually a sign of liver dysfunction or obstruction of the bile ducts. The CF for *yellow* is _____ / _____. The prefix for *excessive, above normal* is _____. The suffix for *blood* is _____.
right upper quadrant (RUQ)	**6-131** Calculi that form in the gallbladder or bile ducts may cause jaund/ice, RUQ pain, obstruction, and inflammation of the gallbladder. *RUQ* means _____ _____ _____.

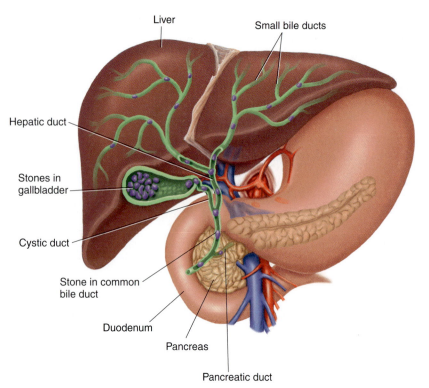

Liver

Small bile ducts

Hepatic duct

Stones in
gallbladder

Cystic duct

Stone in common
bile duct

Duodenum

Pancreas

Pancreatic duct

Figure 6-11 Cholelithiasis and
choledocholithiasis.

cholangi/oma kō-lăn-jē-Ō-mă	**6–132** A bil/i/ary duct, also called *a bile duct,* may become inflamed from a chol/e/lith. The CF *cholangi/o* refers to a bile vessel. A tumor of the bile vessel is called _____ / _____.
cholangi/o/graphy kō-lăn-jē-ŎG-ră-fē	**6–133** The Dx of cholang/itis is determined by ultrasound evaluation and cholangi/o/graphy. The radiographic procedure in this frame for outlining the major bile vessel is _____ / _____ / _____.
bile duct	**6–134** The CF *choledoch/o* means *bile duct.* A choledoch/o/lith is a *stone in the* _____ _____.
choledoch/o	**6–135** Choledoch/o/lith/iasis refers to the *formation of a stone in the common bile duct,* as illustrated in Figure 6-11. The CF for *bile duct* is _____ / _____.
choledoch/o/lith kō-LĔD-ō-kō-lĭth **choledoch/o/rrhaphy** kō-lĕd-ō-KŎR-ă-fē **choledoch/o/tomy** kō-lĕd-ō-KŎT-ō-mē	**6–136** When a stone is trapped in the common bile duct, the duct may require an incision to remove the stone. Once the stone is removed, the duct is sutured. Form medical words that mean *stone in the bile duct:* _____ / _____ / _____. *suture of the bile duct:* _____ / _____ / _____. *incision of the bile duct:* _____ / _____ / _____.

gallbladder	**6-137** Locate the gallbladder, also known as *cholecyst,* in Figure 6-11. This pouch-like structure stores bile, which is produced by the liver. Cholecyst is the medical name for _____.
cholecyst/itis kō-lē-sĭs-TĬ-tĭs	**6-138** Inflammation of the gallbladder may be caused by the presence of gallstones. The Dx *inflammation of the gallbladder* is charted as _____ / _____.
gallstone	**6-139** A *chole/lith* is a _____.
stone, calculus KĂL-kū-lŭs	**6-140** The pancreat/ic duct transports pancreatic juices to the duodenum to help the digestive process. A pancreat/o/lith is a _____, *or* _____, *within the pancreas.*
stone, calculus KĂL-kū-lŭs	**6-141** The suffixes *-osis* and *-iasis* are used to indicate an abnormal or diseased condition. The difference between the two is that *-osis* is used to denote a disorder but does not indicate the specific cause of the abnormality. In contrast, *-iasis* is attached to a WR to identify an abnormal condition produced by something that is specified.* For example, lith/iasis is an abnormal condition produced by a _____, *or* _____.
liver	**6-142** Hepat/osis is an *abnormal or diseased condition of the* _____. The cause of the abnormality is not specified and could be the result of any number of liver diseases.
lith/iasis lĭth-Ĭ-ă-sĭs **pancreat/o/lith/iasis** păn-krē-ă-tō-lĭ-THĬ-ă-sĭs	**6-143** When forming a word that means *abnormal condition of stones, or calculi,* use *-iasis* because the abnormal condition is produced by something specified.* In this case, it is produced by the stones. Use *-iasis* to construct medical words that mean *abnormal condition of stones:* _____ / _____. *pancreat/ic stones:* _____ / _____ / _____ / _____.
chol/e/lith/iasis kō-lē-lĭ-THĬ-ă-sĭs	**6-144** Chol/e/lith/iasis is common in obese women age greater than 40 years. (See Figure 6-11.) A patient with a Dx of an abnormal or diseased condition of gallstones suffers from _____ / _____ / _____ / _____.

 In some instances, you will find that *-osis* and *-iasis* are interchangeable. Whenever you are in doubt about which suffix to use, refer to your medical dictionary.

---

*There are a few exceptions to this rule.

cholecyst/itis
kō-lē-sĭs-TĪ-tĭs

**cholecyst/o/dynia,
cholecyst/algia**
kō-lē-sĭs-tō-DĬN-ē-ă,
kō-lē-sĭs-TĂL-jē-ă

cholecyst/o/lith/iasis
kō-lē-sĭs-tō-lĭ-THĪ-ă-sĭs

6–145 Cholecyst/itis is an inflammation of the gallbladder, usually caused by obstruction of gallstones in the bil/i/ary ducts. The disease is marked by pain in the RUQ of the abdomen. Usually, pain develops shortly after a meal and radiates to the shoulder and back.

Use *cholecyst/o* to form medical words that mean

inflammation of the gallbladder: _____ / _____.

pain in the gallbladder:

_____ / _____ / _____ or _____ / _____.

abnormal condition of gallbladder stone(s):

_____ / _____ / _____ / _____.

cholecyst/ectomy
kō-lē-sĭs-TĔK-tō-mē

bil/i/ary*
BĬL-ē-ār-ē

lapar/o/scop/ic
lăp-ă-rō-SKŎP-ĭk

6–146 Chol/e/cyst/ectomy is performed through lapar/o/scop/ic or open surgery. If bile ducts are obstructed, a classic "gallbladder attack," more properly referred to as *bili/ary* colic, results in pain in the RUQ. Nausea and vomiting may accompany the attack.

Form medical terms that mean

excision of the gallbladder: _____ / _____.

pertaining to bile or gall: _____ / _____ / _____.

pertaining to visual examination of the abdomen:

_____ / _____ / _____ / _____.

Pancreas

pancreat/ectomy
păn-krē-ă-TĔK-tō-mē

6–147 Because of its critical function of producing insulin and digestive enzymes, a complete excision of the pancreas is not usually performed. When excision of the pancreas is indicated, the surgeon performs a _____ / _____.

pancreat/ectomy
păn-krē-ă-TĔK-tō-mē

6–148 Pancreat/ic CA is an extremely lethal disease. Surgery is performed for relief, but it is not a cure for this CA. When part or all of the pancreas is removed, the surgeon performs a _____ / _____.

poison

6–149 Poison is any substance taken into the body by ingestion, inhalation, injection, or absorption that interferes with normal physiological function. Common elements used to refer to poison are *tox/o, toxic/o,* and *-toxic.* Whenever you see any of these elements in a word, you will know that the element refers to _____.

toxic/o/logy
tŏks-ĭ-KŎL-ō-jē

6–150 Virtually any substance can be poisonous if consumed in sufficient quantity. The term *poison* usually implies an excessive degree of a tox/ic dosage, rather than a specific group of substances. Aspirin is not usually thought of as a poison, but overdoses of this drug can result in the accidental death of a child.

Form a word that means *study of poisons.* _____ / _____ / _____

_____
*There are a few exceptions to this rule.

Pink indicates a prefix. Blue indicates a suffix. Boldface indicates a word root or combining form.

abnormal condition, poison **toxic/o, tox/o**	**6-151** *Toxic/osis* literally means _____ _____ of _____. The CF for *poison* is _____ / _____ or _____ / _____.
toxic/o/logy tŏks-ĭ-KŎL-ō-jē	**6-152** Substances that impair health or destroy life when ingested, inhaled, or absorbed by the body in relatively small amounts are considered tox/ic substances. Identifying the tox/ic substance is critical to expeditious treatment. Scientific study of poisons is known as _____ / _____ / _____.
ultra/son/o/graphy ūl-tră-sŏn-ŎG-ră-fē	**6-153** The suffix *-gram* is used in words to mean *record, writing.* The suffix *-graphy* is used in words to mean *process of recording.* Ultra/son/o/graphy (US) is the *process of imaging deep structures of the body by recording reflection of high-frequency sound waves (ultrasound) and displaying the reflected echoes on a monitor.* US is also called *ultrasound and echo.* When confirmation of a suspected disease or tumor is needed, the physician may order the radi/o/graph/ic imaging procedure called *ultrasound,* also known as _____ / _____ / _____ / _____ (US).

SECTION REVIEW 6-6

Using the following table, write the combining form or suffix that matches its definition in the space provided to the left of the definition. There may be more than one word element that matches a definition.

Combining Forms

chol/e	*pancreat/o*
cholecyst/o	*therm/o*
choledoch/o	*toxic/o*
cyst/o	*tox/o*
hepat/o	

Suffixes

-algia	*-graphy*	*-plasty*
-dynia	*-iasis*	*-rrhaphy*
-ectomy	*-lith*	*-stomy*
-emesis	*-megaly*	*-toxic*
-gram	*-oma*	

1. _____ tumor

2. _____ abnormal condition (produced by something specified)

3. _____ bile duct

4. _____ bile, gall

5. _____ bladder

6. _____ enlargement

7. _____ excision, removal

8. _____ forming an opening (mouth)

9. _____ gallbladder

10. _____ heat

11. _____ liver

12. _____ pain

13. _____ pancreas

14. _____ poison

15. _____ process of recording

16. _____ record, writing

17. _____ stone, calculus

18. _____ surgical repair

19. _____ suture

20. _____ vomiting

Competency Verification: Check your answers in Appendix B: Answer Key, page 601. If you are not satisfied with your level of comprehension, go back to Frame 6–112, and rework the frames.

Correct Answers _____ × 5 = _____ % Score

Abbreviations

This section introduces digestive system–related abbreviations and their meanings. Included are abbreviations contained in the medical record activities that follow.

Abbreviation	Meaning	Abbreviation	Meaning
BE	barium enema	IBD	inflammatory bowel disease
BM	bowel movement	IBS	irritable bowel syndrome
BMI	body mass index	IV	intravenous
CA	cancer; chronological age; cardiac arrest	LES	lower esophageal sphincter
CT	computed tomography	MRI	magnetic resonance imaging
Dx	diagnosis	NG	nasogastric
EGD	esophagogastroduodenoscopy	OR	operating room
ESWL	extracorporeal shock-wave lithotripsy	PUD	peptic ulcer disease
FBS	fasting blood sugar	RGB	Roux-en-Y gastric bypass
GERD	gastroesophageal reflux disease	RUQ	right upper quadrant
GI	gastrointestinal	US	ultrasound; ultrasonography

Additional Medical Terms

The following are additional medical terms related to the digestive system. Recognizing and learning these terms will help you understand the connections among a pathological condition, its diagnosis, and the rationale behind the method of treatment selected for a particular disorder.

Diseases and Conditions

ascites ă-SĪ-tēz	Abnormal accumulation of serous fluid in the peritoneal cavity *Ascites may be a symptom of inflammatory disorders in the abdomen, venous hypertension caused by liver disease, or heart failure (HF). (See Figure 6-12.)*
borborygmus bŏr-bō-RĬG-mŭs	Gurgling or rumbling sound heard over the large intestine caused by gas moving through the intestines
cirrhosis sĭ-RŌ-sĭs *cirrh:* yellow *-osis:* abnormal condition; increase (used primarily with blood cells)	Chronic liver disease characterized by destruction of liver cells that eventually leads to ineffective liver function and jaundice *Cirrhosis is most commonly caused by chronic alcoholism. It may also be caused by hepatitis, toxins, infectious agents, and circulatory disorders.*

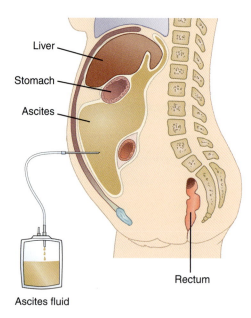

Liver

Stomach

Ascites

Rectum

Ascites fluid

Figure 6-12 Ascites with removal of fluid from the abdominal cavity by using a catheter.

celiac disease SĒ-lē-ăk	Disorder that damages the lining of the small intestine in response to gluten (protein found in barley, oats, and wheat) ingestion, which results in malabsorption of nutrients *Treatment for celiac disease consists of the adoption of a gluten-free diet. Patients generally recover by adhering to strict gluten-free dietary guidelines.*
diverticular disease dī-věr-TĬK-ū-lăr	Condition in which bulging pouches (diverticula) in the gastrointestinal (GI) tract push the mucosal lining through the surrounding muscle *When feces become trapped inside a diverticular sac, it causes inflammation, infection, abdominal pain, and fever, a condition known as diverticulitis. (See Figure 6-13.)*

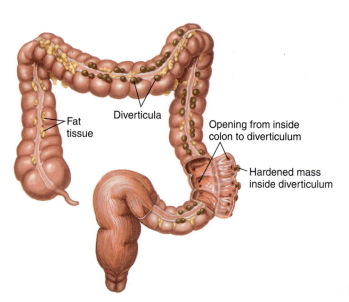

Fat
tissue

Diverticula

Opening from inside
colon to diverticulum

Hardened mass
inside diverticulum

Figure 6-13 Diverticular disease.

dysentery
DĬS-ĕn-tĕr-ē
  dys-: bad; painful;
      difficult
  enter: intestine (usually
      small intestine)
  -y: condition;
      process

Inflammation of the intestine, especially of the colon, which may be caused by chemical irritants, bacteria, protozoa, or parasites

Dysentery is common in underdeveloped areas of the world and in times of disaster and social disorganization when sanitary living conditions, clean food, and safe water are not available. It is characterized by diarrhea, colitis, and abdominal cramps.

---

fistula
FĬS-tū-lă

Abnormal passage from one organ to another or from a hollow organ to the surface

An anal fistula is located near the anus and may open into the rectum.

---

gastroesophageal reflux disease (GERD)
găs-trō-ē-sŏf-ă-JĒ-ăl
RĒ-flŭks dĭ-ZĒZ
  gastr/o: stomach
  esophag: esophagus
  -eal: pertaining to

Backflow (reflux) of gastric contents into the esophagus caused by malfunction of the lower esophageal sphincter (LES)

Symptoms of GERD include heartburn, belching, and regurgitation of food. Treatment includes elevating the head of the bed while sleeping, avoiding alcohol and foods that stimulate acid secretion, and taking drugs to decrease production of acid.

---

hematochezia
hĕm-ă-tō-KĒ-zē-ă

Passage of stools containing bright red blood

---

hemorrhoid
HĔM-ō-royd

Mass of enlarged, twisted varicose veins in the mucous membrane inside (internal) or just outside (external) the rectum; also known as *piles*

---

hernia
HĔR-nē-ă

Protrusion or projection of an organ or a part of an organ through the wall of the cavity that normally contains it (See Figure 6-14.)

---

inflammatory bowel disease (IBD)
ĭn-FLĂM-ă-tŏr-ē BŌWL

Ulceration of the colon mucosa

Crohn disease and ulcerative colitis are forms of IBD.

  Crohn disease
  KRŌN

Chronic IBD that usually affects the ileum but may affect any portion of the intestinal tract; also called *regional enteritis*

Crohn disease is distinguished from closely related bowel disorders by its inflammatory pattern, which tends to be patchy or segmented.

  ulcerative colitis
  ŬL-sĕr-ā-tĭv kō-LĪ-tĭs
    col: colon
    -itis: inflammation

Chronic IBD of the colon characterized by episodes of diarrhea, rectal bleeding, and pain

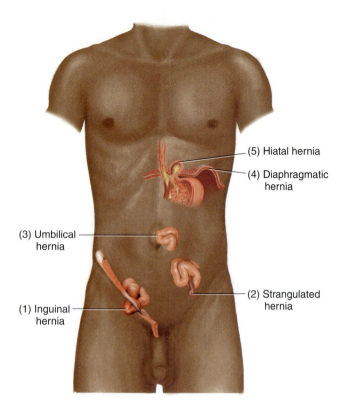

(5) Hiatal hernia

(4) Diaphragmatic hernia

(3) Umbilical hernia

(1) Inguinal hernia

(2) Strangulated hernia

Figure 6-14 Common locations of hernias.

irritable bowel syndrome (IBS) ĬR-ĭ-tă-bl BŎWL SĬN-drōm	Condition characterized by gastrointestinal signs and symptoms, including constipation, diarrhea, gas, and bloating, all in the absence of organic pathology; also called *spastic colon* *Contributing factors of IBS include stress and tension. Treatment consists of dietary modifications, such as avoiding irritating foods or a high-fiber diet, and taking laxatives if constipation is a symptom. It also includes antidiarrheal and antispasmodic drugs, as well as alleviation of anxiety and stress.*
obesity **morbid obesity**	Condition in which a person accumulates an amount of fat that exceeds the body's skeletal and physical standards, usually an increase of 20% or greater than the ideal body weight Severe obesity in which a person has a body mass index (BMI) of 40 or greater, which is generally 100 or more pounds more than the ideal body weight *Morbid obesity is a disease with serious medical, psychological, and social ramifications.*

pancreatitis
păn-krē-ă-TĪ-tĭs
   pancreat: pancreas
     -itis: inflammation
	Inflammation of the pancreas that occurs when pancreatic enzymes that digest food are activated in the pancreas instead of the duodenum and attack pancreatic tissue, causing damage to the gland
	
	Pancreatitis can also be caused by chronic alcoholism, gallstone obstruction, drug toxicity, and viral infections. Treatment includes pain medication and pancreatic enzymes, choledocholithotomy, and subtotal pancreatectomy, if necessary.

peritonitis pĕr-ĭ-tō-NĪ-tĭs	Bacterial or fungal infection of the peritoneum that can result from any rupture (perforation) in the abdomen or as a complication of other medical conditions *Treatment includes antibiotics and, in some cases, surgery. If left untreated, peritonitis can lead to severe, potentially life-threatening infection throughout the body.*

polyp PŎL-ĭp	Small, stalk-like growth that resembles a mushroom and protrudes upward or outward from a mucous membrane surface *Polyps detected during colonoscopy are excised (polypectomy) and the biopsy specimen sent to the laboratory for microscopic tissue examination. This test is used to screen for CA or abnormal cells. (See Figure 6-15.)*
volvulus VŎL-vū-lŭs	Twisting of the bowel on itself, causing obstruction *Volvulus usually requires surgery to untwist the loop of bowel.*

Diagnostic Procedures

barium enema (BE) BĂ-rē-ŭm ĔN-ĕ-mă	Radiographic examination of the rectum and colon after administration of barium (radiopaque contrast medium) into the rectum; also called *lower GI series* *BE is used for diagnosis of obstructions, tumors, and other abnormalities of the colon. (See Figure 6-16.)*

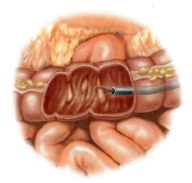

Figure 6-15 Polypectomy.

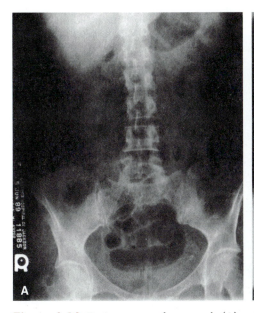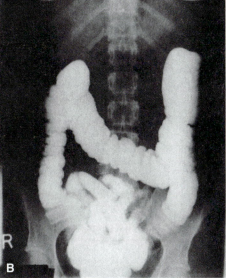

Figure 6-16 Barium enema done poorly (A) and correctly (B).

barium swallow BĂ-rē-ŭm	Radiographic examination of the esophagus, stomach, and small intestine after oral administration of barium (radiopaque contrast medium); also called *upper GI series* *Barium swallow is commonly performed in patients experiencing dysphagia. Structural abnormalities of the esophagus, stomach, and small intestine may also be diagnosed by using this technique.*
computed tomography (CT) kŏm-PŪ-tĕd tō-MŎG-ră-fē *tom/o:* to cut *-graphy:* process of recording	Tomography in which a narrow beam of x-rays rotates in a full arc around the patient to acquire multiple views of the body, which a computer interprets to produce cross-sectional images of an internal organ or tissue; also called *computerized axial tomography (CAT)* *CT scans are used to view the gallbladder, liver, bile ducts, and pancreas and diagnose tumors, cysts, inflammation, abscesses, perforation, bleeding, and obstructions. A contrast material may be used to enhance the structures.*
endoscopy ĕn-DŎS-kō-pē *endo-:* in, within *-scopy:* visual examination	Visual examination of the interior of organs and cavities with a specialized lighted instrument called an *endoscope* *The organ, cavity, or canal being examined dictates the name of the endoscopic procedure. A camera and video recorder are commonly used during the procedure to provide a permanent record.*
capsule	Endoscopy using a tiny, wireless camera the size of a vitamin pill that is swallowed and travels through the digestive tract taking thousands of photos that are transmitted to a recorder worn on a belt around the waist *Capsule endoscopy allows the small intestine to be reached more easily than traditional endoscopy to diagnose gastrointestinal bleeding, cancer, polyps, and inflammatory bowel disease such as Crohn disease. (See Figure 6-17.)*
upper GI	Endoscopy of the esophagus (esophagoscopy), stomach (gastroscopy), and duodenum (duodenoscopy) *Endoscopy of the upper GI tract is performed to identify tumors, esophagitis, gastroesophageal varices, peptic ulcers, and the source of upper GI bleeding. It is also used to confirm the presence and extent of varices in the lower esophagus and stomach in patients with liver disease.*
lower GI	Endoscopy of the colon (colonoscopy), sigmoid colon (sigmoidoscopy), and rectum and anal canal (proctoscopy) *Endoscopy of the lower GI tract is used to identify pathological conditions in the colon. It may also be used to remove polyps. When polyps are discovered in the colon, they are removed and tested for CA.*

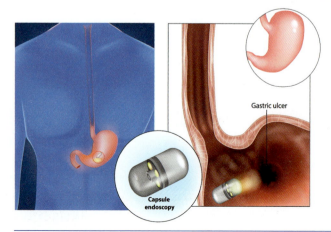

Gastric ulcer

Capsule endoscopy

Figure 6-17 Capsule endoscopy showing gastric ulcer.

magnetic resonance imaging (MRI) măg-NĔT-ĭc RĔZ-ĕn-ăns ĬM-ĭj-ĭng	Radiographic procedure that uses electromagnetic energy to produce multiplanar cross-sectional images of the body *In the digestive system, MRI is particularly useful in detecting abdominal masses and viewing images of abdominal structures.*
stool guaiac GWĪ-ăk	Laboratory test performed on feces to detect the presence of blood in the stool (bowel movement) that is not apparent on visual inspection; also called *hemoccult test*
ultrasonography (US) ŭl-tră-sŏn-ŎG-ră-fē *ultra-:* excess, beyond *son/o:* sound *-graphy:* process of recording	Radiographic procedure in which a small transducer passed over the skin transmits high-frequency sound waves (ultrasound) that bounce off body tissues and are then recorded to produce an image of an internal organ or tissue; also called *echography* *US is used to view the liver, gallbladder, bile ducts, and pancreas, among other structures. It is also used to diagnose digestive disorders, locate cysts and tumors, and guide insertion of instruments during surgical procedures.*

Medical and Surgical Procedures

appendectomy ăp-ĕn-DĔK-tō-mē *cappend:* appendix *-ectomy:* excision, removal	Surgical removal of an infected appendix (appendicitis) *Appendectomy is a common emergency surgery in which the appendix must be removed quickly through a right lower quadrant (RLQ) incision. (See Figure 6-18A.) Delay in treatment may result in rupture of the appendix, causing peritonitis as fecal matter enters the peritoneal cavity. There are two types of appendectomies, but if no rupture has occurred, the less invasive laparoscopic appendectomy is usually performed. (See Figure 6-18B.)*
open	Excision of the appendix through a 2- to 4-inch incision in the RLQ of the abdomen
laparoscopic lăp-ă-rō-SKŎP-ĭk *lapar/o:* abdomen *scopic:* instrument for examining	Less invasive appendectomy performed through small incisions made into the abdomen *(See Figure 6-18B.)* *The laparoscope, which has a small video camera and surgical tools, is placed into one of the incisions while the surgeon looks at a television monitor to guide the tools inside the abdomen. The appendix is removed through one of the incisions. Laparoscopic surgery results in a smaller scar and reduces recovery time. (See Figure 6-19.)*

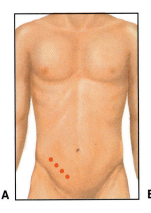 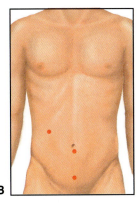

Figure 6-18 Appendectomy incision sites. (A) Open appendectomy. (B) Laparoscopic appendectomy.

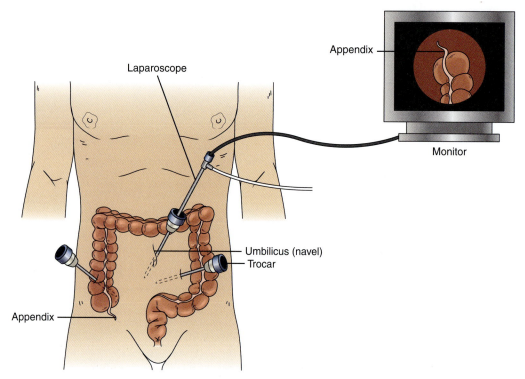

Figure 6-19 Laparoscopic appendectomy with trocars (access devices used to insert laparoscopic instruments).

bariatric surgery BĂR-ē-ă-trĭk	Group of procedures that treat morbid obesity *Commonly employed bariatric surgeries include vertical banded gastroplasty and RGB. (See Figure 6-20.)*
vertical banded gastroplasty găs-trō-PLĂS-tē *gastr/o:* stomach *-plasty:* surgical repair	Bariatric surgery in which the upper stomach near the esophagus is stapled vertically to reduce it to a small pouch and a band is inserted that restricts and delays food from leaving the pouch, causing a feeling of fullness (See Figure 6-20A.)
Roux-en-Y gastric bypass (RGB) rū-ĕn-WĪ GĂS-trĭk	Bariatric surgery in which the stomach is first stapled to decrease it to a small pouch and then the jejunum is shortened and connected to the small stomach pouch, causing the base of the duodenum leading from the nonfunctioning portion of the stomach to form a "Y" configuration, which decreases the pathway of food through the intestine, thus reducing absorption of calories and fats; also called *gastric bypass with gastroenterostomy* *RGB may be performed laparoscopically, or it can be performed as an open procedure (laparotomy), which involves a large incision being made in the middle of the abdomen. RGB is the most commonly performed weight loss surgery today. (See Figure 6-20B.)*

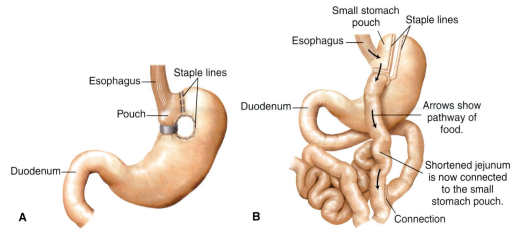

Figure 6-20 Bariatric surgery. (A) Vertical banded gastroplasty. (B) Roux-en-Y gastric bypass.

lithotripsy
LĬTH-ō-trĭp-sē
    lith/o: stone, calculus
  -*tripsy:* crushing
	Procedure for eliminating a stone within the gallbladder or urinary system by crushing the stone surgically or using a noninvasive method, such as ultrasonic shock waves, to shatter it
	
	The crushed fragments may be expelled or washed out.

extracorporeal shock-wave lithotripsy (ESWL)
ĕks-tră-kor-POR-ē-ăl LĬTH-ō-trĭp-sē
    extra-: outside
    corpor: body
      -*eal:* pertaining to
    lith/o: stone, calculus
  -*tripsy:* crushing
	Use of shock waves as a noninvasive method to destroy stones in the gallbladder and biliary ducts
	
	In ESWL, ultrasound is used to locate the stone or stones and monitor their destruction. The patient usually undergoes a course of oral dissolution drugs to ensure complete removal of all stones and stone fragments.

nasogastric (NG) intubation
nā-zō-GĂS-trĭk ĭn-tū-BĀ-shŭn
    nas/o: nose
    gastr: stomach
      -*ic:* pertaining to
	Insertion of a nasogastric tube through the nose into the stomach
	
	Nasogastric intubation is used to relieve gastric distention by removing gas, gastric secretions, or food. It is also used to instill medication, food, or fluids, or to obtain a specimen for laboratory analysis.

Pharmacology

The following table lists common drug categories used to treat gastrointestinal disorders as well as their therapeutic actions.

Drug Category	Action
antacids ănt-ĂS-ĭds	Neutralize acids in the stomach
antidiarrheals ăn-tĭ-dī-ă-RĒ-ăls	Control loose stools and relieve diarrhea by absorbing excess water in the bowel or slowing peristalsis in the intestinal tract
antiemetics ăn-tĭ-ē-MĚT-ĭks	Control nausea and vomiting by blocking nerve impulses to the vomiting center of the brain
H₂ blockers	Block H_2 receptors in the stomach to prevent the release of acid to treat heartburn, peptic ulcers, and GERD
laxatives LĂK-să-tĭvz	Relieve constipation and facilitate passage of feces through the lower GI tract

Pronunciation Help	*Long Sound*	ā in rāte	ē in rēbirth	ī in īsle	ō in ōver	ū in ūnite
	Short Sound	ă in ăpple	ĕ in ĕver	ĭ in ĭt	ŏ in nŏt	ŭ in cŭt

Word Elements Review

This review provides a verification of your knowledge of the word elements covered in this chapter. First, use a slash to break the term into its component parts and identify each element by labeling it P for prefix, WR for word root, CF for combining form, and S for suffix. Then provide the meaning of the medical term. Remember to define the suffix first, define the beginning of the word second, and define the middle part of the term last. The first word is a sample completed for you.

Medical Term	Meaning
colon/o/scope CF S	instrument for examining the colon
1. hepat/itis	
2. lith/iasis	
3. chol/e/cyst/ectomy	
4. cholangi/oma	
5. lapar/o/scop/ic	

Match the following medical terms with the definitions in the numbered list.

biliary	gastroenterologist	pyloromyotomy
choledochoplasty	pancreatectomy	sigmoidoscopy
cholelithiasis	postprandial	sublingual
colonoscope	proctoscope	toxicology

6. _____ surgical repair of the bile duct

7. _____ study of poisons

8. _____ pertaining to after a meal

9. _____ visual examination of the sigmoid colon

10. _____ specialist who treats stomach and intestinal disorders

11. _____ instrument to examine the colon

12. _____ excision of the pancreas

13. _____ pertaining to bile or gall

14. _____ incision of the pylorus muscle (layer)

15. _____ pertaining to under the tongue

Competency Verification: Check your answers in Appendix B: Answer Key, page 602. If you are not satisfied with your level of comprehension, review the vocabulary, and retake the review.

Correct Answers _____ × 6.67 = _____ % Score

Additional Medical Terms Review

Match the following medical term(s) with the definitions in the numbered list.

antiemetics   Crohn disease   IBS
ascites   fistula   jaundice
barium enema   hematochezia   lithotripsy
barium swallow   hemoccult   polyp
cirrhosis   IBD   volvulus

1. _____ is a test performed on feces that detects the presence of blood that is not apparent on visual inspection and is also called *stool guaiac.*

2. _____ control nausea and prevent vomiting.

3. _____ is a small benign growth that projects from a mucous membrane.

4. _____ is an abnormal accumulation of serous fluid in the peritoneal cavity.

5. _____ refers to chronic inflammatory bowel disease, which usually affects the ileum.

6. _____ refers to surgically crushing a stone.

7. _____ is an abnormal, tubelike passage from one organ to another or from one organ to the surface.

8. _____ is a yellow discoloration of the skin caused by hyperbilirubinemia.

9. _____ is a radiographic examination of the rectum and colon after administration of barium sulfate.

10. _____ refers to ulceration of the mucosa of the colon, as seen in Crohn disease.

11. _____ refers to passage of stools containing red blood.

12. _____ means twisting of the bowel on itself, causing obstruction.

13. _____ refers to a chronic liver disease characterized pathologically by destruction of liver cells and jaundice.

14. _____ is a radiographic examination of the esophagus, stomach, and small intestine after oral administration of barium sulfate.

15. _____ is a condition characterized by constipation, diarrhea, gas, and bloating without organic pathology and is also called *spastic colon.*

Competency Verification: Check your answers in Appendix B: Answer Key, page 602. If you are not satisfied with your level of comprehension, review the additional medical terms section, and retake the review.

Correct Answers _____ × 6.67 = _____ % Score

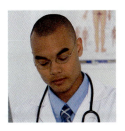

Medical Record Activities

To develop a working vocabulary of medical terms and to understand how those terms are used in the health-care industry, it is important that you complete the following activities.

MEDICAL RECORD ACTIVITY 6-1

PROGRESS NOTE: RECTAL BLEEDING

This activity contains a progress note about rectal bleeding. Read the progress note that follows and underline the medical terms. Then complete the terminology and critical thinking exercises.

PROGRESS NOTE

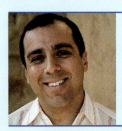

PATIENT NAME: Gomez, Herman
MEDICAL RECORD ID: 60-49229
DATE: May 25, 20xx

CHIEF COMPLAINT: This 50-year-old Hispanic male, a carpenter, states that he has lost approximately 40 pounds since his last examination.

HISTORY: Patient says he has had no dysphagia or postprandial distress, and there is no report of diarrhea, nausea, emesis, hematemesis, or constipation. Patient has had a history of regional enteritis, appendicitis, and colonic bleeding. The regional enteritis resulted in an ileostomy with appendectomy about 6 months ago.

ASSESSMENT: His sigmoidoscopy using a 10-cm scope showed no evidence of bleeding at the anorectal area. A 35-cm scope was then inserted to a level of 13 cm. At this point, angulation prevented further passage of the scope. No abnormalities had been encountered, but dark blood was noted at that level.

IMPRESSION: My impression is that the rectal bleeding could be caused by a polyp, bleeding diverticulum, or rectal carcinoma.

PLAN: Patient has been advised to schedule a colonoscopy next week and to come to the emergency department if symptoms worsen.

Ann Rochet M.D.

Ann Rochet, M.D.

AR:hk
D: 5/25/20xx; T: 5/25/20xx

Terminology 6-1

Terms listed in the following table come from the Progress Note: Rectal Bleeding *from earlier. Use a medical dictionary, such as* Taber's Cyclopedic Medical Dictionary; *the appendices of this book; or other resources to define each term. Then, pronounce the term, and place a ✓ in the box after you do so.*

Term	Definition
angulation ăng-ū-LĂ-shŭn ☐	
anorectal ā-nō-RĔK-tăl ☐	
carcinoma kăr-sĭ-NŌ-mă ☐	
diverticulum dī-vĕr-TĬK-ū-lŭm ☐	
dysphagia dĭs-FĂ-jē-ă ☐	
emesis ĔM-ĕ-sĭs ☐	
enteritis ĕn-tĕr-Ī-tĭs ☐	
hematemesis hĕm-ăt-ĔM-ĕ-sĭs ☐	
ileostomy ĭl-ē-ŎS-tō-mē ☐	
postprandial pōst-PRĂN-dē-ăl ☐	

Critical Thinking 6-1

Review the previous progress note to answer the following questions. Use a medical dictionary, such as Taber's Cyclopedic Medical Dictionary, *and other resources, if needed.*

1. What was the symptom that made the patient seek medical help?

   _____

   _____

2. What surgical procedures were performed on the patient for regional enteritis?

   _____

   _____

3. What abnormality was found with sigmoidoscopy?

   _____

   _____

4. What is causing the rectal bleeding?

   _____

   _____

5. Write the plural form of *diverticulum.*

   _____

   _____

MEDICAL RECORD ACTIVITY 6-2

OPERATIVE REPORT: ESOPHAGEAL CARCINOMA

This activity contains an operative report for esophageal carcinoma. Read the following operative report, and underline the medical terms. Then complete the terminology and critical thinking exercises.

OPERATIVE REPORT

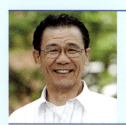

PATIENT NAME: Chin, Arun
MEDICAL RECORD ID: 62-48423
DATE: August 6, 20xx

ADMITTING DIAGNOSIS: Esophageal carcinoma.

DISCHARGE DIAGNOSIS: Esophageal carcinoma.

HISTORY OF PRESENT ILLNESS: Patient had been complaining of dysphagia over the last 4 months with a recent worsening in symptoms.

ESTIMATED BLOOD LOSS: Less than 30 mL.

DESCRIPTION OF PROCEDURE: Under cover of general anesthesia, esophagoscopy was performed, and a small, friable biopsy specimen was obtained. Pathology tests confirmed it to be malignant. A barium x-ray study revealed polypoid, intraluminal, esophageal obstruction. Surgical findings revealed an infiltrating tumor of the middle third of the esophagus with intraluminal, friable, polypoid masses, each 3 cm in diameter. A resection of the esophagus was performed with reanastomosis of the stomach at the aortic arch. An adjacent mediastinal lymph node was excised. There were no complications during the procedure. Patient left the operating room in stable condition.

Katherine Oswald M.D.

Katherine Oswald, M.D.

KO:cm
D: 8/6/20xx; T: 8/6/20xx

Terminology 6-2

Terms listed in the following table come from the Operative Report: Esophageal Carcinoma. *Use a medical dictionary, such as* Taber's Cyclopedic Medical Dictionary; *the appendices of this book; or other resources to define each term. Then pronounce the term, and place a ✓ in the box after you do so.*

Term	Definition
aortic arch ā-OR-tĭk ☐	
carcinoma kăr-sĭ-NŌ-mă ☐	
esophagoscopy ē-sŏf-ă-GŎS-kō-pē ☐	
friable fRĬ-ă-bl ☐	
intraluminal ĭn-tră-LŪ-mĭ-năl ☐	
malignant mă-LĬG-nănt ☐	
mediastinal mē-dē-ăs-TĬ-năl ☐	
OR	
polypoid PŎL-ē-poyd ☐	
reanastomosis rē-ăn-ăs-tō-MŌ-sĭs ☐	

Critical Thinking 6-2

Review the previous operative report to answer the following questions. Use a medical dictionary, such as Taber's Cyclopedic Medical Dictionary, *and other resources, if needed.*

1. What surgery was performed on this patient?

   _____

   _____

2. What diagnostic testing confirmed malignancy?

   _____

   _____

3. Where was the carcinoma located?

   _____

   _____

4. Why was the adjacent lymph node excised?

   _____

   _____

MEDICAL RECORD ACTIVITY 6-3

CLINICAL APPLICATION

This activity is a clinical application that will help you integrate and reinforce your understanding of how the following medical terms are used in the clinical environment. Complete the following clinically related sentences by selecting an appropriate term from the list.

antiemetic	*diverticulitis*	*GERD*	*jaundice*
ascites	*dysentery*	*hepatorrhaphy*	*polypectomy*
cholangiography	*fistula*	*hernioplasty*	*volvulus*

1. A 55-year-old obese male patient is seen with a complaint of left upper quadrant pain and constipation. Abdominal radiograph shows an accumulation of feces in the transverse colon with a twisting of a segment of the descending colon. This twisting of the colon is a condition known as a(n) _____.

2. A 23-year-old male complains of fever, diarrhea, and abdominal cramping for 2 days. He says the symptoms began several hours after drinking stream water while camping. The physician suspects a condition caused by a bacteria or another parasite and diagnoses him with _____.

3. Marlene is a 29-year-old female who presents with a complaint of a pain that begins in her chest, spreads to her throat, and causes a bitter taste in her mouth. Her physician suspects she has a malfunction of the lower esophageal sphincter allowing a backflow of stomach contents into the esophagus. This condition is known as _____.

4. This 63-year-old male is admitted to the hospital with a diagnosis of alcoholic cirrhosis. The physician percusses the abdomen and determines that there is an accumulation of fluid in the peritoneal cavity. The term for accumulation of fluid within the abdomen is _____.

5. While performing a sigmoidoscopy, the physician observes several small, tumorlike projections within the sigmoid colon and rectum. A biopsy is performed to rule out malignancy. The physician excises these growths by using the surgical procedure known as a _____.

6. This 44-year-old male complains of upper abdominal pain that worsens after meals. Palpation of the abdomen causes extreme tenderness. To rule out gallstones, a radiographic examination of the bile ducts with a contrast medium is ordered. This procedure is known as a _____.

7. Jeannie, a 6-year-old girl, is brought in by her mother with complaints of diarrhea and vomiting for 2 days. The physician prescribes an antidiarrheal and administers an _____, which is a medication to help control the vomiting.

8. Ms. E. is a 32-year-old female with a history of intravenous drug use. She tests positive for hepatitis B. This chronic disease is causing a yellow discoloration of the skin and the sclerae of her eyes. Yellowing of the skin and eyes is a condition called _____.

9. After a routine colonoscopy, the patient is advised that he has numerous inflamed bulging pouches throughout his descending colon. This diverticular disease is known as _____.

10. Robert presents with an inguinal hernia. To correct the abnormality, a surgical repair of the hernia will be performed. This surgery is called _____.

Competency Verification: Check your answers in Appendix B: Answer Key, page 603. If you are not satisfied with your level of comprehension, review the material in this chapter, and retake the review.

Correct Answers _____ × 10 = _____ % Score

DIGESTIVE SYSTEM CHAPTER REVIEW

WORD ELEMENTS SUMMARY

The following table summarizes CFs, suffixes, and prefixes related to the digestive system. Study the word elements and their meanings before completing the Vocabulary Review that follows.

Word Element	Meaning	Word Element	Meaning
Combining Forms			
appendic/o	appendix	**jejun/o**	jejunum (second part of the small intestine)
carcin/o	cancer	**lith/o**	stone, calculus
chol/e	bile, gall	**my/o**	muscle
cholecyst/o	gallbladder	**myc/o**	fungus
choledoch/o	bile duct	**nas/o**	nose
cirrh/o, jaund/o	yellow	**or/o, stomat/o**	mouth
col/o, colon/o	colon	**orth/o**	straight
corpor/o	body	**pancreat/o**	pancreas
dent/o, odont/o	teeth	**peritone/o**	peritoneum
duoden/o	duodenum (first part of the small intestine)	**polyp/o**	small growth
enter/o	intestine (usually the small intestine)	**proct/o**	anus, rectum
esophag/o	esophagus	**ptyal/o, sial/o**	saliva, salivary gland
gastr/o	stomach	**pylor/o**	pylorus
gingiv/o	gum(s)	**rect/o**	rectum
gloss/o, lingu/o	tongue	**sigmoid/o**	sigmoid colon
hemat/o, hem/o	blood	**son/o**	sound
hepat/o	liver	**tom/o**	to cut
ile/o	ileum (third part of the small intestine)	**tox/o, toxic/o**	poison
Suffixes			
-algia, -dynia	pain	**-phagia**	swallowing, eating
-ectomy	excision, removal	**-plasty**	surgical repair
-emesis	vomiting	**-rrhaphy**	suture
-gram	record, writing	**-rrhea**	discharge, flow
-graphy	process of recording	**-scope**	instrument for examining
-iasis	abnormal condition (produced by something specified)	**-scopy**	visual examination
-itis	inflammation	**-spasm**	involuntary contraction, twitching

Continued

Word Element	Meaning	Word Element	Meaning
-lith	stone, calculus	-stenosis	narrowing, stricture
-logist	specialist in the study of	-stomy	forming an opening (mouth)
-megaly	enlargement	-tome	instrument to cut
-oma	tumor	-tomy	incision
-osis	abnormal condition; increase (used primarily with blood cells)	-tripsy	crushing
-pepsia	digestion		
Prefixes			
dia-	through, across	hyper-	excessive, above normal
dys-	bad; painful; difficult	hypo-	under, below, deficient
endo-	in, within	peri-	around
epi-	above, upon	sub-	under, below
extra-	outside	ultra-	excess, beyond

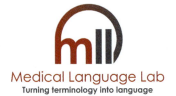

Medical Language Lab
Turning terminology into language

Visit the *Medical Language Lab* at *medicallanguagelab.com*. Use the flash-card–word elements exercise to reinforce your study of word elements. We recommend you complete the flash-card activity before starting the Vocabulary Review that follows.

Vocabulary Review

Match the following medical word(s) with the definitions in the numbered list.

anastomosis	duodenotomy	GERD	peritonitis
bariatric	dyspepsia	H₂ blockers	rectoplasty
celiac disease	dysphagia	hematemesis	sigmoidotomy
cholecystectomy	friable	hepatomegaly	stomatalgia
cholelithiasis	gastroscopy	ileostomy	ultrasound

1. _____ refers to visual examination of the stomach.

2. _____ means bad, painful, difficult digestion.

3. _____ means vomiting blood.

4. _____ refers to high-frequency sound waves that produce internal images of the body.

5. _____ are used to prevent the release of acid to treat heartburn, peptic ulcers, and GERD.

6. _____ damages the lining of the small intestine in response to gluten and results in malabsorption of nutrients.

7. _____ means pain in the mouth.

8. _____ is an incision of the duodenum.

9. _____ means enlargement of the liver.

10. _____ refers to painful swallowing.

11. _____ means removal of the gallbladder.

12. _____ is a surgical connection between two vessels.

13. _____ is an incision of the sigmoid colon.

14. _____ refers to surgical repair of the rectum.

15. _____ is a reflux of gastric contents into the esophagus with heartburn.

16. _____ refers to formation of an opening (mouth) into the ileum.

17. _____ refers to the presence or formation of gallstones.

18. _____ means easily broken or pulverized.

19. _____ is an infection of the lining of the abdomen.

20. _____ is surgery that treats morbid obesity by altering digestive structures to limit food intake.

Competency Verification: Check your answers in Appendix B: Answer Key, page 603. If you are not satisfied with your level of comprehension, review the chapter vocabulary, and retake the review.

Correct Answers: _____ × 5 = _____ % Score

Urinary System

OBJECTIVES

Upon completion of this chapter, you will be able to:

• Describe the type of medical treatment urologists and nephrologists provide.

• Identify urinary structures by labeling the anatomical illustrations.

• Describe the primary functions of the urinary system.

• Describe diseases, conditions, and procedures related to the urinary system.

• Apply your word-building skills by constructing medical terms related to the urinary system.

• Describe common abbreviations and symbols related to the urinary system.

• Recognize, define, pronounce, and spell terms correctly.

• Demonstrate your knowledge of this chapter by successfully completing the frames, reviews, and activities.

MEDICAL SPECIALTIES: UROLOGY AND NEPHROLOGY

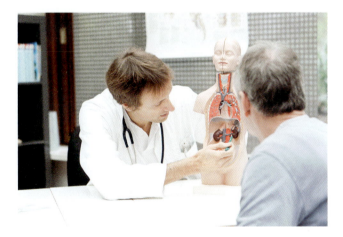

Urology

Urologists are physicians who specialize in the diagnosis and treatment of urinary disorders. Because some urinary structures in the male perform a dual role (both urinary functions and reproductive functions), the urologist also treats male reproductive disorders. These disorders in males include, but are not limited to, treatment of prostate cancer, infertility, and sexual dysfunctions. Generally, the urologist performs surgery and treats urination problems, such as difficulty holding urine (incontinence) and obstruction of urinary flow caused by tumors or stones in the urinary organs. Urologists also manage male reproductive disorders, such as impotence (erectile dysfunction). Some types of urologists include the urogynecologist, who specializes in treating urinary problems involving the female reproductive system, and the pediatric urologist, who specializes in diagnosing and treating urinary problems in children.

Nephrology

The medical specialty of **nephrology** is a subspecialty of internal medicine. **Nephrologists** provide diagnostic evaluation and ongoing care of patients with medical disorders related to the kidneys. These include, but are not limited to, chronic kidney disease; diabetic kidney disease; complicated hypertension; inherited renal diseases, such as polycystic kidney disease; kidney stones; pre- and postkidney transplantation problems; excess fluid accumulation; and problems with electrolyte and mineral metabolism. They also supervise the provision of dialysis services to individuals whose kidneys have deteriorated to the point that their lives would be in jeopardy without renal replacement therapy, a problem commonly known as *end-stage renal disease* (ESRD).

Anatomy and Physiology Overview

The urinary system is composed of the kidneys, ureters, bladder, and urethra. Its purpose is to regulate the volume and composition of fluids in the body and remove waste substances and excess fluid from blood. Waste substances are filtered from blood by the kidneys and excreted in urine, which exits via the ureters into the urinary bladder. Urine is stored in the bladder until the urge to urinate occurs, at which point the muscles at the bladder outlet relax, allowing urine to be expelled through the urethra. Review Figure 7-1 to identify the location of urinary structures within the body.

The kidneys perform the major work of the urinary system. The other parts of the system are mainly passageways and storage areas. The functions of the kidneys include regulating the amount of water in the body and keeping body fluids at a constant concentration and acid–base level. They achieve these functions by filtering blood and excreting waste substances and excess water as urine. Other essential substances are reabsorbed into the bloodstream by the process called **reabsorption.**

The filtering–reabsorption process is necessary to maintain the balance of substances required for a relatively stable internal body environment. This stable internal environment, known as **homeostasis,** is necessary for the cells of the body to survive and carry out their functions effectively. If the kidneys fail, waste substances cannot be eliminated from the body. Thus, waste substances accumulate in blood to toxic levels, and cells can no longer function. Death ultimately results unless impurities are filtered out of blood by means of an artificial filtration system, such as hemodialysis or peritoneal dialysis. Otherwise, the nonfunctioning kidneys may be replaced with donor kidneys from a live or deceased person through kidney transplantation.

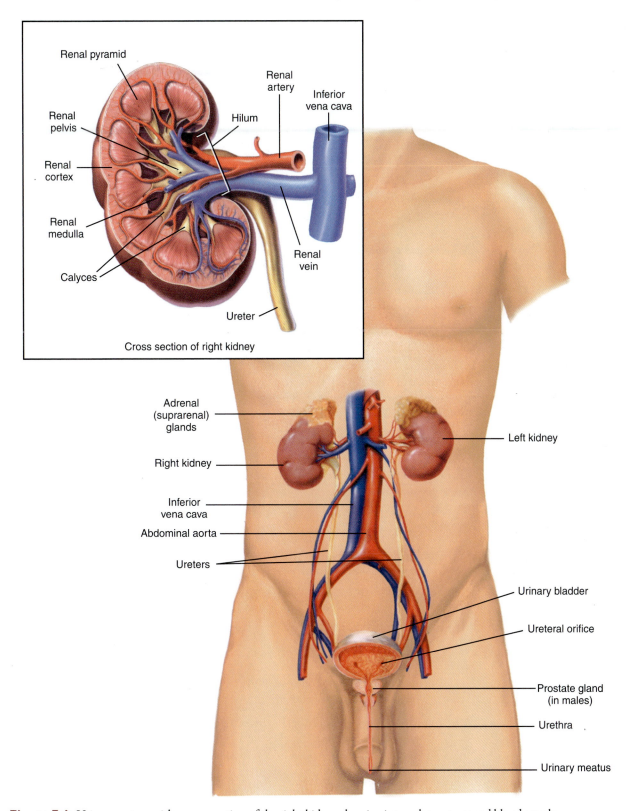

Figure 7-1 Urinary system with a cross section of the right kidney showing internal structures and blood vessels.

WORD ELEMENTS

This section introduces word elements related to the urinary system. Review the word elements and their meanings in the following table. Then, pronounce each term in the word analysis column, and place a ✓ in the box after you do so.

Word Element	Meaning	Word Analysis
Combining Forms		
cyst/o	bladder	**cyst/o**/scopy (sĭs-TŎS-kō-pē ☐) visual examination of the urinary tract using a cystoscope inserted through the urethra *-scopy:* visual examination *Cystoscopy helps diagnose urinary tract disorders, obtain tissue and urine samples, excise tumors, or inject a contrast medium into the bladder.*
vesic/o		**vesic/o**/cele (VĔS-ĭ-kō-sēl ☐) hernial protrusion of the urinary bladder; also called cystocele *-cele:* hernia, swelling
glomerul/o	glomerulus	**glomerul**/ar (glō-MĔR-ū-lăr ☐) pertaining to the glomerulus *-ar:* pertaining to *The glomerulus is a cluster of capillaries forming the structural and functional unit of the kidney known as the nephron. Glomerular capillaries filter blood, the first step in urine formation.*
meat/o	opening, meatus	**meat**/us (mē-Ā-tŭs ☐) opening or tunnel through any part of the body, such as the external opening of the urethra *-us:* condition, structure
nephr/o	kidney	**nephr**/oma (nĕ-FRŌ-mă ☐) tumor of the kidney *oma:* tumor
ren/o		**ren**/al (RĒ-năl ☐) pertaining to the kidney *-al:* pertaining to
pyel/o	renal pelvis	**pyel/o**/plasty (PĪ-ĕ-lō-plăs-tē ☐) surgical repair of the renal pelvis *-plasty:* surgical repair
ur/o	urine, urinary tract	**ur**/emia (ū-RĒ-mē-ă ☐) excessive urea and other nitrogenous waste products in *-emia:* blood condition *Healthy kidneys remove waste and extra water from the blood. Uremia occurs when there are abnormally high levels of waste products due to renal failure.*
urin/o		**urin**/ary (Ū-rĭ-nār-ē ☐) pertaining to urine or the formation of urine or the urinary tract *-ary:* pertaining to
ureter/o	ureter	**ureter/o**/stenosis (ū-rē-tĕr-ō-stě-NŌ-sĭs ☐) narrowing or stricture of a ureter *-stenosis:* narrowing, stricture
urethr/o	urethra	**urethr/o**/cele (ū-RĒ-thrō-sēl ☐) hernial protrusion of the urethra *-cele:* hernia, swelling *Urethrocele may be congenital or acquired and secondary to obesity, childbirth, and poor muscle tone.*
Suffixes		
-emia	blood condition	azot/**emia** (ăz-ō-TĒ-mē-ă ☐) excessive amounts of nitrogenous compounds in blood *azot:* nitrogenous compounds *Azotemia is a toxic condition caused by the kidneys' failure to remove urea from blood.*

Word Element	Meaning	Word Analysis
-iasis	abnormal condition (produced by something specified)	lith/**iasis** (lĭth-Ī-ă-sĭs ☐) abnormal condition of stones or calculi *lith:* stone, calculus *Calculi occur most commonly in the kidney, lower urinary tract, and gallbladder.*
-lysis	separation; destruction; loosening	dia/**lysis** (dī-ĂL-ĭ-sĭs ☐) process of removing toxic wastes from blood when the kidneys are unable to do so *dia-:* through, across
-pathy	disease	nephr/o/**pathy** (nĕ-FRŎP-ă-thē ☐) disease of the kidneys *nephr:* kidney
-pexy	fixation (of an organ)	nephr/o/**pexy** (NĚF-rō-pĕks-ē ☐) surgical procedure to affix a displaced kidney *nephr/o:* kidney
-ptosis	prolapse, downward displacement	nephr/o/**ptosis** (nĕf-rŏp-TŌ-sĭs ☐) downward displacement or dropping of a kidney *nephr/o:* kidney
-tripsy	crushing	lith/o/**tripsy** (LĬTH-ō-trĭp-sē ☐) crushing of a stone *lith/o:* stone, calculus *Lithotripsy is a surgical procedure that employs sound waves to crush a stone in the kidney, ureter, bladder, or gallbladder. The fragments may then be expelled or washed out.*
-uria	urine	poly/**uria** (pŏl-ē-Ū-rē-ă ☐) excessive urination *poly-:* many, much

Pronunciation Help	*Long Sound*	ā in rāte	ē in rēbirth	ī in īsle	ō in ōver	ū in ūnite
	Short Sound	ă in ălone	ĕ in ĕver	ĭ in ĭt	ŏ in nŏt	ŭ in cŭt

Visit the *Medical Terminology Simplified* online resource center at FADavis.com for an audio exercise of the terms in this table. It will help you master pronunciations and meanings of medical terms.

SECTION REVIEW 7-1

For the following medical terms, first, write the suffix and its meaning. Then, translate the meaning of the remaining elements starting with the first part of the word. The first word is completed for you.

Term	Meaning
1. glomerul/o/scler/osis	-osis: abnormal condition, increase (used primarily with blood cells); glomerulus; hardening, sclera (white of the eye)
2. cyst/o/scopy	visual examination of the bladder
3. poly/uria	More urine
4. lith/o/tripsy	Stones / Calculi
5. dia/lysis	Separation
6. ureter/o/stenosis	Ureter
7. meat/us	Opening
8. ur/emia	blood Condition
9. nephr/oma	tumor of the kidney
10. azot/emia	excessive nitrogenous substance in blood

Competency Verification: Check your answers in Appendix B: Answer Key, page 603. If you are not satisfied with your level of comprehension, review the vocabulary, and retake the review.

Correct Answers _____ × 10 = _____ % Score

Macroscopic Structures

The macroscopic structures that make up the urinary system include two kidneys, two ureters, a bladder, and a urethra.

Kidneys

7-1   Label the urinary structures in Figure 7-2 as you read the following material:

The urinary system is composed of a (1) **right kidney** and a left kidney. These are the primary structural units responsible for urine formation. Each kidney is composed of an outer layer, called the (2) **renal cortex,** and an inner region, called the (3) **renal medulla.** Blood enters the kidneys through the (4) **renal artery** and leaves through the (5) **renal vein.** Inside the kidney, the renal artery branches into smaller arteries called arterioles that lead into microscopic filtering units called (6) **nephrons.** Each nephron is designed to filter urea and other waste products effectively from blood.

Pink indicates a prefix. Blue indicates a suffix. Boldface indicates a word root or combining form.

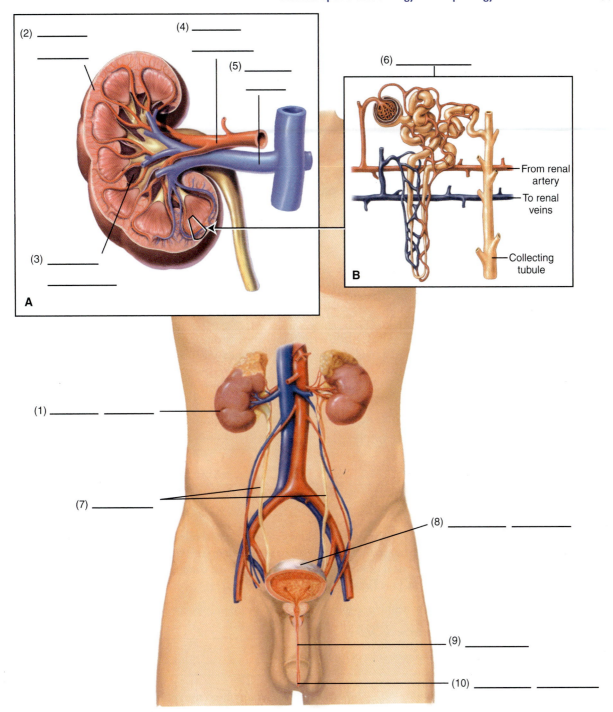

Figure 7-2 Urinary system. (A) Cross section of a right kidney showing internal structures and blood vessels. (B) Single nephron with a collecting duct and associated blood vessels.

---

kidney(s)	**7–2** The combining forms (CFs) **nephr/o** and **ren/o** refer to the kidneys. Whenever you see terms, such as *nephr/itis* and *ren/al,* you will know they refer to the

_____ *nephro* _____.

ren/al RĒ-năl **nephr/ectomy** ně-FRĔK-tō-mē	**7-3** Nephr/ectomy is a surgical procedure to remove a diseased kidney. Alternatively, a healthy kidney may be removed from a donor so that it can be transplanted into a patient with ren/al failure. Identify the terms in this frame that mean *pertaining to a kidney:* <u>ren</u> / <u>al</u>. *excision of a kidney:* <u>nephr</u> / <u>ectomy</u>

nephr/ectomy ně-FRĔK-tō-mē	**7-4** A diseased kidney, such as in ren/al cancer, may necessitate its removal. Use **nephr/o** to form a word that means excision of a kidney. _____ / _____

(!)   If you had difficulty deciding whether to use **nephr/o** or **ren/o** in the previous frames, refer to your medical dictionary. Until you master the language of medicine, the dictionary will help you identify commonly used terms in medicine.

lith/iasis lĭth-Ī-ă-sĭs	**7-5** The CF **lith/o** refers to a stone or calculus; the suffix *-iasis* describes an abnormal condition (produced by something specified). An abnormal condition of stones is called <u>lith</u> / <u>iasis</u>.

nephr/o/lith NĔF-rō-lĭth **nephr/o/lith/iasis** něf-rō-lĭth-Ī-ă-sĭs	**7-6** Use **nephr/o** to construct a medical word that means *stone (in the) kidney:* _____ / _____ / _____. *abnormal condition of kidney stone(s):* _____ / _____ / _____ / _____.

nephr/algia ně-FRĂL-jē-ă **nephr/itis** něf-RĪ-tĭs	**7-7** Formation of a kidney stone, or ren/al calculus, can vary in size from micro/scop/ic (commonly referred to as sand or gravel) to a stone large enough to block the ureter or fill the ren/al pelvis. The stone commonly causes nephr/itis and nephr/algia. (See Figure 7–3 and Figure 7-4.) Use nephr/o to build a word that means *pain in the kidney:* _____ / _____. *inflammation of the kidney:* _____ / _____.

stone	**7-8** *Nephr/o/lith* and *ren/al calculus* mean the patient suffers from a kidney _____.

lith/ectomy lĭ-THĔK-tō-mē **lith/o/tripsy** LĬTH-ō-trĭp-sē	**7-9** Nephr/o/lith/iasis occurs when salts in the urine precipitate (settle out of the solution and grow in size). Elimination of the stone(s) may occur spontaneously, but crushing the stone(s) by means of lith/o/tripsy may sometimes be necessary. Build medical terms that mean *excision of a stone:* _____ / _____. *crushing a stone:* _____ / _____ / _____.

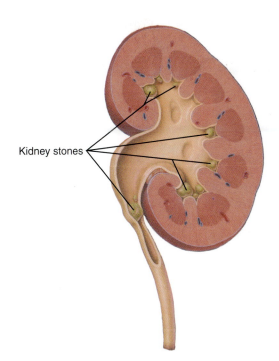

Figure 7-3 Kidney stones shown in the calices and ureter.

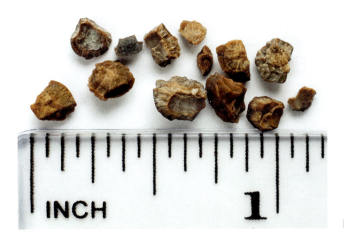

Figure 7-4 Surgically removed kidney stones.

| US | **7-10** Extracorporeal shock-wave lithotripsy (ESWL) is a surgical procedure for treating ren/al calculi. Powerful ultrasound (US) vibrations break up and destroy calculi in the urinary tract. (See Figure 7-5.) The calculi and their fragments are removed during urination and by administration of an oral dissolution drug. |
| ESWL | Write the abbreviation that means |

ultrasound: ___US___.

extracorporeal shock-wave lithotripsy: _ESWL_.

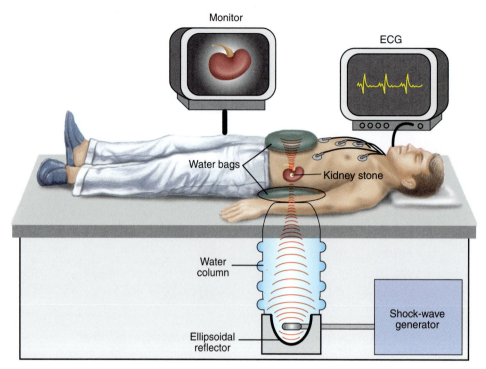

Monitor

ECG

Water bags — Kidney stone

Water column

Shock-wave generator

Ellipsoidal reflector

Figure 7-5 Extracorporeal shock-wave lithotripsy.

7–11 Surgical suffixes *-ectomy, -tomy,* and *-tome* are commonly confusing to beginning medical terminology students. To reinforce your understanding of their meanings, review them in the following chart:

Surgical Suffix	Meaning
-ectomy	excision, removal
-tomy ✓	incision
-tome ✓	instrument to cut

7–12 Stones trapped in the kidney or ureter may be removed surgically. (See Figure 7-4.)

Nephr/o/lith/o/tomy is an _____ to remove a ren/al

incision, stone *or* calculus

_____.

ren/al RĒ-năl **sten/osis** stĕ-NŌ-sĭs **glomerul/o/nephr/itis** glō-mĕr-ū-lō-nĕ-FRĪ-tĭs **hyper/tension** hī-pĕr-TĔN-shŭn	**7-13** Ren/al hyper/tension produced by kidney disease is the most common type of hyper/tension caused by glomerul/o/nephr/itis or ren/al artery sten/osis. Identify terms in this frame that mean *pertaining to the kidney(s):* _____/_____. *narrowing, stricture:* _____·/_____. *inflammation of the glomerulus of the kidney:* _____/_____/_____/_____. *high blood pressure:* _____/_____.
protein/uria prō-tēn-Ū-rē-ă	**7-14** Nephr/o/tic syndrome, a group of symptoms characterized by chronic loss of protein in urine (protein/uria), leads to depletion of body protein, especially albumin. Normally, albumin and other serum proteins maintain fluid levels within the vascular space. When levels of these proteins are low, fluid leaks from blood vessels into tissues, resulting in edema. The syndrome may also occur as a result of other disease processes. Loss of protein in the urine is called _____/_____.
swelling — edema.	**7-15** Many disorders manifest fluid retention (excess fluid in tissues). A characteristic of nephr/o/tic syndrome is edema (swelling), especially around the ankles, feet, and eyes. The term *edema* indicates _____.
diuretic dī-ū-RĔT-ĭc	**7-16** Diuretics are drugs prescribed to control edema and stimulate the flow of urine. Edema around the ankles and feet may also be caused by eating a diet high in sodium. When this condition occurs, the physician may recommend a low-sodium diet and prescribe a drug known as a _____.
supra- **ren** **-al**	**7-17** Supra/ren/al is a directional term that means above the kidney. Identify elements in this frame that mean *above, excessive, superior:* _supra·_____. *kidney:* _ren_____. *pertaining to:* _al_____.
scler/o	**7-18** The CF *scler/o* is used in words to indicate hardening of a body part. It also refers to the sclera (white of the eye). To indicate a hardening, use the CF _____/_____.
hardening	**7-19** *Scler/osis* is an abnormal condition of _____.

nephr/osis
něf-RŌ-sĭs

nephr/o/scler/osis
něf-rō-sklě-RŌ-sĭs

nephr/o/lith
NĚF-rō-lĭth

nephr/o/lith/iasis
něf-rō-lĭth-Ī-ă-sĭs

7-20 Hyper/tension damages kidneys by causing scler/o/tic changes, such as arteri/o/scler/osis with thickening and hardening of ren/al blood vessels (nephr/o/scler/osis). Recall that *-iasis* is used to denote an abnormal condition (produced by something specified).

Use *nephr/o* to form medical words that mean

abnormal condition of a kidney: _____/_____.

abnormal condition of kidney hardening:

_____/_____/_____/_____.

calculus in a kidney: _____/_____/_____.

abnormal condition of kidney stone(s):

_____/_____/_____/_____.

---

nephr/o/megaly
něf-rō-MĔG-ă-lē

nephr/o/rrhaphy
něf-ROR-ă-fē

nephr/o/tomy
ně-FRŎT-ō-mē

nephr/o/lith/o/tomy
něf-rō-lĭth-ŎT-ō-mē

7-21 Many kidney disorders can be treated surgically. Learn these procedures by building surgical terms with *nephr/o* that mean

enlargement of a kidney:

_____/_____/_____.

suture of a kidney: _____/_____/_____.

incision of the kidney: _____/_____/_____.

incision (to remove a) kidney stone:

_____/_____/_____/_____/_____.

---

per/cutane/ous nephr/o/stomy
pĕr-kū-TĀ-nē-ŭs
ně-FRŎS-tō-mē

7-22 When urine cannot pass from the kidney through the ureter because of a blockage, a **per/cutane/ous nephr/o/stomy** may be performed. This surgical procedure creates an opening between the kidney (bypassing the ureters and bladder) and the skin. Its purpose is to drain urine through a **nephrostomy tube** (catheter) and into a collecting receptacle outside the body. (See Figure 7-6.)

What type of surgery is commonly performed to provide urinary drainage when the ureter is obstructed by a calculus?

_____/_____/_____ _____/_____/_____.

---

catheter
KĂTH-ě-tĕr

7-23 The nephrostomy tube is a small, flexible, rubber tube inserted into the skin through the back or flank into the kidney to drain urine into an outside receptacle.

Another term for a nephrostomy tube is _____.

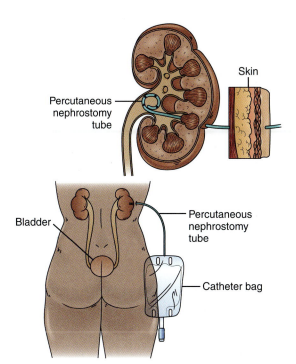

Figure 7-6 Percutaneous nephrostomy.

---

per- **-ous** **cutane** pĕr-kū-TĀ-nē-ŭs **nephr/o** **-stomy**	**7-24** A benefit of **per/cutane/ous nephr/o/stomy** is that it allows the kidney to function properly and protects it from further damage. Identify the word element in this frame that means *through:* __per__ . *pertaining to:* __ous__ . *skin:* __cutane__ . *kidney:* __nephr__ / __o__ . *forming an opening (mouth):* __stomy__ . *(handwritten: percutaneous nephrostomy)*

nephr/o/ptosis nĕf-rŏp-TŌ-sĭs	**7-25** A kidney may prolapse from its normal position because of a birth defect or injury. The downward displacement may occur because the kidney supports are weakened as a result of a sudden strain or blow. This condition is called *nephr/o/ptosis*, or *floating kidney*. A prolapsed kidney is charted in a medical record as _____/_____/_____.

-ptosis **nephr/o**	**7-26** Determine the element in *nephr/o/ptosis* that means *prolapse, downward displacement:* _____. *kidney:* _____/_____.

nephr/o/pexy NĔF-rō-pĕks-ē	**7-27** Nephr/o/ptosis can be treated surgically. Use *-pexy* to build a surgical term that means *fixation of the kidney:* _____/_____/_____.

SECTION REVIEW 7-2

Using the following table, write the CF, suffix, or prefix that matches its definition in the space provided to the left of the definition. There may be more than one word element that matches a definition.

Combining Forms	Suffixes		Prefixes
lith/o	*-iasis*	*-ptosis*	*dia-*
nephr/o	*-megaly*	*-rrhaphy*	*poly-*
ren/o	*-osis*	*-tome*	*supra-*
scler/o	*-pathy*	*-tomy*	
	-pexy		

1. _____ abnormal condition; increase (used primarily with blood cells)
2. __*iasis*__ abnormal condition (produced by something specified)
3. __*supra*__ above; excessive; superior
4. __*pathy*__ disease
5. __*megaly*__ enlargement
6. _____ through, across
7. __*pexy*__ fixation (of an organ)
8. __*scler/o*__ hardening; sclera (white of the eye)
9. __*tome*__ instrument to cut
10. __*tomy*__ incision
11. __*ren/o / nephr/o*__ kidney
12. _____ prolapse, downward displacement
13. __*lith/o*__ stone, calculus
14. __*rrhaphy*__ suture
15. __*poly*__ many, much

Competency Verification: Check your answers in Appendix B: Answer Key, page 603. If you are not satisfied with your level of comprehension, go back to Frame 7–1, and rework the frames.

Correct Answers _____ x 6.67 = _____ % Score

Ureters, Bladder, and Urethra

7-28 The ureters, bladder, and urethra are mainly passageways for transportation, storage, and elimination of urine. Within both kidneys, the renal pelvis narrows to form two muscular tubes called the (7) **ureters.**

Label the ureters in Figure 7-2.

7-29   The contraction of ureteral muscles pushes urine away from the kidneys. It is temporarily stored in the (8) **urinary bladder** until it is expelled from the body through the (9) **urethra** and (10) **urinary meatus** during the process of urination (micturition).

Label Figure 7-2 to locate the urinary structures.

cyst/itis sĭs-TĪ-tĭs **cyst/o/lith/iasis** sĭs-tō-lĭ-THĪ-ă-sĭs **cyst/o/lith/o/tomy** sĭs-tō-lĭth-ŎT-ō-mē	**7-30** The CFs *cyst/o* and *vesic/o* are used in words to refer to the bladder. Use *cyst/o* to form words that mean *inflammation of the bladder:* _____/_____. *abnormal condition of a bladder stone:* _____/_____/_____/_____. *incision of the bladder to remove a stone:* _____/_____/_____/_____/_____.

Competency Verification: Check your labeling of Figure 7-2 in Appendix B: Answer Key, page 603.

py/uria pī-Ū-rē-ă **dys/uria** dĭs-Ū-rē-ă **bacteri/uria** băk-tē-rē-Ū-rē-ă **cyst/itis** sĭs-TĪ-tĭs	**7-31** Cyst/itis is more common in women because of the shorter urethra and the closeness of the urethr/al orifice to the anus. Symptoms of cyst/itis include dys/uria, urgency, and urinary frequency. Urinalysis reveals bacteri/uria and py/uria. *py - pus.* *dys - pain.* Identify the words in this frame that mean *pus in urine:* _____/_____. *painful urination:* _____/_____. *bacteria in urine:* _____/_____. *inflammation of the bladder:* _____/_____.
suture SŪ-chūr	**7-32** The surgical suffix *-rrhaphy* is used in words to mean _____.
ureter/o/rrhaphy ū-rē-tĕr-OR-ră-fē **cyst/o/rrhaphy** sĭs-TOR-ă-fē	**7-33** Construct surgical words that mean *suture of the ureter:* _____/_____/_____. *suture of the bladder:* _____/_____/_____.

bladder

hernia, swelling

rectum
RĔK-tŭm

7–34   A hernia is a protrusion of an anatomical structure through the wall that normally contains it. Hernias may develop in several parts of the body. Examples of hernias are cyst/o/cele and rect/o/cele. (See Figure 7-7.)

A cyst/o/cele is a herniation of part of the urin/ary bladder through the vagin/al wall and is caused by weakened pelv/ic muscles. A rect/o/cele is a herniation of a portion of the rectum toward the vagina through weakened vagin/al muscles.

Define the following word elements in this frame

cyst/o: _____.

-cele: _____, _____.

rect/o: _____.

cyst/o/cele
SĬS-tō-sēl

7–35   Cyst/o/cele develops over years as vaginal muscles weaken and can no longer support the weight of urine in the urinary bladder. This condition usually occurs after a woman has had several deliveries. It also occurs in older people because of weakened pelvic muscles resulting from the aging process.

When the physician diagnoses *herniation of the bladder,* you know the Dx will be charted as a _____ / _____ / _____.

rect/o/cele
RĔK-tō-sēl

7–36   Can you determine the Dx of a patient with a *herniation of the rectum into the vagina?*

_____ / _____ / _____

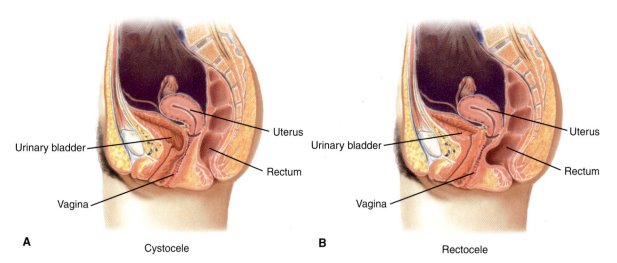

A   Cystocele   **B**   Rectocele

Figure 7-7 Herniations. (A) Cystocele. (B) Rectocele.

cyst/o/scope
SĬST-ō-skōp

cyst/o/scopy,
urethr/o/scopy
sĭs-TŎS-kō-pē, SĬS-tō-ū-rē-THRŎS-kō-pē

7-37 Cyst/o/scopy (cysto), also called *cyst/o/urethr/o/scopy,* is a procedure that uses a rigid or flexible cyst/o/scope inserted into the urinary meatus and through the urethra to examine the urinary bladder. (See Figure 7-8.)

The endo/scope used to perform cyst/o/scopy is called a

_____/_____/_____.

The cyst/o/scope is used to perform the diagnostic procedure called

_____/_____/_____ or

_____/_____/_____/_____/_____.

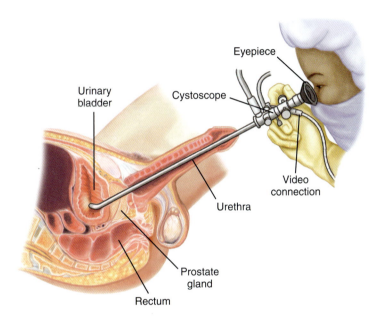

Urinary bladder — Cystoscope — Eyepiece — Video connection — Urethra — Prostate gland — Rectum

Figure 7-8 Cystoscopy of the urinary bladder via the urethra using a cystoscope.

cyst/o/scope
SĬST-ō-skōp

7-38 The cyst/o/scope has an optical lighting system and special lenses and mirrors. It also contains a hollow channel for inserting operative devices to obtain biopsy specimens and remove growths and small stones. A video attachment can be used to create a permanent visual record.

To excise polyps from the bladder, the ur/o/logist uses a special instrument called a

_____/_____/_____.

cyst/o

-scope

radi/o

-graphy

7-39 In addition to inserting operative devices through a cyst/o/scope, the physician may place catheters through the cyst/o/scope to obtain urine samples and to inject a contrast medium into the bladder during radi/o/graphy.

Determine elements in this frame that mean

bladder: _____/_____.

instrument for examining: _____.

radiation, x-ray; radius (lower arm bone on thumb side): _____/_____.

process of recording: _____.

urethr/o	**7-40** The urethra differs in men and women. In men, it serves a dual purpose of conveying sperm and discharging urine from the bladder. The female urethra performs only the latter function. Regardless of the sex, the CF for urethra is _____/_____.
urethr/itis ū-rē-THRĪ-tĭs **urethr/ectomy** ū-rē-THRĔK-tō-mē **urethr/o/pexy** ū-RĒ-thrō-pĕks-ē **urethr/o/plasty** ū-RĒ-thrō-plăs-tē	**7-41** Form medical words that mean *inflammation of the urethra:* _____/_____. *excision of the urethra:* _____/_____. *surgical fixation of the urethra:* _____/_____/_____. *surgical repair of the urethra:* _____/_____/_____.
pain, urethra ū-RĒ-thră	**7-42** *Urethr/algia* and *urethr/o/dynia refer* to _____ in the _____.
urethr/algia ū-rē-THRĂL-jē-ă	**7-43** In addition to *urethr/o/dynia,* construct a word that means *pain in the urethra:* _____/_____.
cyst/itis sĭs-TĪ-tĭs **urethr/itis** ū-rē-THRĪ-tĭs	**7-44** Build words that mean *inflammation of the bladder:* _____/_____. *inflammation of the urethra:* _____/_____.
urinary tract infection	**7-45** Urinary tract infections (UTIs) account for most office visits by patients experiencing urinary tract problems. What does the abbreviation UTI refer to? _____ _____ _____
urethr/al ū-RĒ-thrăl **lumen** LŪ-mĕn **dys/uria** dĭs-Ū-rē-ă	**7-46** *Urethr/al* stricture is a condition of narrowing of the lumen (tubular space within a structure). It is usually caused by infection, cancer, or scar tissue. *Dys/uria* is the primary symptom caused by increased strain from difficulty urinating. Identify the terms in this frame that mean *pertaining to the urethra:* _____/_____. *tubular space within a structure:* _____. *painful urination:* _____/_____.

Pink indicates a prefix. Blue indicates a suffix. Boldface indicates a word root or combining form.

urethr/o/plasty ū-RĒ-thrō-plăs-tē **sten/osis** stĕ-NŌ-sĭs **dys/uria** dĭs-Ū-rē-ă	**7–47** Urethr/al stricture, also called *urethr/al sten/osis,* is treated with the surgical procedure called *urethr/o/plasty.* This procedure is used to relieve dys/uria and recurrent UTIs by restoring unobstructed urine flow. Identify the terms in this frame that mean *surgical repair of the urethra:* _____ / _____ / _____ . *abnormal condition of narrowing or stricture:* _sten_ / _osis_ . *painful urination:* _dys_ / _uria_ .
urethr/o/scope ū-RĒ-thrō-skōp **urethr/o/scopy** ū-rē-THRŎS-kō-pē	**7–48** Form diagnostic terms that mean *instrument for examining the urethra:* _____ / _____ / _____ . *visual examination of the urethra:* _____ / _____ / _____ .
urethr/o/cyst/itis ū-rē-thrō-sĭs-TĪ-tĭs	*-itis urethro cyst* **7–49** Construct a medical word that means *inflammation of urethra and bladder:* _____ / _____ / _____ / _____ . *cystourethritis*
meat/o/tomy mē-ă-TŎT-ō-mē **meat/o/rrhaphy** MĒ-ă-TŎR-ăf-ē	**7–50** The CF *meat/o* means *opening,* or meatus. The urinary meatus is the external opening of the urethra, located at the tip of the penis in males and anterior to the vagina in females. The urinary meatus is where urine is discharged from the body. Use meat/o to construct medical words that mean *incision of the meatus:* _meat_ / _o_ / _tomy_ . *suture of the meatus:* _meat_ / _o_ / _rrhaphy_ .
-ia	**7–51** Identify the element in *-algia, -dynia, -pepsia,* and *-phagia* that means *condition:* _____ .
malignant vmă-LĬG-nănt **benign** bĕ-NĪN	**7–52** Malignant tumors are cancerous; benign tumors are noncancerous. *Use malignant or benign to complete the following statements:* Cancerous tumors are _malignant_ tumors. Noncancerous tumors are _benign_ tumors.
noncancerous	**7–53** Benign tumors do not invade surrounding tissue and are contained within a capsule. They become harmful only when they start placing pressure on adjacent structures. For example, a benign tumor of the uterus may place pressure on the urinary bladder and cause frequent urination. Benign tumors are (cancerous / noncancerous) _____ growths.
cancerous	**7–54** Malignant tumors spread rapidly and are invasive and life-threatening. Malignant tumors are (cancerous / noncancerous) _____ .

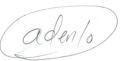

---

pain, gland	**7-55** The CF *aden/o* is used in words to <u>denote</u> a gland. Aden/o/dynia is _____ in a _____.

---

gland **cancer** **tumor**	**7-56** Urin/ary tract tumors may be benign or malignant. The most common malignant ren/al tumor is an aden/o/carcin/oma. Define these elements *aden/o:* _Gland_ *carcin:* _Cancer_ *-oma:* _— tumor_

---

aden/oma văd-ĕ-NŌ-mă **aden/o/carcin/oma** ăd-ĕ-nō-kăr-sĭn-Ō-mă	**7-57** An *aden/oma* is a benign glandular tumor composed of tissue from which it is developing; an *aden/o/carcin/oma* is a <u>malignant glandular tumor</u>. Determine words in this frame that mean *benign glandular tumor:* _aden_ / _oma._ *malignant glandular tumor:* _aden_ / _o_ / _carcin_ / _oma._

adenoma— benign tumor

adenocarcinoma— malignant tumor

SECTION REVIEW 7-3

Using the following table, write the CF or suffix that matches its definition in the space provided to the left of the definition. There may be more than one word element that matches a definition.

Combining Forms

aden/o	ureter/o ✓
carcin/o	urethr/o ✓
cyst/o *bladder*	vesic/o ✗
enter/o	
pyel/o ✓ *renal pelvis*	
rect/o	

Suffixes

-ectomy ✓	-oma ✓
-ectasis ✗	-pathy ✓
-iasis ✓	-plasty ✓
-itis ✓	-rrhaphy ✓
-lith ✓	-scope ✓
-megaly ✓	-tomy ✓

1. ____iasis____ abnormal condition (produced by something specified)
2. ____cyst/o____ bladder
3. ____carcin/o____ cancer
4. ____pnthy____ disease
5. ____megaly____ enlargement
6. ____ectomy____ excision, removal
7. _____ dilation, expansion
8. ____aden____ gland
9. ____tomy____ incision
10. ____-itis____ inflammation
11. ____scope____ instrument for examining
12. _____ intestine (usually small intestine)
13. ____pyel/o____ renal pelvis
14. ____reeto____ rectum
15. ____lith/o____ stone, calculus
16. ____plasty____ surgical repair
17. ____-rrhaphy____ suture
18. ____-oma____ tumor
19. ____ureter/o____ ureter
20. ____urethr/o____ urethra

Competency Verification: Check your answers in Appendix B: Answer Key, page 604. If you are not satisfied with your level of comprehension, go back to Frame 7–28, and rework the frames.

Correct Answers _____ x 5 = _____ % Score

Microscopic Structures

The **nephron** is the functional unit of the kidney. It is the structure that produces urine in the process of removing wastes and excess substances from blood. Each nephron contains a glomerulus and a renal tubule.

7-58 Microscopic examination of the kidney reveals about 1 million nephrons, all of which play a vital role in the maintenance of normal fluid balance (homeostasis) in the body. The nephrons are located within the outer layer of the kidney, called the (1) **renal cortex,** and the inner region, called the (2) **renal medulla.**

The first part of the nephron, the (3) **glomerular capsule,** also called *Bowman* capsule, surrounds a tiny ball of coiled intertwining capillaries known as the (4) **glomerulus. In** the first step of urine production, water, salts, sugar, urea, and other nitrogenous waste products are filtered across the wall of glomerular capillaries and into the glomerular capsule. This waste-containing fluid is known as renal *filtrate.*

Label the structures in Figure 7-9.

7-59 The collection of filtrate in the glomerular capsule flows into the long, twisted tube called the (5) **renal tubule,** where reabsorption of nutrients continues. The reabsorption process ensures that the body retains essential substances, such as glucose, water, and salts. However, waste products of metabolism become toxic if allowed to accumulate in the body. Thus, acids, drugs, and other wastes leave the body in urine. This final process of urine formation occurs in the (6) **collecting tubule** that conveys the newly formed urine to the renal pelvis, which narrows into the ureter. Urine flows through the ureters into the bladder for temporary storage. The bladder eventually expels urine through the urethra during the process of urination.

Label the structures of the nephron in Figure 7-9.

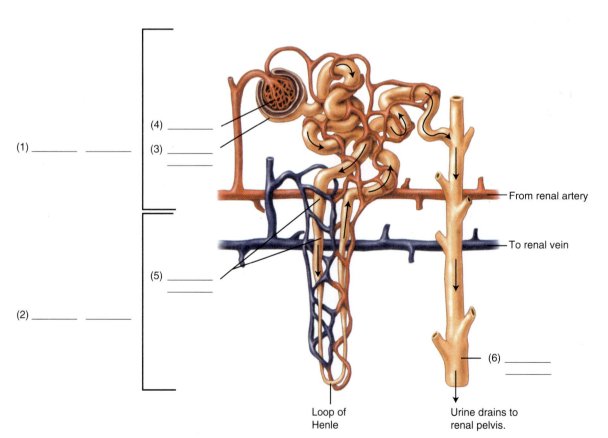

(1) _____ _____

(4) _____

(3) _____
    _____

From renal artery

To renal vein

(5) _____
    _____

(2) _____ _____

(6) _____
    _____

Loop of Henle

Urine drains to renal pelvis.

Figure 7-9 Nephron and associated blood vessels, with arrows indicating the direction of blood flow and flow of renal filtrate.

Pink indicates a prefix. Blue indicates a suffix. Boldface indicates a word root or combining form.

hyper/tension hī-pĕr-TĔN-shŭn	**7-60** Glomerul/o/nephr/itis is an inflammatory disease of the kidney that primarily involves the glomerulus. It is characterized by hyper/tension, olig/uria, electrolyte imbalances, and edema. The CF *olig/o* means *scanty*. Identify terms in this frame that mean *high blood pressure:* _____ / _____. ✓ *diminished capacity to pass urine:* _olig_ / _uria_ . ✓ *swelling (of a body part):* _____. ✓ *inflammation of the glomerulus and kidney:* _____ / ____ / _____ / _____. ✓ ~ itis
olig/uria ŏl-ĭg-Ū-rē-ă	
edema ĕ-DĒ-mă	
glomerul/o/nephr/itis glō-mĕr-ū-lō-nĕ-FRĬ-tĭs	

glomerul/itis glō-mĕr-ū-LĪ-tĭs	**7-61** Use *glomerul/o* to form medical words that mean *inflammation of a glomerulus:* _____ / _____. *disease of a glomerulus:* _____ / ____ / _____.
glomerul/o/pathy glō-mĕr-ū-LŎP-ă-thē	

glomerulus or glomeruli, hardening glō-MĔR-ū-lŭs, glō-MĔR-ū-lī	**7-62** Glomerul/o/scler/osis literally means an abnormal condition of the _____ _____.

Competency Verification: Check your labeling of Figure 7-9 with Appendix B: Answer Key, page 604.

pyel/o/pathy pī-ĕ-LŎP-ă-thē	**7-63** The CF *pyel/o* refers to the renal pelvis, a funnel-shaped chamber that collects urine from the kidney before flowing into the ureter. Use the CF *pyel/o* to construct the word that means *any disease of the renal pelvis:* _____ / ____ / _____.

KUB	**7-64** To determine urinary tract abnormalities, such as tumors, swollen kidneys, and calculi, the physician may order a radi/o/graph/ic examination called *KUB* (kidney, ureter, bladder). The radi/o/graph identifies the location, size, shape, and malformation of the kidneys, ureters, and bladder. Stones and calcified areas may also be detected. The diagnostic test of the kidneys, ureters, and bladder is charted with the abbreviation _____.

renal pelvis—Pyello

7-65   Pyel/o/nephr/itis is a bacterial infection of the ren/al pelvis and kidney caused by bacterial invasion from the middle and lower urinary tract or the bloodstream. Bacteria may gain access to the bladder via the urethra and ascend to the kidney.

pyel/itis
pī-ĕ-LĬ-tĭs

pyel/o/nephr/itis
pī-ĕ-lō-nĕ-FRĪ-tĭs

Form medical words that mean

inflammation of the renal pelvis: _____/_____.

inflammation of the renal pelvis and kidney: _____/_____/_____/

_____.

 Two combining forms that sound alike but have different meanings are **pyel/o** and **py/o**. Here is a useful clarification:

Combining Form	Meaning		Example
pyel/o	renal pelvis		pyel/o/pathy
py/o	pus		py/o/rrhea

pyel/o/plasty
PĪ-ĕ-lō-plăs-tē

pyel/o/gram
PĪ-ĕ-lō-grăm

7-66   Use *pyel/o* (*renal pelvis*) to form medical words that mean

surgical repair of the renal pelvis: _____/_____/_____.

record (x-ray) of the renal pelvis: _____/_____/_____.

py/o/rrhea
pī-ō-RĒ-ă

py/o/nephr/osis
pī-ō-nĕf-RŌ-sĭs

7-67   Use *py/o* (*pus*) to build words that mean

discharge or flow of pus: _____/_____/_____.

abnormal condition of pus from the kidney:

_____/_____/_____/_____.

 Remember not to use *-iasis* because the pus is not produced by something specified; the term just denotes that there is pus in the kidneys.

7-68   An important diagnostic test that provides early detection of ren/al disease is urinalysis (UA). Urine samples are analyzed for abnormalities, such as blood or pus in urine, and other physical and chemical properties. A quick urinalysis can be done with a dipstick test. (See Figure 7-10.)

py/uria
pī-Ū-rē-ă

Hemat/uria is a condition of blood in urine. Form a word that means pus in urine:

_____/_____.

an/uria
ăn-Ū-rē-ă

7-69   The prefixes *a-* and *an-* are used in words to mean without or not. The *a-* is usually used before a consonant; the *an-* is usually used before a vowel.

Construct a word that literally means *without urine:* _____/_____.

Pink indicates a prefix. Blue indicates a suffix. Boldface indicates a word root or combining form.

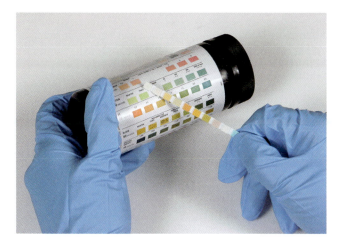

Figure 7-10 Urine dipstick.

rrhea – discharge

---

proxim/al

dist/al

7-70   Hydr/o/nephr/osis is an enlargement of the kidney resulting from constant pressure from backed-up urine in the ureter. It may be caused by a stricture, tumor, or a stone in the proxim/al part of a ureter that obstructs the flow of urine. When obstruction occurs in the dist/al part of the ureter, the condition is called *hydr/o/ureter with hydr/o/nephr/osis.* (See Figure 7-11.)

Identify the terms in this frame that mean

nearest the point of attachment: _____/_____.

farthest from the point of attachment: _____/_____.

---

hydr/o/nephr/osis
hī-drō-něf-RŌ-sĭs

7-71   The presence of ren/al calculi increases the risk of UTIs because they obstruct the free flow of urine. Untreated obstruction of a stone in any of the urin/ary structures can also result in retention of urine and damage to the kidney. (See Figure 7-11.)

Build a word that means *abnormal condition of water (urine) in the kidney:*

_____/_____/_____/_____.

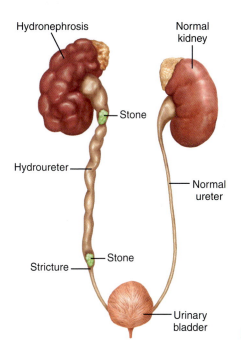

Hydronephrosis

Normal kidney

Stone

Hydroureter

Normal ureter

Stone

Stricture

Urinary bladder

rrhea.

Kidney – nephro

Figure 7-11 Hydronephrosis and hydroureter.

hemat/uria hĕm-ă-TŪ-rē-ă **protein/uria** prō-tēn-Ū-rē-ă	**7–72** A person who suffers from hydr/o/nephr/osis may experience pain, hemat/uria, and py/uria. Blood or pus may be present in urine. Build medical words that mean *blood in urine:* _____/_____. *protein in urine:* _____/_____.
olig/uria ŏl-ĭg-Ū-rē-ă	**7–73** Kidney disease diminishes the kidney's capacity to form urine. Build a word that means *diminished or scanty amount of urine formation.* _____/_____
py/uria pī-Ū-rē-ă	**7–74** *Py/uria* refers to the presence of an excessive number of white blood cells in urine. It is generally a sign of a urinary tract infection. A bacterial infection of the bladder and urethra may result in the condition called _____/_____.
poly/uria pŏl-ē-Ū-rē-ă	**7–75** The prefix *poly-* means many or much. Combine *poly-* and *-uria* to build a word that means excessive urination: _____/_____.
noct/uria nŏk-TŪ-rē-ă	**7–76** Noct/uria refers to frequent, excessive urination at night, and can disrupt sleep. If a person has a tendency to urinate at night during sleep cycle, the condition is known as _____/_____. Nocturia can also be a sign of an underlying condition, such as an infection or diabetes.
urination ū-rĭ-NĀ-shŭn	**7–77** Continence is the ability to retain urine or feces until the proper time for their discharge. A person who has urinary continence is able to control urination. A person with urinary in/continence is not able to control _____.
in/continence ĭn-KŎN-tĭ-nĕns	**7–78** Older patients in nursing homes may experience uncontrolled loss of urine from the bladder. They may suffer from the condition known as urinary _____/_____.
ur/o/logist ū-RŎL-ō-jĭst **nephr/o/logist** nĕ-FRŎL-ō-jĭst	**7–79** Ur/o/logists specialize in treating urin/ary tract disorders; nephr/o/logists specialize in management of kidney disease, kidney transplantation, and dia/lysis. Persons with urin/ary disorders see a medical specialist called a _____/_____/_____. Persons with kidney disorders, including transplantations and dia/lysis, see a medical specialist called a _____/_____/_____.

hemat/uria hĕm-ă-TŪ-rē-ă	**7–80** Cyst/itis, an inflammatory condition of the urin/ary bladder, is commonly caused by bacterial infection and is characterized by pain, frequency of urination, urgency, and, sometimes, hemat/uria. If cyst/itis results in traces of blood in urine, the medical term for this condition is _____/_____.
poly/cyst/ic pŏl-ē-SĬS-tĭk **ren/al** RĒ-năl	**7–81** A healthy kidney eliminates waste from blood and maintains the body's normal chemical balance. An unhealthy kidney causes many different types of diseases. For example, poly/cyst/ic kidney disease (PKD), which is a hereditary disease, is characterized by cysts in the kidney that eventually destroy the nephrons. Ren/al failure commonly develops over time, requiring dialysis or kidney transplantation. (See Figure 7-12.) Identify terms in this frame that mean *pertaining to many cysts:* _____/_____/_____. *pertaining to the kidney:* _____/_____.
hyper/tension hī-pĕr-TĔN-shŭn **poly/cyst/ic** pŏl-ē-SĬS-tĭk	**7–82** In the early stage of PKD, there are few signs. Often, this degenerative disease is not apparent until hyper/tension and enlarged kidneys are detected during a physical examination. The term in this frame that refers to *high blood pressure* is _____/_____. PKD is an abbreviation that means _____/_____/_____ kidney disease.
acute renal failure RĒ-năl	**7–83** Any condition that impairs flow of blood to the kidneys, such as shock, injury, and exposure to toxins, may result in acute renal failure (ARF). The abbreviation ARF refers to _____ _____ _____.

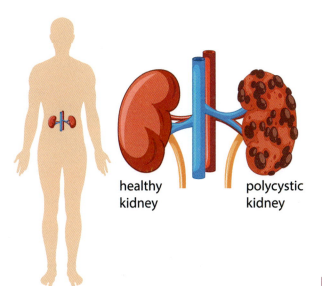

healthy
kidney

polycystic
kidney

Figure 7-12 Polycystic kidney disease.

SECTION REVIEW 7-4

Using the following table, write the CF, suffix, or prefix that matches its definition in the space provided to the left of the definition. There may be more than one word element that matches a definition.

Combining Forms		Suffixes	Prefixes
azot/o	py/o	-cele	a-
cyst/o	ren/o	-ist	an-
glomerul/o	scler/o	-logist	intra-
hemat/o	ureter/o	-ptosis	poly-
nephr/o	urethr/o		
noct/o	ur/o		
olig/o	vesic/o		
pyel/o			

1. _____ bladder

2. _____ blood

3. _____ specialist in the study of

4. _____ glomerulus

5. _____ hardening; sclera (white of the eye)

6. _____ specialist

7. _____ kidney

8. _____ pus

9. _____ nitrogenous compounds

10. _____ renal pelvis

11. _____ scanty

12. _____ ureter

13. _____ urethra

14. _____ urine; urinary tract

15. _____ night

16. _____ hernia, swelling

17. _____ many, much

18. _____ prolapse, downward displacement

19. _____ in, within

20. _____ without, not

Competency Verification: Check your answers in Appendix B: Answer Key, page 604. If you are not satisfied with your level of comprehension, go back to Frame 7–58, and rework the frames.

Correct Answers _____ x 5 =_____ % Score

Abbreviations

This section introduces urinary system–related abbreviations and their meanings. Included are abbreviations contained in the medical record activities that follow.

Abbreviation	Meaning	Abbreviation	Meaning
ARF	acute renal failure	HD	hemodialysis
BNO	bladder neck obstruction	IVP	intravenous pyelogram; intravenous pyelography
BPH	benign prostatic hyperplasia; benign prostatic hypertrophy	IVU	intravenous urogram; intravenous urography
BUN	blood urea nitrogen	KUB	kidney, ureter, bladder (radiographic examination)
C&S	culture and sensitivity	PD	peritoneal dialysis
Cath	catheter, catheterization	PKD	polycystic kidney disease
CRF	chronic renal failure	PSA	prostate-specific antigen
CT	computed tomography	RP	retrograde pyelography
cysto	cystoscopy	TURP	transurethral resection of the prostate
ESRD	end-stage renal disease	UA	urinalysis
ESWL	extracorporeal shock-wave lithotripsy	US	ultrasonography, ultrasound
EU	excretory urography	UTI	urinary tract infection
GFR	glomerular filtration rate	VCUG	voiding cystourethrogram; voiding cystourethrography

Additional Medical Terms

The following are additional terms related to the urinary system. Recognizing and learning these terms will help you understand the connection between a pathological condition, its diagnosis, and the rationale behind the method of treatment selected for a particular disorder.

Diseases and Conditions

azoturia
ăz-ō-TŪ-rē-ă
   azot: nitrogenous
       compounds
   -uria: urine

Increase of nitrogenous substances, especially urea, in urine

diuresis
dī-ū-RĒ-sĭs
   di-: double
   ur: urine
   -esis: condition

Increased formation and secretion of urine

end-stage renal disease (ESRD)
RĒ-năl

Kidney disease that has advanced to the point that the kidneys can no longer adequately filter blood, and ultimately, the patient requires dialysis or renal transplantation for survival; also called *chronic renal failure* (CRF) (See Figure 7-13.)

Common diseases leading to ESRD include malignant hypertension, infections, diabetes mellitus, and glomerulonephritis. Diabetes is the most common cause of kidney transplantation.

enuresis
ĕn-ū-RĒ-sĭs
   en-: in, within
   ur: urine
   -esis: condition

Involuntary discharge of urine after the age at which bladder control should be established; also called *bed-wetting at night* or *nocturnal enuresis*

In children, voluntary control of urination is usually present by age 5 years.

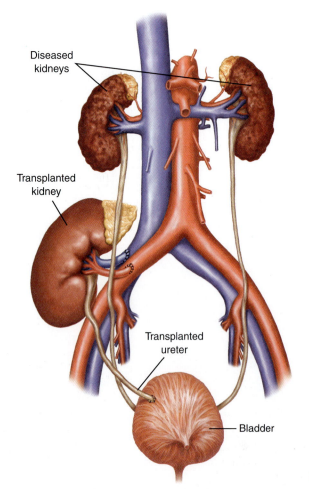

Diseased kidneys

Transplanted kidney

Transplanted ureter

Bladder

Figure 7-13 Renal transplantation.

hypospadias hī-pō-SPĀ-dē-ăs *hypo-:* under, below, deficient *-spadias:* slit, fissure	Abnormal congenital opening of the male urethra on the undersurface of the penis
interstitial nephritis ĭn-tĕr-STĬSH-ăl nĕf-RĪ-tĭs *nephr:* kidney *-itis:* inflammation	Condition associated with pathological changes in the renal interstitial tissue that may be primary or caused by a toxic agent, such as a drug or chemical, which results in the destruction of nephrons and severe impairment in renal function
urgency ĔR-jĕn-sē	Sudden and frequent strong need to urinate *Urgency may be caused by excessive consumption of fluids, alcohol, or caffeine, and pressure on the bladder due to pregnancy or obesity. Urgency may also be a symptom of UTI, enlarged or infected prostate gland, or nerve damage occurring in multiple sclerosis and diabetes.*
Wilms tumor VĬLMZ TOO-mŏr	Malignant neoplasm of the kidney that occurs in young children, usually before the age of 5 years; also called *nephroblastoma* *The most common early signs of Wilms tumor are hypertension, a palpable mass, pain, and hematuria.*

Diagnostic Procedures

blood urea nitrogen (BUN) ū-RĒ-ă NĪ-trō-jĕn	Laboratory test that measures the amount of urea (nitrogenous waste product) in blood and demonstrates the kidneys' ability to filter urea from blood for excretion in urine *An increase in BUN level may indicate impaired kidney function.*
creatinine clearance krē–ĂT-ĭn-ĭn	Laboratory test that measures the rate at which creatinine is cleared from blood by the kidney *Creatinine clearance is the most common, most precise test that uses blood and urine samples to assess kidney function.*
computed tomography (CT) kŏm-PŪ-tĕd tō-MŎG-ră-fē *tom/o:* to cut, slice *-graphy:* process of recording	Tomography in which a narrow beam of x-ray rotates in a full arc around the patient to acquire multiple views of the body, and a computer interprets them to produce cross-sectional images of an internal organ or tissue; also called *computerized axial tomography (CAT) scanning* *CT detects kidney stones, obstructions, renal masses, and other urinary disorders. CT may be performed with or without a contrast medium.*

pyelography pī-ĕ-LŎG-ră-fē 　　*pyel/o:* renal pelvis 　*-graphy:* process of 　　　　　recording	Radiographic study of the kidney, ureters, and, usually, the bladder after injection of a contrast agent *A contrast medium is injected into a vein (intravenous pyelography) or through a catheter placed through the urethra, bladder, or ureter and into the renal pelvis (retrograde pyelography).*
intravenous pyelography (IVP) ĭn-tră-VĒ-nŭs pī-ĕ-LŎG-ră-fē 　　*intra:* in, within 　　*ven:* vein 　　*-ous:* pertaining 　　　　　to 　　*pyel/o:* renal pelvis 　*-graphy:* process of 　　　　　recording	Radiographic imaging in which a contrast medium is injected intravenously and serial x-ray films are taken to provide visualization of the entire urinary tract; also called intravenous urography (IVU) or excretory urography (EU) *In IVP, the x-ray image produced is known as a pyelogram or urogram.*
retrograde pyelography (RP) RĔT-rō-grād pī-ĕ-LŎG-ră-fē 　　*retro-:* backward, 　　　　　behind 　　*-grade:* to go 　　*pyel/o:* renal pelvis 　*-graphy:* process of 　　　　　recording	Radiographic imaging in which a contrast medium is introduced through a cystoscope directly into the bladder and ureters using small-caliber catheters *RP provides detailed visualization of the urinary collecting system (pelvis and calyces of the kidney as well as the ureters). It helps locate any urinary tract obstruction. It may also serve as a substitute for IVP when a patient is allergic to the contrast medium.*
nuclear scan	Radiographic technique that produces images of an organ or area of the body by introducing a radionuclide substance (tracer or radiopharmaceutical) that releases a low level of radiation; also called nuclear scanning, radionuclide imaging, and nuclear medicine scan *The amount of radioactivity used in a nuclear scan is very small and is not known to cause harm.*
renal RĒ-năl 　　*ren:* kidney 　　*-al:* pertaining to	Nuclear scan that determines renal function and shape
ultrasonography (US) ŭl-tră-sŏn-ŎG-ră-fē 　　*-ultra:* excess, beyond 　　*son/o:* sound 　*-graphy:* process of 　　　　　recording	Radiographic procedure in which a small transducer passed over the skin transmits high-frequency sound waves (ultrasound) that bounce off body tissues and are then recorded to produce an image of an internal organ or tissue (See Figure 7-14.) *US provides images of urinary tract structures and detects such abnormalities as tumors, obstructions, and polycystic kidney disease. It also helps measure postvoid residual urine (urine that remains in the bladder after urinating).*

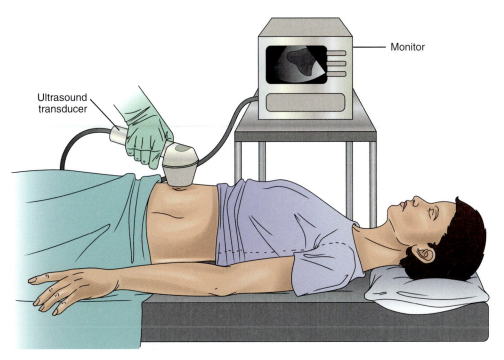

Monitor

Ultrasound transducer

Figure 7-14 Ultrasonography of the bladder.

voiding cystourethrography (VCUG) sĭs-tō-ū-rē-THRŎG-ră-fē *cyst/o:* bladder *urethr/o:* urethra *-graphy:* process of recording	Radiography of the bladder and urethra while the bladder fills and empties *VCUG involves placement of a radiopaque liquid (that can be seen on a radiograph) in the bladder through a catheter. Radiographs taken before, during, and after voiding reveal interior abnormalities of the urethra and bladder and help determine whether urine flow is normal when the bladder empties.*

Medical and Surgical Procedures

catheterization (Cath) kăth-ĕ-tĕr-ĭ-ZĀ-shŭn	Insertion of a catheter (hollow flexible tube) into a body cavity or organ to instill a substance or remove fluid, most commonly through the urethra into the bladder to drain urine *Catheters are available as two basic types: a straight catheter, which is used only for immediate drainage, and a Foley catheter, which is used for short-term and long-term (indwelling) drainage. An inflated balloon keeps the catheter in place. (See Figure 7-15.)*

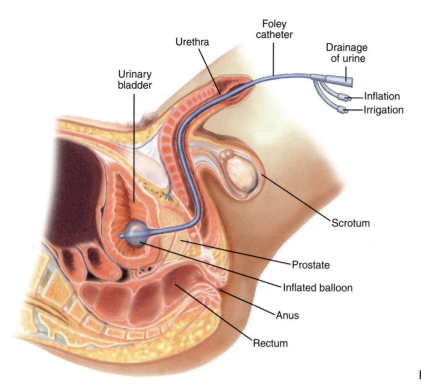

Figure 7-15 Catheterization.

dialysis dī-ĂL-ĭ-sĭs *dia-:* through, across *-lysis:* separation; destruction; loosening	Mechanical filtering process used to clean blood of high concentrations of metabolic waste products, draw off excess fluids, and regulate body chemistry when kidneys fail to function properly *Two primary methods of dialysis are used to dialyze blood: hemodialysis and peritoneal dialysis.*
hemodialysis (HD) hē-mō-dī-ĂL-ĭ-sĭs	Process of removing excess fluids and toxins from blood by continually shunting (diverting) the patient's blood from the body into a dialysis machine for filtering, and then returning the clean blood to the patient's body via tubes connected to the circulatory system (See Figure 7-16.)
peritoneal dialysis (PD) pĕr-ĭ-tō-NĒ-ăl dī-ĂL-ĭ-sĭs	Type of dialysis that uses the peritoneum in a person's abdomen as the membrane through which fluid and dissolved substances are exchanged with the blood (See Figure 7-17.) *It is used to remove excess fluid, correct electrolyte problems, and remove toxins in patients with kidney failure.*

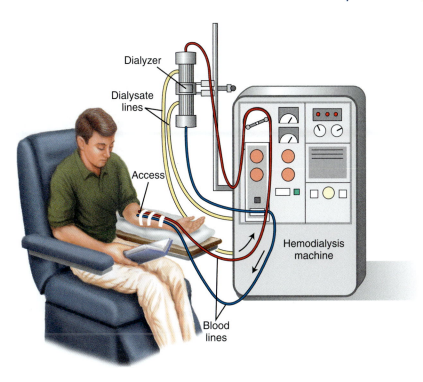

Figure 7-16 Hemodialysis.

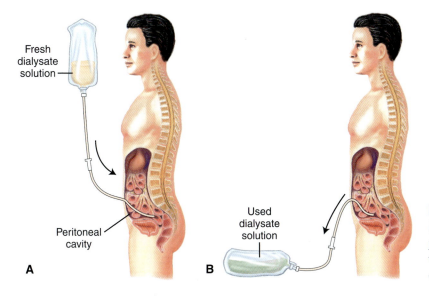

Figure 7-17 Peritoneal dialysis. (A) Introducing dialysis fluid into the peritoneal cavity. (B) Draining dialysate with waste products from the peritoneal cavity.

ureteral stent	Placement of a thin tube into the ureter to prevent or treat obstruction of flow of urine from the kidney
ū-RĒ-tĕr-ăl *ureter:* ureter *-al:* pertaining to	*Indwelling stents require constant monitoring because they may lead to infection, blockage, or stone formation. To avoid complications, they must be removed or changed periodically. (See Figure 7-18.)*

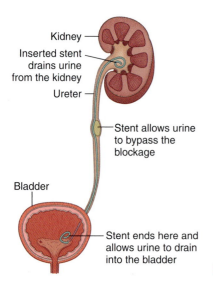

Kidney

Inserted stent drains urine from the kidney

Ureter

Stent allows urine to bypass the blockage

Bladder

Stent ends here and allows urine to drain into the bladder

Figure 7-18 Ureteral stent placement.

Pharmacology

The following table lists common drug categories used to treat urinary disorders, as well as their therapeutic actions.

Drug Category	Action
antibiotics ăn-tĭ-bī-ŎT-ĭks	Kill bacteria that commonly cause urinary tract infections (UTIs) *Most antibiotics come in pill or liquid form. Some may be administered as an injection or intravenously if the patient has a severe kidney infection.*
antidiuretic ăn-tĭ-dī-ū-RĔT-ĭks	Controls fluid balance in the body by reducing urination *Effects of antidiuretic are opposite of diuretics.*
antispasmodics ăn-tĭ-spăz-MŌT-ĭks	Suppress spasms of the ureter, bladder, and urethra by relaxing the smooth muscles lining their walls, thus allowing normal emptying of the bladder
diuretics dī-ū-RĔT-ĭks	Block reabsorption of sodium by the kidneys, thereby increasing the amount of salt and water excreted in the urine *Diuretics promote reduction of fluid retained in body tissues and also prevent edema.*
potassium supplements pō-TĂS-ē-ŭm	Replace potassium loss caused by diuretic drugs *Diuretics increase sodium excretion and also potassium excretion.*

Pronunciation Help	*Long Sound*	ā in rāte	ē in rēbirth	ī in īsle	ō in ōver	ū in ūnite
	Short Sound	ă in ălone	ĕ in ĕver	ĭ in ĭt	ŏ in nŏt	ŭ in cŭt

Word Elements Review

This review provides a verification of your knowledge of the word elements covered in this chapter. First, use a slash to break the term into its component parts, and identify each element by labeling it P for prefix, WR for word root, CF for combining form, or S for suffix. Then, provide the meaning of the medical term. Remember to define the suffix first, define the beginning of the word next, and define the middle part of the term last. The first word is a sample completed for you.

Medical Term	Meaning
nepr/o/lith/o/tomy CF CF S	incision of the kidney to remove a stone or calculus
1. lithotripsy	
2. nephromegaly	
3. uremia	
4. ureterostenosis	
5. vesicocele	

Match the following medical terms with the definitions in the numbered list.

adenocarcinoma   glomerulonephritis   nephroptosis   pyeloplasty
benign   nephralgia   nephrosclerosis   pyuria
cystocele   nephropexy   pyelography   urethroplasty

6. _____pyuria_____ presence of pus in urine, typically from bacterial infection
7. _____nephralgia_____ pain in the kidneys
8. _____cystocele_____ hernial protrusion of the urinary bladder   *cele·*
9. _____nephrosclerosis_____ abnormal hardening of the kidneys
10. _____pyeloplasty·_____ surgical repair of the renal pelvis
11. _____adenocarcinoma·_____ cancerous tumor of a gland
12. _____pyelography_____ radiography or process of recording the renal pelvis
13. _____benign·_____ noncancerous tumor   *its·*
14. _____glomerulonephritis_____ inflammation of the glomerulus
15. _____nephroptosis_____ prolapse, downward displacement of kidneys

---

Competency Verification: Check your answers in Appendix B: Answer Key, page 604. If you are not satisfied with your level of comprehension, review the vocabulary, and retake the review.

Correct Answers _____ x 6.67 = _____ % Score

Additional Medical Terms Review

Match the following medical term(s) with the definitions in the numbered list.

antibiotics	*dialysis*	*hemodialysis*	*uremia*
azoturia	*diuresis*	*interstitial nephritis*	*US*
BUN	*diuretics*	*renal hypertension*	*VCUG*
catheterization	*enuresis*	*retrograde pyelography*	*Wilms tumor*

1. _____ prevent edema by blocking reabsorption of sodium in the kidneys.

2. _____ is a malignant neoplasm in the kidney that occurs in young children.

3. _____ is an increase in nitrogenous compounds in urine.

4. _____ are used in the treatment and prevention of bacterial infections.

5. _____ means increased formation and secretion of urine.

6. _____ is a radiological technique in which a contrast medium is introduced through a cystoscope to provide detailed visualization of the urinary collecting system.

7. _____ uses an artificial kidney machine to filter blood when the kidneys fail to function.

8. _____ is associated with pathological changes in the renal tissue, which may be primary or caused by a toxic agent.

9. _____ is a test that measures the amount of urea excreted by kidneys into blood.

10. _____ means urinary incontinence, including bed-wetting.

11. _____ refers to insertion of a hollow, flexible tube into a body cavity or organ to instill a substance or remove fluid.

12. _____ is radiography of the bladder and urethra after introduction of a contrast medium and during the process of urination.

13. _____ refers to an elevated level of urea and other nitrogenous waste products in blood.

14. _____ refers to high blood pressure that results from kidney disease.

15. _____ is the mechanical filtering process used to remove high concentrations of metabolic waste products from blood.

Competency Verification: Check your answers in Appendix B: Answer Key, page 604. If you are not satisfied with your level of comprehension, review the pathological, diagnostic, and therapeutic terms, and retake the review.

Correct Answers _____ × 6.67 = _____ % Score

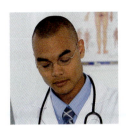

Medical Record Activities

To develop a working vocabulary of medical terms and understand how those terms are used in the health-care industry, it is important that you complete the following activities.

MEDICAL RECORD ACTIVITY 7-1

HOSPITAL ADMISSION: BENIGN PROSTATIC HYPERTROPHY, CARCINOMA OF THE COLON

This activity contains a hospital report in which a patient is admitted for a colectomy. Read the hospital report that follows, and underline the medical terms. Then, complete the terminology and critical thinking exercises.

HOSPITAL ADMISSION

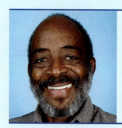

PATIENT NAME: Jenkins, James
MEDICAL RECORD ID: 34-220987
DATE: September 5, 20xx

HISTORY OF PRESENT ILLNESS: Patient is a 65-year-old black male with symptoms of dysuria and urinary frequency before this admission. He recently was found to have colon cancer and is being admitted for colectomy. Preoperative catheterization was not possible, and consultation with Dr. Moriarty was obtained.

PAST HISTORY: Negative for transurethral resection of the prostate or any urological trauma or venereal disease. Past medical history includes hemorrhoid symptoms, bilateral inguinal hernia repair, high cholesterol, retinal surgery, spontaneous pneumothorax ×2 requiring chest tube insertion. He also had a basal cell carcinoma.

PHYSICAL EXAMINATION: Head: Normocephalic. **Eyes, Ears, Nose, and Throat:** Within normal limits. **Neck:** No nodes. No bruits over carotids. **Chest:** Clear to auscultation and percussion.

Heart: Normal heart sounds. No murmur. **Abdomen:** Soft and nontender. No masses palpable. Very distended.

Genitalia: Normal. **Rectal:** Examination revealed benign prostatic hypertrophy.

ASSESSMENT: 1. Mild to moderate benign prostatic hypertrophy.
2. Status post colon resection for carcinoma of the colon.

PLAN: Admit patient to surgery for a colectomy.

Anthony D'Augustino, M.D.

Anthony D'Augustino, M.D.

AD: br

D: 9-5-20xx; T: 9-5:20xx

Terminology 7-1

Terms listed in the following table come from the previous hospital admission report. Use a medical dictionary, such as Taber's Cyclopedic Medical Dictionary; the appendices of this book; or other resources to define each term. Then, pronounce the term, and place a checkmark (✓) in the box after you do so.

Term	Definition
auscultation aws-kŭl-TĀ-shŭn ☐	
basal cell carcinoma BĀ-săl SĔL kăr-sĭ-NŌ-mă ☐	
benign prostatic hypertrophy bē-NĪN prŏs-TĂT-ĭk hī-PĔR-trŏ-fē ☐	
bruits BRWĒZ ☐	
catheterization kăth-ĕ-tĕr-ĭ-ZĀ-shŭn ☐	
impotence ĬM-pō-tĕns ☐	
inguinal hernia ĬNG-gwĭ-năl HĔR-nē-ă ☐	
normocephalic nor-mō-sĕ-FĂL-ĭk ☐	
palpable PĂL-pă-bl ☐	
percussion pĕr-KŬSH-ŭn ☐	
pneumothorax nū-mō-THŌ-răks ☐	

Critical Thinking 7-1

Review the hospital admission report to answer the following questions. Use a medical dictionary, such as Taber's Cyclopedic Medical Dictionary, *and other resources, if needed.*

1. What prompted the consultation with the urologist, Dr. Moriati?

_____

_____

2. What abnormality did the urologist discover?

_____

_____

3. Did the patient have any previous surgery on his prostate?

_____

_____

4. Where was the patient's hernia?

_____

_____

5. What in the patient's past medical history contributed to his present urological problem?

_____

_____

MEDICAL RECORD ACTIVITY 7-2

PROGRESS NOTE: CYSTITIS

This activity describes an outpatient clinical visit in which the patient is diagnosed with cystitis. Read the progress note that follows, and underline the medical terms. Then, complete the terminology and critical thinking exercises.

PROGRESS NOTE

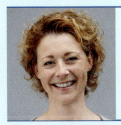

PATIENT NAME: Huggins, Rosa
MEDICAL RECORD ID: 79-15892
DATE: May 25, 20xx

CHIEF COMPLAINT: This 52-year-old white woman has been complaining of diffuse pelvic pain with urinary bladder spasm since cystoscopy 10 days ago, at which time marked cystitis was noted.

PAST HISTORY: The patient reports nocturia three to four times, urinary frequency, urinary urgency, and epigastric discomfort. She has a history of polyuria, hematuria, and urinary incontinence. There is a history of numerous stones, large and small, in the gallbladder. In 20xx, she was admitted to the hospital with cholecystitis, chronic and acute; cholelithiasis; and choledocholithiasis. Subsequently, cholecystectomy, choledocholithotomy, and incidental appendectomy were performed.

IMPRESSION: Urinary incontinence is caused by cystitis and is temporary in nature.

PLAN: 1. Ciprofloxacin 250 mg for 7 days.
      2. Patient instructed to call if symptoms persist.

Stanley Josephson, M.D.

Stanley Josephson, M.D.

SJ: ba
D: 05//25/20xx; T: 05//25/20xx

Terminology 7-2

Terms listed in the following table come from the previous progress note. Use a medical dictionary, such as Taber's Cyclopedic Medical Dictionary; *the appendices of this book; or other resources to define each term. Then, pronounce the term, and place a checkmark (✓) in the box after you do so.*

Term	Definition
cholecystectomy kō-lē-sĭs-TĔK-tō-mē ☐	
choledocholithiasis kō-lĕd-ō-kō-lĭ-THĪ-ă-sĭs ☐	
choledocholithotomy kō-lĕd-ō-kō-lĭth-ŎT-ō-mē ☐	
cholelithiasis kō-lē-lĭ-THĪ-ă-sĭs ☐	
cystoscopy sĭs-TŎS-kō-pē ☐	
hematuria hĕm-ă-TŪ-rē-ă ☐	
nocturia nŏk-TŪ-rē-ă ☐	
polyuria pŏl-ē-Ū-rē-ă ☐	
urinary incontinence Ū-rĭ-nār-ē ĭn-KŎNT-ĭn-ĕns ☐	

Visit the *Medical Terminology Simplified* online resource center at FADavis.com to hear pronunciation and meanings of selected terms in this medical report.

Critical Thinking 7-2

Review the previous progress note to answer the following questions. Use a medical dictionary, such as Taber's Cyclopedic Medical Dictionary, *and other resources, if needed.*

1. What was found when the patient had a cystoscopy?

_____

_____

2. What are the symptoms of cystitis?

_____

_____

3. What is the patient's past surgical history?

_____

_____

4. What is the treatment for cystitis?

_____

_____

5. What are the dangers of untreated cystitis?

_____

_____

6. What instrument is used to perform a cystoscopy?

_____

_____

MEDICAL RECORD ACTIVITY 7-3

CLINICAL APPLICATION

This activity is a clinical application that will help you integrate and reinforce your understanding of how the following medical terms are used in the clinical environment.

Azoturia	cystoscopy	enuresis	nephrolithiasis
BUN	cystourethrography	hypertension	uremia
Catheterization	dialysis	hypospadias	Wilms tumor

Complete the clinically related sentences by selecting a medical term from the previous list.

1. Elliott, a 68-year-old male, presents with complaints of dysuria, hematuria, urinary urgency, and urinary frequency. The physician inserts a tube through the urethra to visualize the bladder and obtain specimens for biopsy. This procedure is called a(n) ___Cystoscopy___.

2. Joseph, a 6-year-old boy, is brought to the clinic by his mother. She tells the physician that Joseph wets his bed several times a week and that many nights he wakes her up to take him to the toilet. This involuntary discharge of urine is known as ___Enuresis___.

3. This 74-year-old female nursing home patient is seen with complaints of nausea, vomiting, lack of appetite, and itching of the skin. She has a history of chronic renal failure. Her physician orders a blood test to determine the level of urea. This laboratory test is called a(n) _____.

4. Mike is a 58-year-old male who is diagnosed with urine retention caused by benign prostatic hypertrophy. To withdraw urine from his bladder, the physician performs a procedure in which a hollow flexible tube is inserted into the bladder through his urethra. This procedure is known as a(n) _____.

5. Betty is a 55-year-old female who presents with a history of diabetic nephropathy. While reviewing her laboratory test results, the physician notes a decrease in renal function that has resulted in elevated levels of waste products in her blood. The physician diagnoses this condition as _____.

6. A 44-year-old male presents with a complaint of left flank pain that comes on suddenly and spreads to the groin. After the examination, the physician orders additional tests to confirm a diagnosis of stones in the kidneys, a condition called _____.

7. Ms. L is a 38-year-old female who suffers from type 2 diabetes and stage 2 chronic kidney disease. The physician notes her blood pressure is elevated and explains it is the result of her kidney disease. The high blood pressure is a condition called renal _____.

8. Jenny, 3 years old, is brought to the clinic with fever, abdominal pain, and urine with a pink tint. The pediatrician detects a palpable abdominal mass and elevated blood pressure. She suspects a neoplasm of the kidney. More tests are ordered to confirm the suspected diagnosis of _____.

9. Mrs. K, a 66-year-old female, presents with end-stage renal disease. Her physician explains that her kidneys are no longer able to remove metabolic waste products from her blood. He tells her that she needs to have the waste products removed from her kidneys by a mechanical filtering process known as _____.

10. Mrs. M presents with complaints of chronic urinary tract infections. A test is ordered to assess her bladder function. During the test, a contrast medium will be administered and the physician will observe the flow of urine while she is voiding. This radiographic procedure is known as voiding _____.

Competency Verification: Check your answers in Appendix B: Answer Key, page 605. If you are not satisfied with your level of comprehension, review the material in this chapter, and retake the review.

Number of correct responses: _____ × 10 = _____ % Score

URINARY SYSTEM CHAPTER REVIEW

WORD ELEMENTS SUMMARY

The following table summarizes CFs, suffixes, and prefixes related to the urinary system. Study the word elements and their meanings before completing the Vocabulary Review that follows.

Word Element	Meaning	Word Element	Meaning
Combining Forms			
aden/o	gland	**nephr/o, ren/o**	kidney
azot/o	nitrogenous compounds	**noct/o**	night
carcin/o	cancer	**olig/o**	scanty
cyst/o, vesic/o	bladder	**py/o**	pus
erythr/o	red	**pyel/o**	renal pelvis
glomerul/o	glomerulus	**scler/o**	hardening; sclera (white of the eye)
hemat/o	blood	**ureter/o**	ureter
lith/o	stone, calculus	**urethr/o**	urethra
meat/o	opening, meatus	**ur/o, urin/o**	urine
Suffixes			
-al, -ic, -ous	pertaining to	-megaly	enlargement
-algia, -dynia	pain	-oma	tumor
-cele	hernia, swelling	-osis	abnormal condition; increase (used primarily with blood cells)
-ectasis	dilation, expansion	-pathy	disease
-ectomy	excision, removal	-pepsia	digestion
-edema	swelling	-pexy	fixation (of an organ)
-emesis	vomiting	-phagia	swallowing, eating
-grade	to go	-phobia	fear
-gram	record, writing	-plasty	surgical repair
-graphy	process of recording	-ptosis	prolapse, downward displacement
-ia	condition	-rrhaphy	suture
-iasis	abnormal condition (produced specified)	-rrhea	discharge, flow by something
-ist	specialist	-stomy	forming an opening (mouth)
-lith	stone, calculus	-tome	instrument to cut
-logist	specialist in the study of	-tomy	incision
-logy	study of	-tripsy	crushing
-lysis	separation; destruction; loosening	-uria	urine

Continued

Word Element	Meaning	Word Element	Meaning
Prefixes			
a-, an-	without; not	**intra-**	in, within
dia-	through; across	**poly-**	many, much
dys-	bad; painful; difficult	**retro-**	backward; behind
in-	in; not	**supra-**	above; excessive; superior

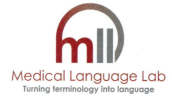

Medical Language Lab
Turning terminology into language

Visit the *Medical Language Lab* at the website *medicallanguagelab.com.* Use the flash-card exercise for this chapter to reinforce your study of word elements. We recommend you complete the flash-card exercise before starting the Vocabulary Review that follows.

Vocabulary Review

Match the medical term(s) with the definitions in the numbered list.

acute renal failure   cystocele   malignant   oliguria
anuria   diuretics   nephrolithotomy   polyuria
benign   edema   nephrons   renal pelvis
bilateral   hematuria   nephroptosis   ureteropyeloplasty
cholelithiasis   IVP   nocturia   urinary incontinence

1. _____ refers to cancerous growths.

2. _____ are microscopic filtering units in the kidney that are responsible for keeping body fluids in balance.

3. _____ refers to formation of gallstones.

4. _____ is a funnel-shaped reservoir that is the basin of the kidney.

5. _____ is an x-ray film of the kidneys after injection of dye.

6. _____ are drugs that stimulate the flow of urine.

7. _____ means swelling (of body tissues).

8. _____ refers to noncancerous growths.

9. _____ is an incision into a kidney to remove a stone.

10. _____ is a condition that results from lack of blood flow to the kidneys.

11. _____ is downward displacement of a kidney.

12. _____ is surgical repair of a ureter and renal pelvis.

13. _____ means pertaining to two sides.

14. _____ means excessive urination at night.

15. _____ refers to the inability to hold urine.

16. _____ refers to the presence of red blood cells in urine.

17. _____ means excessive discharge of urine.

18. _____ is a diminished amount of urine formation.

19. _____ is an absence of urine formation.

20. _____ is a herniation of the urinary bladder.

Competency Verification: Check your answers in Appendix B: Answer Key, page 605. If you are not satisfied with your level of comprehension, review the chapter vocabulary, and retake the review.

Correct Answers _____ × 5 = _____ % Score

Reproductive Systems

OBJECTIVES

Upon completion of this chapter, you will be able to:

- Describe the type of medical treatment gynecologists and obstetricians provide.
- Identify female and male reproductive structures by labeling them on the anatomical illustrations.
- Describe primary functions of the female and male reproductive systems.
- Describe diseases, conditions, and procedures related to the female and male reproductive systems.
- Apply your word-building skills by constructing medical terms related to the female and male reproductive systems.
- Describe common abbreviations and symbols related to the female and male reproductive systems.
- Recognize, define, pronounce, and spell terms correctly.
- Demonstrate your knowledge of this chapter by successfully completing the frames, reviews, and activities.

MEDICAL SPECIALTIES: OBSTETRICS, GYNECOLOGY, AND UROLOGY

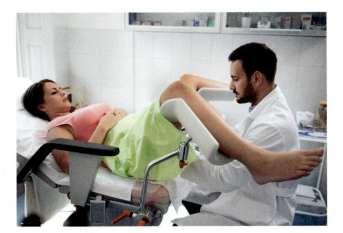

Obstetrics and Gynecology (OB-GYN) is a branch of medicine that specializes in the care of women during pregnancy and childbirth and in the diagnosis and treatment of diseases of the female reproductive organs. The OB-GYN physician also specializes in other women's health issues, such as menopause, hormone disorders, contraception (birth control), and infertility. The OB-GYN physician combines two specialties and is known as an *obstetrician/ gynecologist.*

The branch of medicine that specializes in the birth of children and with the care of women before, during, and after they give birth to a child is a single specialty called *obstetrics* and the physician is known as an *obstetrician.* The branch of medicine that specializes in health care for women, especially the diagnosis and treatment of disorders affecting the female reproductive system, is a single specialty called *gynecology,* and the physician is known as a *gynecologist.*

Urology

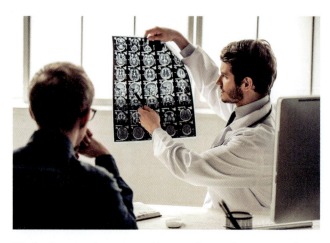

Urologists are physicians who specialize in diagnosis and treatment of urinary disorders. Because some urinary structures in the male perform a dual role (both urinary functions and reproductive functions), the urologist also treats male reproductive disorders, also known as urogenital disorders. These male disorders include, but are not limited to, treatment of bladder cancer, infertility, and sexual dysfunctions. Generally, the urologist performs surgery and treats urination problems, such as difficulty holding urine (incontinence) and obstruction of urinary flow caused by tumors or stones in the urinary organs. Urologists also manage male reproductive disorders, such as impotence (erectile dysfunction).

Anatomy and Physiology Overview

Although structures of the female and male reproductive systems differ, both have a common purpose. They are specialized to produce and unite gametes (reproductive cells) and transport them to sites of fertilization. Reproductive systems of both sexes are designed specifically to perpetuate the species and pass genetic material from generation to generation. In addition, both sexes produce hormones, which are vital in the development and maintenance of sexual characteristics and regulation of reproductive physiology.

Female Reproductive System

The female reproductive system is composed of internal organs of reproduction and external genitalia. The internal organs are the ovaries, fallopian tubes (oviducts, uterine tubes), uterus, and vagina. External organs, also called the **genitalia,** are known collectively as the **vulva.** Included in the vulva are the mons pubis, labia majora, labia minora, clitoris, and Bartholin glands. (See Figure 8-1.) The combined organs of the female reproductive system are designed to produce and transport ova (female sex cells), discharge ova from the body if fertilization does not occur, and nourish and provide a place for the developing fetus throughout pregnancy when fertilization occurs. The female reproductive system also produces the female sex hormones estrogen and progesterone, which are responsible for development of secondary sex characteristics, such as breast development and regulation of the menstrual cycle.

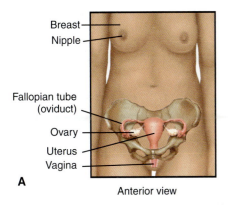

Breast
Nipple

Fallopian tube
(oviduct)

Ovary

Uterus

Vagina

A

Anterior view

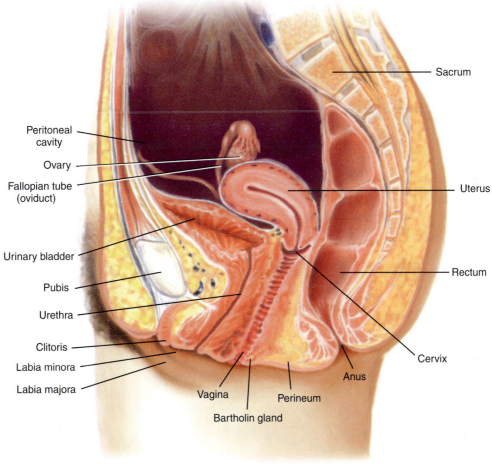

Sacrum

Peritoneal
cavity

Ovary

Fallopian tube
(oviduct)

Urinary bladder

Pubis

Urethra

Clitoris

Labia minora

Labia majora

Uterus

Rectum

Cervix

Anus

Vagina

Perineum

Bartholin gland

B

Lateral view

Figure 8-1 Female reproductive system. (A) Anterior view. (B) Lateral view.

WORD ELEMENTS

This section introduces word elements related to the female reproductive system. Review the word elements and their meanings in the following table, then pronounce each term in the word analysis column, and place a ✓ in the box after you do so.

Word Element	Meaning	Word Analysis
Combining Forms		
amni/o	amnion (amniotic sac)	**amni/o**/centesis (ăm-nē-ō-sĕn-TĒ-sĭs ☐): surgical puncture of the amniotic sac *-centesis:* surgical puncture *The sample of amniotic fluid obtained in amniocentesis is studied chemically and cytologically to detect genetic abnormalities, biochemical disorders, and maternal–fetal blood incompatibility.*
cervic/o	neck; cervix uteri (neck of the uterus)	**cervic**/it is (sĕr-vĭ-SĪ-tĭs ☐): inflammation of the cervix uteri *-it is:* inflammation *Cervicitis often results from a sexually transmitted infection (STI). It may also become chronic because, unlike the uterine lining, the cervical lining is not renewed each month during menstruation.*
colp/o	vagina	**colp/o**/scopy (kŏl-PŎS-kō-pē ☐): examination of the vagina and cervix with an optical magnifying instrument (colposcope) *-scopy:* visual examination *Colposcopy is commonly performed after a Papanicolaou ("Pap") test for treatment of cervical dysplasia and to obtain biopsy specimens of the cervix.*
vagin/o		**vagin/o**/cele (VĂJ-ĭn-ō-sēl ☐): herniation into the vagina; also called a colpocele *-cele:* hernia; swelling
galact/o	milk	**galact/o**/rrhea (gă-lăk-tō-RĒ-ă ☐): discharge or flow of milk *-rrhea:* discharge, flow
lact/o		**lact/o**/gen (LĂK-tō-jĕn ☐): production and secretion of milk *-gen:* forming, producing, origin
gynec/o	woman, female	**gynec/o**/logist (gī-nĕ-KŎL-ō-jĭst ☐): physician specializing in treating disorders of the female reproductive system *-logist:* specialist in the study of
hyster/o	uterus (womb)	**hyster**/ectomy (hĭs-tĕr-ĔK-tō-mē ☐): excision of the uterus *-ectomy:* excision, removal

uter/o		**uter/o**/vagin/al (ū-tĕr-ō-VĂJ-ĭ-năl ☐): pertaining to the uterus and vagina
		  vagin: vagina
		    -al: pertaining to

mamm/o	breast	**mamm/o**/gram (MĂM-ō-grăm ☐): radiograph of the breast *-gram:* record, writing
mast/o		**mast/o**/pexy (MĂS-tō-pĕks-ē ☐): surgical fixation of the breast(s) *-pexy:* fixation (of an organ) *Mastopexy is a cosmetic surgery to affix sagging breasts in a more elevated position, commonly improving their shape.*
men/o	menses, menstruation	**men/o**/rrhagia (mĕn-ō-RĀ-jē-ă ☐): excessive amount of menstrual flow over a longer duration than normal *-rrhagia:* bursting forth (of)

metr/o	uterus (womb); measure	endo/**metr**/it is (ĕn-dō-mē-TRĪ-tĭs ☐): inflammation of the endometrium
		  endo-: in, within
		    -it is: inflammation

nat/o	birth	pre/**nat**/al (prē-NĀ-tl ☐): pertaining to (the period) before birth
		  pre-: before, in front of
		    -al: pertaining to

Word Element	Meaning	Word Analysis
oophor/o	ovary	**oophor/oma** (ō-ŏf-or-Ō-mă ☐): ovarian tumor *-oma:* tumor
ovari/o		**ovari/o/rrhexis** (ō-văr-rē-ō-RĔK-sĭs ☐): rupture of an ovary *-rrhexis:* rupture
perine/o	perineum	**perine/o/rrhaphy** (pĕr-ĭ-nē-OR-ă-fē ☐): suture of the perineum *-rrhaphy:* suture *Perineorrhaphy is performed to repair a laceration that occurs spontaneously or is made surgically during the delivery of the fetus.*
salping/o	tube (usually fallopian or eustachian [auditory] tubes)	**salping/ectomy** (săl-pĭn-JĔK-tō-mē ☐): excision of a fallopian tube *-ectomy:* excision
vulv/o	vulva	**vulv/o/pathy** (vŭl-VŎP-ă-thē ☐): disease of the vulva *-pathy:* disease
episi/o		**episi/o/tomy** (ĕ-pēs-ē-ŎT-ō-mē ☐): incision of the perineum *-tomy:* incision *Episiotomy is performed to enlarge the vaginal opening for delivery of the fetus. The perineum is the region between the vaginal orifice and the anus.*

Suffixes

Word Element	Meaning	Word Analysis
-arche	beginning	men/**arche** (mĕn-ĂR-kē ☐): initial menstrual period *men:* menses, menstruation *Menarche usually occurs between ages 9 and 17 years.*
-gravida	pregnant woman	primi/**gravida** (prī-mĭ-GRĂV-ĭ-dă ☐): woman during her first pregnancy *primi-:* first
-para	to bear (offspring)	multi/**para** (mŭl-TĬP-ă-ră ☐): woman who has delivered more than one viable infant *multi-:* many, much
-salpinx	tube (usually fallopian or eustachian [auditory] tubes)	**hemat/o/salpinx** (hĕm-ă-tō-SĂL-pinks ☐): collection of blood in a fallopian tube; also called hemosalpinx *hemat/o:* blood *Hematosalpinx is commonly associated with a tubal pregnancy.*
-tocia	childbirth, labor	dys/**tocia** (dĭs-TŌ-sē-ă ☐): childbirth that is painful and difficult *dys-:* bad; painful; difficult *Dystocia may be caused by an obstruction or constriction of the birth passage or abnormal size, shape, position, or condition of the fetus.*
-version	turning	retro/**version** (rĕt-rō-VĔR-shŭn ☐): tipping back of an organ *retro-:* backward, behind *Uterine retroversion is measured as first-, second-, or third-degree, depending on the angle of tilt in relationship to the vagina.*

Pronunciation Help	*Long Sound*	ā in rāte	ē in rēbirth	ī in īsle	ō in ōver	ū in ūnite
	Short Sound	ă in ăpple	ĕ in ĕver	ĭ in ĭt	ŏ in nŏt	ŭ in cŭt

 Visit the *Medical Terminology Simplified* online resource center at FADavis.com for an audio exercise of the terms in this table to help master pronunciations and meanings of the selected medical terms.

SECTION REVIEW 8-1

For the following medical terms, first, write the suffix and its meaning. Then, translate the meaning of the remaining elements starting with the first part of the word. The first word is completed for you.

Term	Meaning
1. primi/gravida	-gravida: pregnant woman; first
2. colp/o/scopy	Visual examination of vagina.
3. gynec/o/logist	Physician who specializes in women health
4. perine/o/rrhaphy	Suture of perineum.
5. hyster/ectomy	removal /excision of uterus.
6. oophor/oma	tumor of the ovary.
7. (dys)/tocia to bear/give birth	
8. endo/metr/it is	
9. mamm/o/gram	breast recording.
10. amni/o/centesis	

Competency Verification: Check your answers in Appendix B: Answer Key, page 606. If you are not satisfied with your level of comprehension, review the vocabulary, and retake the review.

Correct Answers _____ x 10 = _____ % Score

Internal Structures

8-1 The female reproductive system is composed of internal and external organs of reproduction. (See Figure 8-2 and Figure 8-3.) The internal reproductive organs are the (1) **ovaries**, (2) **fallopian tubes**, (3) **uterus**, and (4) **vagina.** Label these organs in Figures 8-2 and 8-3 as you learn the names of the internal reproductive organs.

tumor TOO-mŏr	**8-2** An oophor/oma is an ovarian _____. Pronounce the initial *o* and the second *o* in words with *oophor/o.*

Pink indicates a prefix. Blue indicates a suffix. Boldface indicates a word root or combining form.

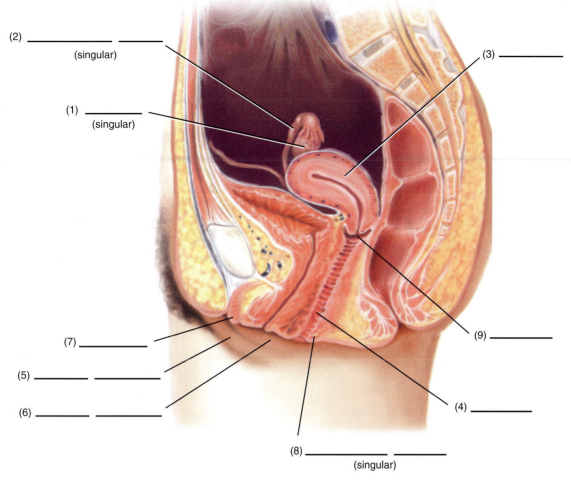

(2) _____ _____
(singular)

(1) _____
(singular)

(3) _____

(7) _____

(5) _____ _____

(6) _____ _____

(9) _____

(4) _____

(8) _____ _____
(singular)

Figure 8-2 Lateral view of the female reproductive system.

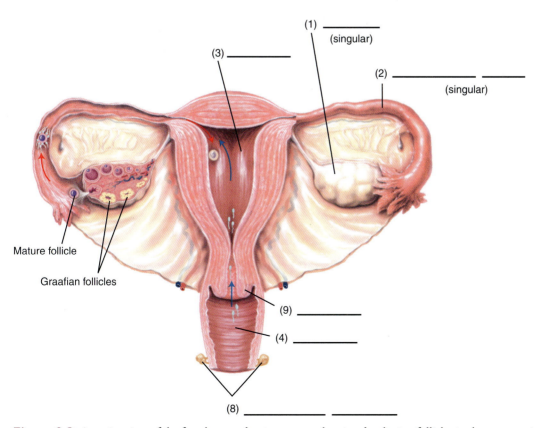

(1) _____
(singular)

(3) _____

(2) _____ _____
(singular)

Mature follicle

Graafian follicles

(9) _____

(4) _____

(8) _____ _____

Figure 8-3 Anterior view of the female reproductive system, showing developing follicles in the cross section of the right ovary with red arrows indicating movement of the ovum toward the uterus and *blue arrows* indicating movement of sperm toward the fallopian tube.

oophor/o/pathy
ō-ŏf-ŏr-ŎP-ă-thē

oophor/o/plasty
ō-ŎF-ŏr-ō-plăs-tē

oophor/o/pexy
ō-ŏf-ō-rō-PĔK-sē

8–3   The main purpose of the ovaries is to produce an ovum, the female reproductive cell. This process is called *ovulation*. Another important function of the ovaries is to produce the hormones estrogen and progesterone.

Use *oophor/o* to build medical words that mean

disease of the ovaries: _____/_____/_____.

surgical repair of an ovary:

_____/_____/_____.

fixation of a displaced ovary:

_____/_____/_____.

---

salping/o/plasty
săl-PĬNG-gō-plăs-tē

8–4   The CF *salping/o* means tube (usually *fallopian or eustachian [auditory] tube*) and is related to the female reproductive system. Eustachian (auditory) tubes are related to the sense of hearing and are discussed in Chapter 11.

Surgical repair of a fallopian tube (also known as an *oviduct*) is called

_____/_____/_____.

---

salping/o

8–5   Approximately once per month, maturation of the ovum, or *ovulation*, occurs when the egg leaves the ovary and slowly travels down the fallopian tube to the uterus. (See Figure 8-3.) If union of the ovum with sperm takes place during this time, fertilization (pregnancy) results.

To form words for the fallopian tube(s), uterine tube(s), or oviduct(s), use the CF

_____/_____.

---

salping/ectomy
săl-pĭn-JĔK-tō-mē

8–6   If the fertilized egg attaches to the wall of the fallopian tube (instead of the uterus), the tube must be removed to prevent serious bleeding or possible death of the mother.

When a fallopian tube is removed, the surgical procedure is called

_____/_____.

---

instrument

8–7   A salping/o/scope is an _____ for viewing the fallopian tube(s).

---

salping/o/scopy
săl-pĭng-GŎS-kō-pē

8–8   Visual examination of the fallopian tube(s) is called

_____/_____/_____.

Pink indicates a prefix. Blue indicates a suffix. Boldface indicates a word root or combining form.

salping/o/cele săl-PĬNG-ō-sēl	**8-9** Herniation of a fallopian tube(s) is known as _____/_____/_____.
oviducts Ŏ-vĭ-dŭkts	**8-10** Locate the two small tubes in Figure 8-3 that lead to each ovary. They are called *fallopian tubes, uterine tubes,* or _____.
hernia *or* herniation, uterus HĔR-nē-ă, hĕr-nē-Ā-shŭn, Ū-tĕr-ŭs	**8-11** The uterus, also called the womb, is the organ that contains and nourishes the embryo and fetus from the time the fertilized egg is implanted to the time of birth. The CF ***hyster/o*** is used to form words about the uterus as an organ. A hyster/o/cele is a _____ of the _____.
hyster/o/pathy hĭs-tēr-ŎP-ă-thē **hyster/algia, hyster/o/ dynia** hĭs-tĕr-ĂL-jē-ă, hĭs-tĕr-ō- DĬN-ē-ă **hyster/o/spasm** HĬS-tĕr-ō-spăzm	**8-12** Use *hyster/o* to build medical words that mean *disease of the uterus:* _____/_____/_____. *pain in the uterus:* _____/_____ or _____/_____/_____. *involuntary contraction, twitching of the uterus:* _____/_____/_____.
hyster/ectomy hĭs-tĕr-ĔK-tō-mē **hyster/o/tomy** hĭs-tĕr-ŎT-ō-mē	**8-13** Presence of one or more tumors (either benign or malignant) in the uterus may necessitate its removal. (See Figure 8-4.) Use *hyster/o* to form surgical terms that mean *excision of the uterus:* _____/_____. *incision of the uterus:* _____/_____/_____.

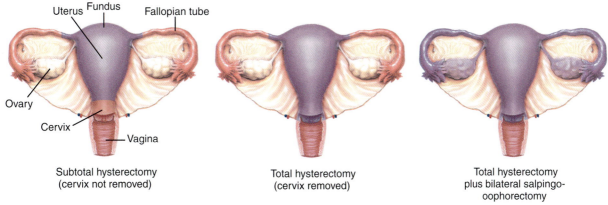

Uterus Fundus   Fallopian tube

Ovary

Cervix   Vagina

Subtotal hysterectomy
(cervix not removed)

Total hysterectomy
(cervix removed)

Total hysterectomy
plus bilateral salpingo-
oophorectomy

Figure 8-4 Hysterectomy, showing the excised structure shaded in purple.

dictionary	**8-14** Besides *hyster/o,* the CFs *metr/o* and *uter/o* are also used to denote the uterus. When in doubt about forming medical words with *hyster/o, uter/o,* or *metr/o,* refer to your medical _____.
hyster/o/scopy hĭs-tĕr-ŎS-kō-pē **uter/o/scopy** Ū-tĕr-ŏs-kō-pē	**8-15** The uterus is a muscular, hollow, pear-shaped structure located in the pelvic area between the bladder and the rectum. (See Figure 8-1.) Use *hyster/o* to form a word that means visual *examination of the uterus.* _____/_____/_____ Use *uter/o* to form another word that means *visual examination of the uterus.* _____/_____/_____
hyster/o/ptosis hĭs-tĕr-ŏp-TŌ-sĭs	**8-16** The uterus is supported and held in place by ligaments. Weakening of these ligaments may cause a downward displacement, or *prolapse,* of the uterus. Combine *hyster/o* and *-ptosis* to form a word that means prolapse or *downward displacement of the uterus.* _____/_____/_____
hyster/o, uter/o **-pexy**	**8-17** A prolapsed uterus may be caused by heavy physical exertion, pregnancy, or an inherent weakness. The surgical procedure to correct a prolapsed uterus is known as *hyster/o/pexy* or *uter/o/pexy.* Write the elements in this frame that mean *uterus:* _____ _____/_____, _____/_____. *fixation (of an organ):* _____.
estrogen, progesterone ĔS-trō-jĕn, prō-JĔS-tĕr-ōn	**8-18** The ovaries secrete two important hormones: estrogen and progesterone. These hormones play an important role in the processes of menstruation and pregnancy, as well as the development of secondary sex characteristics. When ovaries are diseased and necessitate removal, the body becomes deficient in the hormones known as _____ and _____.
men/o/pause MĔN-ō-pawz **trans/derm/al** trănz-DĔR-măl	**8-19** Men/o/pause, a natural process, is the gradual ending of the menstrual cycle, which also results in an estrogen hormone deficiency. Hormone replacement therapy (HRT) given orally or as a trans/derm/al patch may be used to relieve uncomfortable symptoms of men/o/pause. Identify terms in this frame that mean *cessation of the menses:* _____/_____/_____. *through, across the skin:* _____/_____/_____.
post/men/o/pause PŌST-mĕn-ō-pawz	**8-20** The term *pre/men/o/pause* refers to a period before men/o/pause. Can you build a word that refers to a period *after* men/o/pause? _____/_____/_____/_____

Pink indicates a prefix. Blue indicates a suffix. Boldface indicates a word root or combining form.

blood **blood**	**8-21** The elements **hemat/o, hem/o,** and *-emia* mean _____. Hemat/o/logy is the study of _____.
hemat/o/logist hē-mă-TŎL-ō-jĭst **hemat/o/pathy** hē-mă-TŎP-ă-thē **hemat/emesis** hĕm-ăt-ĔM-ĕ-sĭs	**8-22** Use **hemat/o** to build medical words that mean *specialist in the study of blood:* _____/_____/_____. *disease of the blood:* _____/_____/_____. *vomiting blood:* _____/_____.
curet kū-RĚT	**8-23** Dilation and curettage (D&C) is a surgical procedure to widen (dilate) the cervic/al canal of the uterus and scrape (curet) the endo/metri/um of the uterus. The uterine cavity is examined with a uterine sound to prevent perforation during dilation and to measure the depth of the uterus. The instrument used to scrape the endo/metri/um is known as a _____. (See Figure 8-5.)
uterine sound **serrated**	**8-24** Review Figure 8-5 to learn about the surgical procedure and instruments used to perform D&C. The instrument that is used to measure the uterus and prevent perforation during dilation is called a _____ _____. Scraping the uterine lining requires the use of a _____ curet.
inflammation, vagina vă-JĪ-nă	**8-25** The vagina is a muscular tube that extends from the cervix (neck of the uterus) to the exterior of the body. (See Figure 8-3.) In addition to serving as the organ of sexual intercourse and the receptor of semen, the vagina discharges menstrual flow and acts as a passageway for the delivery of the fetus. The CFs *colp/o* and *vagin/o* refer to the vagina. Colp/itis is an _____ of the _____.
vagin/itis văj-ĭn-Ī-tĭs	**8-26** Form another word in addition to *colp/itis* that means *inflammation of the vagina.* _____/_____
colp/algia kŏl-PĂL-jē-ā	**8-27** Colp/o/dynia denotes a *pain in the vagina.* Use *colp/o* to build another term for *pain in the vagina.* _____/_____

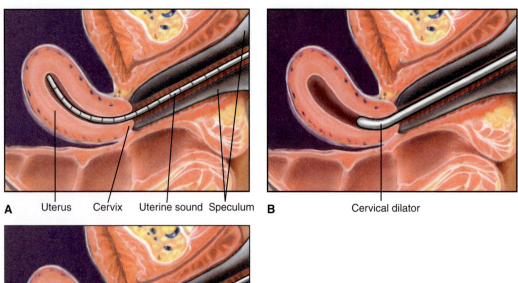

A   Uterus   Cervix   Uterine sound   Speculum   **B**   Cervical dilator

C   Serrated curette

Figure 8-5 Dilation and curettage of the uterus. (A) Examination of the uterine cavity with a uterine sound. (B) Dilation of the cervix using dilators of increasing size to allow insertion of a curet. (C) Curettage of the uterine lining with a serrated uterine curet.

---

colp/o/spasm
KŎL-pō-spăzm

colp/o/ptosis
kŏl-pŏp-TŌ-sĭs

colp/o/pexy
KŎL-pō-pĕk-sē

8–28 Use *colp/o* to construct medical words that mean

spasm or twitching of the vagina: _____/ _____/ _____.

prolapse or downward displacement of the vagina:

_____/ _____/ _____.

fixation of the vagina: _____/ _____/ _____.

---

vagin/o/plasty
VĂJ-ĭ-nō-plăs-tē

vagin/o/scope
VĂJ-ĭn-ō-skōp

vagin/o/tomy
văj-ĭ-NŎT-ō-mē

8–29 Use *vagin/o* to form medical words that mean

surgical repair of the vagina: _____/ _____/ _____.

instrument to view the vagina: _____/ _____/ _____.

incision of the vagina: _____/ _____/ _____.

Pink indicates a prefix. Blue indicates a suffix. Boldface indicates a word root or combining form.

vesic/o/vagin/al fistula
věs-ĭ-kō-VĂJ-ĭ-năl,
FĬS-tū-lă

8-30   A vesic/o/vagin/al fistula is another type of path/o/logy that can develop in the female reproductive system. This is an abnormal passage between the urinary bladder and the vagina. (See Figure 8-6.)

An abnormal connection that develops between the bladder and the vagina is known

as a _____/_____/_____/_____

_____.

vagina
vă-JĬ-nă

8-31   The term *fistula* refers to an abnormal passage from one epithelial surface to another epithelial surface. It can occur in any body system. Thus, a vesic/o/vagin/al fistula is only one type of fistula. A ureter/o/vagin/al fistula occurs between the lower

ureter and the _____.

vagina
vă-JĬ-nă

8-32   A rect/o/vagin/al fistula is one that develops between the rectum and the

_____.

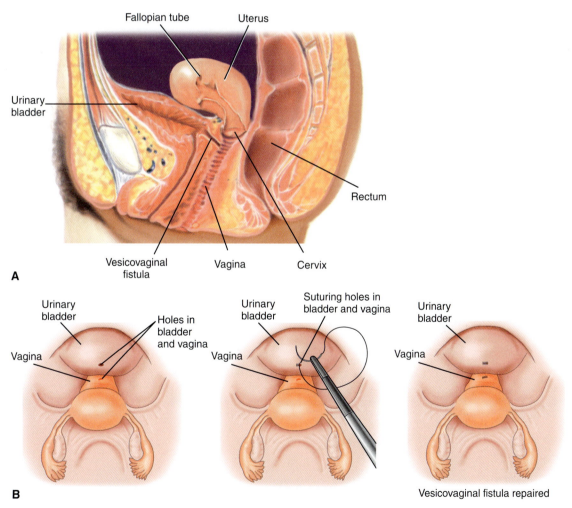

Figure 8-6 Vesicovaginal fistula. (A) Lateral view of female reproductive system with vesicovaginal fistula. (B) Frontal view of the urinary bladder and vagina with vesicovaginal fistula repair.

-rrhagia, -rrhage	**8-33** Colp/o/rrhagia refers to a *vagin/al hem/o/rrhage*. The elements in these words that mean *bursting forth (of)* are _____ and _____.

hem/o/rrhage HĔM-ĕ-rĭj	**8-34** Form a word that means *bursting forth (of) blood*. _____/____/_____

vagina vă-JĪ-nă **bladder** **hernia, swelling** HĔR-nē-ă	**8-35** Women who have had several vagin/al childbirths may suffer from herniation of the bladder, or colp/o/cyst/o/cele. Identify the elements in colp/o/cyst/o/cele. *colp/o:* _____ *cyst/o:* _____ *-cele:* _____ or _____

vagin/al VĂJ-ĭn-ăl **hyster/ectomy** hĭs-tĕr-ĔK-tō-mē	**8-36** When the uterus is removed through the vagina, the surgical procedure is known as a *vagin/al hyster/ectomy or a colp/o/hyster/ectomy*. Identify words in this frame that mean *pertaining to the vagina:* _____/_____. *excision of the uterus:* _____/_____.

SECTION REVIEW 8-2

Using the following table, write the CF and suffix that matches its definition in the space provided to the left of the definition. There may be more than one word element that matches a definition.

Combining Forms

colp/o	oophor/o
cyst/o	ovari/o
hemat/o	salping/o
hem/o	uter/o
hyster/o	vagin/o
metr/o	
muc/o	

Suffixes

-arche	-ptosis
-cele	-rrhage
-logist	-rrhagia
-logy	-salpinx
-oid	-scope
-pexy	-tome
-plasty	-tomy

1. _____ bladder

2. _____ blood

3. _____ bursting forth (of)

4. _____ uterus (womb)

5. _____ hernia; swelling

6. _____ incision

7. _____ instrument to cut

8. _____ instrument for examining

9. _____ tube (usually fallopian or eustachian [auditory] tubes)

10. _____ fixation (of an organ)

11. _____ mucus

12. _____ ovary

13. _____ beginning

14. _____ uterus (womb); measure

15. _____ prolapse, downward displacement

16. _____ resembling

17. _____ specialist in the study of

18. _____ study of

19. _____ surgical repair

20. _____ vagina

Competency Verification: Check your answers in Appendix B: Answer Key, page 606. If you are not satisfied with your level of comprehension, go back to Frame 8–1, and rework the frames.

Correct Answers _____ x 5 = _____ % Score

External Structures

8-37   The external structures, or *genitalia,* include the (5) **labia majora** (the outer lips of the vagina), (6) **labia minora** (the smaller, inner lips of the vagina), (7) **clitoris,** and (8) **Bartholin glands.** Label Figures 8-2 and 8-3 to locate the structures of the genitalia.

---

vulva
VŬL-vă

8-38   The CF *vulv/o* refers to the vulva, the combined external structures of the female reproductive system. *Vulv/o/uter/ine* refers to the uterus and

_____.

---

clitoris, Bartholin glands
KLĬT-ō-rĭs, BĂR-tō-lĭn

8-39   The external structures, or *genitalia* (also known as the *vulva*), include the labia majora, labia minora, _____, and _____

_____.

---

muc/ous
MŪ-kŭs

8-40   Mucus secretions from Bartholin glands help keep the vagina moist and lubricated, facilitating intercourse.

Use *-ous* to build a word that means *pertaining to mucus.*

_____/_____ (adjective ending)

8-41   The (9) **cervix** is the neck of the uterus and extends into the upper portion of the vagina. Examine the position of the cervix in the lateral and anterior view as you label Figures 8-2 and 8-3.

---

cervic/itis
sĕr-vĭ-SĪ-tĭs

8-42   The CF *cervic/o* refers to the neck or the cervix uteri (neck of the uterus). Inflammation of the cervix uteri is called _____/_____.

---

vagina, uteri
vă-JĪ-nă, Ū-tĕ-rī

8-43   When *cervic/o* is used in a word, you can determine whether it refers to the neck or the cervix uteri by reviewing the other parts of the word. For example, colp/o/cervic/al refers to the _____ and cervix

_____.

---

colp/o/scopy
kŏl-PŎS-kō-pē

8-44   A *colp/o/scope* is an instrument with a magnifying lens that is used to examine vagin/al and cervic/al tissue. Visual examination of vagin/al and cervic/al tissue using a colposcope is called _____/_____/_____.

---

colp/o/scope
KŎL-pō-skōp

colp/o/scopy
kŏl-PŎS-kō-pē

vagin/al
VĂJ-ĭn-ăl

cervic/al
SĔR-vĭ-kăl

8-45   Determine the words in Frame 8–44 that mean

instrument for examining the vagina and cervix uteri:

_____/_____/_____.

visual examination of the vagina and cervix uteri by using a colp/o/scope:

_____/_____/_____.

pertaining to the vagina: _____/_____.

pertaining to the cervix uteri: _____/_____.

Pink indicates a prefix. Blue indicates a suffix. Boldface indicates a word root or combining form.

uterus Ū-těr-ŭs	**8-46** *Cervix uteri* refers to the neck of the _____.

Competency Verification: Check your labeling of Figures 8-2 and 8-3 in Appendix B: Answer Key, page 606.

gynec/o/logist gī-ně-KŎL-ō-jĭst	**8-47** The term *gynec/o/logy* means *study of females* or *women* and is the medical specialty for treating female reproductive disorders. A specialist in the study of female reproductive disorders is called a _____/_____/_____ _____.
gynec/o	**8-48** The CF in *gynec/o/logy* that means *woman* or *female* is _____/_____.
gynec/o/pathy gī-ně-KŎP-ă-thē	**8-49** Use *-pathy* to form a word that means *disease of a female*. _____/_____/_____
gynec/o/logy gī-ně-KŎL-ō-jē	**8-50** *GYN* is the abbreviation for *gynec/o/logy*. *OB-GYN* refers to *obstetrics and* _____/_____/_____.
menses, menstruation MĚN-sēz, měn-stroo-Ā-shŭn	**8-51** The CF **men/o** means menses or *menstruation,* which is the monthly flow of blood and tissue from the uterus. Men/o/rrhea is a flow of _____ or _____.
dys/men/o/rrhea dĭs-měn-ō-RĒ-ă	**8-52** Use *dys-* and *men/o/rrhea* to develop a word that means *painful or difficult menstrual flow*. _____/_____/_____/_____
dys/men/o/rrhea dĭs-měn-ō-RĒ-ă	**8-53** Dys/men/o/rrhea is pain associated with menstruation. Primary dys/men/o/rrhea is menstrual pain that results from factors intrinsic to the uterus and the process of menstruation. It is extremely common, occurring at least occasionally in almost all women. If the painful episode is mild and brief, it is considered functional and normal and requires no treatment. The symptomatic term that literally means *bad, painful, difficult menstruation* is _____/_____/_____/_____.
menstruation měn-stroo-Ā-shun	**8-54** Men/o/pause terminates the reproductive period of life and is a permanent cessation of menses, or _____.

menstruation mĕn-stroo-Ā-shun	**8-55** A/men/o/rrhea is the *absence or abnormal stoppage of menstruation.* Men/o/rrhea is a *flow of the menses, or* _____.
olig/o/men/o/rrhea ŏl-ĭ-gō-mĕn-ō-RĒ-ă *olig/o:* scanty *men/o:* menses, menstruation *-rrhea:* discharge, flow	**8-56** Use the prefix *oligo-* to build a word that means scanty or infrequent menstrual flow: _____/_____/_____/_____/_____.

Breasts

mamm/o, mast/o	**8-57** The breasts, also called *mamm/ary glands,* are present in both sexes but they normally function only in females. The biological role of the mammary glands is to secrete milk for the nourishment of the infant, a process called *lactation.* The CFs that refer to the breast are _____/_____ and _____/_____.
mast/o/dynia, mast/algia măst-ō-DĬN-ē-ă, măst-ĂL-jē-ă	**8-58** Use *mast/o* to form a word that means *pain in the breast.* _____/_____/_____ or _____/_____
mast/ectomy măs-TĔK-tō-mē	**8-59** To prevent the spread of cancer (CA), a malignant breast tumor may be treated with a partial or complete excision. When a breast has to be removed, the patient undergoes a _____/_____.
	8-60 During puberty, the female's breasts develop as a result of periodic stimulation of the ovarian hormones estrogen and progesterone. (See Figure 8-7.) Estrogen is responsible for the development of (1) **adipose tissue,** which enlarges the size of the breasts until they reach full maturity around age 16 years. Breast size is primarily determined by the amount of fat around the (2) **glandular tissue,** but it is not a factor in the ability to produce and secrete milk. Label the adipose and glandular tissues in Figure 8-7.
	8-61 During pregnancy, high levels of estrogen and progesterone prepare the mammary glands for milk production. Each breast has approximately 20 lobes. Each (3) **lobe** is drained by a (4) **lactiferous duct** that opens on the tip of the raised (5) **nipple.** Circling the nipple is a border of slightly darker skin called the (6) **areola.** Label the structures of the mammary glands in Figure 8-7.
lactation lăk-TĀ-shŭn	**8-62** During pregnancy, the breasts enlarge and remain so until lactation ceases. At menopause, breast tissue begins to atrophy. The ability of mammary glands to secrete milk for the nourishment of the infant is a process called _____.

Pink indicates a prefix. Blue indicates a suffix. Boldface indicates a word root or combining form.

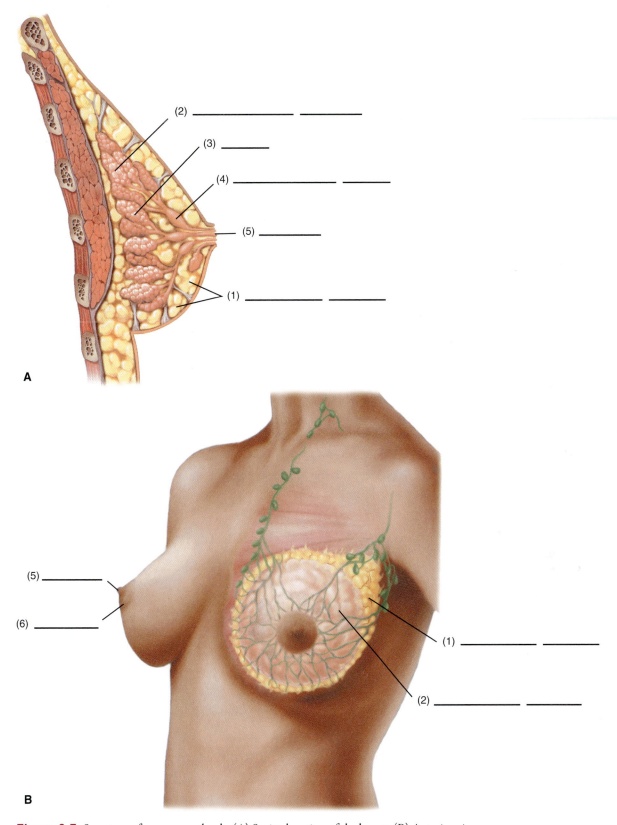

(2) _____ _____

(3) _____

(4) _____ _____

(5) _____

(1) _____ _____

A

(5) _____

(6) _____

(1) _____ _____

(2) _____ _____

B

Figure 8-7 Structure of mammary glands. (A) Sagittal section of the breast. (B) Anterior view showing lymph nodes and structures of the breast.

-graphy **mamm/o**	**8–63**　Mamm/o/graphy, an x-ray examination of the breast, is used in the diagnosis (Dx) of CA. Determine the elements in this frame that mean *process of recording:* _____. *breast:* _____/_____.
mamm/o/plasty MĂM-ō-plăs-tē	**8–64**　Use ***mamm/o*** to construct a word that means *surgical reconstruction or repair of a breast.* _____/_____/_____
mast/o/plasty MĂS-tō-plăs-tē **mast/o/pexy** MĂS-to-pĕk-sē	**8–65**　Correction of pendulous breasts can be performed by reconstructive cosmetic surgery to lift the breasts. Use ***mast/o*** to develop surgical terms that mean *surgical repair of the breast:* _____/_____/_____. *fixation of the breast:* _____/_____/_____.

8–66　When a small primary tumor is localized, the surgeon performs a lump/ectomy. In these instances, the tumor and some of the normal tissue surrounding it are excised. All tissue removed from the breast via biopsy is subjected to analysis to determine whether CA cells are present in the normal tissue surrounding the tumor. (See Figure 8-8.)

Competency Verification: Check your labeling of Figure 8-7 in Appendix B: Answer Key, page 607.

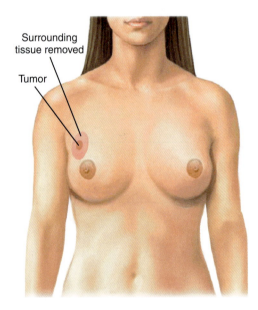

Surrounding tissue removed

Tumor

Figure 8-8　Lumpectomy, with the primary tumor in red and the surrounding tissue removed during lumpectomy highlighted pink.

before, after	**8-67**　The term *nat/al* means *pertaining to birth. Pre/nat/al* refers to the period _____ birth; *post/nat/al* refers to the period _____ birth.
neo- **nat/o** **-logy**	**8-68**　Identify elements in neo/nat/o/logy that mean *new:* _____ *birth:* _____/_____ *study of:* _____
neo/nat/o/logist nē-ō-nā-TŎL-ō-jĭst	**8-69**　Neo/nat/o/logy is the *study and treatment of the neonate (newborn infant).* A physician who specializes in the care and treatment of the neonate is called a _____/_____/_____/_____.
woman	**8-70**　*Gravida* is used to describe a pregnant woman, as is the suffix *-gravida*. A *primi/gravida* is a woman pregnant for the first time; a *multi/gravida* is a woman who has been pregnant more than once. Whenever you see gravida in a word, you will know it denotes a pregnant _____.
fourth **second**	**8-71**　*Gravida* may also be followed by numbers to denote the number of pregnancies, as in *gravida 1, gravida 2, gravida 3,* and *gravida 4* (or *gravida I, II, III,* and *IV*). *Gravida 4* is a woman in her _____ pregnancy. *Gravida 2* is a woman in her _____ pregnancy.
gravida 3 GRĂV-ĭ-dă **gravida 5** GRĂV-ĭ-dă	**8-72**　A woman in her third pregnancy is described as _____ _____. A woman in her fifth pregnancy is described as _____ _____.
two, five	**8-73**　The word *para* refers to a woman who has given birth to an infant, whether or not the offspring was alive at birth. It also may be followed by numbers to indicate the number of deliveries, as in *para 1, 2, 3,* or *4* (or *I, II, III,* or *IV*). *Para 2* means _____ deliveries; *para 5* means _____ deliveries.
para 6 PĂR-ă	**8-74**　A woman who has delivered three infants would be described as para 3. A woman who has delivered six infants would be described as _____ _____.
PID	**8-75**　*Pelvic inflammatory disease* (PID) is a collective term for inflammation of the uterus, fallopian tubes, ovaries, and adjacent pelvic structures. This disease is usually caused by bacterial infection. The abbreviation for pelvic inflammatory disease is _____.

path/o/gen PĂTH-ō-jĕn	**8-76** In the female reproductive system, an infection may be confined to a single organ, or it may involve all of the internal female reproductive organs. Path/o/gens generally enter through the vagina during coitus, induced abortion, childbirth, or the postpartum period. As an ascending infection, pathogens spread from the vagina and cervix to the upper structures of the female reproductive tract. A term in this frame that means *forming, producing, or origin of disease* is _____ / _____ / _____ .
sexually transmitted infection (STI) **pelvic inflammatory disease**	**8-77** The two most common causes of PID are gonorrhea and chlamydia, both of which are STIs. Unless treated promptly, PID may result in sterility because the fallopian tubes and ovaries become scarred. Widespread infection of reproductive structures may also lead to fatal septicemia. The abbreviation STI refers to _____ _____ _____ . The abbreviation PID refers to _____ _____ _____ .
pelvic inflammatory disease	**8-78** Because some regions of the fallopian tubes have an internal diameter as small as that of a human hair, the scarring and closure of the tubes caused by PID is one of the major causes of female sterility (infertility). Chlamydia and gonorrhea are two main causes of PID. The abbreviation PID means _____ _____ .
oophor/itis ō-ŏf-ō-RĪ-tĭs **oophor/oma** ō-ŏf-ō-RŌ-mă	**8-79** A pelvic infection that involves the ovaries is known as *oophor/itis.* Use *oophor/o* to build a term that means *inflammation of the ovaries:* _____ / _____ . *tumor of the ovaries:* _____ / _____ .
salping/ectomy săl-pĭn-JĔK-tō-mē	**8-80** The CF *salping/o* means tube (*usually fallopian or eustachian [auditory] tubes*). A tumor or cyst in a fallopian tube may necessitate the removal of the fallopian tube. Build a surgical term that means excision of a fallopian tube. _____ / _____
incision, uterus	**8-81** Abdominal incision of the uterus (hyster/o/tomy) is performed to remove the fetus during a cesarean section (CS), also called *C-section.* Hyster/o/tomy is an _____ into the _____ .
CS, C-section	**8-82** Abbreviations for *cesarean section* are _____ and _____ .

SECTION REVIEW 8-3

Using the following table, write the CF, suffix, or prefix that matches its definition in the space provided to the left of the definition. There may be more than one word element that matches a definition.

Combining Forms		Suffixes		Prefixes
cervic/o	men/o	-algia	-ous	dys-
colp/o	salping/o	-ary	-pathy	post-
episi/o	vagin/o	-dynia	-rrhea	pre-
gynec/o	vulv/o	-ectomy	-scope	
mamm/o		-itis	-scopy	
mast/o		-logist	-tome	

1. _____ after; behind

2. _____ woman, female

3. _____ before; in front of

4. _____ breast

5. _____ disease

6. _____ excision, removal

7. _____ discharge, flow

8. _____ inflammation

9. _____ instrument to cut

10. _____ instrument for examining

11. _____ visual examination

12. _____ menses, menstruation

13. _____ neck; cervix uteri (neck of uterus)

14. _____ pain

15. _____ pertaining to

16. _____ specialist in the study of

17. _____ tube (usually fallopian or eustachian [auditory] tubes)

18. _____ vagina

19. _____ vulva

20. _____ bad; painful; difficult

Competency Verification: Check your answers in Appendix B: Answer Key, page 607. If you are not satisfied with your level of comprehension, go back to Frame 8–37, and rework the frames.

Correct Answers _____ x 5 = _____ % Score

Male Reproductive System

The primary sex organs of the male are called **gonads,** specifically the **testes** (singular, **testis**). Gonads produce gametes (sperm) and secrete sex hormones. The remaining accessory reproductive organs are the structures that are essential in caring for and transporting sperm. All of these organs and structures are designed to accomplish the male's reproductive role of producing and delivering sperm to the female reproductive tract, where fertilization can occur.

These structures can be divided into three categories:

1. **Sperm-transporting ducts,** which include the epididymis, vas deferens (or ductus deferens), ejaculatory duct, and urethra.
2. **Accessory glands,** which include the seminal vesicles, prostate gland, and bulbourethral glands.
3. **Copulatory organ,** called the **penis,** which contains erectile tissue. (See Figure 8-9.)

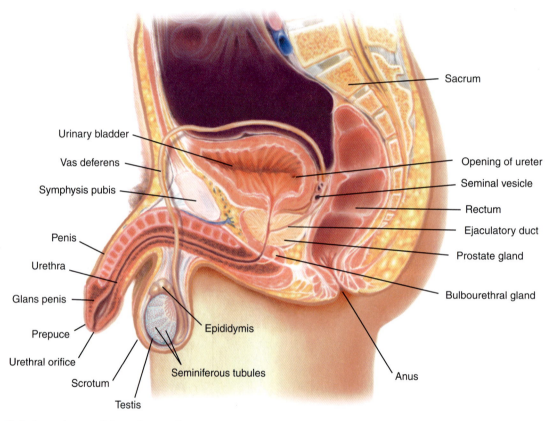

Figure 8-9 Lateral view of the male reproductive system.

WORD ELEMENTS

This section introduces word elements related to the male reproductive system. Review the word elements and their meanings in the following table, then pronounce each term in the word analysis column, and place a ✓ in the box after you do so.

Word Element	Meaning	Word Analysis
Combining Forms		
andr/o	male	**andr/o/gen** (ĂN-drō-jĕn ☐): forming or producing male (hormones) *-gen:* forming, producing, origin *The hormones testosterone and androsterone produce or stimulate the development of male characteristics (masculinization).*
balan/o	glans penis	**balan/itis** (băl-ă-NĪ-tĭs ☐): inflammation of the glans penis *-itis:* inflammation

Word Element	Meaning	Word Analysis
gonad/o	gonads, sex glands	**gonad/o/tropin** (gŏn-ă-dō-TRŌ-pĭn ☐): hormone that stimulates the gonads *-tropin:* stimulate *Gonadotropin is a hormone that stimulates the function of the testes and ovaries (gonads).*

orch/o	testis (plural, *testes*)	**crypt/orch/ism** (krĭpt-OR-kĭzm ☐): condition of undescended testicles; also called *cryptorchidism*
		  crypt: hidden
		   -ism: condition
		
		In cryptorchism, the testicles are retained in the abdomen or inguinal canal. If spontaneous descent does not occur by age 1 year, hormone therapy or surgery may be performed.

orchi/o		**orchi/o/pexy** (OR-kē-ō-pĕk-sē ☐): surgical fixation of a testis *-pexy:* fixation (of an organ) *An orchiopexy is performed to mobilize an undescended testis, bring it into the scrotum, and attach it so that it will not retract.*
orchid/o		**orchid/ectomy** (or-kĭ-DĔK-tō-mē ☐): excision of one or both testes *-ectomy:* excision, removal
test/o		**test/algia** (tĕs-TĂL-jē-ă ☐): pain in the testes *-algia:* pain
prostat/o	prostate gland	**prostat/itis** (prŏs-tă-TĪ-tĭs ☐): inflammation of the prostate gland, usually as a result of infection *-itis:* inflammation
spermat/o	spermatozoa, sperm cells	**spermat/o/cyte** (spĕr-MĂT-ō-sīt ☐): sperm cell *cyte:* cell
sperm/i*		**sperm/i/cide** (SPĔR-mĭ-sīd ☐): agent that kills spermatozoa; also called spermatocide *-cide:* killing

sperm/o		**a/sperm/ia** (ă-SPĔR-mē-ă ☐): without spermatozoa; sperm cells
		  a-: without, not
		  -ia: condition
		
		In aspermia, semen fails to form or be ejaculated.

varic/o	dilated vein	**varic/o/cele** (VĂR-ĭ-kō-sēl ☐): dilated or enlarged vein of the spermatic cord *-cele:* hernia; swelling
vas/o	vessel; vas deferens; duct	**vas/ectomy** (văs-ĔK-tō-mē ☐): removal of all or part of the vas deferens *-ectomy:* excision, removal

Pronunciation Help	Long Sound	ā in rāte	ē in rēbirth	ī in īsle	ō in ōver	ū in ūnite
	Short Sound	ă in ăpple	ĕ in ĕver	ĭ in ĭt	ŏ in nŏt	ŭ in cŭt

*Using the combining vowel *i* instead of *o* is an exception to the rule.

Visit the *Medical Terminology Simplified* online resource center at FADavis.com for an audio exercise of the terms in this table. It will help you master pronunciations and meanings of medical terms.

SECTION REVIEW 8-4

For the following medical terms, first, write the suffix and its meaning. Then, translate the meaning of the remaining elements starting with the first part of the word. The first word is completed for you.

Term	Meaning
1. vas/ectomy	–ectomy: excision, removal; vessel, vas deferens, duct
2. balan/it is	
3. spermat/i/cide	
4. gonad/o/tropin	
5. orchi/o/pexy	
6. a/sperm/ia	
7. vesicul/itis	
8. orchid/ectomy	
9. andr/o/gen	
10. crypt/orch/ism	

Competency Verification: Check your answers in Appendix B: Answer Key, page 607. If you are not satisfied with your level of comprehension, review the word elements tables, and retake the review.

Correct Answers _____ x 10 = _____ % Score

8–83   Label Figure 8-10 as you learn about the male organs of reproduction. The (1) **testes** (singular, *testis*), also called *testicles* (singular, *testicle*), are paired oval glands that descend into the (2) **scrotum.** At the onset of puberty, the testes produce the hormone testosterone.

testis
TĔS-tĭs

testicle
TĔS-tĭ-kl

8–84   The male hormone testosterone stimulates and promotes the growth of secondary sex characteristics in the male. This hormone is produced by the testes (plural).

The singular form of testes is _____.

The singular form of testicles is _____.

test/itis
tĕs-TĪ-tĭs

test/ectomy
tĕs-TĔK-tō-mē

test/o/pathy
tĕs-TŎP-ă-thē

8–85   Use *test/o* to form medical words that mean

inflammation of the testis: _____/_____.

excision of the testis: _____/_____.

disease of the testis: _____/_____/_____.

Pink indicates a prefix. Blue indicates a suffix. Boldface indicates a word root or combining form.

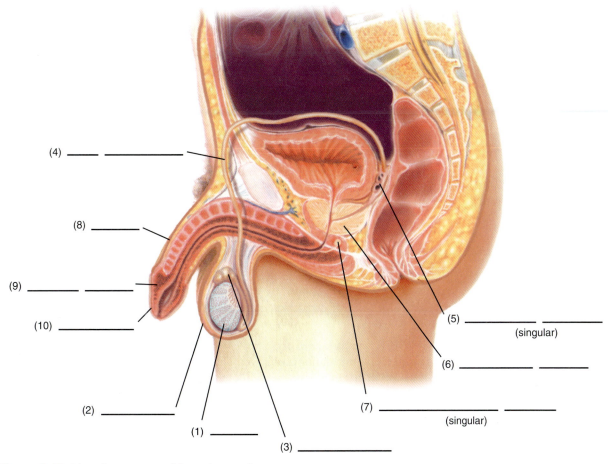

Figure 8-10 Identifying organs of the male reproductive system.

---

spermatozoa spěr-măt-ō-ZŌ-ă	**8–86** The CF *spermat/o* means *spermatozoa, sperm cells,* which are the male sex cell produced by the testes. *Spermat/o/genesis is the beginning or formation of sperm cells, or* _____.
stone, calculus KĂL-kū-lŭs	**8–87** A spermat/o/lith is a _____, or _____, in the spermatic duct.
spermat/o/genesis spěr-măt-ō-JĚN-ě-sĭs	**8–88** The suffix *-genesis* is used in words to mean *forming, producing, and origin.* Construct a word that means *producing or forming sperm.* _____ / _____ / _____
spermat/o/cyte spěr-MĂT-ō-sīt **spermat/oid** SPĚR-mă-toyd	**8–89** Use *spermat/o* to form a word that means *spermatozoa, or sperm cell:* _____ / _____ / _____. *resembling spermatozoa, or sperm:* _____ / _____.

spermat/uria spĕr-mă-TŪ-rē-ă	**8-90** Spermat/uria is a condition in which there is sperm in the urine. A discharge of semen in urine is also called _____/_____.
without	**8-91** *A/spermat/ism* is a condition in which a male lacks sperm. A/spermat/ism literally means _____ sperm.
olig/o/sperm/ia ŏl-ĭ-gō-SPĔR-mē-ă	**8-92** Olig/o/sperm/ia, also known as a *low sperm count,* is a condition in which there are fewer sperm cells in the ejaculate than normal. It is one of the main causes of male infertility. Use *olig/o* to build a word that means *condition of scanty sperm.* _____/_____/_____/_____
olig/o/sperm/ia ŏl-ĭ-gō-SPĔR-mē-ă	**8-93** When the physician detects a low sperm count, the Dx is noted in the medical record as _____/_____/_____/_____.
	8-94 A comma-shaped organ, the (3) **epididymis,** stores and propels sperm toward the urethra during ejaculation. The (4) **vas deferens,** also called *ductus deferens,* is a duct that transports sperm from the testes to the urethra. Sperm is excreted in semen, or the seminal fluid. Semen is a mixture of secretions from the (5) **seminal vesicles,** (6) **prostate gland,** and (7) **bulbourethral glands,** also known as *Cowper glands.* Label Figure 8-10 as you continue to learn about the male reproductive organs.
muc/o	**8-95** Ducts of bulbourethral (Cowper) glands open into the urethra and secrete thick mucus, which acts as a lubricant during sexual stimulation. Write the CF that refers to mucus. _____/_____
adjective	**8-96** Muc/us is a noun. Muc/ous is a(n) (noun, adjective) _____.
orchi/o/plasty OR-kē-ō-plăs-tē **orchi/o/rrhaphy** or-kē-OR-ă-fē **orchi/o/pexy** or-kē-ō-PĔK-sē	**8-97** In addition to *test/o,* two other CFs that refer to the testes are *orchi/o* and *orchid/o.* Use *orchi/o* to develop medical words that mean *surgical repair of the testicle:* _____/_____/_____. *suture of a testicle:* _____/_____/_____. *fixation of a testicle:* _____/_____/_____.
enlargement	**8-98** The CF *prostat/o* means *prostate gland.* The prostate gland secretes a thick fluid, which, as part of semen, helps sperm to move spontaneously. Prostat/o/megaly is a(n) _____ of the prostate gland.

prostat/o/megaly prŏs-tă-tō-MĔG-ă-lē	**8–99** Benign prostatic hyperplasia (BPH), also called *benign prostatic hypertrophy,* is a gradual enlargement of the prostate gland that normally occurs as a man ages. It is a common disorder in men over the age of 60 years. The enlarged prostate compresses the urethra and causes the bladder to retain urine. Symptoms include an inability to empty the bladder completely and a weak urine stream. (See Figure 8-11.) Construct a medical word that means *enlargement of the prostate gland.* _____ / _____ / _____
growth, nourishment	**8–100** The abbreviation BPH refers *to benign prostat/ic hyper/plasia,* or *benign prostat/ic hyper/trophy.* The suffix *-plasia* means *formation,* _____. The suffix *-trophy* means *development,* _____.
trans/urethr/al trăns-ū-RĒ-thrăl	**8–101** Common symptoms of BPH include hesitancy and dribbling on urination and a weak urine stream. Treatment includes drugs to decrease prostate size or a trans/urethr/al resection of the prostate (TURP), in which the obstructing tissue is removed. TURP makes it possible to perform surgery on certain organs that lie near the urethra without having an abdominal incision. (See Figure 8-12.) Because this surgery is performed by passing a resect/o/scope through the urethra, it is called _____/_____/_____ *resection of the prostate.*

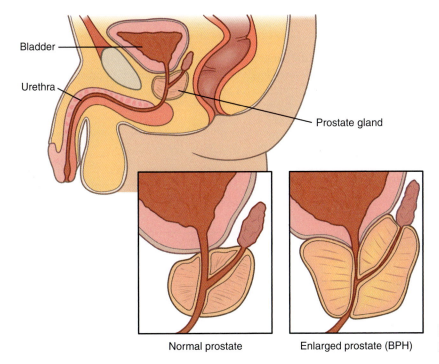

Bladder

Urethra

Prostate gland

Normal prostate   Enlarged prostate (BPH)

Figure 8-11 Benign prostatic hyperplasia.

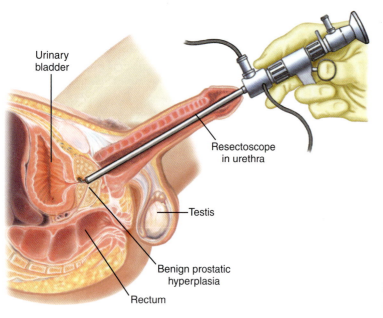

Urinary
bladder

Resectoscope
in urethra

Testis

Benign prostatic
hyperplasia

Rectum

Figure 8-12 Transurethral resection of the prostate (TURP).

---

resect/o/scope
rē-SĚK-tō-skōp

8–102   The resect/o/scope (special type of endoscope) contains a light, valves for controlling irrigating fluid, and an electrical loop that cuts tissue and seals blood vessels. The wire loop is used to remove obstructing tissue piece by piece through the resectoscope. The chips of tissue are irrigated into the bladder and then flushed out at the end of the surgical procedure.

The endo/scop/ic instrument used by the urologist to perform TURP is called a

_____/_____/_____.

PSA

8–103   The prostate-specific antigen (PSA) test is a blood test that screens for prostate abnormalities. Elevated levels of PSA are associated with prostate enlargement and CA. The abbreviation for *prostate-specific antigen* is

_____.

---

prostat/itis
prŏs-tă-TĪ-tĭs

prostat/o/cyst/itis
prŏs-tă-tō-sĭs-TĪ-tĭs

8–104   Build medical words that mean

inflammation of the prostate gland: _____/_____.

inflammation of the prostate gland and bladder:

_____/_____/_____/_____.

8–105   The (8) **penis** is the male sex organ that transports sperm into the female's vagina. A slightly enlarged region at the tip of the penis is the (9) **glans penis.** The tip of the penis is covered by a fold of skin called the (10) **foreskin,** or *prepuce.* Label Figure 8-10 as you learn the names of organs of reproduction.

Pink indicates a prefix. Blue indicates a suffix. Boldface indicates a word root or combining form.

water **hernia, swelling** HĔR-nē-ă	**8-106** Hydr/o/cele is a collection of fluid in a saclike cavity, specifically the testis. Analyze hydr/o/cele by defining the elements. *hydr/o:* _____ *-cele:* _____ , _____

Competency Verification: Check your labeling of Figure 8-10 in Appendix B: Answer Key, page 607.

prostat/ectomy prŏs-tă-TĔK-tō-mē	**8-107** Prostate CA is the third leading cause of cancer-related deaths in men (after lung and colon CAs). Surgery may be performed to remove the prostate and adjacent affected tissues. Develop a surgical term that means *excision of the prostate gland.* _____ / _____
cancer (CA)	**8-108** Currently, PSA is considered the most sensitive tumor marker for prostate _____ .
threatening	**8-109** Tumors may be benign or malignant. Benign tumors are not malignant (cancerous) and not life-threatening. A malignant tumor, however, is cancerous and life- _____ .
benign bē-NĬN	**8-110** Tumors are also called *neo/plasms* (new growths or formations). Similar to tumors, neo/plasms can be malignant or _____ .
cancer/ous KĂN-sĕr-ŭs	**8-111** A benign tumor is non/cancer/ous. A malignant tumor is _____ / _____ .
neo/plasm NĒ-ō-plăzm	**8-112** A new growth in any body system or organ is called a _____ / _____ .
prostat/itis prŏs-tă-TĪ-tĭs	**8-113** Prostat/itis, an acute or chronic inflammation of the prostate gland, is usually the result of infection. The patient usually complains of burning, urinary frequency, and urgency. Build a symptomatic term that means *inflammation of the prostate gland.* _____ / _____
growth	**8-114** The suffixes *-plasm* and *-plasia* refer to formation or _____ .

dys- **-plasia**	**8–115** Dys/plasia is an abnormal development of tissue. Identify the element in dys/plasia that means *bad, painful, or difficult:* _____. *formation, growth:* _____.
without, not **formation, growth**	**8–116** *A/plasia means without formation* and is a condition that is caused by failure of an organ to develop or form normally. Analyze *a/plasia* by defining the elements. *a-:* _____, _____ *-plasia:* _____, _____
hyper- **-plasia**	**8–117** Hyper/plasia is an excessive increase in the number of cells in a tissue or organ, as shown in Figure 8-11. Determine the element in *hyper/plasia* that means *excessive:* _____. *formation or growth:* _____.
vas/o	**8–118** Vas/ectomy, a sterilization procedure, involves bi/later/al cutting and tying of the vas deferens to prevent the passage of sperm. This sterilization procedure is most commonly performed at an outpatient surgery center by using local an/esthesia. (See Figure 8-13.) From the term *vas/ectomy,* construct the CF that means *vessel, vas deferens, or duct.* _____ / _____

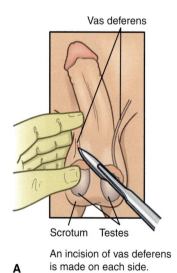

A An incision of vas deferens is made on each side.

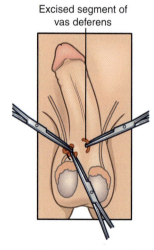

B The excised segment of vas deferens is withdrawn and ends are tied (ligation).

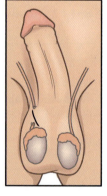

C Vas deferens is returned and scrotum incision is closed with sutures. This procedure is performed for both the right and left vas deferens.

Figure 8-13 Vasectomy.

an/esthesia
ăn-ĕs-THĒ-zē-ă

bi/later/al
bī-LĂT-ĕr-ăl

vas/ectomy
văs-ĔK-tō-mē

8-119   Identify the terms in Frame 8–118 that mean

without feeling: _____/_____.

pertaining to two sides: _____/_____/_____.

excision of the vas deferens: _____/_____.

---

prostat/itis
prŏs-tă-TĪ-tĭs

8-120   Vas/ectomy is also performed routinely before removal of the prostate gland to prevent inflammation of the testes and epididymides. Potency is not affected.

Inflammation of the prostate gland is called _____/_____.

---

vas/ectomy reversal
văs-ĔK-tō-mē

8-121   Vas/o/vas/o/stomy, also called vas/ectomy reversal, is a surgical procedure in which the function of the vas deferens on each side of the testes is restored after having been cut and ligated in a preceding vasectomy.

Another term for *vas/o/vas/o/stomy* is

_____/_____ _____.

---

patency
PĀ-tĕn-sē

vas/o/vas/o/stomy
văs-ō-vă-SŎS-tō-mē

8-122   Vas/o/vas/o/stomy may be performed if a man wants to regain his fertility. In most cases, patency (opening up) of the canals is achieved, but fertility is not always regained.

The term in this frame that refers to *the state of being open* is

_____.

The surgical term in this frame that is synonymous with vas/ectomy reversal is

_____/_____/_____/_____/_____.

SECTION REVIEW 8-5

Using the following table, write the CF, suffix, or prefix that matches its definition in the space provided to the left of the definition. There may be more than one word element that matches a definition.

Combining Forms		Suffixes		Prefixes
carcin/o	*prostat/o*	*-cele*	*-pexy*	*dys-*
cyst/o	*spermat/o*	*-cyte*	*-rrhaphy*	*hyper-*
muc/o	*sperm/o*	*-genesis*	*-tome*	*neo-*
olig/o	*test/o*	*-itis*		
orchid/o	*vas/o*	*-megaly*		
orchi/o		*-pathy*		

1. _____ suture

2. _____ bad; painful; difficult

3. _____ bladder

4. _____ cancer

5. _____ cell

6. _____ disease

7. _____ enlargement

8. _____ hernia; swelling

9. _____ inflammation

10. _____ instrument to cut

11. _____ vessel; vas deferens; duct

12. _____ mucus

13. _____ new

14. _____ forming, producing; origin

15. _____ prostate gland

16. _____ testes

17. _____ scanty

18. _____ spermatozoa, sperm cells

19. _____ fixation (of an organ)

20. _____ excessive; above normal

Competency Verification: Check your answers in Appendix B: Answer Key, page 607. If you are not satisfied with your level of comprehension, go back to Frame 8–83, and rework the frames.

Correct Answers _____ x 5 = _____ % Score

Abbreviations

This section introduces reproductive system–related abbreviations and their meanings. Included are abbreviations contained in the medical record activities that follow.

Abbreviation	Meaning	Abbreviation	Meaning
Female Reproductive System			
CS, C-section	cesarean section	OB-GYN	obstetrics and gynecology
D&C	dilation and curettage	OCP	oral contraceptive pill
Dx	diagnosis	Pap	Papanicolaou (test)
G	gravida (pregnant)	para 1, 2, 3	unipara, bipara, tripara (number of viable births)
GYN	gynecology	PID	pelvic inflammatory disease
HRT	hormone replacement therapy	TAH	total abdominal hysterectomy
IVF	in vitro fertilization	TRAM	transverse rectus abdominis muscle
LMP	last menstrual period	TSS	toxic shock syndrome
OB	obstetrics	TVH	total vaginal hysterectomy
Male Reproductive System			
ED	erectile dysfunction	PSA	prostate-specific antigen
BPH	benign prostatic hyperplasia, benign prostatic hypertrophy	TURP	transurethral resection of the prostate
DRE	digital rectal examination	TRUS	transrectal ultrasonography
Sexually Transmitted Infections			
GC	gonorrhea	STD	sexually transmitted disease
HPV	human papillomavirus	STI	sexually transmitted infection
HSV	herpes simplex virus	VD	venereal disease

Additional Medical Terms

The following are additional terms related to the female and male reproductive systems. Recognizing and learning these terms will help you understand the connections among a pathological condition, its diagnosis, and the rationale behind the method of treatment selected for a particular disorder.

Diseases and Conditions

Female Reproductive System

candidiasis kăn-dĭ-DĪ-ă-sĭs	Vaginal fungal infection caused by *Candida albicans* and characterized by a curdy, or cheeselike, discharge and extreme itching

cervical cancer SĔR-vĭ-kăl	Malignancy that occurs in the lower part of the uterus that is strongly associated with human papillomavirus (HPV) infection, a sexually transmitted infection; other risk factors include early onset of sexual activity, multiple sexual partners, having other STIs, weak immune system, and smoking *Early-stage cervical cancer usually has no signs or symptoms, but late-stage symptoms include vaginal bleeding and pelvic pain. Treatment depends on the stage of CA and includes hysterectomy, radiation, chemotherapy, or a combination of the three. (See Figure 8-14.)*
ectopic pregnancy ĕk-TŎP-ik	Implantation of the fertilized ovum outside of the uterine cavity, such as a fallopian tube, an ovary, the abdomen, or the cervix uteri (See Figure 8-15.) *Ectopic pregnancy occurs in approximately 1% of pregnancies, most commonly in the oviducts (tubal pregnancy). Some types of ectopic pregnancies include ovarian, interstitial, and isthmic.*

Cervical Cancer

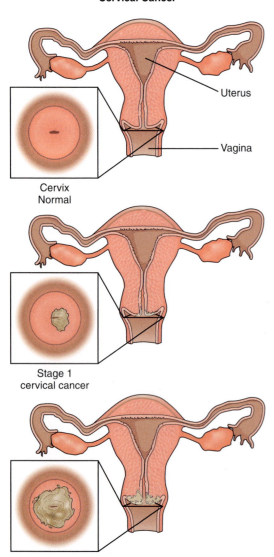

Cervix
Normal

Stage 1
cervical cancer

Stage 2
cervical cancer

Uterus

Vagina

Figure 8-14 Stages of cervical cancer.

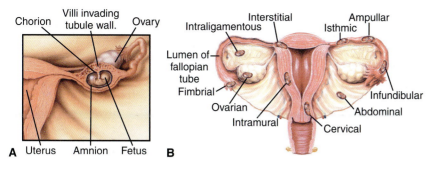

Figure 8-15 Tubal pregnancy (A) and other sites of ectopic pregnancy (B).

endometriosis
ĕn-dō-mē-trē-Ō-sĭs
  endo: in, within
  metri: uterus (womb)
  -osis: abnormal condition; increase (used primarily with blood cells)
	Painful disorder in which tissue that normally lines the inside of the uterus (endometrium) grows outside the uterine cavity (See Figure 8-16.)
	
	Endometriosis most commonly involves the ovaries, fallopian tubes, and the tissue lining the pelvis.

fibroid
FĪ-broyd
  fibr: fiber, fibrous tissue
  -oids: resembling
	Benign neoplasm in the uterus that is composed largely of fibrous tissue; also called *leiomyoma*
	
	Uterine fibroids are the most common tumors in women. If fibroids grow too large and cause symptoms, such as pelvic pain or menorrhagia, hysterectomy may be indicated.

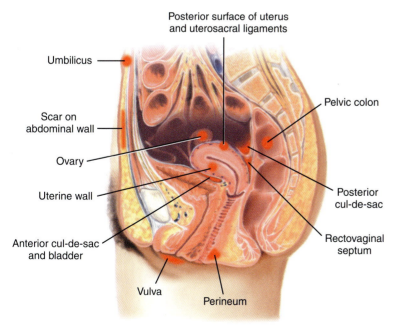

Figure 8-16 Endometriosis.

gestational hypertension
jĕs-TĀ-shŭn-ăl
hī-pĕr-TĔN-shŭn

Potentially life-threatening disorder that usually develops after the 20th week of pregnancy and is characterized by edema and proteinuria

Gestational hypertension may occur in nonconvulsive or convulsive forms.

preeclampsia
prē-ē-KLĂMP-sē-ă

Nonconvulsive form of gestational hypertension, which, if left untreated, may progress to eclampsia

Treatment includes bedrest and blood pressure monitoring.

eclampsia
ē-KLĂMP-sē-ă

Convulsive form of gestational hypertension that is a medical emergency and life-threatening to the mother and baby

Treatment includes bedrest, blood pressure monitoring, and antiseizure drugs.

leukorrhea
loo-kō-RĒ-ă
  leuk/o: white
  -rrhea: discharge, flow

White discharge from the vagina

A greater than usual amount of leukorrhea is normal in pregnancy, and a decrease is to be expected after delivery, during lactation, and after menopause. Leukorrhea is the most common reason women seek gynecological care.

sterility
stĕr-ĬL-ĭ-tē

Inability of a woman to become pregnant or for a man to impregnate a woman

toxic shock syndrome (TSS)
TŎK-sĭk SHŎK
SĬN-drōm
  tox: poison
   -ic: pertaining to

Rare and sometimes fatal *Staphylococcus* infection that generally occurs in menstruating women, most of whom use vaginal tampons for menstrual protection

In TSS, the normally harmless vaginal bacterium Staphylococcus aureus multiplies in the old blood in the tampon and releases toxins. The tampon itself creates small tears in the vaginal wall that allow the toxins to enter the bloodstream.

Male Reproductive System

anorchism
ăn-ŎR-kĭzm
  an: without, not
  orch: testis (plural, testes)
  -ism: condition

Congenital absence of one or both testes; also called *anorchidism* or anorchia

balanitis
băl-ă-NĪ-tĭs
  balan: glans penis
   -itis: inflammation

Inflammation of the skin covering the glans penis

Balanitis is caused by irritation and invasion of microorganisms. It is commonly associated with inadequate hygiene of the prepuce and phimosis.

cryptorchism
krĭpt-OR-kĭ-zm
   crypt: hidden
    orch: testis (plural,
         testes)
   -ism: condition
	Failure of one or both testicles to descend into the scrotum; also called *cryptorchidism*
	
	Cryptorchism is associated with a high risk of sterility, causing a low sperm count and male infertility. If the testes do not descend on their own at an early age, orchiopexy is performed to bring the testicles into the scrotum.

epispadias
ĕp-ĭ-SPĀ-dē-ăs
      epi-: above, upon
   -spadias: slit, fissure
	Congenital defect in which the urethra opens on the upper side of the penis near the glans penis instead of the tip

hypospadias
hī-pō-SPĀ-dē-ăs
    hypo: under, below,
        deficient
   -spadias: slit, fissure
	Congenital defect in which the male urethra opens on the undersurface of the penis instead of the tip

impotence ĬM-pŏ-tĕns	Inability of a man to achieve or maintain a penile erection; commonly called erectile *dysfunction (ED)*

phimosis
fĭ-MŌ-sĭs
   phim: muzzle
   -osis: abnormal
        condition;
        increase (used
        primarily with
        blood cells)
	Stenosis or narrowness of the preputial orifice so that the foreskin cannot be pushed back over the glans penis

sexually transmitted infections (STIs)	Any disease that may be acquired as a result of sexual intercourse or other intimate contact with an infected individual and affects the male and female reproductive systems; also called *sexually transmitted diseases (STDs)*
chlamydia klă-MĬD-ē-ă	Sexually transmitted bacterial infection that causes cervicitis in women and urethritis and epididymitis in men
	Chlamydial infection is now highly prevalent and is among the most potentially damaging of all STIs. Antibiotics are prescribed to cure the infection. If left untreated, chlamydia can cause PID and infertility in women.
gonorrhea gŏn-ō-RĒ-ă *gon/o:* seed (ovum or spermatozoon) *-rrhea:* discharge, flow	Sexually transmitted bacterial infection of the mucous membrane of the genital tract in men and women
	Gonorrheal infection results from anal, vaginal, or oral sex with an infected partner. It can also be passed on from an infected mother to her infant during the birth process (as the baby passes through the vaginal canal). Gonorrhea and chlamydia commonly occur together. Both partners are treated for these infections with antibiotics.
herpes genitalis HĔR-pēz jĕn-ĭ-TĂL-ĭs	Highly contagious viral infection of the male and female genitalia that is transmitted by direct contact with infected body secretions (usually through sexual intercourse) and differs from other STIs in that it can recur spontaneously once the virus has been acquired; also called *venereal herpes*
	Herpes genitalis is most commonly caused by herpes simplex virus (HSV) type 2. Treatment is symptomatic, which means that medications are given to reduce the symptoms of swelling and pain. There is no cure for genital herpes. A particularly life-threatening form of the disease can occur in infants infected by the virus during vaginal birth.
human papillomavirus (HPV)	Infection of the genital areas of men and women, including the penis, vulva, and anus, as well as the rectal, cervical, and vaginal linings
	There are over 40 types of HPV infections. One type, genital warts, causes CA of the cervix in females and penile cancer in males. A vaccine that protects against four types of HPV is available for young males and females at age 11 years.
syphilis SĬF-ĭ-lĭs	Infectious, chronic STI characterized initially by skin lesions (chancres), typically on the genitals, rectum, or mouth
	Syphilis may exist without symptoms for years and cause long-term complications, including death, if not treated. It can also be transmitted from mother to fetus, causing multiple, severe health problems for the baby, and is known as congenital syphilis. Penicillin, intramuscularly or intravenously, is the antibiotic of choice for the treatment of all stages of syphilis.
trichomoniasis trĭk-ō-mō-NĪ-ă-sĭs	Infection of the vagina or male genital tract that commonly causes vaginitis, urethritis, and cystitis
	Trichomoniasis is the most common asymptomatic STI. Treatment consists of a single oral dose of a combined antibacterial and antiprotozoal medication.

Diagnostic Procedures

Female Reproductive System

amniocentesis ăm-nē-ō-sĕn-TĒ-sĭs *amni/o:* amnion 　　　　(amniotic sac) *-centesis:* surgical 　　　　puncture	Obstetric procedure that involves surgical puncture of the amniotic sac under ultrasound guidance to remove amniotic fluid *In amniocentesis, cells of the fetus found in the fluid are cultured and studied to detect genetic abnormalities and maternal–fetal blood incompatibility. (See Figure 8-17.)*

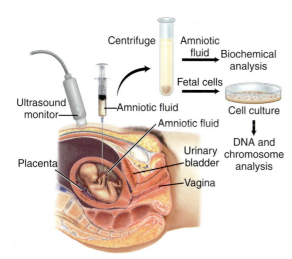

Figure 8-17 Amniocentesis.

colposcopy kŏl-PŎS-kō-pē *colp/o:* vagina *-scopy:* visual 　　　　examination	Examination of the vagina and the cervix with an optical magnifying instrument (colposcope) *Colposcopy is commonly performed after a Pap test to obtain biopsy specimens of the cervix and identify abnormal cervical tissue. (See Figure 8-18.)*

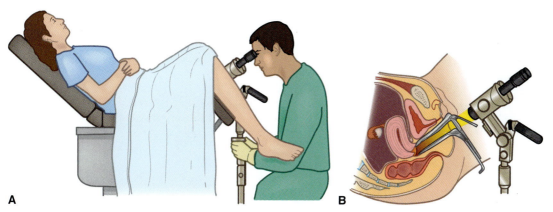

A　　　　　　　　　　　　　　　　　　　　**B**

Figure 8-18 Colposcopy. (A) Woman in dorsal lithotomy position for examination. (B) Colposcope illuminating the cervix for biopsy.

laparoscopy
lăp-ăr-ŎS-kō-pē
  lapar/o: abdomen
  -scopy: visual
          examination
	Visual examination of the abdominal cavity with a laparoscope through one or more small incisions in the abdominal wall, usually at the umbilicus (See Figure 8-19.)
	
	Laparoscopy is used for inspection of the ovaries and the fallopian tubes, diagnosis of endometriosis, destruction of uterine leiomyomas, myomectomy, and gynecological sterilization.

mammography
măm-ŎG-ră-fē
  mamm/o: breast
  -graphy: process of
          recording
	Radiography of the breast used to diagnose benign and malignant tumors

Papanicolaou (Pap) test pă-pă-NĬ-kō-lŏw	Microscopic analysis of cells taken from the cervix and vagina to detect the presence of carcinoma *Cells are obtained for a Pap test via insertion of a vaginal speculum and the use of a swab to scrape a small tissue sample from the cervix and vagina. (See Figure 8-20.)*

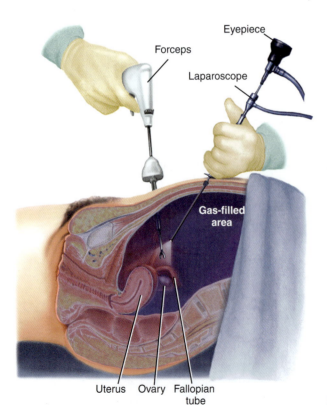

Figure 8-19 Laparoscopy.

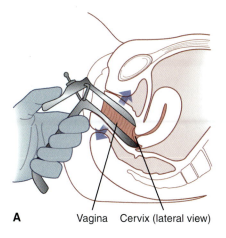
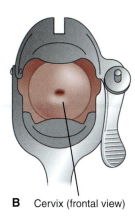

A   Vagina   Cervix (lateral view)   **B**   Cervix (frontal view)

Figure 8-20 Papanicolaou (Pap) test. (A) Insertion of speculum to expand the vaginal walls and reveal the cervix. (B) Cervix exposed to obtain cells for Pap test. *From Dillon PM: Nursing Health Assessment, 2nd ed. FA Davis, Philadelphia, 2007, pp 634–635, with permission.*

ultrasonography (US)
ŭl-tră-sŏn-ŎG-ră-fē
   ultra-: excess, beyond
   son/o: sound
   -graphy: process of recording
	Radiographic procedure in which a small transducer passed over the skin transmits high-frequency sound waves (ultrasound) that bounce off body tissues and are then recorded to produce an image of an internal organ or tissue
	
	Pelvic US is used to evaluate the female reproductive organs and the fetus during pregnancy. Transvaginal US places the sound probe in the vagina, instead of across the pelvis or the abdomen, producing a sharper examination of normal and pathological structures within the pelvis.

Male Reproductive System

digital rectal examination (DRE)
DĬJ-ĭ-tăl RĔK-tăl
   rect: rectum
   -al: pertaining to
	Examination of the prostate gland by finger palpation through the anal canal and the rectum
	
	DRE is usually performed during physical examination to detect prostate enlargement. It is also used to check for problems with organs or other structures in the pelvis and lower abdomen. (See Figure 8-21.)

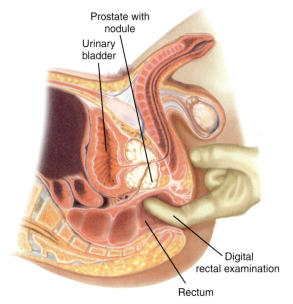

Prostate with nodule

Urinary bladder

Digital rectal examination

Rectum

Figure 8-21 Digital rectal examination.

| **transrectal ultrasound (TRUS) and biopsy of the prostate**
trans: across, through
rect: rectum
al: pertaining to
bi-: two
-opsy: view of | An ultrasound probe is inserted into the rectum to obtain an image of the prostate gland and collect multiple needle biopsy specimens of the prostate gland tissues where abnormalities are detected

High-frequency sound waves are recorded and transformed into video or photographic images of the prostate gland. If CA is identified, the physician will be able to grade the CA and determine its aggressiveness or likelihood of spreading. (See Figure 8-22.) |

Medical and Surgical Procedures

Female Reproductive System

| **cerclage**
sār-KLŎZH | Obstetric procedure in which a nonabsorbable suture is used for holding the cervix closed to prevent spontaneous abortion in a woman who has an incompetent cervix |

| **episiotomy**
ĕ-pĭs-ē-ŎT-ō-mē
episi/o: vulva
-tomy: incision | Surgical incision of the perineum to enlarge the vaginal opening for obstetrical purposes during the birth process

Episiotomy is used to aid a difficult delivery and prevent rupture of tissues. (See Figure 8-23.) |

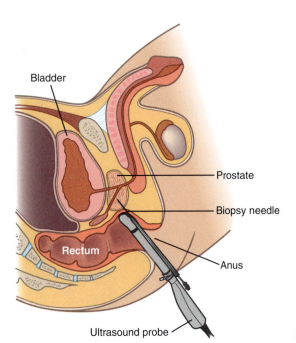

Bladder

Prostate

Biopsy needle

Rectum

Anus

Ultrasound probe

Figure 8-22 Transrectal ultrasound and biopsy of the prostate.

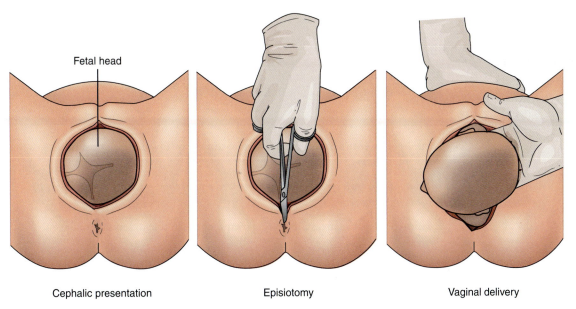

Fetal head

Cephalic presentation   Episiotomy   Vaginal delivery

Figure 8-23 Episiotomy.

---

hysterosalpingo-oophorectomy hĭs-tĕr-ō-săl-pĭng-gō-ō-ŏ-for-ĔK-tō-mē *hyster/o:* uterus (womb) *salping/o:* tube (usually fallopian or eustachian [auditory] tube) *oophor:* ovary *-ectomy:* excision	Surgical removal of a uterus, a fallopian tube, and an ovary

---

lumpectomy lŭm-PĔK-tō-mē	Excision of a small, primary breast tumor ("lump") and some of the normal tissue that surrounds it *In lumpectomy, lymph nodes may also be removed because they are located within the breast tissue taken during surgery. All tissue is removed from the breast via biopsy to determine whether cancer cells are present in the normal tissue surrounding the tumor. Lumpectomy is the most common form of breast CA surgery today. (See Figure 8-8.)*

mastectomy
măs-TĔK-tō-mē
    mast: breast
    -ectomy: excision,
            removal
	Complete or partial excision of one or both breasts, most commonly performed to remove a malignant tumor
	
	Mastectomy may be simple, radical, or modified, depending on the extent of the malignancy and amount of breast tissue excised.

total	Excision of an entire breast, nipple, areola, and the involved overlying skin; also called *simple mastectomy* *In total mastectomy, lymph nodes are removed only if they are included in the breast tissue being removed.*
modified radical	Excision of an entire breast, including lymph nodes in the underarm (axillary dissection) *Most women who have mastectomies today have modified radical mastectomies. (See Figure 8-24.)*
radical	Excision of an entire breast, all underarm lymph nodes, and chest wall muscles under the breast

Entire breast and underarm lymph nodes removed, chest muscles left intact

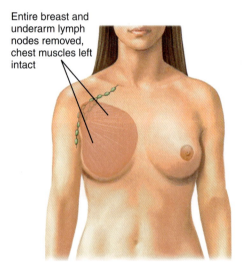

Figure 8-24 Modified radical mastectomy.

reconstructive breast surgery	Reconstruction of a breast that has been removed because of CA or other disease *Reconstruction is commonly possible immediately after mastectomy so that the patient awakens from anesthesia with a breast mound already in place.*
tissue (skin) expansion	Common breast reconstruction technique in which a balloon expander is inserted beneath the skin and chest muscle; saline solution is gradually injected to increase size, and the expander is then replaced with a more permanent implant (see Figure 8-25.)
transverse rectus abdominis muscle (TRAM) flap	Surgical creation of a skin flap (using skin and fat from the lower half of the abdomen), which is passed under the skin to the breast area, shaped into a natural-looking breast, and sutured into place *The TRAM flap procedure is one of the most popular reconstruction options. (See Figure 8-26.)*

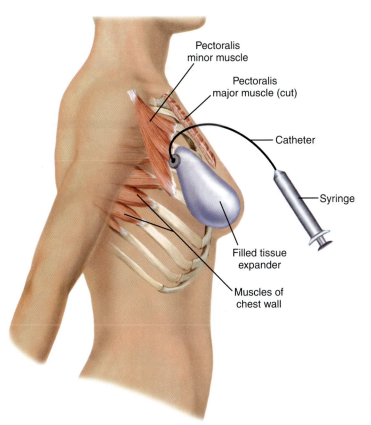

Pectoralis
minor muscle

Pectoralis
major muscle (cut)

Catheter

Syringe

Filled tissue
expander

Muscles of
chest wall

Figure 8-25 Tissue expander for breast reconstruction.

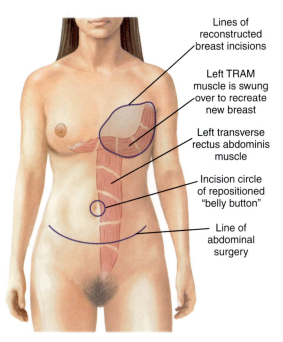

Lines of
reconstructed
breast incisions

Left TRAM
muscle is swung
over to recreate
new breast

Left transverse
rectus abdominis
muscle

Incision circle
of repositioned
"belly button"

Line of
abdominal
surgery

Figure 8-26 TRAM flap.

tubal ligation TŪ-băl lī-GĀ-shŭn	Sterilization procedure that involves blocking both fallopian tubes by cutting or burning them and tying them off

Male Reproductive System

brachytherapy brăk-ē-THĔR-ă-pē *brachy:* short (distance) *-therapy:* treatment	Radiation oncology procedure where radioactive "seeds" are placed directly within or near a tumor in the prostate to destroy malignant cells (See Figure 8-27.)

circumcision sĕr-kŭm-SĬ-zhŭn	Surgical removal of the foreskin, or prepuce, of the penis, usually performed on the male as an infant

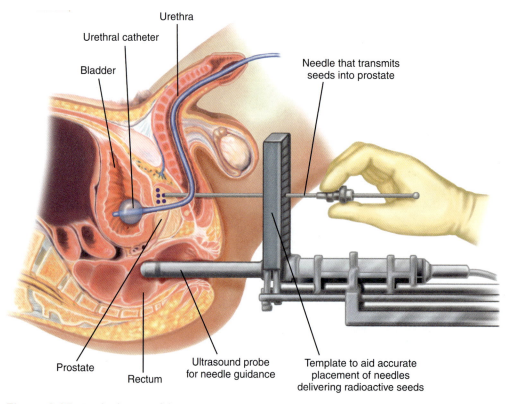

Figure 8-27 Brachytherapy of the prostate.

transurethral resection of the prostate (TURP)	Surgical procedure to relieve obstruction caused by BPH (excessive overgrowth of normal tissue) by insertion of a resectoscope into the penis and through the urethra to "chip away" at prostatic tissue and flush out chips using an irrigating solution
	The pieces of prostatic tissue obtained through TURP are sent to the laboratory to be analyzed for possible evidence of CA. Although TURP relieves the obstruction, overgrowth of tissue may recur over several years. Lasers may also be used to destroy prostatic tissue and relieve obstruction. (See Figure 8-12.)

Pharmacology

The following table lists common drug categories used to treat reproductive disorders, as well as their therapeutic actions.

Drug Category	Action
Female Reproductive System	
antifungals ăn-tĭ-FŬN-găplz	Treat vaginal fungal infection, such as candidiasis
estrogens ĔS-trō-jĕnz	Treat symptoms of menopause (hot flashes, vaginal dryness) through HRT
contraceptives kŏn-tră-SĔP-tĭvz	Prevent ovulation to avoid pregnancy *The most common female contraceptives are oral contraceptive pills (OCPs), also known as birth control pills.*
oxytocics ŏk-sē-TŌ-sĭks	Induce labor at term by increasing the strength and frequency of uterine contractions
spermicides SPĔR-mĭ-sīdz	Destroy sperm by creating a highly acidic environment in the uterus *Spermicides are used as a method of birth control.*
Male Reproductive System	
erectile agents ĕ-RĔK-tīl	Treat erectile dysfunction (impotence) by increasing blood flow to the penis, resulting in an erection
gonadotropins gŏn-ă-dō-TRŌ-pĭnz	Increase sperm count in infertility cases

Pronunciation Help	*Long Sound*	ā in rāte	ē in rēbirth	ī in īsle	ō in ōver	ū in ūnite
	Short Sound	ă in ăpple	ĕ in ĕver	ĭ in ĭt	ŏ in nŏt	ŭ in cŭt

Word Elements Review

This review provides a verification of your knowledge of the word elements covered in this chapter. First, use a slash to break the term into its component parts and identify each element by labeling it P for prefix, WR for word root, CF for combining form, or S for suffix. Then, provide the meaning of the medical term. Remember to define the suffix first, define the beginning of the word second, and define the middle part of the term last. The first word is a sample completed for you.

Medical Term	Meaning
muc/oid *WR S*	*resembling mucus*
1. vas/ectomy	
2. amni/o/centesis	
3. mast/o/plasty	
4. oophor/oma	
5. crypt/orchid/ism	

Match the medical terms below with the definitions in the numbered list.

balanitis   hysterectomy   primigravida
colposcopy   mastopexy   prostatocystitis
cervicitis   oligospermia   spermatozoa
galactorrhea   perineorrhaphy   testopathy

6. _____ inflammation of the prostate gland and bladder

7. _____ fixation of the breast

8. _____ visual examination of the vagina

9. _____ condition of scanty spermatozoa or sperm cells

10. _____ excision or removal of the uterus

11. _____ inflammation of the glans penis

12. _____ disease of the testes or testicles

13. _____ discharge or flow of milk

14. _____ suture of the perineum

15. _____ woman during her first pregnancy

Competency Verification: Check your answers in Appendix B: Answer Key, page 608. If you are not satisfied with your level of comprehension, review the vocabulary, and retake the review.

Correct Answers _____ × 6.67 = _____ % Score

Additional Medical Terms Review

Match the medical term(s) below with the definitions in the numbered list.

anorchism	*cryptorchidism*	*gonorrhea*	*phimosis*
candidiasis	*D&C*	*impotence*	*sterility*
cerclage	*endometriosis*	*leukorrhea*	*syphilis*
chlamydia	*fibroid*	*mammography*	*toxic shock syndrome*
circumcision	*gonadotropins*	*oligomenorrhea*	*trichomoniasis*

1. _____ refers to the failure of the testicles to descend into the scrotum.

2. _____ is a benign neoplasm in the uterus composed largely of leiomyomas.

3. _____ refers to the inability of a woman to become pregnant or for a man to impregnate a woman.

4. _____ refers to the congenital absence of one or both testes.

5. _____ is a vaginal fungal infection caused by *Candida albicans* and is characterized by a curdy discharge and extreme itching.

6. _____ is a sexually transmitted bacterial infection that causes cervicitis in women and urethritis and epididymitis in men.

7. _____ is the surgical removal of the foreskin, or *prepuce,* of the penis.

8. _____ is an obstetric procedure to prevent spontaneous abortion in a woman who has an incompetent cervix.

9. _____ is a discharge from the vagina and a common reason for women to seek gynecological care.

10. _____ is a condition in which endometrial tissue is found in various abnormal sites throughout the pelvis or in the abdominal wall.

11. _____ refers to radiography of the breast and is used to diagnose benign and malignant tumors.

12. _____ is a sexually transmitted bacterial infection that most commonly affects the genitourinary tract and, occasionally, the pharynx or rectum.

13. _____ is a sexually transmitted infection that is characterized by lesions that change to a chancre and, eventually, serious organ damage.

14. _____ is a rare and sometimes fatal staphylococcal infection that occurs in menstruating women who use vaginal tampons.

15. _____ is an infection of the vagina or male genital tract that commonly causes vaginitis, urethritis, and cystitis.

16. _____ refers to a widening of the uterine cervix so that the surface lining of the uterus can be scraped.

17. _____ means stenosis of the preputial orifice so that the foreskin does not retract over the glans penis.

18. _____ refers to the inability of a man to achieve a penile erection.

19. _____ refers to scanty or infrequent menstrual flow.

20. _____ are hormonal preparations used to increase the sperm count in cases of infertility.

Competency Verification: Check your answers in Appendix B: Answer Key, page 608. If you are not satisfied with your level of comprehension, review the pathological, diagnostic, and therapeutic terms, and retake the review.

Correct Answers _____ × 5 = _____ % Score

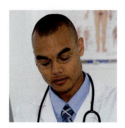

Medical Record Activities

To develop a working vocabulary of medical terms and to understand how those terms are used in the health-care industry, it is important that you complete the following activities.

MEDICAL RECORD ACTIVITY 8-1

EMERGENCY DEPARTMENT REPORT: PELVIC INFLAMMATORY DISEASE

This activity contains an emergency department report for pelvic inflammatory disease. Read the report that follows, and underline the medical terms. Then, complete the terminology and critical thinking exercises.

EMERGENCY DEPARTMENT REPORT

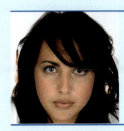

PATIENT NAME: Roman, Mona
Medical Record ID: 79-7435098671
DATE: April 1, 20xx

DATE OF VISIT: 04/01/20

CHIEF COMPLAINT: Vaginal irritation and drainage.

HISTORY OF PRESENT ILLNESS: This is a 20-year-old female who says that for the past weeks she has had lower abdominal pressure, a lot of vaginal discharge, and burning with urination. Her last menstrual period was March 13. She says it was normal in duration and intensity. No other specific complaints, except that she states that her boyfriend said that he might have gonorrhea, and she wants to be checked.

REVIEW OF SYSTEMS: No fever or chills, vomiting, diarrhea, or rashes.

MEDICATIONS: She says that she has been using an over-the-counter medication (Monistat) without improvement.

PHYSICAL EXAMINATION: A well-developed 20-year-old female who is in no apparent distress. Her vitals are stable. She is afebrile. Her skin is without cyanosis or rashes. Chest is clear. Heart rate and rhythm are regular. Her abdomen is soft, with active bowel sounds. She has tenderness in the suprapubic area. Pelvic examination reveals normal external genitalia, although the vaginal mucosa is markedly erythematous, and she has a lot of foul-smelling, purulent drainage. There is no gross ulceration. Cervical cultures were obtained. Wet mount was prepared and showed some trichomonads. Bimanual examination shows uterine motion tenderness. There is no adnexal mass or tenderness.

DIAGNOSIS: Probable pelvic inflammatory disease. Trichomoniasis. Possible gonorrhea exposure.

PLAN: She was given 400 mg Suprax here, 1 g Zithromax, and a prescription for Flagyl 250 mg t.i.d. for 10 days, as well as doxycycline 100 mg b.i.d. for 10 days. She should follow up with the clinic in 2 to 3 days and return if any problems occur.

M. Wolf M.D.
_____
M. Wolf, M.D.

MW:js
D: 04/01/xx ; T: 04/01/xx

Terminology 8-1

Terms listed in the table below come from the emergency department report Pelvic Inflammatory Disease. *Use a medical dictionary, such as* Taber's Cyclopedic Medical Dictionary; *the appendices of this book; or other resources to define each term. Then, pronounce the term, and place a ✓ in the box after you do so.*

Term	Definition
adnexal ăd-NĚK-săl ☐	
afebrile ā-FĚB-rĭl ☐	
cyanosis sī-ă-NŌ-sĭs ☐	
doxycycline dăwk-sē-SĪ-klēn ☐	
erythematous ĕr-ĭ-THĚM-ă-tŭs ☐	
Flagyl FLĂ-jĭl ☐	
gonorrhea gŏn-ō-RĒ-ă ☐	
Monistat MŎN-ĭh-stăt ☐	
pelvic inflammatory disease PĚL-vĭk ĭn-FLĂM-ă-tōr-ē dĭ-ZĒZ ☐	
purulent PŪR-ū-lĕnt ☐	
suprapubic soo-pră-PŪ-bĭk ☐	
Suprax SOO-prăks ☐	

Term	Definition
trichomonads trĭk-ō-MŌ-nădz ☐	
Trichomoniasis trĭk-ō-mō-NĪ-ă-sĭs ☐	
Zithromax ZĬ-thrō-măx ☐	

Visit the *Medical Terminology Simplified* online resource center at FADavis.com to hear pronunciation and meanings of terms in this medical report.

Critical Thinking 8-1

Review the emergency department report above to answer the following questions. Use a medical dictionary, such as Taber's Cyclopedic Medical Dictionary, *and other resources, if needed.*

1. What conditions are treated with the over-the-counter medication Monistat?

   _____

   _____

2. Place a "+" in the space provided for positive findings and a "–" for negative findings. A positive finding indicates the patient had these symptoms; a negative finding indicates the patient did not have the symptoms.

   hematuria _____   skin rash _____

   vaginal irritation _____   vaginal drainage _____

   fever _____   foul-smelling drainage _____

3. What were the diagnoses for this patient?

   _____

   _____

4. What is trichomoniasis, and how is it treated?

   _____

   _____

5. What are the possible complications if the patient does not treat her sexually transmitted infection (STI)?

   _____

   _____

MEDICAL RECORD ACTIVITY 8-2

OPERATIVE REPORT: BILATERAL VASECTOMY

This activity contains an operative report for a bilateral vasectomy. Read the report that follows, and underline the medical terms. Then, complete the terminology and critical thinking exercises.

OPERATIVE REPORT

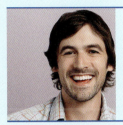

PATIENT NAME: Drummond, Neil
Medical Record Id: 89-93284670
Date: April 20, 20xx

PROCEDURE: Bilateral vasectomy

SUMMARY: Under adequate IV sedation, the patient was placed on the table in the supine position and prepped, his scrotum was shaved, and he was draped in the usual fashion. The right testicle was grasped and brought to skin level. This area was injected with 1% xylocaine anesthesia. After a few minutes, a small incision was made, and the right vas was located. A hemostat was used and clamped on the right and left vas. A segment of the right vas was removed, and both ends were cauterized and tied independently with 3-0 silk suture. The skin was closed with 2-0 chromic suture. The same procedure was performed on the left side. The hemostats were removed and sterile dressings were applied. There were no complications or bleeding. Patient was transferred to recovery in a satisfactory condition.

DISCHARGE: Patient was discharged to his home to the care of his wife. Postoperative care instruction sheet was given, along with prescription of Darvocet-N 100 mg, 1 q4h, as required, for pain. Patient will be seen for follow-up semen analysis in 6 weeks.

Peter Falk, M.D.

Peter Falk, M.D.

PF:sr
D: 4/20/20xx; T: 4/20/20xx

TERMINOLOGY 8-2

Terms listed in the table below come from the operative report Bilateral Vasectomy. *Use a medical dictionary, such as* Taber's Cyclopedic Medical Dictionary; *the appendices of this book; or other resources to define each term. Then, pronounce the term, and place a ✓ in the box after you do so.*

Term	Definition
bilateral bī-LĂT-ĕr-ăl ☐	
cauterized KAW-tĕr-īzd ☐	
Darvocet-N DĂHR-vō-sĕt ☐	
hemostat HĒ-mō-stăt ☐	
semen SĒ-mĕn ☐	
supine sū-PĪN ☐	
vasectomy văs-ĔK-tō-mē ☐	
Xylocaine ZĪ-lō-kān ☐	

 Visit the *Medical Terminology Simplified* online resource center at FADavis.com to hear pronunciation and meanings of terms in this medical report.

Critical Thinking 8-2

Review the operative report above to answer the following questions. Use a medical dictionary, such as Taber's Cyclopedic Medical Dictionary, *and other resources, if needed.*

1. What is the end result of a bilateral vasectomy?

   _____

   _____

2. Was the patient awake during the surgery? What type of anesthesia was used?

   _____

   _____

3. What was used to prevent bleeding?

   _____

   _____

4. What type of suture material was used to close the incision?

   _____

   _____

5. What was the patient given for pain relief at home?

   _____

   _____

6. Why is it important for the patient to go for a follow-up visit?

   _____

   _____

MEDICAL RECORD ACTIVITY 8-3

CLINICAL APPLICATION

This activity is a clinical application that will help you integrate and reinforce your understanding of how the following medical terms are used in the clinical environment. Complete the following clinically related sentences by selecting an appropriate term from the list.

brachytherapy	cryptorchidism	fibroid	orchidoplasty
candidiasis	ectopic pregnancy	herpes genitalis	preeclampsia
colposcopy	endometriosis	lumpectomy	TURP

1. A 65-year-old male with urinary obstruction has benign prostatic hyperplasia. His physician recommends surgery to remove prostatic tissue and improve urinary flow. The surgeon inserts an endoscope through the urethra and removes prostatic tissue in a procedure called a(n) _____.

2. Cecilia, a 25-year-old gravida 1, para 0 in her 22nd week of gestation, complains of edema of her hands and feet. Her urinalysis is positive for proteinuria and her blood pressure is elevated at 148/96 mm Hg. She is advised that she may have a form of pregnancy-induced hypertension called _____.

3. An 18-year-old female complains of a white, cheesy, vaginal discharge and extreme itching of the vagina and vulva. During the gynecological examination, swabs of the discharge are obtained for laboratory testing. The nurse practitioner suspects a fungal infection called _____.

4. Michael is a 5-day-old neonate born 4 weeks premature. His mother is concerned because she can only locate one of Michael's testicles. Her physician explains that Michael has a condition in which one or both testicles fail to descend into the scrotum. This condition is known as _____.

5. A 26-year-old male complains of burning and tingling at the head of his penis. He is also concerned about a small cluster of blisters on the shaft. The physician suspects the patient has a sexually transmitted infection caused by the herpes simplex virus type 2, which she charts as _____.

6. A 39-year-old female complains of severe right-sided abdominal pain that radiates to her pelvis. She states her last menstrual period was about 8 weeks ago. During the pelvic examination, she expresses tenderness of the uterus and fallopian tubes. The physician suspects an implantation of the fertilized ovum outside of the uterine cavity and diagnoses a(n) _____.

7. This 30-year-old female is seen today for a follow-up visit after an abnormal Pap test result. The gynecologist uses an optical magnifying instrument to visualize the interior of the vagina and the cervix. This procedure is known as a(n) _____.

8. Mrs. J. is a 40-year-old female with a complaint of pelvic pain and heavy menstrual flow. While performing the pelvic examination, her physician feels lumps behind the uterus. He suspects the presence of endometrial tissue outside of the uterus, known as _____.

9. A 33-year-old male sustains a severe laceration of the left testicle in a construction accident. The urologist decides the patient must undergo surgical repair of the testicle, commonly referred to as _____.

10. A 60-year-old female is diagnosed with early-stage cancer of the left breast. The gynecologist finds there is only one tumor with no metastasis and recommends removal of the primary tumor along with some of the surrounding tissue. This surgical procedure is known as a(n) _____.

Competency Verification: Check your answers in Appendix B: Answer Key, page 609. If you are not satisfied with your level of comprehension, review the material in this chapter, and retake the review.

Correct Answers: _____ × 10 = _____ % Score

REPRODUCTIVE SYSTEMS CHAPTER REVIEW

WORD ELEMENTS SUMMARY

The following table summarizes CFs, suffixes, and prefixes related to the reproductive systems. Study the word elements and their meanings before completing the Vocabulary Review that follows.

Word Element	Meaning	Word Element	Meaning
Combining Forms			
Female Reproductive System			
amni/o	amnion (amniotic sac)	**metr/o**	uterus (womb); measure
cervic/o	neck; cervix uteri (neck of the uterus)	**mamm/o, mast/o**	breast
colp/o, vagin/o	vagina	**men/o**	menses, menstruation
episi/o, vulv/o	vulva	**nat/o**	birth
galact/o, lact/o	milk	**oophor/o, ovari/o**	ovary
gynec/o	woman, female	**path/o**	disease
hyster/o, uter/o	uterus (womb)	**perine/o**	perineum
lapar/o	abdomen	**salping/o**	tube (usually fallopian or eustachian [auditory] tubes)
Male Reproductive System			
andr/o	male	**orchid/o, orchi/o, orch/o, test/o**	testis (plural, testes)
balan/o	glans penis	**prostat/o**	prostate gland
gonad/o	gonads, sex glands	**spermat/o, sperm/i, sperm/o**	spermatozoa, sperm cells
muc/o	mucus	**varic/o**	dilated vein
olig/o	scanty	**vas/o**	vessel; vas deferens; duct
Suffixes			
-al, -ic, -ous	pertaining to	**-para**	to bear (offspring)
-algia, -dynia	pain	**-pathy**	disease
-arche	beginning	**-pexy**	fixation (of an organ)
-cele	hernia; swelling	**-plasia, -plasm**	formation, growth
-cyesis	pregnancy	**-plasty**	surgical repair
-ectomy	excision, removal	**-ptosis**	prolapse, downward displacement
-genesis	forming, producing, origin	**-rrhage, -rrhagia**	bursting forth (of)
-gravida	pregnant woman	**-rrhaphy**	suture
-ia	condition	**-rrhea**	discharge, flow
-ist	specialist	**-salpinx**	tube (usually fallopian or eustachian [auditory] tubes)

Continued

Word Element	Meaning	Word Element	Meaning
-itis	inflammation	-scope	instrument for examining
-lith	stone, calculus	-spasm	involuntary contraction, twitching
-logist	specialist in the study of	-tocia	childbirth, labor
-logy	study of	-tome	instrument to cut
-megaly	enlargement	-tomy	incision
-oid	resembling	-uria	urine
-oma	tumor	-version	turning
Prefixes			
a-, an-	without, not	neo-	new
dys-	bad; painful; difficult	post-	after; behind
hyper-	excessive, above normal	pre-	before; in front of

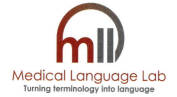

Medical Language Lab
Turning terminology into language

Visit the *Medical Language Lab* at the website *medicallanguagelab.com.* Use the flash-card exercise to reinforce your study of word elements. We recommend you complete the flash-card exercise before starting the following vocabulary Review.

Vocabulary Review

Match the medical terms with the definitions in the numbered list.

amenorrhea	estrogen	para 4	testopathy
aspermatism	gravida 4	PID	testosterone
cervix uteri	hydrocele	postmenopausal	uterus
dysmenorrhea	oophoritis	prostatic cancer	vas deferens
epididymis	oxytocics	prostatomegaly	vasectomy

1. _____ means enlargement of the prostate gland.

2. _____ refers to a disease of the testes.

3. _____ is a male hormone produced by the testes.

4. _____ is an absence or abnormal stoppage of the menses.

5. _____ is a female hormone produced by the ovaries.

6. _____ is an inflamed condition of the ovaries.

7. _____ is a condition in which there is a lack of male sperm.

8. _____ refers to a woman in her fourth pregnancy.

9. _____ is an organ that nourishes the embryo.

10. _____ is a malignant neoplasm of the prostate.

11. _____ is a tube that temporarily stores sperm.

12. _____ is a collection of fluid in a saclike cavity.

13. _____ is a duct that transports sperm from the testes to the urethra.

14. _____ refers to a woman who has delivered four infants.

15. _____ means *neck of the uterus.*

16. _____ refers to painful menstruation.

17. _____ means *occurring after menopause.*

18. _____ are used to induce labor by increasing the strength and frequency of uterine contractions.

19. _____ is a procedure to sterilize a man by cutting the vas deferens, preventing the release of sperm.

20. _____ is a collective term for any extensive bacterial infection of the pelvic organs, especially the uterus, uterine tubes, or ovaries.

Competency Verification: Check your answers in Appendix B: Answer Key, page 609. If you are not satisfied with your level of comprehension, review the chapter vocabulary, and retake the review.

Correct Answers: _____ × 5 = _____ % Score

Endocrine and Nervous Systems

OBJECTIVES

Upon completion of this chapter, you will be able to:

- Describe the type of medical treatment endocrinologists and neurologists provide.
- Identify the structures of the endocrine and nervous systems by labeling them on the anatomical illustrations.
- Describe the primary functions of the endocrine and nervous systems.
- Describe diseases, conditions, and procedures related to the endocrine and nervous systems.
- Apply your word-building skills by constructing medical terms related to the endocrine and nervous systems.
- Describe common abbreviations and symbols related to the endocrine and nervous systems.
- Recognize, define, pronounce, and spell terms correctly.
- Demonstrate your knowledge of this chapter by successfully completing the frames, reviews, and activities.

MEDICAL SPECIALTIES: ENDOCRINOLOGY AND NEUROLOGY

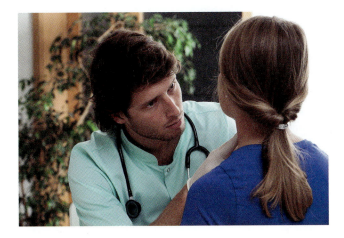

Endocrinology

Endocrinology is the medical specialty concerned with the diagnosis and treatment of endocrine gland disorders. **Endocrinologists** evaluate the body's overall metabolic function and diagnose and treat hormone imbalances caused by underproduction or overproduction of hormones. Endocrinologists treat such disorders as diabetes, osteoporosis, and other disorders of the endocrine glands. When surgery is required, the endocrinologist works closely with the surgeon to provide the most beneficial patient care. Endocrinologists also play important roles related to their field of expertise in university academic research and in the pharmaceutical industry.

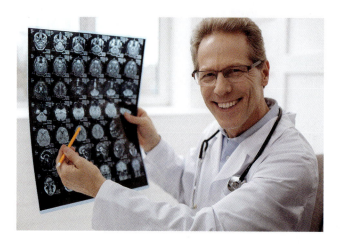

Neurology

Neurology is the medical specialty concerned with the diagnosis and treatment of diseases of the nervous system, which includes the brain, spinal cord, and peripheral nerves. **Neurologists** use specialized examination procedures and employ diagnostic tests, medical and surgical procedures, and drugs to treat nervous system diseases. The branch of surgery involving the nervous system, including the brain and the spinal cord, is called **neurosurgery.** The physician who specializes in neurosurgery is a **neurosurgeon.**

Anatomy and Physiology Overview

The endocrine and nervous systems work together like interlocking supersystems to control many intricate activities of the body. The endocrine system consists of a network of glandular structures that produces hormones and discharges them slowly into the bloodstream. The hormones then enter the bloodstream to circulate throughout the body and activate target cells. In contrast, the nervous system produces electrical messages that are designed to act instantaneously by transmitting electrical impulses to specific body locations. The instantaneous transmissions help control all critical body activities and reactions.

Together, the endocrine and nervous systems monitor changes in the body and external environment, interpret these changes, and coordinate appropriate responses to reestablish and maintain equilibrium in the internal environment of the body (**homeostasis**).

Endocrine System

The hormones secreted by the endocrine glands are chemical messengers carried by the bloodstream to other tissues or organs in the body. The tissues or organs that respond to the effects of a hormone are called **target tissues,** or **target organs.** The chemical messages they deliver tell these tissues or organs to increase or decrease their activity. The hormones act only on target tissues or organs that have the appropriate receptor sites for that given hormone. Review Figure 9-1, which lists the major endocrine glands and their locations in the human body.

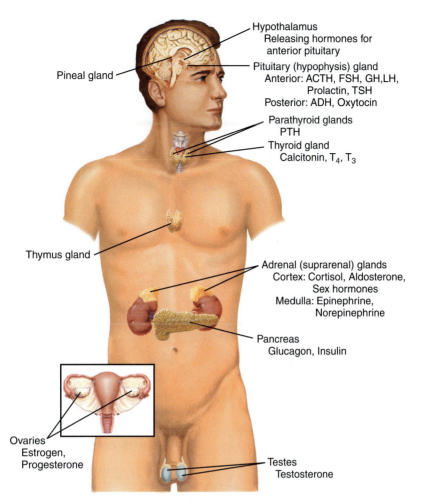

Hypothalamus
  Releasing hormones for
  anterior pituitary

Pituitary (hypophysis) gland
  Anterior: ACTH, FSH, GH,LH,
    Prolactin, TSH
  Posterior: ADH, Oxytocin

Pineal gland

Parathyroid glands
  PTH

Thyroid gland
  Calcitonin, T_4, T_3

Thymus gland

Adrenal (suprarenal) glands
  Cortex: Cortisol, Aldosterone,
    Sex hormones
  Medulla: Epinephrine,
    Norepinephrine

Pancreas
  Glucagon, Insulin

Ovaries
  Estrogen,
  Progesterone

Testes
  Testosterone

Figure 9-1   Locations of major endocrine glands.

WORD ELEMENTS

This section introduces word elements related to the endocrine system. Review the following table. Then, pronounce each term in the word analysis column, and place a ✓ in the box upon completion.

Word Element	Meaning	Word Analysis
Combining Forms		
aden/o	gland	**aden**/oma (ăd-ĕ-NŌ-mă ☐): tumor composed of glandular tissue *-oma:* tumor

adren/o
 	
adrenal/o
	adrenal glands	**adren**/al (ăd-RĒ-năl ☐): pertaining to the adrenal glands
		   -al: pertaining to
		adrenal/ectomy (ăd-rē-năl-ĔK-tō-mē ☐): excision of the adrenal gland(s)
		   -ectomy: excision, removal
		
		Adrenalectomy involves surgical removal of one or both adrenal glands to remove a tumor, aid in correcting a hormone imbalance, or prevent metastasis.

calc/o	calcium	hypo/**calc**/emia (hī-pō-kăl-SĒ-mē-ă ☐): deficiency of calcium in blood
		   hypo-: under, below, deficient
		   -emia: blood condition

gluc/o
 	
glyc/o
	sugar, sweetness	**gluc**/o/genesis (gloo-kō-JĔN-ĕ-sĭs ☐): formation of glucose
		   -genesis: forming, producing, origin
		hyper/**glyc**/emia (hī-pĕr-glī-SĒ-mē-ă ☐): excessive glucose in blood
		   hyper-: excessive, above normal
		   -emia: blood condition
		
		Hyperglycemia is most commonly associated with diabetes mellitus.

pancreat/o	pancreas	**pancreat**/itis (păn-krē-ă-TĪ-tĭs ☐): inflammation of the pancreas *itis:* inflammation *The two most common causes of pancreatitis are alcoholism and biliary tract disease, such as a gallstone that blocks the lower common bile duct. Treatment includes abstaining from alcohol, taking medication to relieve pain and infection, and undergoing choledocholithotomy to remove the gallstones.*
parathyroid/o	parathyroid glands	**parathyroid**/ectomy (păr-ă-thī-royd-ĔK-tō-mē ☐): excision of the parathyroid gland(s) *-ectomy:* excision, removal

pituitar/o	pituitary gland	hypo/**pituitar**/ism (hī-pō-pĭ-TŪ-ĭ-tă-rĭzm ☐): condition of inadequate levels of pituitary hormone in the body
		   hypo-: under, below; deficient
		   -ism: condition

thym/o	thymus gland	**thym**/oma (thī-MŌ-mă ☐): tumor of the thymus gland *-oma:* tumor

thyr/o
 	
thyroid/o
	thyroid gland	**thyr**/o/megaly (thī-rō-MĔG-ă-lē ☐): enlargement of the thyroid gland
		   -megaly: enlargement
		thyroid/o/tomy (thī-royd-ŎT-ō-mē ☐): incision of the thyroid gland
		   -tomy: incision

toxic/o	poison	**toxic**/o/logist (tŏks-ĭ-KŎL-ō-jĭst ☐): specialist in the study of poisons (toxins) *-logist:* specialist in study of *The toxicologist studies the effects that poisons or chemicals have on humans, animals, plants, and other living organisms, as well as subsequent treatments.*

Word Element	Meaning	Word Analysis
Suffixes		
-dipsia	thirst	poly/**dipsia** (pŏl-ē-DĬP-sē-ă ☐): excessive thirst *poly-:* many, much *Polydipsia is a characteristic symptom of diabetes mellitus.*
-trophy	development, nourishment	hyper/**trophy** (hī-PĔR-trŏ-fē ☐): increase in the size of an organ *hyper-:* excessive, above normal *Hypertrophy is caused by an increase in the size of the cells of an organ, rather than an increase in the number of cells, as in carcinoma.*
Pronunciation Help	*Long Sound* *Short Sound*	ā in rāte ē in rēbirth ī in īsle ō in ōver ū in ūnite ă in ăpple ĕ in ĕver ĭ in ĭt ŏ in nŏt ŭ in cŭt

Visit the *Medical Terminology Simplified* online resource center at FADavis.com for an audio exercise of the terms in this table. It will help you master pronunciations and meanings of medical terms.

SECTION REVIEW 9-1

For the following medical terms, first, write the suffix and its meaning. Then, translate the meaning of the remaining elements, starting with the first part of the word. The first word is completed for you.

Term	Meaning
1. toxic/o/logist	–logist: specialist in the study of poison
2. pancreat/itis	_____
3. thyr/o/megaly	_____
4. hyper/trophy	_____
5. gluc/o/genesis	_____
6. hypo/calc/emia	_____
7. adrenal/ectomy	_____
8. poly/dipsia	_____
9. aden/oma	_____
10. thyroid/ectomy	_____

Competency Verification: Check your answers in Appendix B: Answer Key, page 609. If you are not satisfied with your level of comprehension, review the vocabulary, and retake the review.

Correct Answers _____ x 10 = _____ % Score

Hormones

9-1 Hormones are chemical substances produced by specialized cells of the body. Because they travel in blood, hormones reach all body tissues. However, only target organs contain receptors that recognize a particular hormone. The receptors maintain the tissue's responsiveness to hormonal stimulation.

Review Figure 9-2, which illustrates hormones of the pituitary gland and their target organs. The organs shown in Figure 9-2 are directly affected by the amounts of hormones released into the bloodstream by the pituitary gland. For example, underproduction of growth hormone (GH) in children results in dwarfism.

hyper/secretion
hī-pĕr-sē-KRĒ-shŭn

hypo/secretion
hī-pō-sē-KRĒ-shŭn

9-2 Hormone secretion to a target organ is determined by the body's need for the hormone at any given time. These secretions are regulated by the body to prevent overproduction (hyper/secretion) or underproduction (hypo/secretion). When the body's regulating mechanism dysfunctions, hormone levels become deficient or excessive. These types of hormone imbalance cause various endocrine disorders.

List the term in this frame that is synonymous with

overproduction: _____ / _____ .

underproduction: _____ / _____ .

Pink indicates a prefix. Blue indicates a suffix. Boldface indicates a word root or combining form.

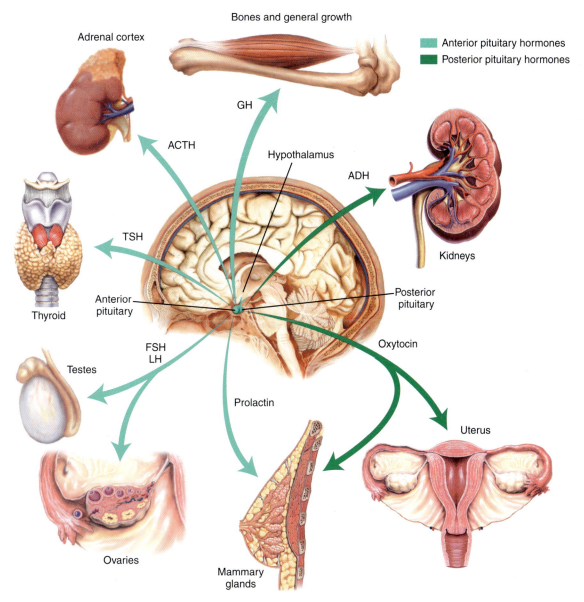

Figure 9-2 Hormones secreted by the anterior and posterior pituitary glands and their target organs.

---

heart

9–3 Although all major hormones circulate to virtually all tissues, each hormone exerts specific effects on its target organ. If a hormone has a specific effect on the stomach, that hormone's target organ is the stomach. If the hormone has a specific effect on the heart, the target organ is the _____.

9–4 Hormones have four key characteristics:
- Chemical substances produced by specialized cells of the body
- Released slowly in minute amounts directly into the bloodstream
- Produced primarily by the endocrine glands
- Almost all inactivated or excreted by the liver and kidneys

9–5 Refer to Frame 9–4 to complete this frame.

List four common characteristics of hormones.

1. _____

_____

_____

2. _____

_____

_____

3. _____

_____

_____

4. _____

_____

_____

To check answers, refer to Frame 9–4.

---

hyper/secretion
hī-pĕr-sē-KRĒ-shŭn

hypo/secretion
hī-pō-sē-KRĒ-shŭn

9–6 Endo/crine gland dysfunction may result in hypo/secretion or hyper/secretion of its hormones. The prefix *hyper-* means *excessive, above normal.* The prefix *hypo-* means *under, below, deficient.*

Build medical terms that mean

excessive secretion: _____/_____.

deficient secretion: _____/_____.

Pituitary Gland

9–7 The tiny (1) **pituitary gland,** also called the *hypophysis,* secretes at least eight major hormones. It is one of the most important endocrine glands because its secretions influence the functions of many organs in the body. Located below the brain, it is no larger than a pea. Label the pituitary gland in Figure 9-3.

---

anter/ior
ăn-TĒ-rē-or

poster/ior
pŏs-TĒ-rē-or

9–8 The pituitary gland consists of two distinct portions: an anter/ior lobe and a poster/ior lobe.

The front lobe is called the _____ / _____ lobe.

The back lobe is called the _____ / _____ lobe.

---

anter/o

poster/o

9–9 Identify the CFs that mean

anterior, front: _____/_____.

back (of body), behind, posterior: _____/_____.

Pink indicates a prefix. Blue indicates a suffix. Boldface indicates a word root or combining form.

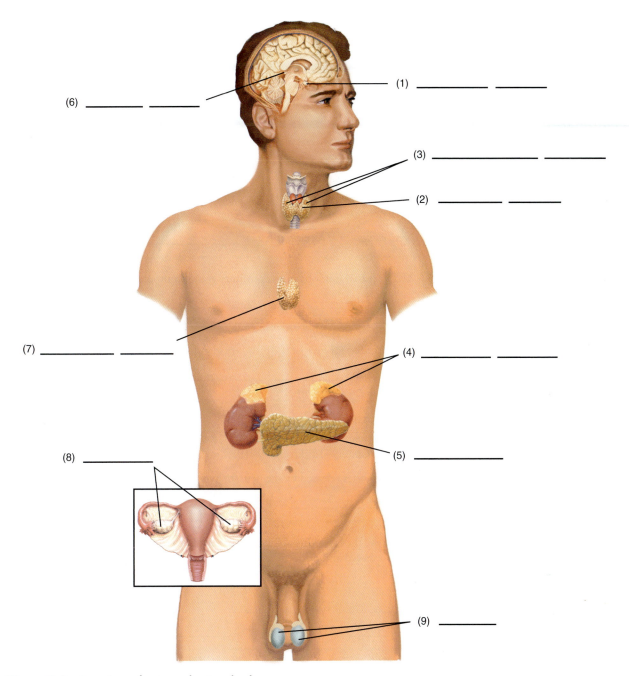

Figure 9-3 Locations of major endocrine glands.

<table>
<tr><td>gland</td><td>

9-10 The anterior lobe of the pituitary gland is called the *aden/o/hypophysis;* the poster/ior lobe is called the *neur/o/hypophysis.* **Neur/o** is also used to form words that refer to mental disorders and is discussed in the nervous system section of this chapter.

The CF *neur/o* means nerve; the CF *aden/o* means _____.

</td></tr>
</table>

anter/ior
ăn-TĒ-rē-or

poster/ior
pŏs-TĒ-rē-or

neur/o/hypophysis
nū-rō-hī-PŎF-ĭ-sĭs

aden/o/hypophysis
ăd-ĕ-nō-hī-PŎF-ĭ-sĭs

9–11 The aden/o/hypophysis is composed of glandular tissue that produces and releases several hormones. The neur/o/hypophysis is composed of nerve fibers and releases neurohormones that it receives from the hypothalamus. Thus, the neur/o/hypophysis merely acts as a storage site until the hormones are released. As such, it is not a true endocrine gland in the precise sense. Refer to Figure 9-2 for a summary of hormones secreted by the pituitary gland and their target organs.

Identify the words in this frame that mean

in front of: _____/_____.

behind, back (of the body): _____ /_____.

hypophysis composed of nervous tissue: _____/_____/ _____.

hypophysis composed of glandular tissue: _____/_____/ _____.

---

neur/o/hypophysis
nū-rō-hī-PŎF-ĭ-sĭs

9–12 The poster/ior lobe of the pituitary gland, composed primarily of nervous tissue, is called the _____/_____/ _____.

---

aden/o/hypophysis
ăd-ĕ-nō-hī-PŎF-ĭ-sĭs

9–13 The anter/ior lobe of the pituitary gland, composed primarily of glandular tissue, is called the _____/_____/ _____.

9–14 Table 9-1 outlines pituitary hormones, along with their target organs and functions and selected associated disorders. Refer to Table 9-1 on pages 416 and 417 to complete Frames 9–14 through 9–19.

The two hormones released by the neur/o/hypophysis are

_____ _____ and _____.

9–15 Define the following abbreviations related to the anterior pituitary gland (adenohypophysis) and posterior pituitary gland (neurohypophysis).

ACTH: _____ LH: _____

FSH: _____ TSH: _____

GH: _____ ADH (vasopressin): _____

9–16 Briefly state the important function of ADH (posterior pituitary hormone) in the kidneys. (See Table 9-1.)

_____

_____

9–17 Write the abbreviation of the anterior pituitary hormone that initiates sperm production in men.

_____

9–18 What is the posterior pituitary hormone that causes contraction of the uterus during childbirth?

_____

Pink indicates a prefix. Blue indicates a suffix. Boldface indicates a word root or combining form.

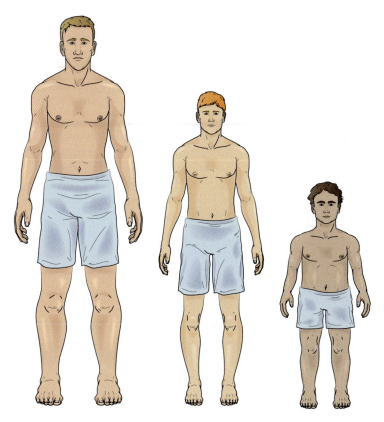

Figure 9-4   Gigantism and dwarfism.

To check answers for
Frames 9–14 through 9–19,
refer to Table 9-1 on
pages 416 and 417.

9–19 Briefly state two functions of GH (anterior pituitary hormone).

_____

_____

_____

_____

---

dwarf/ism

gigant/ism

9–20 Overproduction of GH in children produces an exceptionally large person, a condition known as *gigant/ism*. Underproduction of GH in children is likely to produce an exceptionally small person, a condition called *dwarf/ism*. (See Table 9-1 and Figure 9-4.)

Identify the clinical term for the *condition of an abnormally*

short or undersized person: _____/ _____.

tall or oversized person: _____/ _____.

9–21 Cushing syndrome is a condition in which there is excessive cortisol (a hormone produced by the outer layer of the adren/al gland) in the body. This occurs when an aden/oma (benign tumor) in the pituitary gland produces excessive amounts of adrenocorticotropic hormone (ACTH). Extreme secretions of ACTH then trigger the adren/al gland to secrete excessive amounts of cortisol.

Review Table 9-1 to understand how the hormone ACTH produced in the pituitary gland promotes secretions of cortisol by the adrenal cortex.

---

cortisol KOR-tĭ-sŏl **Cushing**	**9–22** Excessive amounts of ACTH produced by the pituitary gland triggers the adren/al gland to produce excessive amounts of the hormone _____, which, in turn, results in the condition known as _____ syndrome.
adren/al ăd-RĒ-năl hyper/plasia hī-pĕr-PLĀ-zē-ă	**9–23** Cushing syndrome, also known as *adren/al hyper/plasia,* results from overproduction of ACTH. It may also be caused from the use of oral corticosteroid medication. Symptoms of Cushing syndrome include a round face, thin arms and legs, severe fatigue and muscle weakness, high blood pressure and high blood sugar, purple or pink stretch marks on the skin, and weight gain, especially in the abdomen. (See Figure 9-5.) Identify the terms in this frame that mean *pertaining to the adrenal gland:* _____/_____. *excessive formation or growth:* _____/_____.

TABLE 9-1 PITUITARY HORMONES

This table identifies pituitary hormones, their target organs and functions, and associated disorders.

Hormone	Target Organ and Functions	Disorders
Anterior Pituitary (Adenohypophysis) Hormones		
Adrenocorticotropic hormone (ACTH)	• Adrenal cortex—promotes secretions of some hormones by the adrenal cortex, especially cortisol	• Hyposecretion is rare. • Hypersecretion causes Cushing disease. (See Figure 9-5.)
Follicle-stimulating hormone (FSH)	• Ovaries in females—stimulates egg production; increases secretion of estrogen • Testes in males—stimulates sperm production	• Hyposecretion causes failure of sexual maturation. • Hypersecretion has no known significant effects.
Growth hormone (GH), or somatotropin	• Bone, cartilage, liver, muscle, and other tissues—stimulates somatic growth; increases use of fats for energy	• Hyposecretion in children causes pituitary dwarfism. • Hypersecretion in children causes gigantism; hypersecretion in adults causes acromegaly. (See Figure 9-6.)
Luteinizing hormone (LH)	• Ovaries in females—promotes ovulation; stimulates production of estrogen and progesterone • Testes in males—promotes secretion of testosterone	• Hyposecretion causes failure of sexual maturation. • Hypersecretion has no known significant effects.
Prolactin	• Breast—promotes lactation in conjunction with other hormones	• Hyposecretion in nursing mothers causes poor lactation. • Hypersecretion in nursing mothers causes galactorrhea.
Thyroid-stimulating hormone (TSH)	• Thyroid gland—stimulates secretion of thyroid hormone	• Hyposecretion in infants causes cretinism; hyposecretion in adults causes myxedema. • Hypersecretion causes hyperthyroidism.

Pink indicates a prefix. Blue indicates a suffix. Boldface indicates a word root or combining form.

TABLE 9-1 PITUITARY HORMONES—cont'd

Hormone	Target Organ and Functions	Disorders
Posterior Pituitary (Neurohypophysis) Hormones		
Antidiuretic hormone (ADH)	• Kidney—increases water reabsorption (water returns to blood)	• Hyposecretion causes diabetes insipidus. • Hypersecretion causes syndrome of inappropriate antidiuretic hormone (SIADH).
Oxytocin	• Uterus—stimulates uterine contractions; initiates labor • Breast—promotes milk secretion from the mammary glands	• Unknown

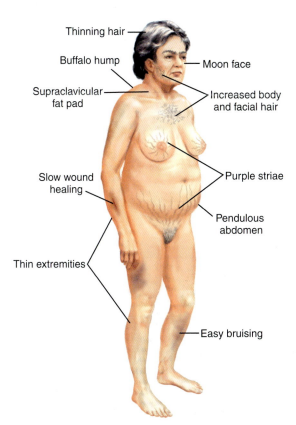

Thinning hair

Buffalo hump

Supraclavicular fat pad

Moon face

Increased body and facial hair

Slow wound healing

Purple striae

Pendulous abdomen

Thin extremities

Easy bruising

Figure 9-5   Physical manifestations seen in Cushing syndrome.

---

acr/o/megaly
ăk-rō-MĔG-ă-lē

9-24 The CF *acr/o* means *extremity.* Acr/o/megaly, a chronic metabolic condition, is characterized by a gradual, marked enlargement and thickening of the bones of the face and jaw. (See Figure 9-6.) This condition, which afflicts middle-aged and older persons, is caused by overproduction of growth hormone and is treated with radiation, pharmacological agents, or surgery, commonly involving partial resection of the pituitary gland.

A term that literally means *enlargement of the extremities is*

_____/_____/_____.

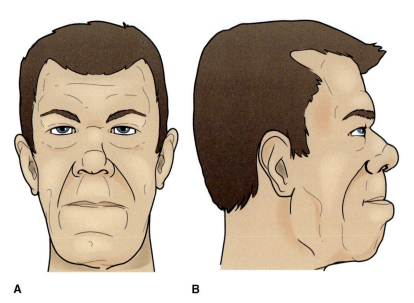

A   **B**

Figure 9-6   Acromegaly. (A) Frontal view. (B) Lateral view.

Thyroid Gland

thyroid/ectomy thī-royd-ĔK-tō-mē	**9–25** The CFs for thyroid gland are ***thyr/o*** and ***thyroid/o.*** Use ***thyroid/o*** to form a word that means *excision of the thyroid gland.* _____/_____
thyr/o/megaly thī-rō-MĔG-ă-lē **thyr/o/pathy** thī-RŎP-ă-thē **thyr/o/tomy** thī-RŎT-ō-mē	**9–26** Use ***thyr/o*** to construct words that mean *enlargement of the thyroid gland:* _____/_____/_____. *disease of the thyroid gland:* _____/_____/_____. *incision of the thyroid gland:* _____/_____/_____.
To check answers for Frames 9–27 through 9–29, refer to Table 9-2 on page 419.	**9–27** Table 9-2 on page 419 outlines thyroid hormones along with their functions and selected associated disorders. Refer to the table to complete Frames 9–27 through 9–29. The thyroid gland secretes three hormones, two of which regulate the body's metabolism (rate at which food is converted into heat and energy). These hormones are called _____ and _____.
	9–28 In conjunction with parathyroid hormone (PTH), calcium levels in blood are regulated by secretion of the thyroid hormone called _____.

9–29 When does calcitonin exert its most important effects in the body?

_____

_____

_____

hypo/thyroid/ism
hī-pō-THĪ-royd-ĭzm

myx/edema
mĭks-ĕ-DĒ-mă

a/trophy
ĂT-rō-fē

9–30 Myx/edema is a condition resulting from advanced hypo/thyroid/ism in the adult. Deficiency of thyroxine hormone occurs as a result of a/trophy of the thyroid gland. Symptoms include the accumulation of mucus-like material, causing skin to be puffy and dry. Review this disorder in Table 9-1.

Identify the terms in this frame that mean

condition of insufficient thyroid (hormone):

_____/_____/_____.

swelling due to mucus: _____/_____.

without development or nourishment: _____/_____.

TABLE 9-2 THYROID HORMONES

This table identifies thyroid hormones, their functions, and associated disorders.

Hormone	Functions	Disorders
Calcitonin	• Regulation of calcium levels in blood in conjunction with parathyroid hormone • Secreted to maintain homeostasis when calcium levels in blood are high	• The most significant effects are exerted in childhood when bones are growing and changing dramatically in mass, size, and shape. • At best, calcitonin is a weak hypocalcemic agent in adults.
Thyroxine (T_4) and triiodothyronine (T_3)	• Increased energy production from all food types • Increased rate of protein synthesis	• Hyposecretion in infants causes cretinism; hyposecretion in adults causes myxedema. • Hypersecretion causes Graves disease (the most common form of hyperthyroidism), indicated by exophthalmos and goiter. (See Figure 9-7.)

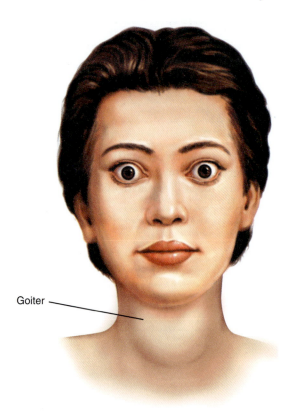

Goiter —

Figure 9-7   Graves disease.

---

excessive, above normal **thyroid gland** THĪ-royd **condition**	**9–31** Hyper/thyroid/ism is caused by hypersecretion of thyroxine by the thyroid gland. High levels of thyroxine accelerate the body's metabolism significantly, causing rapid or irregular heartbeat, sweating, nervousness, and sudden weight loss, among other symptoms. (See Table 9-2.) Analyze *hyper/thyroid/ism* by defining the elements. *hyper-:* _____, _____ _____ *thyroid:* _____ _____ *-ism:* _____

	9–32 The most common form of hyper/thyroid/ism is Graves disease, which is characterized by enlargement of the thyroid gland (goiter), bulging of the eyes (exophthalmos), or both. (See Table 9-2 and Figure 9-7.)

---

thyroid/ectomy thī-royd-ĔK-tō-mē	**9–33** Treatment for hyper/thyroid/ism may involve drug therapy to block production of thyroid hormones or surgical removal of all or part of the thyroid gland with radiation therapy, including radioactive iodine to destroy the remaining thyroid gland. Build a word that means *excision of the thyroid gland:* _____/ _____.

Pink indicates a prefix. Blue indicates a suffix. Boldface indicates a word root or combining form.

toxic/o/logist tŏks-ĭ-KŎL-ō-jĭst	**9-34** Toxic/o/logy is the scientific study of poisons and treatment of conditions produced by them. A specialist in the study of poisons is called a _____/_____/_____.
poison	**9-35** Toxic/o/pathy is any disease caused by _____.
blood	**9-36** The combining form (CF) *calc/o* means *calcium*. *Calc/emia* indicates an abnormal presence of calcium in the _____.
hyper/calc/emia hī-pĕr-kăl-SĒ-mē-ă	**9-37** Hypo/calc/emia is a condition of abnormally low blood calcium. A person with excessively high blood calcium is diagnosed with _____/_____/_____.

SECTION REVIEW 9-2

Using the following table, write the CF, suffix, or prefix that matches its definition in the space provided to the left of the definition. There may be more than one word element that matches a definition.

Combining Forms		Suffixes		Prefixes
acr/o	poster/o	-emia	-tome	dys-
aden/o	radi/o	-logist	-tomy	hyper-
anter/o	thyr/o	-megaly		hypo-
calc/o	thyroid/o	-osis		poly-
neur/o	toxic/o	-pathy		

1. _____ abnormal condition; increase (used primarily with blood cells)

2. _____ excessive, above normal

3. _____ back (of body), behind, posterior

4. _____ bad; painful; difficult

5. _____ blood condition

6. _____ calcium

7. _____ disease

8. _____ enlargement

9. _____ extremity

10. _____ anterior, front

11. _____ gland

12. _____ incision

13. _____ instrument to cut

14. _____ nerve

15. _____ poison

16. _____ radiation, x-ray; radius (lower arm bone on thumb side)

17. _____ specialist in the study of

18. _____ many, much

19. _____ thyroid gland

20. _____ under, below, deficient

Competency Verification: Check your answers in Appendix B: Answer Key, page 610. If you are not satisfied with your level of comprehension, go back to Frame 9–1, and rework the frames.

Correct Answers _____ x 5 = _____% Score

Pink indicates a prefix. Blue indicates a suffix. Boldface indicates a word root or combining form.

Parathyroid Glands

9–38 The (3) **parathyroid glands** are located on the posterior surface of the thyroid gland. The parathyroid glands are so called because they are located around the thyroid gland. Label the parathyroid glands in Figure 9-3.

---

para/thyr/oid glands
păr-ă-THĪ-royd

9–39 The para/thyr/oid glands secrete para/thyr/oid hormone (PTH), which helps regulate the amount of calcium in blood.

When we discuss the two pairs of glands located in the posterior aspect of the

thyr/oid glands, we are talking about the _____ / _____ / _____ glands.

---

para-

9–40 Identify the element in the previous frame that means *located near, beside; beyond.*

_____

PTH

9–41 The hormone produced by the parathyroid glands is called para/thyr/oid hormone (PTH).

The abbreviation for para/thyr/oid hormone is _____.

To check answers for this frame, refer to Table 9-3 below.

9–42 Table 9-3 below outlines the parathyroid hormone along with its target organs and functions and associated disorders. Refer to the table to complete this frame.

The major function of PTH is to regulate levels of _____ and _____.

---

hyper/para/thyr/oid/ism
hī-pĕr-păr-ă-THĪ-roy-dĭzm

9–43 Oste/itis fibrosa cystica is an inflammatory degenerative condition in which cysts and fibrous tissue replace normal bone. It is usually associated with hyper/para/thyr/oid/ism.

The term in this frame that means *abnormal condition characterized by hypersecretion of* PTH is _____ / _____ / _____ / _____.

TABLE 9-3 PARATHYROID HORMONE

This table identifies parathyroid hormone along with its target organs and functions and associated disorders.

Hormone	Target Organ and Functions	Disorder
Parathyroid hormone (PTH)	• Bones—increased reabsorption of calcium and phosphate from bone to blood • Kidneys—increased calcium absorption and phosphate excretion • Small intestine—increased absorption of calcium and phosphate	• Hyposecretion causes tetany. • Hypersecretion causes osteitis fibrosa cystica.

Adrenal Glands

9–44   The (4) **adrenal glands,** also known as the *supra/ren/al glands,* are paired structures located super/ior to the kidneys. Label Figure 9-3 as you continue to learn about the endocrine system.

---

supra/ren/al
soo-pră-RĒ-năl

super/ior

9–45   Indicate the words in Frame 9–44 that mean

above or superior to a kidney: _____/_____/_____.

pertaining to upper or above: _____/_____.

---

enlargement, adrenal

adrenal/ectomy
ăd-rē-năl-ĔK-tō-mē

9–46   *Adren/o* and *adrenal/o* are CFs for the adrenal glands. Adren/o/megaly is an

_____ of the _____ glands.

Use *adrenal/o* to form a word that means *excision of an adrenal gland.*

_____/_____

---

kidneys

9–47   Each adrenal gland is structurally and functionally differentiated into two sections: the outer adrenal cortex, which comprises the bulk of the gland, and the inner portion, the adrenal medulla. The hormones produced by each part have different functions.

The adrenal glands are perched atop the _____.

9–48   Table 9-4 outlines adrenal hormones, along with their target organs and functions and selected associated disorders. Review the table to learn about hormones and their effects on target organs.

To check answers for Frames 9–49 through 9–54, refer to Table 9-4 on page 425.

9–49   To complete Frames 9–49 through 9–54, refer to Table 9-4 on page 425.

Three hormones produced by the adrenal cortex are _____, _____, and

_____.

9–50   Identify two hormones produced by the adrenal cortex that maintain secondary sex characteristics.

_____ and _____

9–51   Epinephrine helps the body cope with dangerous situations. Nerves transmit the message of fear to the glands, which react by rushing adrenaline to all parts of the system. Epinephrine is also called _____.

9–52   When a person is experiencing a stressful situation, the adrenal medulla produces adrenaline, which is also called _____.

9–53   Hormones produced by the adrenal medulla that increase blood pressure are _____ and _____.

Pink indicates a prefix. Blue indicates a suffix. Boldface indicates a word root or combining form.

TABLE 9-4 ADRENAL HORMONES

This table identifies adrenal hormones, their target organs and functions, and associated disorders.

Hormone	Target Organ and Functions	Disorders
Adrenal Cortex Hormones		
Glucocorticoids (mainly cortisol)	• Body cells—promotion of gluconeo-genesis; regulation of carbohydrate, protein, and fat metabolism; aid in depression of inflammatory and immune responses	• Hyposecretion causes Addison disease. • Hypersecretion causes Cushing syndrome. (See Figure 9-5.)
Mineralocorticoids (mainly aldosterone)	• Kidneys—increased blood levels of sodium and decreased blood levels of potassium in the kidney	• Hyposecretion causes Addison disease. • Hypersecretion causes aldosteronism.
Sex hormones (any of the androgens, estrogens, or related steroid hormones) produced by the ovaries, testes, and adrenal cortices	• In females, possibly responsible for female libido. Otherwise insignificant effects in female adults.	• Hyposecretion has no known significant effects. • Hypersecretion of adrenal androgen in females leads to virilism (development of male characteristics). • Hypersecretion of adrenal estrogen and progestin secretion in males leads to feminization (development of feminine characteristics).
Adrenal Medullary Hormones		
Epinephrine (adrenaline) and norepinephrine	• Sympathetic nervous system target organs—hormone effects that mimic sympathetic nervous system activation (sympathomimetic), increase metabolic rate and heart rate, and raise blood pressure by promoting vasoconstriction	• Hyposecretion has no known significant effects. • Hypersecretion causes prolonged "fight-or-flight" reaction and hypertension.

9–54 The main glucocorticoid hormone secreted by the adrenal cortex is

_____.

Pancreas (Islets of Langerhans)

9–55 The (5) **pancreas** is located posterior to the stomach. Hormone-producing cells of the pancreas are called *islets of Langerhans*. The islets produce two distinct hormones: alpha cells, which produce glucagons, and beta cells, which produce insulin. Both hormones play an important role in the proper metabolism of sugars and starches in the body. Label the pancreas in Figure 9-3.

pancreat/oma
păn-krē-ă-TŌ-mă

pancreat/o/lith
păn-krē-ĂT-ō-lĭth

pancreat/o/lith/iasis
păn-krē-ă-tō-lĭ-THĪ-ă-sĭs

pancreat/o/pathy
păn-krē-ă-TŎP-ă-thē

9–56 Use *pancreat/o* (pancreas) to build medical words that mean

tumor of the pancreas: _____/_____.

calculus or stone in the pancreas: _____/_____/_____.

abnormal condition of a pancreatic stone:

_____/_____/_____/_____.

disease of the pancreas: _____/_____/_____.

---

pancreas
PĂN-krē-ăs

9–57 The suffix *-lysis* is used in words to mean *separation, destruction, loosening.*

Pancreat/o/lysis is a destruction of the _____.

To check answers to Frames 9–58 through 9–60, refer to Table 9-5 on page 427.

9–58 Refer to Table 9-5 on page 427 to complete Frames 9–58 through 9–60.

Two hormones produced by the pancreas are _____ and _____.

9–59 Determine the pancreat/ic hormone that

lowers blood glucose: _____.

increases blood glucose: _____.

9–60 How does insulin lower blood glucose?

_____

_____

_____

---

glyc/o/gen
GLĪ-kō-jĕn

9–61 Gluc/ose is the chief source of energy for living organisms. *Gluc/o* and *glyc/o* are CFs that mean sugar, sweetness. The suffixes *-gen* and *-genesis* mean *forming, producing, origin.*

Combine *glyc/o* and *-gen* to form a word that means *forming or producing sugar.*

_____/_____/_____

---

gluc/o/genesis
gloo-kō-JĔN-ĕ-sĭs

glyc/o/genesis
glī-kō-JĔN-ĕ-sĭs

9–62 Use *-genesis* to build words that mean *forming, producing, or origin of sugar.*

_____/_____/_____

_____/_____/_____

---

gluc/o/meter
gloo-KŎM-tĕr

9-63 Diabetes is a general term that, when used alone, refers to diabetes mellitus (DM), a disease that occurs in two primary forms: type 1 diabetes and type 2 diabetes. Diabetes requires continuous monitoring and medication. A gluc/o/meter helps determine the approximate concentration of glucose in blood by withdrawing a drop of blood with a lancet. (See Figure 9-8 and Table 9-5.) An insulin injection can be administered by the patient if the glucose level is high. The instrument used by patients with diabetes to monitor their blood glucose levels is

known as a _____/_____/_____.

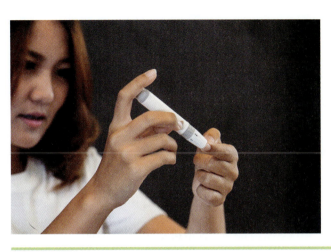

Figure 9-8 Finger lancet and glucometer used for checking blood glucose level.

poly/dipsia
pŏl-ē-DĬP-sē-ă

poly/uria
pŏl-ē-Ū-rē-ă

poly/phagia
pŏl-ē-FĀ-jē-ă

9-64 The suffix *-dipsia* denotes *a condition of thirst*. Poly/dipsia, poly/uria, and poly/phagia are three cardinal signs of diabetes mellitus.

Write the words in this frame that mean

excessive thirst: _____/_____.

excessive urination: _____/_____.

excessive eating: _____/_____.

poly/uria
pŏl-ē-Ū-rē-ă

9-65 When a person drinks too much water, he or she may experience a condition of excessive urine production (urination). The medical term for this condition is:

_____/_____.

TABLE 9-5 PANCREATIC HORMONES

This table identifies pancreatic hormones, their target organs and functions, and associated disorders.

Hormone	Target Organs and Functions	Disorders
Glucagon	• Liver and blood—increased blood glucose level from accelerated conversion of glycogen into glucose in the liver (glycogenolysis) and conversion of other nutrients into glucose in the liver (gluconeogenesis), as well as release of glucose into blood	• Persistently low blood sugar levels (hypoglycemia) may be caused by a deficiency in glucagon.
Insulin	• Tissue cells—lower blood glucose levels from accelerated glucose transport into cells; conversion of glucose to glycogen	• Hyposecretion of insulin causes diabetes mellitus. • Hypersecretion of insulin causes hyperinsulinism.

Pineal and Thymus Glands

9–66 The (6) **pineal gland** and (7) **thymus gland** are classified as endocrine glands, but little is known about their endocrine function. Label these structures in Figure 9-3.

thym/ectomy thī-MĔK-tō-mē	**9–67** The CF *thym/o* means *thymus gland.* Build medical words that mean *excision of the thymus gland:* _____ / _____ . *tumor of the thymus gland:* _____ / _____ . *disease of the thymus gland:* _____ / _____ / _____ . *destruction of the thymus gland:* _____ / _____ / _____ .
thym/oma thī-MŌ-mă	
thym/o/pathy thī-MŎP-ă-thē	
thym/o/lysis thī-MŎL-ĭ-sĭs	

Ovaries and Testes

9–68 The (8) **ovaries** are a pair of small, almond-shaped glands positioned in the upper pelvic cavity, one on each side of the uterus. The (9) **testes** are paired oval glands surrounded by the scrotal sac. The functions of the ovaries and testes are covered in Chapter 8. Label the ovaries and testes in Figure 9-3.

oophor/o, ovari/o **orchid/o, orchi/o, orch/o, test/o**	**9–69** Recall the CFs for *ovaries:* _____ / _____ or _____ / _____ . *testes:* _____ / _____ , _____ / _____ , _____ / _____ , or _____ / _____ .
oophor/o/pathy ō-ŏf-or-ŎP-ă-thē	**9–70** Use *oophor/o* to construct medical words that mean *disease of an ovary:* _____ / _____ / _____ . *incision of an ovary:* _____ / _____ / _____ .
oophor/o/tomy ō-ŏf-or-ŎT-ō-mē	
orchid/o/pexy OR-kĭd-ō-pĕk-sē	**9–71** Use *orchid/o* to form a word that means *surgical fixation of a testis.* _____ / _____ / _____

Competency Verification: Check your labeling of Figure 9-3 in Appendix B: Answer Key, page 610.

Pink indicates a prefix. Blue indicates a suffix. Boldface indicates a word root or combining form.

SECTION REVIEW 9-3

Using the following table, write the CF, suffix, or prefix that matches its definition in the space provided to the left of the definition. There may be more than one word element that matches a definition.

Combining Forms		Suffixes		Prefixes
adrenal/o	orch/o	-dipsia	-pathy	hypo-
adren/o	pancreat/o	-gen	-pexy	para-
gluc/o	thym/o	-genesis	-phagia	poly-
glyc/o	toxic/o	-iasis	-rrhea	supra-
orchid/o		-lith	-uria	
orchi/o		-lysis		

1. _____ abnormal condition (produced by something specified)

2. _____Supra_____ above; excessive; superior

3. _____adren/o_____ adrenal glands

4. _____pathy_____ disease

5. _____-pexy_____ fixation (of an organ)

6. _____-rrhea_____ discharge, flow

7. _____poly_____ many, much

8. _____ near, beside; beyond

9. _____pancreat/o_____ pancreas

10. _____-genesis_____ forming, producing; origin

11. _____-iasis_____ separation; destruction; loosening

12. _____-lith/o_____ stone, calculus

13. _____gluc/o_____ sugar, sweetness

14. _____phagia_____ swallowing, eating

15. _____ testis (plural, *testes*)

16. _____-dipsia_____ thirst

17. _____thym/o_____ thymus gland

18. _____hypo_____ under, below, deficient

19. _____-uria_____ urine

20. _____toxic/o_____ poison

Competency Verification: Check your answers in Appendix B: Answer Key, page 610. If you are not satisfied with your level of comprehension, go back to Frame 9–38, and rework the frames.

Correct Answers _____ x 5 = _____ % Score

Nervous System

The nervous system is an extensive, intricate network of structures that activates, coordinates, and controls the functions of all other body systems. It can be grouped into two main divisions: the **central nervous system (CNS)** and the **peripheral nervous system (PNS)**. The CNS consists of the brain and spinal cord and is the control center of the body. The PNS consists of the peripheral nerves, which include the cranial nerves (emerging from the base of the skull) and the spinal nerves (emerging from the spinal cord). The PNS connects the CNS to remote body parts to relay and receive messages, and its autonomic nerves regulate involuntary functions of the internal organs.

Despite the complex organization of the nervous system, it consists of only two principal types of cells: **neurons** and **neuroglia.** Neurons are the basic structural and functional units of the nervous system. (See Figure 9-9.) They are specialized to respond to physical and chemical stimuli, conduct electrochemical impulses, and release specific chemical regulators. Through these activities, neurons perform such functions as perceiving sensory stimuli, learning, remembering, and controlling muscles and glands. Neuroglia do not carry impulses but perform the functions of support and protection. Many neuroglial (glial) cells form a supporting network by twining around nerve cells or lining certain structures in the brain and the spinal cord. Others bind nervous tissue to supporting structures and attach the neurons to their blood vessels. Specialized glial cells are phagocytic. In other words, they protect the CNS from disease by engulfing invading microbes and clearing away debris. Neuroglia are of clinical interest because they are a common source of tumors (gliomas) of the nervous system.

As illustrated in Figure 9-9, the (1) **dendrites** are branching processes (extensions) that transmit impulses toward the (2) **cell body,** which contains the (3) **nucleus.** The integrated signals in the cell body are then transmitted to the (4) **axon,** a single projection that extends to the neuron's target cell or tissue. Surrounding the axon is a fatty coating called the (5) **myelin sheath.** The sheath insulates the axon and speeds the transmission of electrical impulses. Because of their fatty coating, myelinated axons take on a whitish appearance. As a result, groups of myelinated axons constitute the "white matter" of the brain and spinal cord, whereas cell bodies of neurons that are not covered by a myelin sheath appear gray and are referred to as the "gray matter."

The axon of one neuron does not actually touch the dendrite of the next neuron. Instead, there is a space, or (6) **synapse,** between the two neurons. The transmission of nerve impulses across the synapse depends on the release of a chemical substance called a (7) **neurotransmitter.** Neurotransmitters are chemical messengers that

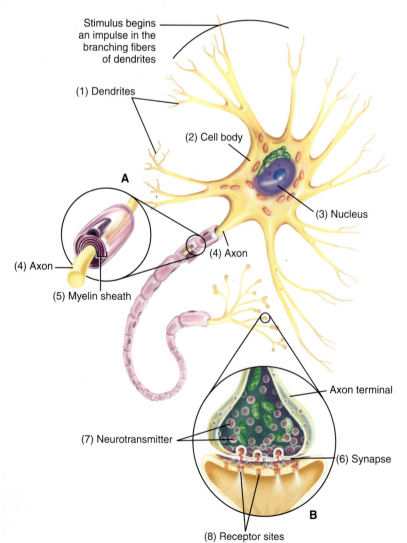

Figure 9-9   Neuron. (A) Myelin sheath. (B) Axon terminal synapse.

allow signals to cross the synapse and bind to (8) **receptor sites** on the dendrites of the next neuron. In this way, the neurotransmission creates another electrical impulse that continues through the next neuron until it reaches the target cell. Examples include neurotransmission to an endocrine gland to make it secrete a hormone and neurotransmission to a set of muscles to make them contract. In the previous two examples, the connection points are called *neuromuscular* and *neuroglandular junctions.* All of these transmissions occur within a fraction of a second. Neurotransmitters play a major role in shaping everyday life and functions.

WORD ELEMENTS

This section introduces word elements related to the nervous system. Review the word elements and their meanings in the following table. Then, pronounce each term in the word analysis column, and place a ✓ in the box after you do so.

Word Element	Meaning	Word Analysis
Combining Forms		
cephal/o	head	**hydro/cephal/us** (hī-drō-SĔF-ă-lŭs ☐): condition of an enlarged cranium (portion of the skull that encloses the brain) *hydro:* water *-us:* condition; structure *Hydrocephalus is caused by accumulation of fluid within the ventricles of the brain.*
cerebr/o	cerebrum	**cerebr/o/spin/al** (sĕr-ĕ-brō-SPĪ-năl ☐): pertaining to the brain and spinal cord *spin:* spine *-al:* pertaining to
encephal/o	brain	**encephal/itis** (ĕn-sĕf-ă-LĪ-tĭs ☐): inflammation of the brain (tissue) *-itis:* inflammation
gli/o	glue; neuroglial tissue	**gli/oma** (glī-Ō-mă ☐): tumor composed of neuroglial tissue (supportive tissue of the nervous system) *-oma:* tumor
mening/o	meninges (membranes covering the brain and spinal cord)	**mening/o/cele** (mĕn-ĬN-gō-sēl ☐): saclike protrusion of the meninges through the skull or vertebral column *-cele:* hernia, swelling *Meningocele is a congenital defect (occurs at birth) and can be repaired by surgery.*
meningi/o		**meningi/oma** (mĕn-ĭn-jē-Ō-mă ☐): tumor composed of meninges *-oma:* tumor
myel/o	bone marrow; spinal cord	**myel/algia** (mī-ĕl-ĂL-jē-ă ☐): pain in the spinal cord or its membranes *-algia:* pain
neur/o	nerve	**neur/o/lysis** (nū-RŎL-ĭs-ĭs ☐): destruction of a nerve *-lysis:* separation; destruction; loosening
Suffixes		
-paresis	partial paralysis	**hemi/paresis** (hĕm-ē-pă-RĒ-sĭs ☐): paralysis of one half of the body (right half or left half) *hemi-:* one half
-phasia	speech	**a/phasia** (ă-FĀ-zē-ă ☐): absence of speech *a-:* without, not *Aphasia is an abnormal neurological condition in which language function is defective or absent because of an injury to certain areas of the cerebral cortex.*
-plegia	paralysis	**quadri/plegia** (kwŏd-rĭ-PLĒ-jē-ă ☐): paralysis of all four extremities *quadri-:* four

Pronunciation Help					
	Long Sound	ā in rāte	ē in rēbirth	ī in īsle	ō in ōver	ū in ūnite
	Short Sound	ă in ăpple	ĕ in ĕver	ĭ in ĭt	ŏ in nŏt	ŭ in cŭt

SECTION REVIEW 9-4

For the following medical terms, first, write the suffix and its meaning. Then, translate the meaning of the remaining elements starting with the first part of the word. The first word is completed for you.

Term	Meaning
1. meningi/oma	–oma: tumor; meninges
2. neur/o/lysis	
3. hemi/paresis	
4. myel/algia	
5. cerebr/o/spin/al	
6. a/phasia	
7. mening/o/cele	
8. encephal/it is	
9. gli/oma	
10. quadri/plegia	

Competency Verification: Check your answers in Appendix B: Answer Key, page 610. If you are not satisfied with your level of comprehension, review the terms in the word elements table, and retake the review.

Correct Answers _____ x 10 = _____ % Score

Brain

The brain is one of the most complex organs in the human body because it coordinates almost all physical and mental activities of the body. Although little is known about the mechanisms by which the brain regulates and coordinates all of the body's voluntary and involuntary activities, it is clear that the primary control over various functional activities is localized to different areas of the brain.

encephal/itis
ĕn-sĕf-ă-LĪ-tĭs

encephal/oma
ĕn-sĕf-ă-lō-mă

9–72 The CF *encephal/o* refers to the brain. Build a word that means

inflammation of brain (tissue): _____ / _____.

tumor of the brain: _____ / _____.

9–73 The brain is divided into three major divisions for discussion. The first is the (1) **cerebrum,** which is the largest and uppermost portion of the brain. A thin layer known as the *cerebral cortex* covers the entire cerebrum and is composed of gray matter. Different areas of the cerebral cortex are responsible for most of the higher mental functions, including vision, speech, voluntary movements, memory, and reasoning. Label the cerebrum in Figure 9-10.

Pink indicates a prefix. Blue indicates a suffix. Boldface indicates a word root or combining form.

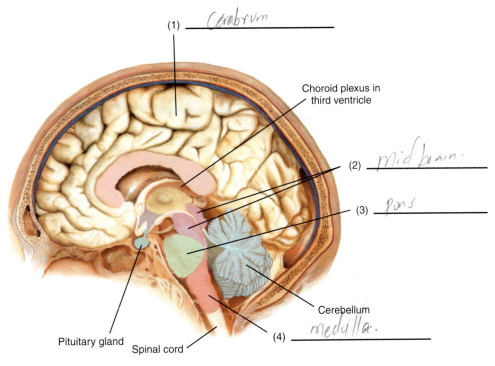

(1) _Cerebrum_

Choroid plexus in
third ventricle

(2) _mid brain._

(3) _pons_

Cerebellum

(4) _medulla._

Pituitary gland   Spinal cord

Figure 9-10   Structures of the brain.

---

cerebr/al
sĕ-RĒ-brăl

9-74 The CF *cerebr/o* refers to the largest and uppermost portion of the brain. Build a word that means *pertaining to the cerebrum.*

_____/_____

---

cerebr/o/tomy
sĕr-ĕ-BRŎT-ō-mē

9-75 Combine *cerebr/o* and *-tomy* to form a surgical procedure that means *incision of the cerebrum.*

_____/_____/_____

9-76 The more rudimentary processes are regulated by the brainstem, which consists of (2) the **midbrain,** (3) the **pons,** and (4) the **medulla.** Attached to the brainstem is (5) the **cerebellum,** which plays a role in equilibrium, posture, and muscular coordination. Locate and label these structures in Figure 9-10.

---

inferior

9-77 The brainstem is the site where motor neurons cross from one side of the body to the other, so the right half of the brain controls movement involving the left side of the body, and vice versa. Locate the brainstem in Figure 9-10.

The brainstem lies (inferior or superior) _____ to the cerebrum.

---

superior

9-78 The pons is part of the brainstem and literally means *bridge.* It contains nerve tracts that connect the cerebellum and the cerebrum with the rest of the brain. Nerves to the eyes and face lie in the pons. Locate the pons in Figure 9-10.

The pons lies (inferior or superior) _____ to the spinal cord.

---

vasomotor
VĂ-sō-mō-tor

cardiac
KĂR-dē-ăk

respiratory
RĔS-pĭ-ră-tor-ē

9–79 The medulla contains three vital centers that regulate the internal activities of the body. The cardiac center slows heart rate when the heart is beating too rapidly; the respiratory center controls the muscles of respiration in response to chemicals or other stimuli; and the vasomotor center affects (constricts or dilates) the muscles in the walls of blood vessels, thus influencing blood pressure.

The vital center that influences blood pressure by dilating or constricting blood vessel

walls is the _____ center.

The _____ center slows heart rate when it is beating too rapidly.

The _____ center controls respiratory muscles in response to chemicals or other stimuli.

Competency Verification: Check your labeling of Figure 9-10 in Appendix B: Answer Key, page 610.

Spinal Cord

The spinal cord is a long, narrow cable of nervous tissue within the spinal canal and is part of the CNS. It descends from the brainstem to the lumbar part of the back and contains about 100 million neurons. Thirty-one pairs of spinal nerves originate from the spinal cord. (See Figure 9-11.) Each pair of nerves serves a specific region on the right or left side of the body. Spinal nerves are mixed nerves that provide a two-way communication between the spinal cord and the parts of the upper and lower limbs, neck, and trunk.

9–80 Spin/al nerves are named according to locations of their respective vertebrae. As shown in Figure 9-11, there are eight pairs of cervic/al nerves, identified as C1–C8; 12 pairs of thorac/ic nerves, identified as T1–T12; five pairs of lumb/ar nerves, identified as L1–L5; five pairs of sacr/al nerves, identified as S1–S5; and one pair of coccyg/eal nerves, identified as Co1.

In Figure 9-11, label the (1) **cervical nerves,** (2) **thoracic nerves,** (3) **lumbar nerves,** (4) **sacral nerves,** and (5) **coccygeal nerve.**

cervic/al nerves
SĔR-vĭ-kăl

thorac/ic nerves
thō-RĂS-ĭk

sacr/al nerves
SĀ-krăl

9–81 Build medical words that mean *pertaining to nerves*

of the neck: ___Cervic___ / ___al___ ___nerve___.

in back of the chest: ___Thorac___ / ___ic___ _____.

of the sacrum: _____ / _____ _____.

spin/al
SPĪ-năl

cerebr/o/spin/al
sĕr-ē-brō-SPĪ-năl

9–82 The spin/al cord, like the brain, is protected and nourished by the meninges, which consist of three layers: dura mater, the outermost membrane; arachnoid membrane, the middle layer, which surrounds the brain and spin/al cord; and pia mater, the inner layer, which is closest to the brain and spinal cord. Additional protection is provided by cerebr/o/spin/al fluid (CSF) circulating in the subarachnoid space. (See Figure 9-11.)

Identify terms in this frame that mean *pertaining to the spine:*
___Spin___ / ___al___.

cerebrum and the spine: ___Cerebr___ / ___o___ / ___spi___.

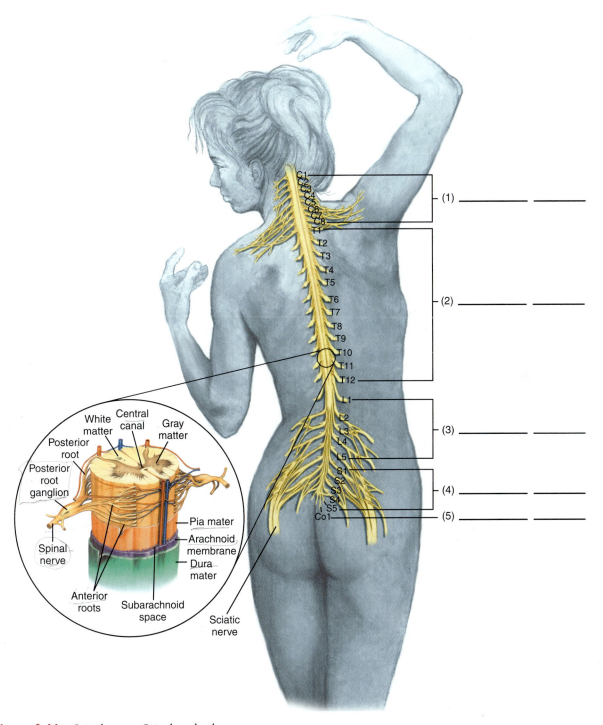

Figure 9-11 Spinal nerves. Spinal cord enlargement.

mening/itis
měn-ĭn-JĪ-tĭs

mening/o/cele
měn-ĬN-gō-sēl

meningi/oma
měn-ĭn-jē-Ō-mă

9-83 *Mening/o* and *meningi/o* refer to the meninges (membranes covering the brain and spinal cord).

Use *mening/o* to build a word that means

inflammation of the meninges: _____ / _____ .

hernia or swelling of the meninges: _____ / _____ / _____ .

Use *meningi/o* to build a word that means

tumor of the meninges: _____ / _____

---

cerebr/o/spin/al
sĕr-ē-brō-SPĪ-năl

9-84 The dura mater, the outer layer of the spinal cord, is a tough, fibrous membrane that covers the entire length of the spinal cord and contains channels for blood to enter brain tissue. The arachnoid, the middle layer, runs across the space known as the sub/dur/al space, which contains cerebr/o/spin/al fluid (CSF). The pia mater, the innermost layer, is a thin membrane containing many blood vessels that nourish the spinal cord.

The fluid that circulates in the subarachnoid space and protects the brain and spinal cord is known as _____ / _____ / _____ / _____ fluid.

---

epi-

dur

-al

9-85 The space between the pia mater and the bones of the spinal cord is called the *epi/dur/al space.* It is the space into which a provider may safely inject anesthetics to offer substantial pain relief without surgery. Nerve blocks treat pain and help manage other nerve disorders. The injection of this nerve-numbing substance is called a *nerve block.* (See Figure 9-12.)

Identify the elements in this frame that mean

above, upon: _*epi*_ .

dura mater; hard: _*dur*_ .

pertaining to: _*al*_ .

(handwritten) epidural pertaining. above dura.

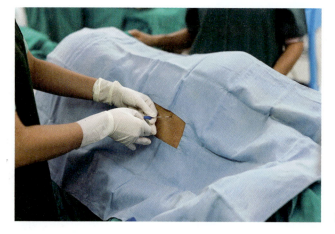

Figure 9-12   Epidural nerve block.

Spinal — myel/o

mening/o/cele měn-ĬN-gō-sēl	**9-86** Herniation of the meninges may occur through a defect in the skull or spinal cord. When herniation of the meninges occurs, the condition is called _____/_____/_____.
myel/itis mī-ě-LĪ-tĭs **myel/o/pathy** mī-ě-LŎP-ă-thē **myel/o/tome** mī-ĔL-ō-tōm	**9-87** The CF *myel/o* means *bone marrow; spinal cord.* Build medical words that mean *inflammation of the spinal cord:* _____/_____. *any disease of the spinal cord:* _myel_ / _o_ / _pathy_. *instrument to cut or dissect the spinal cord:* _myel_ / _o_ / _tome_.

Competency Verification: Check your labeling of Figure 9-11 in Appendix B: Answer Key, page 611.

back (of body) **nerve** **belly, belly side**	**9-88** Each spin/al nerve has two roots, which are neurons entering or leaving the spinal cord. The dors/al root is made of sensory neurons that carry impulses into the spinal cord. The ventr/al root is the motor root. It is made of motor neurons carrying impulses from the spin/al cord to muscles or glands. The cell bodies of these motor neurons are in the gray matter of the spin/al cord. When the two nerve roots merge, the spin/al nerve formed is a mixed nerve. Provide the meaning for the following CFs. *dors/o:* _back_ (_____ _____) *neur/o:* _nerve_ *ventr/o:* _____, _____ _____
neur/algia nū-RĂL-jē-ă **neur/itis** nū-RĪ-tĭs **neur/oma** nū-RŌ-mă **neur/o/pathy** nū-RŎP-ă-thē	**9-89** Use *neur/o* to form medical terms that mean *pain in a nerve:* _n_____/_____. *pain—algia* *inflammation of a nerve:* _____/_____. *nerve—neuritis* *tumor of nerve (tissue):* _____/_____. *neuroma* *any disease of nerves:* _____/_____/_____. *neuropathy*
myel/itis mī-ě-LĪ-tĭs **myel/o/malacia** mī-ě-lō-mă-LĀ-shē-ă **myel/oma** mī-ě-LŌ-mă	**9-90** Use *myel/o* to form medical words that mean *inflammation of the spinal cord:* _myel_ / _itis_. *neuro* *softening of the spinal cord:* _____/_____/_____. *malacia—softening* *tumor of bone marrow:* _____/_____. *myel oma*

cell **thromb/o/cyte** THRŎM-bō-sīt	**9-91** The CF *thromb/o* refers to a blood clot. A thromb/o/cyte is a blood clotting _____. A thromb/o/cyte (platelet) promotes the formation of clots and prevents bleeding. Another name for platelet is _____/_____/_____.
clot	**9-92** Although the terms *embolus* and *thrombus* denote a disorder related to a clot, they both have different meanings. An *embolus* is a clot present in blood vessels or lymphatic vessels and brought there by blood or lymph. A *thrombus* is a clot that adheres to the wall of a blood vessel or organ and may obstruct the vessel or organ in which it resides, preventing the flow of blood. The term *thromb/o/lysis* refers to the destruction or loosening of a blood _____.
thromb/o/genesis thrŏm-bō-JĔN-ĕ-sĭs	**9-93** Use *-genesis* to form a word that means *producing, forming, or origin of a blood clot.* _____/_____/_____
hem/o/rrhage HĔM-ĕ-rĭj **cerebr/o/vascul/ar** sĕr-ĕ-brō-VĂS-kū-lăr **thrombus** THRŎM-bŭs	**9-94** A stroke, also called *cerebr/o/vascul/ar accident* (CVA), is the rapid loss of brain function resulting from disturbance of the normal blood supply (ischemia) to the brain. This can be caused by occlusion by an embolus or a thrombus (ischemic stroke) or by a ruptured blood vessel (hemorrhagic stroke). The resulting neur/o/logic/al symptoms vary according to the location of the obstruction and extent of brain tissue affected. Write the terms in this frame that mean *bursting forth (of) blood:* _____/_____/_____. *pertaining to the cerebrum and blood vessels:* Cerebr / o / Vascul / ar . *stationary blood clot:* _____.
aneurysm/ectomy ăn-ū-rĭz-MĔK-tō-mē	**9-95** Stroke caused by hem/o/rrhage from a cerebral artery is commonly fatal. It usually results from high blood pressure, atherosclerosis, or the bursting of an arterial aneurysm (localized dilation of the blood vessel wall). The CF *aneurysm/o* means *a widening or a widened blood vessel.* Use *aneurysm/o* to construct a medical word that means *excision of an aneurysm.* aneurym / etomy
neur/o/glia nū-RŎG-lē-ă	**9-96** As discussed earlier, the entire nervous system is composed of two principal types of cells, neurons and neuroglia. The supporting cells in the CNS collectively are called *neur/o/glia.* A term that literally means *nerve glue* is _____/_____/_____.
neur/o/cyte NŪ-rō-sīt	**9-97** A neur/o/cyte, commonly called a *neuron,* is a nerve cell. A term that literally means *nerve cell* is _____/_____/_____.

Pink indicates a prefix. Blue indicates a suffix. Boldface indicates a word root or combining form.

Mental Disorders

Mental disorders, also called *mental illnesses, or psychiatric disorders,* are health conditions involving changes in thinking, emotion, behavior, or a combination of these. Although many individuals do experience disturbances in these areas, it only becomes a disorder when everyday life tasks become problematic with distress and resulting impairment in social, occupational, and relationship functioning. The spectrum severity for mental disorders ranges from mild to severe. Addiction to alcohol and drugs is included in this area, and when accompanied by a mental illness, it is referred to as a dual diagnosis. A **dual diagnosis** is a mental illness with some type of drug addiction such as alcohol, heroine, or pain killers. Numerous psychiatric disorders have been identified and are categorized in the DSM V (Diagnostic and Statistic Manual of Mental Disorders 5th edition) and are the recognized standard throughout the healthcare system. The DSM V classifies all mental disorders and is used to improve diagnoses, treatment, research, as well as payment by health-care providers. Mental illness is treatable. In most cases, symptoms can be managed with a combination of medications and talk therapy (psychotherapy). Family support is of vital importance for recovery.

an- -orexia	**9-98** An/orexia nervosa is a potentially life-threatening eating disorder characterized by self-starvation, excessive weight loss, and negative body image and its incidence is most common among females. Onset usually occurs during adolescence. This eating disorder is the third most common chronic illness among adolescents in the United States. (See Figure 9-13.) Provide the word elements in this frame that mean *without, not:* ___*an-*___ . *appetite:* ___*-orexia*___ .

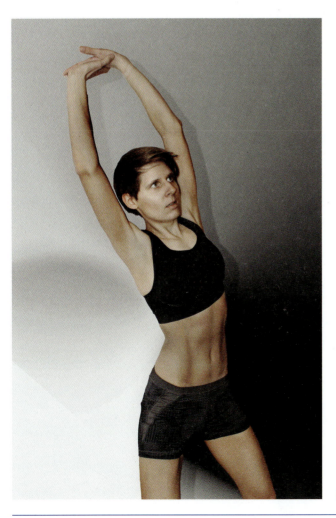

Figure 9-13   Anorexia nervosa.

carcin/o/phobia KĂR-sĭn-ō-fō-bē-ă	**9–99** Besides path/o/logical conditions, which were discussed earlier in this chapter, some CFs and suffixes are used to identify mental disorders. For example, phob/ic disorders are anxiety disorders characterized by extreme, irrational fears. The suffix *-phobia,* which means *fear,* is a general suffix used to describe all types of fears. A person who has an extreme fear of cancer suffers from a phobia known as _____/_____/_____.
xen/o/phobia zĕn-ō-FŌ-bē-ă	**9–100** The CF *xen/o* means *foreign* or *strange.* Combine *xen/o* and *-phobia* to identify the disorder of a person who has a fear of strangers. _Xen_/_o_/_phbia_
necr/o/phobia nĕk-rō-FŌ-bē-ă	**9–101** The CF *necr/o* means *death* or *necrosis.* A person who has a fear of corpses or death suffers from the phobia known as _necr_/_o_/_phb._ .
fear	**9–102** Whenever you see *-phobia* in a term, you will know it means _____ and refers to an anxiety disorder.
neur/osis nū-RŌ-sĭs **neur/oses** nū-RŌ-sēz	**9–103** Earlier in this chapter, you learned that *neur/o* refers to nerves. The CF *neur/o* is also used to form words that refer to mental disorders. For example, *neur/osis* is an emotional disorder that involves an ineffective way of coping with anxiety or inner conflict. Build a word that means *abnormal condition of nerves:* _____/_____ The plural form of *neur/osis* is _____/_____.
psych/iatry sī-KĪ-ă-trē	**9–104** The CF *psych/o* means *mind;* the suffix *-iatry* means *physician, treatment.* The medical specialty concerned with diagnosis and treatment of disorders of the mind, or mental disorders, is _____/_____.
psych/o/therapy sī-kō-THĔR-ă-pē	**9–105** *Psych/o* is used to form words about mental conditions. Psych/osis is a mental disorder with severe impairment of thoughts and emotions that result in loss of contact with reality. Combine *psych/o* and *-therapy* to form a word that means *treatment of the mind (mental condition).* _____/_____/_____
psych/oses sī-KŌ-sēz	**9–106** What is the plural form of psych/osis? _____/_____/_____

megal/o/mania	**9-107** Some psychoses are identified with the suffix *-mania,* which means a *state of mental disorder or frenzy*. Examples include *klept/o/mania* (the urge to steal items you do not need and that usually have little value) and *pyr/o/mania* (the urge to start fires). Use **megal/o** and the suffix -mania to form a mental disorder characterized by the delusion of power, wealth, or extravagant things or actions.
schiz/o/phren/ia skĭz-ō-FRĔN-ē-ă	**9-108** Schiz/o/phren/ia is a psych/osis that commonly involves delusions, such as believing that someone or something is controlling your thoughts. Another of its manifestations is hallucinations, most commonly "hearing" voices or other sounds. Use the CF *schiz/o,* meaning *split,* and **phren/o,** meaning *mind,* along with the suffix *-ia* to build the term for a *psychiatric disorder characterized by delusions, hallucinations, or both*. _____/ ___/ _____/ _____

SECTION REVIEW 9-5

Using the following table, write the CF, suffix, or prefix that matches its definition in the space provided to the left of the definition. There may be more than one word element that matches a definition.

Combining Forms

cerebr/o	myel/o
encephal/o	neur/o
gli/o	scler/o
meningi/o	thromb/o
mening/o	vascul/o

Suffixes

-glia	-rrhagia
-malacia	
-osis	
-phasia *speech*	
-rrhage	

Prefixes

a-
dys-

1. _____ abnormal condition; increase (used primarily with blood cells)

2. _____ bad; painful; difficult

3. ___-rrhagia._____ blood clot

4. ___vascul/o_____ vessel

5. ___cephal/o_____ brain

6. ___-rrhage_____ bursting forth (of)

7. ___-glia._____ glue; neuroglial tissue

8. ___scler/o_____ hardening; sclera (white of the eye)

9. ___menen/o_____ meninges (membranes covering the brain and spinal cord)

10. ___neur/o_____ nerve

11. ___cerebr/o_____ cerebrum

12. ___malacia._____ softening

13. ___-phasia_____ speech

14. ___myel/o_____ bone marrow; spinal cord

15. ___a_____ without, not

Competency Verification: Check your answers in Appendix B: Answer Key, page 611. If you are not satisfied with your level of comprehension, go back to Frame 9–72, and rework the frames.

Correct Answers _____ x 6.67 = _____ % Score

Abbreviations

This section introduces endocrine and nervous system–related abbreviations and their meanings.

Abbreviation	Meaning	Abbreviation	Meaning
Endocrine System			
ADH	antidiuretic hormone	GTT	glucose tolerance test
ACTH	adrenocorticotropic hormone	HRT	hormone replacement therapy
BMI	body mass index	LH	luteinizing hormone
BG	blood glucose	OGTT	oral glucose tolerance test
DM	diabetes mellitus	PGH	pituitary growth hormone
FBG	fasting blood glucose	PTH	parathyroid hormone
FSH	follicle-stimulating hormone	RAIU	radioactive iodine uptake
GH	growth hormone	TSH	thyroid-stimulating hormone
Nervous System			
ALS	amyotrophic lateral sclerosis	DSM V	Diagnostic and Statistic Manual of Mental Disorders 5 *(5th edition)*
C1, C2, and so on	first cervical vertebra, second cervical vertebra, and so on	L1, L2, and so on	first lumbar vertebra, second lumbar vertebra, and so on
CNS	central nervous system	LP	lumbar puncture
CP	cerebral palsy	MS	mitral stenosis; musculoskeletal; multiple sclerosis; mental status; magnesium sulfate
CSF	cerebrospinal fluid	S1, S2, and so on	first sacral vertebra, second sacral vertebra, and so on
CVA	cerebrovascular accident; costovertebral angle	T1, T2, and so on	first thoracic vertebra, second thoracic vertebra, and so on
EEG	electroencephalography	TIA	transient ischemic attack
Radiographic Procedures			
AP	anteroposterior	MRI	magnetic resonance imaging
CT	computed tomography	MSI	magnetic source imaging
IV	intravenous	PA	posteroanterior
MEG	magnetoencephalography	PET	positron emission tomography

Additional Medical Terms

The following are additional terms related to the endocrine and nervous systems. Recognizing and learning these terms will help you understand the connections among a pathological condition, its diagnosis, and the rationale behind the method of treatment selected for a particular disorder.

Diseases and Conditions

Endocrine System

Addison disease Ă-dĭ-sŭn	Hyposecretion of cortisol that results when the adrenal cortex is damaged or atrophied; also called *corticoadrenal insufficiency* *Addison disease is a possibly life-threatening autoimmune disorder in which the body produces antibodies that slowly destroy the adrenal cortex. Patients experience a low level of blood glucose, fatigue, weight loss, and decreased ability to tolerate stress, disease, or surgery. Treatment includes replacement corticosteroids to control the symptoms of this disease. These medicines usually need to be taken for life.*
diabetes mellitus (DM) dī-ă-BĒ-tēz MĔ-lĭ-tŭs	Chronic metabolic disorder of impaired carbohydrate, protein, and fat metabolism caused by insufficient production of insulin or the body's inability to use insulin properly *When used alone, the term diabetes refers to diabetes mellitus. Hyperglycemia and ketosis are responsible for its host of troubling and commonly life-threatening symptoms. Diabetes mellitus occurs in two primary forms: type 1 diabetes and type 2 diabetes.*
type 1 diabetes	Form of diabetes mellitus that is abrupt in onset and is caused by the failure of the pancreas to produce insulin, making this type of disease difficult to regulate *Type 1 diabetes is usually diagnosed in children and young adults. Treatment includes insulin injections to maintain a normal level of glucose in blood.*
type 2 diabetes	Form of diabetes mellitus that is gradual in onset and results from the body's deficiency in producing enough insulin or resistance to the action of insulin by the body's cells *Type 2 is the most common form of diabetes. It is usually diagnosed in adults older than age 40 years. Management of this disease is less problematic than that of type 1. Treatment includes diet, weight loss, and exercise. It may also include insulin or oral antidiabetic agents, which activate the release of pancreatic insulin and improve the body's sensitivity to insulin.*
panhypopituitarism păn-hī-pō-pĭ-TŪ-ĭ-tăr-ĭzm *pan-:* all *hyp/o:* under, below, deficient *pituitar:* pituitary gland *-ism:* condition	Total pituitary impairment that brings about a progressive and general loss of hormone activity

| **pheochromocytoma** fē-ō-krō-mō-sī-TŌ-mă | Rare adrenal gland tumor that causes excessive release of epinephrine (adrenaline) and norepinephrine (hormones that regulate heart rate and blood pressure) and induces severe blood pressure elevation |

Nervous System

| **Alzheimer disease** ĂLTS-hī-měr | Most common form of dementia that is a progressive disease causing a decline in memory, thinking, social, and behavioral skills, leading to the inability to function independently; also called *cerebral degeneration* |
| | *The onset of Alzheimer disease usually occurs in the mid-60s. It involves progressive irreversible loss of memory, deterioration of judgement and reasoning functions, apathy, speech and gait disturbances, and disorientation. These changes occur as amyloid plaques (abnormal deposits of protein) produce damage and destruction to neurons. The course of disease varies and may take months to years and ultimately leads to death.* |

| **amyotrophic lateral sclerosis (ALS)** ă-mī-ō-TRŌ-fĭk, sklĕ-RŌ-sĭs | Degenerative disorder in which the progressive loss of motor neurons in the spinal cord and brainstem leads to muscle weakness and paralysis; also called *Lou Gehrig disease* (named after the baseball player who became afflicted with ALS) |
| | *ALS manifests in adulthood with symptoms of weakness and atrophy of muscles in the hands, forearms, and legs; difficulty in swallowing and talking; and dyspnea as the throat and respiratory muscles become affected. As yet, the cause of and cure for ALS remain unknown.* |

| **epilepsy** ĔP-ĭ-lĕp-sē | Neurological disorder in which the nerve cell activity in the brain is disturbed, causing a seizure, including loss of consciousness |
| | *Epilepsy has many possible causes, including illness, brain injury, and abnormal brain development. Seizure symptoms vary. Some people with epilepsy simply stare blankly for a few seconds during a seizure, whereas in others, epilepsy causes repeated twitching of the arms or legs.* |

| **Huntington chorea** HŬN-tĭng-tŭn kō-RĒ-ă | Hereditary nervous disorder caused by the progressive loss of brain cells, leading to bizarre, involuntary, dancelike movements; also called *neurodegenerative genetic disorder* |

| **multiple sclerosis (MS)** MŬL-tĭ-pl sklĕ-RŌ-sĭs *scler:* hardening; sclera (white of the eye) *-osis:* abnormal condition; increase (used primarily with blood cells) | Progressive degenerative disease of the CNS characterized by inflammation, hardening, and loss of myelin throughout the spinal cord and brain, which produces weakness and other muscle symptoms |

neuroblastoma
nū-rō-blăs-TŌ-mă
   neur/o: nerve
    blast: embryonic cell
    -oma: tumor
	Malignant tumor composed principally of cells resembling neuroblasts
	
	Neuroblastoma occurs most commonly in infants and children.

palsy PAWL-zē	Partial or complete loss of motor function
Bell palsy	Facial paralysis on one side of the face because of inflammation of a facial nerve (cranial nerve VII), most likely caused by a viral infection; also called *facial nerve palsy* *Bell palsy commonly results in grotesque facial disfigurement and facial spasms. Treatment includes corticosteroid drugs to decrease nerve swelling. Ordinarily, the condition lasts a month and resolves by itself.*

cerebral palsy (CP)
SĔR-ĕ-brăl
  cerebr: cerebrum
    -al: pertaining to
	Bilateral, symmetrical, nonprogressive motor dysfunction and partial paralysis, which is usually caused by damage to the cerebrum during gestation or by birth trauma, but can also be hereditary

paralysis pă-RĂL-ĭ-sĭs	Loss of voluntary motion caused by inability to contract one or more muscles *Paralysis may be caused by a variety of problems, such as head trauma, spinal cord injury, and stroke. Paralysis may be classified according to the cause, muscle tone, distribution, or body part affected. (See Figure 9-14.)*

paraplegia
păr-ă-PLĒ-jē-ă
  para: near, beside;
      beyond
  -plegia: paralysis
	Paralysis of the lower portion of the body and both legs
	
	Paraplegia results in loss of sensory and motor control below the level of injury. Other common problems occurring with spinal cord injury to the lumbar and thoracic regions include loss of bladder, bowel, and sexual control.

quadriplegia
kwŏd-rĭ-PLĒ-jē-ă
  quadri: four
  -plegia: paralysis
	Paralysis of all four extremities and, usually, the trunk
	
	Quadriplegia generally results in loss of motor and sensory functions below the level of injury. Paralysis includes the trunk, legs, and pelvic organs, with partial or total paralysis in the upper extremities. The higher the trauma, the more debilitating are the motor and sensory impairments.

Parkinson disease PĂR-kĭn-sŭn	Progressive, degenerative neurological disorder affecting the portion of the brain responsible for controlling movement; also called *paralysis agitans* *The unnecessary skeletal muscle movements of Parkinson disease commonly interfere with voluntary movement—for example, causing the hand to shake (called "tremor"), the most common symptom of Parkinson disease.*

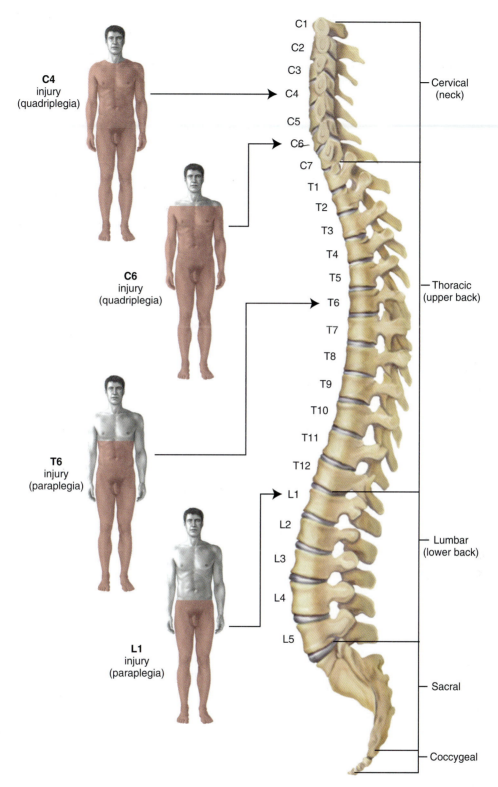

Figure 9-14 Spinal cord injuries showing extent of paralysis.

poliomyelitis
pō-lē-ō-mī-ĕl-Ī-tĭs
  poli/o: gray; gray matter
      (of the brain or
      spinal cord)
  myel: bone marrow;
      spinal cord
  -itis: inflammation

Disease in which the gray matter of the spinal cord is destroyed by a slow-acting virus, eventually leading to paralysis and muscular atrophy

Vaccines have made poliomyelitis, commonly known as polio, *relatively uncommon in the United States. Nevertheless, postpolio syndrome is a complication that develops in some patients, usually 30 or more years after they were first infected. Muscles that were already weak may get weaker. Weakness may also develop in muscles that were not affected before.*

---

sciatica
sī-ĂT-ĭ-kă

Severe pain in the leg along the course of the sciatic nerve, which travels from the hip to the foot

---

seizure
SĒ-zhūr

Abnormal, uncontrolled discharge of electrical activity in the brain, which is commonly a symptom of underlying brain pathology; also called *convulsion*

Chronic, recurrent seizures are a characteristic symptom of epilepsy.

  tonic-clonic
  (grand mal)

Seizure characterized by unconsciousness with excessive motor activity and the body alternating between excessive muscle tone with rigidity (tonic) and involuntary muscular contractions (clonic) in the extremities

Tonic-clonic seizures last about 1 to 2 minutes. Other symptoms include tongue biting, difficulty breathing, and incontinence. The recovery after a seizure is known as the postictal *period.*

  absence (petit mal)

Seizure characterized by a brief, sudden, loss of consciousness lasting only a few seconds

A person can have many absence seizures during the course of the day.

---

shingles
SHĬNG-lz

Eruption of acute, inflammatory, herpetic vesicles on the trunk of the body along a peripheral nerve that is caused by *herpes zoster virus*

Shingles is a viral infection that causes a painful rash and is the same virus that causes chickenpox. (See Figure 9-15.)

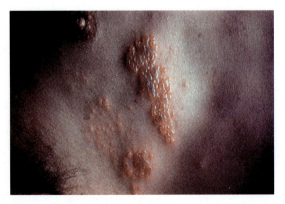

Figure 9-15 Shingles. From Goldsmith, Lazarus, and Tharp: *Adult and Pediatric Dermatology: A Color Guide to Diagnosis and Treatment.* FA Davis, Philadelphia, 1997, p 307, used with permission.

spina bifida SPĪ-nă BĬF-ĭ-dă	Congenital neural tube defect characterized by <u>incomplete</u> closure of the <u>spinal</u> <u>canal</u>; the spinal cord and <u>meninges</u> may or may not protrude through the defect *Spina bifida usually occurs in the lumbosacral area and has several forms. (See Figure 9-16.)*
spina bifida occulta SPĪ-nă BĬF-ĭ-dă ŏ-KŬL-tă	Most common and least severe form of spina bifida without protrusion of the spinal cord or meninges
spina bifida cystica SPĪ-nă BĬF-ĭ-dă SĬS-tĭk-ă	More severe type of spina bifida that <u>involves</u> <u>protrusion</u> of the meninges (meningocele), spinal cord (myelocele), or both (meningomyelocele) *The severity of neurological dysfunction in spina bifida cystica is directly related to the degree of nerve involvement.*

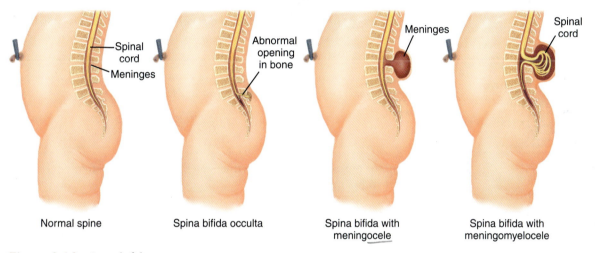

Normal spine   Spina bifida occulta   Spina bifida with meningocele   Spina bifida with meningomyelocele

Figure 9-16   Spina bifida.

transient ischemic attack (TIA) TRĂN-zhĕnt ĭs-KĒ-mĭk *ischem:* to hold back; block *-ic:* pertaining to	Short episodes of neurological dysfunction caused by temporary interference with blood supply to the brain, lasting a few minutes to a few hours; also called *ministroke* *TIAs may recur, and each TIA increases the risk of a stroke. The neurological symptoms vary, depending on the amount of ischemia and the location of the vessels involved. However, a TIA does not destroy brain cells or cause permanent disability.*

Diagnostic Procedures

Endocrine System

fasting blood glucose (FBG) GLOO-kōs	Test that measures glucose levels in blood after the patient has fasted (not eaten) for at least 8 hours; also called *fasting blood sugar (FBS)* *FBG helps determine whether the pancreas is secreting a normal amount of insulin and diagnose other pancreatic disorders, such as diabetes and hypoglycemia.*

glucose tolerance test (GTT)
GLOO-kōs

Screening test in which a patient fasts for 8 to 12 hours, ingests glucose, and then undergoes blood draws to determine how quickly the glucose is cleared from blood; also called *oral glucose tolerance test (OGTT)*

GTT helps diagnose diabetes with higher accuracy compared with other blood glucose tests. It also helps diagnose gestational diabetes or rarer disorders of carbohydrate metabolism.

radioactive iodine uptake (RAIU) test

Imaging procedure that measures levels of radioactivity in the thyroid gland after oral or intravenous administration of radioactive iodine

RAIU helps determine thyroid function by monitoring the thyroid's ability to take up (uptake) iodine from blood.

Nervous System

cerebrospinal fluid (CSF) analysis
sĕr-ĕ-brō-SPĪ-năl
  cerebr/o: cerebrum
  spin: spine
  -al: pertaining to

Laboratory test in which CSF obtained through a lumbar puncture is evaluated macroscopically for clarity and color, microscopically for cells, and chemically for proteins and other substances

CSF analysis helps detect bacteria, viruses, and tumor cells. The analysis also helps diagnose tumors, infection, or multiple sclerosis (MS).

electroencephalography (EEG)

Diagnostic procedure in which electrodes on the scalp record patterns of electrical activity within the brain

EEG helps evaluate seizure disorders, periods of unconsciousness, and sleep disorders; monitors the brain during brain surgery; and determines whether a person is in a coma or is brain dead. (See Figure 9-17.)

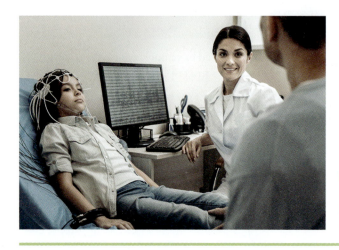

Figure 9-17 Electroencephalography (EEG). Young girl is accompanied by father, while the doctor views electrical brain activity on the monitor to diagnose the presence of seizure activity.

lumbar puncture (LP)
LŬM-băr
  lumb: loins (lower back)
  -ar: pertaining to

Insertion of a needle into the subarachnoid space of the spinal column at the level of the fourth intervertebral space to withdraw CSF to perform various diagnostic and therapeutic procedures; also called *spinal tap* or *spinal puncture*

In lumbar puncture, CSF flows through the needle and is collected and sent to the laboratory for analysis. Therapeutic procedures include withdrawing CSF to reduce intracranial pressure, introducing a local anesthetic to induce spinal anesthesia, and administering intrathecal medications. (See Figure 9-18.)

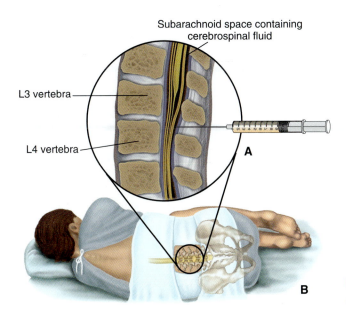

Subarachnoid space containing cerebrospinal fluid

L3 vertebra

L4 vertebra

A

B

Figure 9-18 Lumbar puncture. (A) Collection of cerebrospinal fluid. (B) Position for lumbar puncture.

magnetoencephalography (MEG) măg-nĕt-ō-ĕn-cĕf-ă-LŎG-ră-fē	Noninvasive functional imaging technique in which magnetic forces associated with the electrical activity of the brain are recorded externally on the scalp *When the data from MEG are superimposed on an anatomical image of the brain, typically an MRI scan, it produces a functional, anatomical image of the brain called magnetic source imaging (MSI). MSI aids in presurgical evaluation of patients with epilepsy to identify and localize areas of epileptic activity. MSI results in a high-resolution image that provides a direct measure of brain function.*
magnetic resonance imaging (MRI) măg-NĔT-ĭc RĔZ-ĕn-ăns ĬM-ĭj-ĭng	Radiographic technique that uses electromagnetic energy to produce multiplanar cross-sectional images of the body *MRI of the brain produces cross-sectional, frontal, and sagittal plane views of the brain. It is considered superior to CT for detecting most CNS abnormalities, particularly those of the brainstem and spinal cord. A contrast medium is not required but may be used to enhance visualization of internal structures.*
positron emission tomography (PET) PŎZ-ĭ-trŏn ē-MĬSH-ŭn tō-MŎG-ră-fē *tom/o:* to cut *-graphy:* process of recording	Radiographic technique that combines CT with radiopharmaceuticals to produce a cross-sectional (transverse) image of the distribution of radioactivity (through emission of positrons) in a section of the body, revealing areas where the radiopharmaceutical is metabolized and where metabolism is deficient *PET aids in the diagnosis of neurological disorders, such as brain tumors, epilepsy, stroke, and Alzheimer disease, as well as abdominal and pulmonary disorders.*

Medical and Surgical Procedures

Endocrine System

insulin pump therapy

A small, computerized device continuously delivering precise doses of insulin through a catheter placed under the skin

The pump replaces the need for frequent injections by delivering precise doses of insulin 24 hours per day to match the body's needs closely. A health-care professional determines the programmed rate. (See Figure 9-19.)

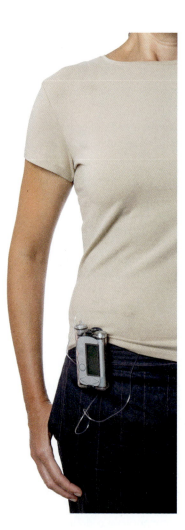

Figure 9-19   Insulin pump therapy.

transsphenoidal hypophysectomy
trăns-sfē-NOY-dăl
hī-pō-fĭ-SĔK-tō-mē

Minimally invasive endoscopic surgery that removes pituitary tumors through the nasal cavity via the sphenoid sinus (transsphenoidal) without affecting brain tissue

Although most tumors can be removed via transsphenoidal hypophysectomy, some large tumors may need to be removed via transfrontal craniotomy (entry through the frontal bone of the skull). (See Figure 9-20.)

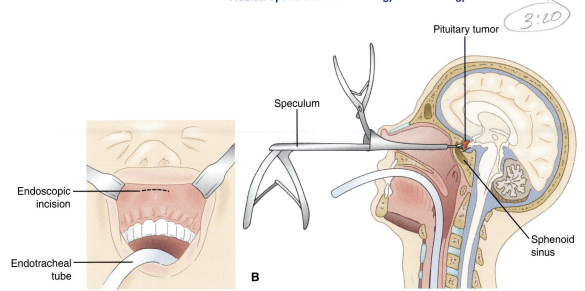

3:20

Figure 9-20 Transsphenoidal hypophysectomy. (A) Incision beneath the upper lip to enter the nasal cavity and gain access to the pituitary gland. (B). Insertion of a speculum and special forceps to remove the pituitary tumor.

Nervous System

craniotomy krā-nē-ŎT-ō-mē *crani/o:* cranium (skull) *-tomy:* incision	Surgical procedure that creates an opening in the skull to gain access to the brain during neurosurgical procedures *A craniotomy is also performed to relieve intracranial pressure, control bleeding, or remove a tumor.*
thalamotomy thăl-ă-MŎT-ō-mē	Partial destruction of the thalamus to treat psychosis, intractable pain, or involuntary movements, including tremors in Parkinson disease
trephination trĕf-ĭn-Ā-shŭn	Excision of a circular disk of bone using a specialized saw, called a *trephine,* to reveal brain tissue during neurosurgery or to relieve intracranial pressure

Pharmacology

The following table lists common drug categories used to treat reproductive disorders and their therapeutic actions.

Drug Category	Action
Endocrine System	
hormone replacement therapy (HRT)	Correct a deficiency in hormones, such as estrogen, testosterone, or thyroid hormone *HRT may include oral administration or injection of synthetic hormones.*
oral hypoglycemics hī-pō-glī-SĒ-mĭcs	Stimulate insulin secretion from pancreatic cells in patients with non–insulin-dependent diabetes, with some pancreatic function
Nervous System	
anesthetics ăn-ĕs-THĔT-ĭks	Produce partial or complete loss of sensation, with or without loss of consciousness *General anesthetics act on the brain to produce complete loss of feeling with loss of consciousness. Local anesthetics act on nerves or nerve tracts to affect only a local area.*
anticonvulsants ăn-tĭ-kŏn-VŬL-sănts	Prevent or reduce the severity of epileptic or other convulsive seizures; also called *antiepileptics*
antiparkinsonian agents ăn-tĭ-păr-kĭn-SŌN-ē-ăn	Control tremors and muscle rigidity associated with Parkinson disease by increasing dopamine levels in the brain
antipsychotics ăn-tĭ-sī-KŎT-ĭkz	Alter neurotransmitters in the brain to alleviate symptoms of psychosis, paranoia, and schizophrenia

Pronunciation Help	Long Sound	ā in rāte	ē in rēbirth	ī in īsle	ō in ōver	ū in ūnite
	Short Sound	ă in ăpple	ĕ in ĕver	ĭ in ĭt	ŏ in nŏt	ŭ in cŭt

Word Elements Review

This review provides a verification of the word elements covered in this chapter. First, use a slash to break the term into its component parts, and identify each element by labeling it P *for prefix,* WR *for word root,* CF *for combining form, and* S *for suffix. Then provide the meaning of the medical term. Remember to define the suffix first, define the beginning of the word next, and define the middle part of the term last. The first word is a sample completed for you.*

Term	Meaning
pancreat/o/lith/iasis CF WR S	*abnormal condition (produced by something specified) of calculus or stone in the pancreas*
1. hemi/paresis	
2. hyper/glycem/ia	
3. hypo/pituitar/ism	
4. meningi/oma	
5. poly/dipsia	
6. quadri/plegia	
7. thyr/omegaly	
8. toxic/o/logist	

Match the following medical terms with the definitions in the numbered list.

acromegaly   encephalitis   hypertrophy   myelitis   pancreatolithiasis   thymoma
adrenalectomy   glioma   hypocalcemia   neuralgia   thalamotomy   thyropathy
aphasia   hemiparesis   meningocele   neurolysis   thrombogenesis

9. _____ tumor composed of neuroglial tissue

10. _____ enlargement of the extremities

11. _____ formation of a blood clot

12. _____ tumor of the thymus gland

13. _____ disease of the thyroid gland

14. _____ pain in the nerve(s)

15. _____ absence of speech

16. _____ protrusion of the meninges through the skull or the vertebral column

17. _____ excision of the adrenal gland

18. _____ destruction of a nerve

19. _____ paralysis of one half of the body (right half or left half)

20. _____ incision of the thalamus

21. _____ inflammation of the spinal cord

22. _____ deficiency of calcium in blood

23. _____ abnormal condition of a pancreatic stone

24. _____ inflammation of the brain

25. _____ increase in the size of an organ

Competency Verification: Check your answers in Appendix B: Answer Key, page 611. If you are not satisfied with your level of comprehension, review the vocabulary, and retake the review.

Correct Answers _____ × 4 = _____ % Score

Additional Medical Terms Review

Match the following medical terms with the definitions in the numbered list.

Alzheimer disease	*Huntington chorea*	*panhypopituitarism*	*sciatica*
antipsychotics	*hypophysectomy*	*Parkinson disease*	*shingles*
Bell palsy	*lumbar puncture*	*PET*	*spina bifida*
EEG	*MRI*	*pheochromocytoma*	*TIA*
epilepsy	*myxedema*	*poliomyelitis*	*thalamotomy*
exophthalmos	*neuroblastoma*	*quadriplegia*	*type 1 diabetes*
Graves disease			

1. _____ is facial paralysis on one side of the face because of inflammation of a facial nerve.

2. _____ describes short episodes of neurological dysfunction resulting from temporary interference with blood supply to the brain.

3. _____ are used to alter symptoms of psychosis and schizophrenia.

4. _____ is abnormal protrusion of the eyeball, possibly caused by thyrotoxicosis.

5. _____ means hyperthyroidism and is also called *toxic goiter,* which is characterized by exophthalmos.

6. _____ is a surgical procedure to remove a pituitary tumor.

7. _____ is advanced hypothyroidism in adults that results from hypofunction of the thyroid gland and causes edema and increased blood pressure.

8. _____ is a small chromaffin cell tumor, usually located in the adrenal medulla.

9. _____ is a progressive degenerative neurological disorder that causes hand tremors.

10. _____ refers to inflammation of the gray matter caused by a virus, commonly resulting in spinal and muscle deformities and paralysis.

11. _____ refers to severe pain in the leg along the course of the sciatic nerve.

12. _____ is a congenital defect characterized by incomplete closure of the spinal canal through which the spinal cord and meninges may or may not protrude.

13. _____ is a diagnostic procedure in which electrodes placed on the scalp record electrical activity within the brain.

14. _____ is a malignant tumor composed principally of cells resembling neuroblasts and occurs chiefly in infants and children.

15. _____ is a brain disorder marked by amyloid plaques that lead to deterioration of mental capacity, total disability, and death.

16. _____ is a radiographic technique that uses electromagnetic energy to produce cross-sectional, frontal, and sagittal views of the brain.

17. _____ is a chronic disease caused by insufficient production of insulin or the body's inability to use insulin properly.

18. _____ refers to eruption of acute, inflammatory, herpetic vesicles on the trunk of the body along a peripheral nerve.

19. _____ is a paralysis of four extremities and usually the trunk.

20. _____ refers to total pituitary impairment that brings about progressive and general loss of hormone activity.

21. _____ is a hereditary nervous disorder caused by progressive loss of brain cells that leads to bizarre, involuntary, dancelike movements.

22. _____ is the withdrawal of spinal fluid for diagnostic or therapeutic purposes.

23. _____ is a neurological disorder in which the nerve cell activity in the brain is disturbed, causing a seizure.

24. _____ refers to partial destruction of the thalamus to treat psychosis or intractable pain.

25. _____ produces a cross-sectional image of radioactivity in a section of the body to reveal areas where the radiopharmaceutical is metabolized and where metabolism is deficient.

Competency Verification: Check your answers in Appendix B: Answer Key, page 611. If you are not satisfied with your level of comprehension, review the additional medical terms and retake the review.

Correct Answers _____ × 4 = _____ % Score

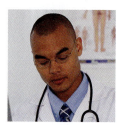

Medical Record Activities

To develop a working vocabulary of medical terms and to understand how those terms are used in the health-care industry, it is important that you complete the following activities.

MEDICAL RECORD ACTIVITY 9-1

DISCHARGE SUMMARY: DIABETES MELLITUS

This activity contains a discharge summary in which a patient is diagnosed with diabetes mellitus. Read the discharge summary that follows and underline the medical terms. Then, complete the terminology and critical thinking exercises.

DISCHARGE SUMMARY

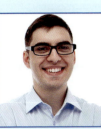

PATIENT NAME: Gutierrez, Ramon
MEDICAL RECORD ID: 27-14821
DATE: April 27, 20xx

ADMITTED: 4/27/xx

DISCHARGED: 5/2/xx

ADMITTING DIAGNOSIS: Diabetes mellitus, new onset.

DISCHARGE DIAGNOSIS: Type 1 diabetes mellitus, new onset.

HISTORY OF PRESENT ILLNESS: Patient is a 15-year-old white male who presented in the office complaining of increased appetite, polydipsia, and polyuria and was found to have elevated blood glucose of 400 and glycosuria. He was sent to the hospital for further evaluation and treatment.

HOSPITAL COURSE: Upon admission, laboratory tests showed electrolytes WNL (within normal limits), and ketones were negative. Urinalysis showed a trace of glucose (blood glucose [BG] 380), and there was no evidence of acidosis. Metabolically, the patient was stable. Patient was started on split-mixed insulin dosing. The patient and his family received full diabetes instruction during his hospitalization, and they seemed to understand this well. The patient picked up on all of this information quickly, asked appropriate questions, and appeared to be coping well with his new condition. By day 5, his polyuria and polydipsia resolved. When the patient was able to draw up and self-administer insulin and perform his own fingersticks, he was discharged.

DISCHARGE INSTRUCTIONS: The patient was discharged to home with his parents with a prescription for a mixture of Humulin L 12 units and Humulin R 6 units each morning and Humulin L 5 units and Humulin R 6 units each afternoon. He will continue with fingerstick blood glucose four times daily at home until seen in the office for follow-up. I warned him of all glycemic symptoms to watch for, and he is to call the office with any problems that may occur. Patient is to follow an ADA 2,000-calorie diet.

DISCHARGE CONDITION: The patient's overall condition was much improved, and at the time of discharge, BG levels were stabilized, and he was doing well.

Justin R. Henderson, M.D.
_____
Justin R. Henderson, M.D.

JRH:ls

D: 5/2/20xx; T:05/2/20xx

Terminology 9-1

Terms listed in the following table come from the previous Discharge Summary: Diabetes Mellitus. Use a medical dictionary, such as Taber's Cyclopedic Medical Dictionary; *the appendices of this book; or other resources to define each term. Then, pronounce the term, and place a checkmark (✓) in the box after you do so.*

Term	Definition
acidosis ăs-ĭ-DŌ-sĭs ☐	
ADA	
BG	
diabetes mellitus dī-ă-BĒ-tēz MĔ-lĭ-tŭs ☐	
electrolytes ē-LĔK-trō-līts ☐	
glycemic glī-SĒ-mĭk ☐	
glycosuria glĭ-kō-SŪ-rē-ă ☐	
Humulin L HŪ-mū-lĭn ☐	
Humulin R HŪ-mū-lĭn ☐	
ketones KĒ-tōnz ☐	
metabolically mĕt-ă-BŎL-ĭk-ă-lē ☐	

Term	Definition
polydipsia pŏl-ē-DĬP-sē-ă ☐	
polyuria pŏl-ē-Ū-rē-ă ☐	
type 1 diabetes mellitus dī-ă-BĒ-tēz MĔ-lĭ-tŭs ☐	
WNL	

Visit the *Medical Terminology Simplified* online resource center at FADavis.com to hear pronunciation and meanings of terms in this medical report.

Critical Thinking 9-1

Review the previous Discharge Summary: Diabetes Mellitus to answer the following questions. Use a medical dictionary, such as Taber's Cyclopedic Medical Dictionary, *and other resources, if needed.*

1. What symptoms of diabetes mellitus (DM) did the patient experience before his office visit?

   _____

   _____

2. What confirmed the patient's new diagnosis of DM?

   _____

   _____

3. What conditions had to be met before the patient could be discharged from the hospital?

   _____

   _____

4. How many times a day does the patient have to take insulin?

   _____

   _____

5. Why does the patient have to perform finger sticks four times a day?

   _____

   _____

6. What is an ADA 2,000-calorie diet? Why is it important?

   _____

   _____

MEDICAL RECORD ACTIVITY 9-2

CHART NOTE: PERIPHERAL NEUROPATHY

This activity contains a chart note in which a patient on disability is diagnosed with peripheral neuropathy. Read the chart note that follows, and underline the medical terms. Then, complete the terminology and critical thinking exercises.

CHART NOTE

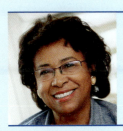

PATIENT NAME: Worther, Christine
MEDICAL RECORD ID: 28-65491
DATE: January 5, 20xx

PAST HISTORY: This 62-year-old black female complains of prolonged pain and burning in her feet, more on the left than on the right, as well as diminished proprioception and difficulty walking, particularly in the dark. The history of her present condition began 2½ to 3 years ago. Additionally, she had been diagnosed with systemic lupus erythematosus by a military physician, who had referred her to Dr. Reed, who reportedly confirmed it in 20xx. The patient has moderate intermittent lower back pain and currently experiences less burning in the lower extremities, but there is still some numbness, which is increased by sitting, driving, or walking for a long time. She has no history of head or neck injury, meningitis, or encephalitis. The only family history of neurological illness is that her maternal grandmother had some type of seizure disorder, and presently the patient is on disability.

NEUROLOGICAL EXAMINATION

HEAD AND NECK: Normal configuration, full range of head and neck movements, and no audible bruits.

CRANIAL NERVE EXAMINATION: Revealed symmetrical function of cranial nerves II through XII, except for hearing loss.

MOTOR SYSTEM EXAMINATION: Reveals normal gait and station and generally good strength, coordination, and reflexes. Forward flexion brings her fingertips down to her toes, but when the patient tries to straighten up, she bends her legs at the knees, and she says that she is not able to get up otherwise.

SENSORY EXAMINATION: Reveals decreased position and vibratory sense as well as pinprick sensation in the lower extremities, much more on the right up to the upper third of the shin and just in the foot and ankle on the left.

IMPRESSION: Peripheral neuropathy of unknown cause, possibly related to lupus, but she does not seem to have other major clinical manifestations at this time. There is nothing that suggests central nervous system lupus at this juncture either. She also has low back pain, intermittent diffuse arthralgias easily controlled by minimal medication, and otosclerosis with hearing loss.

PLAN: Patient should undergo EMG and nerve conduction studies of the lower extremities to further characterize the nature and progression of her neuropathy. I will arrange for this study.

Gene R. Kingston, M.D.

Gene R. Kingston, M.D.

GRK:mlo

D: 1/5/20xx; T: 1/5/20

Terminology 9-2

Terms listed in the following table are taken from the previous Chart Note: Peripheral Neuropathy. Use a medical dictionary, such as Taber's Cyclopedic Medical Dictionary; the appendices of this book; or other resources to define each term. Then, pronounce the term, and place a checkmark (✓) in the box after you do so.

Term	Definition
arthralgias ăr-THRĂL-jē-ăz ☐	
EMG	
encephalitis ĕn-sĕf-ă-LĪ-tĭs ☐	
gait GĀT ☐	
meningitis mĕn-ĭn-JĪ-tĭs ☐	
otosclerosis ō-tō-sklĕ-RŌ-sĭs ☐	
peripheral neuropathy pĕr-ĬF-ĕr-ăl nū-RŎP-ă-thē ☐	
proprioception prō-prē-ō-SĔP-shŭn ☐	

Critical Thinking 9-2

Review the previous Chart Note: Peripheral Neuropathy to answer the following questions. Use a medical dictionary, such as Taber's Cyclopedic Medical Dictionary, *and other resources, if needed.*

1. What are the patient's presenting complaints?

   _____

   _____

2. Are the patient's cranial nerves intact?

   _____

   _____

3. How was the motor system examination described?

   _____

   _____

4. How extensive is the patient's sensory loss?

   _____

   _____

5. What test(s) did the doctor order to further understand the extent of her peripheral neuropathy?

   _____

   _____

MEDICAL RECORD ACTIVITY 9-3

CLINICAL APPLICATION

This activity is a clinical application that will help you integrate and reinforce your understanding of how the following endocrine terms are used in a clinical environment. Complete the following clinically related sentences by selecting an appropriate term from the list.

Addison disease	*Graves disease*	*sciatica*
Alzheimer disease	*myxedema*	*shingles*
epilepsy	*Parkinson disease*	*TIA*
glucose tolerance test	*pheochromocytoma*	*type 1 diabetes mellitus*

1. A 50-year-old female complains of extreme fatigue, depression, sluggishness, and intolerance to cold. The physician suspects thyroid hormone deficiency and orders tests to confirm hypothyroidism. When hypothyroidism develops during adulthood, it is known as _____.

2. An 18-year-old male is brought to the emergency department by his mother, who says that her son lost consciousness, became stiff, and had convulsions. These symptoms lasted only a few seconds, and he appeared confused afterward. The physician orders tests to confirm the diagnosis of a seizure disorder known as _____.

3. This 38-year-old female complains of weight loss and profuse sweating and expresses concern that her eyes seem to be bulging from the sockets. The physician finds that her thyroid gland is enlarged. His initial impression is that she suffers from a form of hyperthyroidism called _____.

4. John is a 29-year-old male who is obese and has an elevated level of blood glucose. The physician suspects type 2 diabetes mellitus. He has John schedule a follow-up visit to take a test that will measure blood glucose levels at regular intervals over a 3-hour period. This test is called a(n) _____.

5. A 44-year-old male presents with a complaint of pain in his lower back extending through his buttocks to his left leg and foot. He says the pain is worsened when rising to stand from a sitting position or after prolonged sitting. The physician explains that his condition is caused by a compressed nerve and diagnoses this pain as _____.

6. Mr. K. complains of muscle weakness, chronic fatigue, and hyperpigmentation of the skin. After reviewing his medical history and laboratory tests, the endocrinologist suspects that Mr. K. suffers from a deficiency of cortical hormones. This rare illness is marked by gradual, progressive failure of the adrenal glands to produce sufficient amounts of cortical hormones and is known as _____.

7. A 56-year-old female presents to the physician's office with multiple painful, itchy vesicles along the right side of her chest and abdomen. The physician diagnoses her with a condition that is caused by the herpes zoster virus and is called _____.

8. Joe is a 68-year-old male admitted to the hospital with complaints of sudden weakness of his left leg and arm, diplopia, slurred speech, and difficulty walking. After examination, the physician concludes that Joe has suffered a "ministroke," also known as a(n) _____.

9. Mr. J., a 75-year-old male, is accompanied by his daughter for his appointment. She tells the physician that her father has been experiencing memory loss, confusion, and difficulty speaking. The physician orders tests to rule out neurological disorders but suspects the patient suffers from a type of dementia known as _____.

10. A 26-year-old male presents with complaints of headaches, high blood pressure, anxiety, and excessive sweating. The physician orders urine and blood tests to measure levels of epinephrine and norepinephrine to rule out an adrenal tumor, a condition known as _____.

Competency Verification: Check your answers in Appendix B: Answer Key, page 612. If you are not satisfied with your level of comprehension, review the material in this chapter, and retake the review.

Correct Answers: _____ × 10 = _____ % Score

ENDOCRINE AND NERVOUS SYSTEMS CHAPTER REVIEW

WORD ELEMENTS SUMMARY

The following table summarizes CFs, suffixes, and prefixes related to the endocrine and nervous systems. Study the word elements and their meanings before completing the Vocabulary Review that follows.

Word Element	Meaning	Word Element	Meaning
Combining Forms			
Endocrine System			
aden/o	gland	pituitar/o	pituitary gland
adren/o, adrenal/o	adrenal glands	thym/o	thymus gland
pancreat/o	pancreas	thyroid/o	thyroid gland
parathyroid/o	parathyroid glands		
Nervous System			
cephal/o	head	mening/o, meningi/o	meninges (membranes covering the brain and spinal cord)
cerebr/o	cerebrum	myel/o	bone marrow; spinal cord
encephal/o	brain	neur/o	nerve
gli/o	glue; neuroglial tissue	spin/o	spine
Other			
cyst/o	bladder orch/o	orchid/o, orchi/o,	testis (plural, *testes*)
enter/o	intestine (usually small intestine)	scler/o	hardening; sclera (white of the eye)
gluc/o, glyc/o	sugar, sweetness	thromb/o	blood clot
hem/o	blood	toxic/o	poison
nephr/o, ren/o	kidney	vascul/o	blood vessel
Suffixes			
-algia, -dynia	pain	-oid	resembling
-dipsia	thirst	-osis	abnormal condition; increase (used primarily with blood cells)
-emia	blood condition	-pathy	disease
-gen, -genesis	forming, producing; origin	-penia	decrease, deficiency
-glia	glue; neuroglial tissue	-phagia	swallowing, eating
-iasis	abnormal condition (produced by something specified)	-phasia	speech
-ism	condition	-plegia	paralysis
-lith	stone, calculus	-rrhagia	bursting forth (of)

Continued

Word Element	Meaning	Word Element	Meaning
-logist	specialist in the study of	-rrhea	discharge, flow
-logy	study of	-tome	instrument to cut
-malacia	softening	-tomy	incision
-megaly	enlargement	-uria	urine
Prefixes			
a-	without, not	hyper-	excessive, above normal
dys-	bad; painful; difficult	hypo-	under, below, deficient
endo-	within	para-	near, beside; beyond

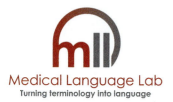

Medical Language Lab
Turning terminology into language

Visit the *Medical Language Lab* at *medicallanguagelab.com.* Use the flash-card–word elements exercise to reinforce your study of word elements. We recommend you complete the flash-card activity before starting the following Vocabulary.

Vocabulary Review

Match the following medical term(s) with the definitions in the numbered list.

acromegaly	deglutition	hyperglycemia	neurohypophysis	polydipsia
adenohypophysis	diabetes mellitus	insulin	neuromalacia	polyphagia
adrenalectomy	glycogenesis	jaundice	pancreatolith	pruritus
adrenaline	hormone	meningocele	pancreatolysis	thyrotoxicosis
cerebral palsy	hypercalcemia	metastasis	pancreatopathy	vertigo

1. _____ is an enlargement of the extremities.

2. _____ is the destruction of the pancreatic tissue caused by a pathological condition.

3. _____ is the anterior lobe of the pituitary gland, composed of glandular tissue.

4. _____ refers to partial paralysis and lack of muscular coordination caused by damage to the cerebrum before or during the birth process.

5. _____ refers to excessive amounts of calcium in blood.

6. _____ is a pancreatic hormone that decreases the blood glucose level.

7. _____ is the posterior lobe of the pituitary, composed primarily of nerve tissue.

8. _____ is a disease of the pancreas.

9. _____ refers to excessive consumption of food.

10. _____ is a chronic metabolic disorder marked by hyperglycemia.

11. _____ is an increase of blood glucose, as in diabetes.

12. _____ is a calculus or stone in the pancreas.

13. _____ refers to excessive thirst.

14. _____ is a toxic condition resulting from hyperactivity of the thyroid gland.

15. _____ is the excision of an adrenal gland.

16. _____ is a hormone secreted by the adrenal medulla that causes some of the physiological expressions of fear and anxiety and is also called *epinephrine*.

17. _____ is the production or formation of sugar.

18. _____ refers to protrusion of the membranes of the brain or spinal cord through a defect in the skull or spinal column.

19. _____ is the softening of nerve tissue.

20. _____ refers to severe itching.

21. _____ refers to the act of swallowing.

22. _____ is an illusion of movement.

23. _____ is a yellowish discoloration of skin and eyes.

24. _____ refers to the spread of a malignant tumor beyond its primary site to a secondary organ or location.

25. _____ is a chemical substance produced by specialized cells of the body and released slowly into the bloodstream.

Competency Verification: Check your answers in Appendix B: Answer Key, page 612. If you are not satisfied with your level of comprehension, review the chapter vocabulary, and retake the review.

Correct Answers: _____ × 5 = _____ % Score

Musculoskeletal System

OBJECTIVES

Upon completion of this chapter, you will be able to:

• Describe the type of medical treatments that orthopedists, rheumatologists, and chiropractors provide.

• Identify skeletal structures by labeling them on anatomical illustrations.

• Describe the primary functions of the musculoskeletal system.

• Describe diseases, conditions, and procedures related to the musculoskeletal system.

• Apply your word-building skills by constructing medical terms related to the musculoskeletal system.

• Describe common abbreviations and symbols related to the musculoskeletal system.

• Recognize, define, pronounce, and spell terms correctly.

• Demonstrate your knowledge of this chapter by successfully completing the frames, reviews, and activities.

MEDICAL SPECIALTIES: ORTHOPEDICS, RHEUMATOLOGY, AND CHIROPRACTIC MEDICINE

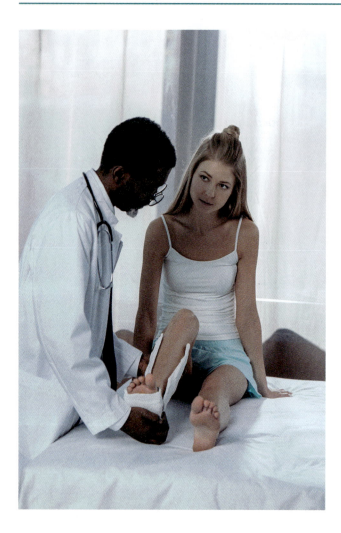

Orthopedics and Rheumatology

Orthopedics is the branch of medicine concerned with prevention, diagnosis, care, and treatment of musculoskeletal disorders. These disorders include injuries to or diseases of the body's bones, joints, ligaments, muscles, and tendons. **Orthopedists** are surgeons who specialize in orthopedics. They employ medical, physical, and surgical methods to restore function that is lost as a result of injury or disease to the musculoskeletal system. Orthopedists coordinate their treatments with other health-care providers, such as physical therapists, occupational therapists, and sports medicine physicians. In addition to the orthopedist, who treats bone and joint diseases, the **rheumatologist** is a board-certified internist who has undergone additional training in diseases and conditions affecting the bones, joints, and muscles. These diseases include treatment of various types of arthritis, such as osteoarthritis and rheumatoid arthritis.

Chiropractic Medicine

Another health-care provider who treats musculoskeletal disorders is the **chiropractor.** Unlike medical doctors, chiropractors are not physicians. They do not employ drugs or surgery, the primary basis of treatment used by medical physicians. Chiropractic medicine is a form of alternative medicine, in which the chiropractor diagnoses and treats many different spinal disorders that cause musculoskeletal or nerve pain. Similar to other types of doctors, the chiropractor performs a physical and neurological examination as part of the process of providing an accurate diagnosis. Radiographic or computed tomographic studies may also be ordered to confirm a diagnosis and to determine the most effective type of treatment.

Anatomy and Physiology Overview

The musculoskeletal system includes muscles, bones, joints, and related structures, such as tendons and connective tissue, which function in the movement of body parts and organs.

Muscles have four key functions: producing body movements, stabilizing body positions, storing and moving substances within the body, and generating heat. Through contraction, muscles cause motion and help maintain body posture. Less apparent motions that muscles are responsible for include the passage and elimination of food through the digestive system, propulsion of blood through the arteries, and contraction of the bladder to eliminate urine. Muscles are named for their location in the body, the type of movement they cause, or their size or shape. In addition, some muscles are named for the number of components that make up the muscle. Examples of component muscles are triceps, which are muscles with *three heads;* biceps, which are muscles with *two heads;* and deltoids, which are muscles that resemble a triangle. To illustrate these conventions, examine the muscles in Figure 10-1.

The main function of bones is to form a skeleton to support and protect the body and serve as storage areas for mineral salts, especially calcium and phosphorus. Joints, also called **articulations,** are the places where two bones connect. Joints vary widely in the degree of movement they afford. Some joints, such as suture joints between the skull bones, are constructed in such a way that no movement is possible. Most joints, however, allow a wide range of motion, for example, finger, elbow, and knee joints. Because bones cannot move without the help of muscles, muscle tissue must provide contraction.

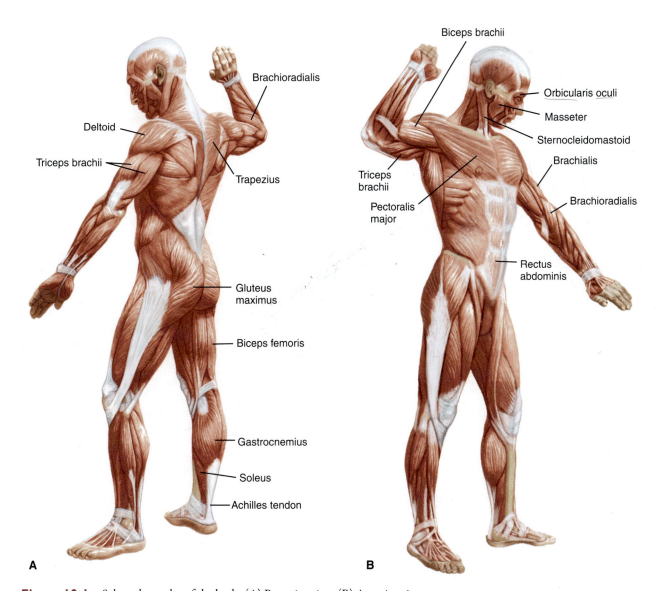

Figure 10-1   Selected muscles of the body. (A) Posterior view. (B) Anterior view.

WORD ELEMENTS

This section introduces word elements related to the muscles of the body. Review the word elements and their meanings in the following table. Then, pronounce each term in the word analysis column and place a ✓ in the box after you do so.

Word Element	Meaning	Word Analysis
Combining Forms		
fasci/o	band, fascia (fibrous membrane supporting and separating muscles)	**fasci/o**/plasty (FĂSH-ē-ō-plăs-tē ☐): surgical repair of fascia *-plasty:* surgical repair
fibr/o	fiber, fibrous tissue	**fibr**/oma (fĭ-BRŌ-mă ☐): tumor of fibrous tissue *-oma:* tumor
leiomy/o	smooth muscle (visceral)	**leiomy**/oma (lī-ō-mī-Ō-mă ☐): tumor of smooth muscle *-oma:* tumor

lumb/o	loins (lower back)	**lumb/o**/cost/al (lŭm-bō-KŎS-tăl ☐): pertaining to the loins (lower back)
		  cost: ribs
		   -al: pertaining to

muscul/o	muscle	**muscul**/ar (MŬS-kū-lăr ☐): pertaining to muscles *-ar:* pertaining to
my/o		**my/o**/rrhexis (mī-or-ĔK-sĭs ☐): rupture of a muscle *-rrhexis:* rupture
ten/o	tendon	**ten/o**/tomy (tĕn-ŎT-ō-mē ☐): incision of a tendon *-tomy:* incision *Tenotomy is performed to correct muscle imbalance, as in the correction of strabismus of the eye or clubfoot.*
tend/o		**tend/o**/plasty (TĔN-dō-plăs-tē ☐): surgical repair of a tendon *-plasty:* surgical repair
tendin/o		**tendin**/itis (tĕn-dĭn-Ī-tĭs ☐): inflammation of a tendon, usually resulting from strain; also called tendonitis *-itis:* inflammation *Tendinitis usually results from an injury or strain; also called* tendonitis.
Suffixes		
-algia	pain	**my**/**algia** (mī-ĂL-jē-ă ☐): pain or tenderness in muscles *my:* muscle
-dynia		lumb/o/**dynia** (LŬM-bō-dĭn-ē-ă ☐): pain in the lumbar region of the back *lumb/o:* loins (lower back)
-asthenia	weakness, debility	my/**asthenia** (mī-ăs-THĒ-nē-ă ☐): weakness of muscle (and abnormal fatigue) *my:* muscle
-pathy	disease	my/o/**pathy** (mī-ŎP-ă-thē ☐): disease of muscle tissue *my/o:* muscle *Myopathy is a disease that commonly indicates a skeletal muscle disorder.*
-plegia	paralysis	hemi/**plegia** (hĕm-ē-PLĒ-jē-ă ☐): paralysis of one side of the body *hemi-:* one half *Types of hemiplegia include cerebral hemiplegia and facial hemiplegia.*

Word Element	Meaning	Word Analysis
-rrhaphy	suture	my/o/**rrhaphy** (mī-OR-ă-fē ☐): suture of muscle, usually in the treatment of a muscle wound *my/o:* muscle
-sarcoma	malignant tumor of connective tissue	my/o/**sarcoma** (mī-ō-sar-KŌ-mă ☐): malignant tumor of muscle tissue *my/o:* muscle
Pronunciation Help	*Long Sound* *Short Sound*	ā in rāte ē in rēbirth ī in īsle ō in ōver ū in ūnite ă in ăpple ĕ in ĕver ĭ in ĭt ŏ in nŏt ŭ in cŭt

 Visit the *Medical Terminology Simplified* online resource center at FADavis.com for an audio exercise of the terms in this table. It will help you master pronunciations and meanings of medical terms.

SECTION REVIEW 10-1

For the following medical terms, first, write the suffix and its meaning. Then, translate the meaning of the remaining elements starting with the first part of the word. The first word is completed for you.

Term	Meaning
1. chondr/itis	–itis: inflammation; cartilage
2. my/o/rrhaphy	Suture of the muscle
3. hemi/plegia	Paralysis of the side of the body
4. ten/o/tomy	Incision of tendon
5. leiomy/oma	tumor of smooth muscle
6. tend/o/lysis	
7. my/o/pathy	
8. lumb/o/cost/al	
9. tendin/it is	
10. my/algia	

Competency Verification: Check your answers in Appendix B: Answer Key, page 613. If you are not satisfied with your level of comprehension, review the vocabulary, and retake the review.

Correct Answers _____ x 10 = _____ % Score

Muscles

There are three types of muscular fibers or tissue:

- **Skeletal muscle fibers** are composed of striations that move bones of the skeleton and work mainly in a voluntary manner. Muscle fibers contract in response to stimulation and then relax when the stimulation ends. Their activity can be consciously controlled by neurons that are part of the somatic (voluntary) division of the nervous system. To some extent, skeletal muscles are also controlled subconsciously. For example, the diaphragm continues to alternately contract and relax without conscious control so that breathing does not stop.
- **Cardiac muscle fibers,** also composed of striations, are found only in the heart and form most of the heart wall. The alternating contraction and relaxation of the heart is involuntary and is not consciously controlled. Rather, the heart beats because it has a pacemaker that initiates each contraction. This built-in rhythm is called **autorhythmicity.** Several hormones and neurotransmitters can adjust heart rate by speeding or slowing the pacemaker.
- **Smooth muscle fibers** are shorter and lack the striations of skeletal and cardiac muscle tissue. For this reason, the tissue has a smooth appearance, which gives the tissue its name. The action of smooth muscle is usually involuntary, and some smooth muscle tissues, such as the muscles that propel food through the gastrointestinal tract, have autorhythmicity. Smooth muscle and cardiac muscle are regulated by neurons that are part of the autonomic (involuntary) division of the nervous system and hormones released by endocrine glands.

Pink indicates a prefix. Blue indicates a suffix. Boldface indicates a word root or combining form.

muscle(s)	**10-1** Fibers within each muscle are characteristically arranged into specific patterns that provide specific functional capabilities. Most skeletal muscles lie between the skin and the skeleton. My/o/genesis is the embryonic formation of _____.
my/o/plasty MĪ-ō-plăs-tē **my/o/rrhaphy** mī-OR-ă-fē	**10-2** Practice building medical words that mean *surgical repair of muscle:* _____ / _____ / _____. *suture of muscle:* _____ / _____ / _____.
my/o/rrhexis mī-or-ĔK-sĭs	**10-3** Sports-related injuries are commonly caused by the tremendous stress exerted on certain parts of musculoskeletal structures. In many instances, these types of athletic injuries may result in a torn muscle. Form a word that means *rupture (tear) of a muscle.* _____ / _____ / _____
my/algia mī-ĂL-jē-ă	**10-4** My/o/dynia refers to muscle pain. Form another word that means *muscle pain.* _____ / _____
my/o/pathy mī-ŎP-ă-thē	**10-5** Form a medical term that means disease of *muscle.* _____ / _____ / _____
hardening, sclera	**10-6** The CF *scler/o* refers to _____; _____ (white of the eye).
scler/osis sklĕ-RŌ-sĭs **my/o/scler/osis** mī-ō-sklĕr-Ō-sĭs	**10-7** An abnormal condition of hardening is called ___Scler___ / _osis_ . An abnormal condition of muscle hardening is called _my_ / _o_ / _sclerxis_ / _____ .
triceps brachii TRĪ-cĕps brā-kē **biceps femoris** BĪ-sĕps FĔM-or-ĭs **biceps brachii** BĪ-sĕps BRĀ-kē	**10-8** To become familiar with the names of the major muscles of the body, study Figure 10-1, and name the muscles that mean *three heads:* _____ / _____. *two heads:* _____ _____ and _____ _____.
pectoralis major pĕk-tō-RĂ-lĭs	**10-9** The CF **pector/o** means *chest.* Identify the muscles that refer to the chest in Figure 10-1. _____ _____

deltoid dĕlt-oyd	**10-10** Recall the suffix that means *resembling*. Identify the uppermost part of the arm muscle that means resembling a triangle. _____
tendon	**10-11** The CF **tend/o** means *tendon,* which is fibrous connective tissue that attaches muscles to bone. Tend/o/plasty is a surgical repair of a _____.
tend/o/tome TĔN-dō-tōm **tend/o/tomy** tĕn-DŎT-ō-mē **tend/o/plasty** TĔN-dō-plăs-tē	**10-12** Use **tend/o** to form words that mean *instrument to cut a tendon:* _____ / _____ / _____. *incision of a tendon:* _____ / _____ / _____. *surgical repair of a tendon:* _____ / _____ / _____.
inferior ✓	**10-13** The Achilles tendon is attached to a muscle in the lower leg. Locate the Achilles tendon in Figure 10-1A. It is located (superior, inferior) _____ to the gastrocnemius muscle.
paralysis pă-RĂL-ĭ-sĭs	**10-14** The prefix *quadri-* refers to four. Quadri/plegia is a _____ of all four extremities.
paralysis pă-RĂL-ĭ-sĭs	**10-15** The prefix *hemi-* means one half. Hemi/plegia is a _____ of half the body.
	10-16 With the exception of rotations of the body, other types of body movements occur in pairs, as summarized in Figure 10-2.

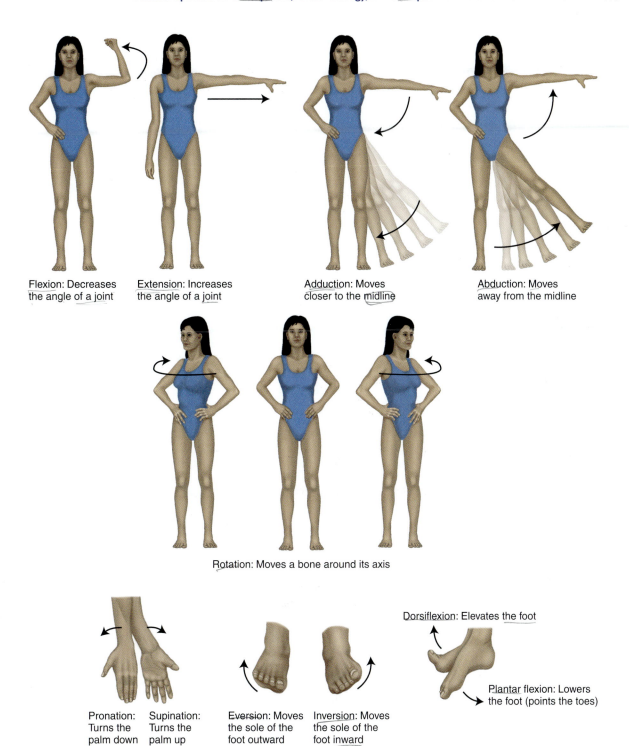

Flexion: Decreases the angle of a joint

Extension: Increases the angle of a joint

Adduction: Moves closer to the midline

Abduction: Moves away from the midline

Rotation: Moves a bone around its axis

Pronation: Turns the palm down

Supination: Turns the palm up

Eversion: Moves the sole of the foot outward

Inversion: Moves the sole of the foot inward

Dorsiflexion: Elevates the foot

Plantar flexion: Lowers the foot (points the toes)

Figure 10-2 Body movements generated by muscles.

SECTION REVIEW 10-2

Using the following table, write the combining form, suffix, or prefix that matches its definition in the space provided to the left of the definition. There may be more than one word element that matches a definition.

Combining Forms		Suffixes		Prefixes
chondr/o	tendin/o	-cyte	-rrhaphy	hemi-
cyst/o	tend/o	-genesis	-rrhexis	quadri-
enter/o	ten/o	-lysis	-sarcoma	
hepat/o		-osis	-tome	
my/o		-plasty	-tomy	
scler/o		-plegia		

1. _____ abnormal condition; increase (used primarily with blood cells)

2. _____ bladder

3. ___Cyte___ cell

4. ___quadri___ four

5. ___hemi___ one half

6. ___scler/o___ hardening; sclera (white of eye)

7. ___tomy___ incision

8. _____ intestine (usually small intestine)

9. ___hepatic___ liver

10. ___my/o___ muscle

11. ___plegia___ paralysis

12. ___-genesis___ forming, producing; origin

13. ___-rrhexis___ rupture

14. ___plasty___ surgical repair

15. ___-rrhaphy___ suture

16. ___ten/o / tend/o___ tendon

17. ___-tome___ instrument to cut

18. ___Chondr/o___ cartilage

19. ___sarcoma___ malignant tumor of connective tissue

20. ___-lysis___ separation; destruction; loosening

Competency Verification: Check your answers in Appendix B: Answer Key, page 613. If you are not satisfied with your level of comprehension, go back to Frame 10–1, and rework the frames.

Correct Answers _____ x 5 = _____ % Score

Skeletal System

The skeleton of a human adult consists of 206 individual bones, but this chapter covers only the major bones. For anatomical purposes, the human skeleton is divided into the axial skeleton (distinguished by bone color in Figure 10-3) and the appendicular skeleton (distinguished by blue color in Figure 10-3). The axial skeleton protects internal organs and provides central support around which other parts of the body move. It consists of the bones of the head, chest, and spine. The appendicular skeleton enables the body to move. It consists of the bones of the shoulders, arms, hips, and legs. The ability to walk, run, or catch a ball is possible because of the movable joints of the limbs.

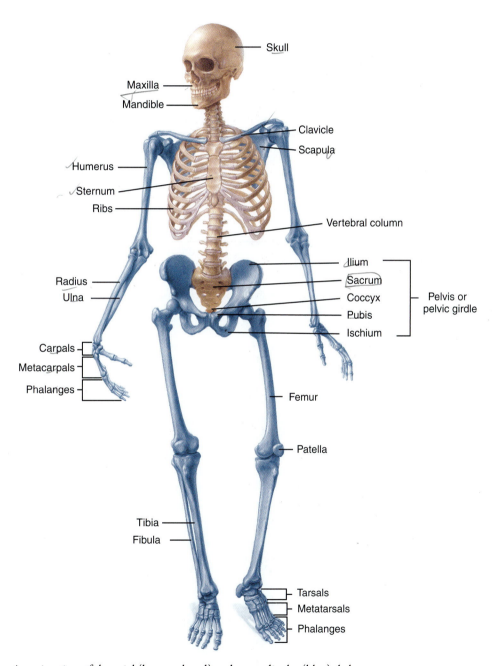

Figure 10-3   Anterior view of the axial (bone-colored) and appendicular (blue) skeleton.

WORD ELEMENTS

This section introduces word elements related to specific bones of the upper extremities. Review the word elements and their meanings in the following table. Then pronounce each term in the word analysis column and place a ✓ after you do so.

Word Element	Meaning	Word Analysis
Combining Forms		
Specific Bones of the Upper Extremities		
carp/o	carpus (wrist bones)	**carp/o/ptosis** (kăr-pŏp-TŌ-sĭs ☐): downward displacement of the wrist; also called *dropped wrist* *-ptosis:* prolapse, downward displacement
cervic/o	neck; cervix uteri (neck of the uterus)	**cervic/al** (SĔR-vĭ-kăl ☐): pertaining to the neck *-al:* pertaining to *The term cervical is also used to denote the region of the neck or a constricted area of a necklike structure, such as the neck of a tooth or the cervix uteri.*

cost/o	ribs	**sub/cost/al** (sŭb-KŎS-tăl ☐): beneath the ribs
		  sub-: under, below
		   -al: pertaining to

crani/o	cranium (skull)	**crani/o/tomy** (krā-nē-ŎT-ō-mē ☐): incision through the cranium, usually to gain access to the brain during neurosurgical procedures *-tomy:* incision *Craniotomy is performed to relieve intracranial pressure, control bleeding, or remove a tumor.*
humer/o	humerus (upper arm bone)	**humer/al** (HŪ-mĕr-ăl ☐): pertaining to the humerus *-al:* pertaining to
metacarp/o	metacarpus (hand bones)	**metacarp/ectomy** (mĕt-ă-kăr-PĔK-tō-mē ☐): excision of one or more metacarpal bones *-ectomy:* excision, removal
phalang/o	phalanges (bones of the fingers and toes)	**phalang/itis** (făl-ăn-JĪ-tĭs ☐): inflammation of one or more phalanges *-itis:* inflammation
spondyl/o*	vertebra (backbone)	**spondyl/itis** (spŏn-dĭl-Ī-tĭs ☐): inflammation of any of the vertebrae (plural), usually characterized by stiffness and pain *-itis:* inflammation *Ankylosing spondylitis is a form of arthritis that may eventually cause the spine to fuse in a fixed, immobile position. Spondylitis may result from a traumatic injury to the spine, infection, or rheumatoid disease.*
vertebr/o*		**vertebr/al** (VĔR-tĕ-brăl): pertaining to a vertebra or the vertebral column *-al:* pertaining to

stern/o	sternum (breastbone)	**stern/o/cost/al** (stĕr-nō-KŎS-tăl ☐): pertaining to the sternum and ribs
		  cost: ribs
		  -al: pertaining to

Specific Bones of the Lower Extremities		
calcane/o	calcaneum (heel bone)	**calcane/o/dynia** (kăl-kăn-ē-ō-DĬN-ē-ă ☐): painful condition of the heel *-dynia:* pain
femor/o	femur (thigh bone)	**femor/al** (FĔM-or-ăl ☐): pertaining to the femur *-al:* pertaining to

3.50 · AAAAA

Word Element	Meaning	Word Analysis
fibul/o	fibula (smaller, outer bone of the lower leg)	**fibul**/ar (FĬB-ū-lăr ☐): pertaining to the fibula -*ar:* pertaining to
patell/o	patella (kneecap)	**patell**/ectomy (păt-ĕ-LĔK-tō-mē ☐): excision of the patella -*ectomy:* excision, removal
pelv/i†	pelvis	**pelv/i**/metry (pĕl-VĬM-ĕ-trē ☐): measurement of the pelvic dimensions or proportions -*metry:* act of measuring *Pelvimetry helps determine whether or not it will be possible to deliver a fetus through the normal route.*
pelv/o		**pelv**/is (PĔL-vĭs ☐): pertaining to the pelvis -*is:* noun ending *A woman's pelvis is usually less massive but wider and more circular than a man's pelvis.*
radi/o	radiation, x-ray; radius (lower arm bone on the thumb side)	**radi/o**/graph (RĀ-dē-ō-grăf ☐): x-ray image -*graph:* instrument for recording
tibi/o	tibia (larger bone of the lower leg)	**tibi**/al (TĬB-ē-ăl ☐): pertaining to the tibia (shin bone) -*al:* pertaining to
Other Related Structures		
ankyl/o	stiffness; bent, crooked	**ankyl**/osis (ăng-kĭ-LŌ-sĭs ☐): immobility of a joint -*osis:* abnormal condition; increase (used primarily with blood cells) *Ankylosis may be congenital or it may be caused by disease, trauma, surgery, or contractures resulting from immobility.*
arthr/o	joint	**arthr**/itis (ăr-THRĪ-tĭs ☐): inflammation of a joint -*itis:* inflammation *Arthritis is commonly accompanied by pain, swelling, stiffness, and deformity.*
chondr/o	cartilage	**cost/o/chondr**/itis (kŏs-tō-kŏn-DRĪ-tĭs ☐): inflammation of cartilage of the anterior chest wall (ribs) *cost/o:* ribs -*itis:* inflammation *Costochondritis is characterized by pain and tenderness that may radiate from the initial site of inflammation.*
lamin/o	lamina (part of the vertebral arch)	**lamin**/ectomy (lăm-ĭ-NĔK-tō-mē ☐): excision of the lamina (bony arches of one or more vertebrae) -*ectomy:* excision, removal
myel/o	bone marrow; spinal cord	**myel/o**/cele (MĪ-ĕ-lō-sēl ☐): herniation of the spinal cord -*cele:* hernia, swelling *Swelling of the spinal cord* *Myelocele is a saclike protrusion of the spinal cord through a congenital defect in the vertebral column.*
orth/o	straight	**orth/o**/ped/ics (or-thō-PĒ-dĭks ☐): branch of medicine concerned with the prevention and correction of musculoskeletal system disorders *ped:* foot; child -*ics:* pertaining to
oste/o	bone	**oste**/itis (ŏs-tē-Ī-tĭs ☐): inflammation of bone -*itis:* inflammation

-itis — inflammation g

Continued

Word Element	Meaning	Word Analysis
Suffixes		
-clast	to break; surgical fracture	oste/o/**clast** (ŎS-tē-ō-klăst ☐): (mononucleated cell that) breaks down bone *oste/o:* bone *An osteoclast destroys the matrix of bone. The term osteoclast also refers to an instrument used to surgically fracture a bone (osteoclasis).*
-cyte	cell	oste/o/**cyte** (ŎS-tē-ō-sīt ☐): bone cell *oste/o:* bone
-desis	binding, fixation (of a bone or joint)	arthr/o/**desis** (ăr-thrō-DĒ-sĭs ☐): surgical immobilization of a joint *arthr/o:* joint
-malacia	softening	oste/o/**malacia** (ŏs-tē-ō-mă-LĀ-shē-ă ☐): softening and bending of bones *oste/o:* bone *Osteomalacia is caused by vitamin D deficiency that results in shortage or loss of calcium salts, causing bones to become increasingly soft, flexible, brittle, and deformed.*
-physis	growth	dia/**physis** (dī-ĂF-ĭ-sĭs ☐): shaft or middle region of a long bone *dia-:* through, across
-porosis	porous	oste/o/**porosis** (ŏs-tē-ō-por-Ō-sĭs ☐): porous bones *oste/o:* bone *Osteoporosis is characterized by decrease in bone density and increase in porosity, causing bones to become brittle and increasing the risk of fractures.*

| **Pronunciation Help** | *Long Sound*
Short Sound | ā in rāte
ă in ăpple | ē in rēbirth
ĕ in ĕver | ī in īsle
ĭ in ĭt | ō in ōver
ŏ in nŏt | ū in ūnite
ŭ in cŭt |

*The CF spondyl/o is used to form words about the condition of a structure. The CF vertebr/o is used to form words that describe a structure.

†Using the combining vowel *i* instead of *o* is an exception to the rule.

Visit the *Medical Terminology Simplified* online resource center at FADavis.com for an audio exercise of the terms in this table. It will help you master pronunciations and meanings of medical terms.

Pink indicates a prefix. Blue indicates a suffix. Boldface indicates a word root or combining form.

SECTION REVIEW 10-3

For the following medical terms, first, write the suffix and its meaning. Then, translate the meaning of the remaining elements starting with the first part of the word. The first word is completed for you.

Term | **Meaning**

1. dia/physis — -physis: growth; through, across

2. sub/cost/al — beneath the ribs

3. oste/o/malacia — softening of bone

4. lamin/ectomy — Removal of lamina

5. pelv/i/metry — measurement of pelvic

6. myel/o/cele

7. oste/o/porosis

8. ankyl/osis

9. carp/o/ptosis

10. crani/o/tomy

Competency Verification: Check your answers in Appendix B: Answer Key, page 613. If you are not satisfied with your level of comprehension, review the vocabulary, and retake the review.

Correct Answers _____ x 10 = _____ % Score

Structure and Function of Bones

oste/o

10-17 To understand the skeletal system, it is important to know the types and names of major bones, their functions, and where they are located. Regardless of the size or shape of a bone, the CF used to designate bone is _____/_____.

10-18 There are four basic types of bones: long, short, flat, and irregular. Long bones are longer than they are wide and are slightly curved for strength. Long bones vary tremendously in size and include those in the thigh (femur), leg (tibia and fibula), arm (humerus), and fingers and toes (phalanges). Short bones are somewhat cube shaped and are nearly equal in length and width. Examples of short bones are the carpal (wrist) bones and the tarsal (ankle) bones. Flat bones are broad and thin. They cover and protect soft body parts; examples are the cranial bones, which protect the brain, and the sternum and ribs, which protect organs in the thorax. Irregular bones, such as the bones of the vertebrae and certain bones of the ears and face, have varied shapes and sizes and are commonly clustered.

Refer to Figure 10-3 to review the different types of bones.

short bones

flat bones

irregular bones

long bones

10–19 Identify the four types of bones described in Frame 10–18.

Cube-shaped bones of the wrists and ankles are the

_____ _____.

Broad bones in the shoulders and ribs are the

_____ _____.

Certain bones of the ears and the bones of the vertebrae are the

_____ _____.

Type of bones that are longer than they are wide and slightly curved are known as

_____ _____.

10–20 Most long bones are located in the extremities of the body. (See Figure 10–4.) The main elongated portion of such a bone, the (1) **diaphysis,** is composed of several tissue layers: the thin fibrous outer membrane, the (2) **periosteum,** the thick layer of hard (3) **compact bone,** and the inner (4) **medullary cavity.** Label the parts of the long bone in Figure 10-4.

10–21 The two ends of bones, the (5) **distal epiphysis** and (6) **proximal epiphysis,** have a bulbous shape to provide space for muscle and ligament attachments near the joints. Label these structures in Figure 10-4.

10–22 There are two kinds of bone tissue based on porosity, and most bones have both types. Compact (dense) bone tissue is the hard, outer layer; (7) **spongy (cancellous) bone** tissue is the porous, highly vascular inner portion. Compact bone tissue is covered by the periosteum, which serves as a place of attachment for muscles, provides protection, and gives durable strength to the bone. The spongy bone tissue makes the bone lighter and provides a space for bone marrow, where blood cells are produced. Label the spongy bone in Figure 10-4, and note the position and structure of compact and spongy bone.

10–23 In Figure 10-4, observe how the diaphysis forms a cylinder that surrounds the medullary cavity. In adults, the medullary cavity is filled with yellow bone marrow, so named because of the large amounts of fatty tissue it contains.

oste/o/blasts
ŎS-tē-ō-blăstz

peri/oste/um
pĕr-ē-ŎS-tē-ŭm

10–24 The peri/oste/um, as illustrated in Figure 10-4, covers the entire surface of the bone. Its blood vessels supply nutrients, and its nerves signal pain. In growing bones, the inner layer contains bone-forming cells known as oste/o/blasts. Because blood vessels and oste/o/blasts are located in the peri/oste/um, this site provides a means for bone repair and general bone nutrition. The peri/oste/um also provides a point of attachment for muscles.

Identify terms in this frame that mean

embryonic cell (that develops into) bone:

_____ / _____ / _____.

structure around bone: _____ / _____ / _____.

Pink indicates a prefix. Blue indicates a suffix. Boldface indicates a word root or combining form.

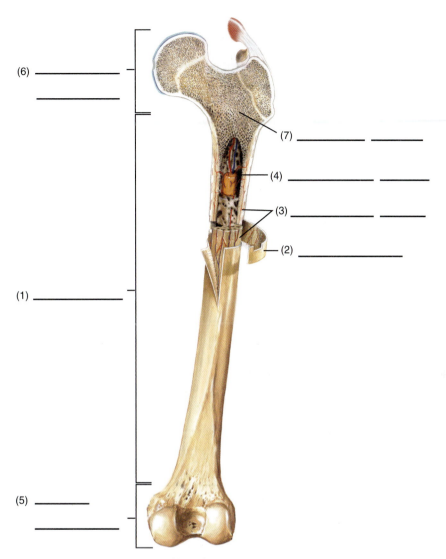

(6) _____

_____

(7) _____ _____

(4) _____ _____

(3) _____ _____

(2) _____

(1) _____

(5) _____

_____

Figure 10-4   Longitudinal section of a long bone (femur) and interior bone structure.

-genesis

oste/o

oste/o/cytes
ŎS-tē-ō-sītz

10–25 Oste/o/genesis is the formation or development of bones.

Identify elements in this frame that mean

forming, producing, origin: _____.

bone: _____/_____.

When talking about bone cells, the medical term to use is

_____/_____/_____.

leuk/o/poiesis
loo-kō-poy-Ē-sĭs

erythr/o/poiesis
ĕ-rĭth-rō-poy-Ē-sĭs

10–26   In an adult, production of red blood cells (erythr/o/poiesis) occurs in red bone marrow. Red bone marrow is also responsible for the formation of white blood cells (leuk/o/poiesis) and platelets.

Identify terms in this frame that mean

formation or production of white blood cells:

_____/_____/_____.

formation or production of red blood cells:

_____/_____/_____.

Competency Verification: Check your labeling of Figure 10-4 in Appendix B: Answer Key, page 614.

oste/o/cytes
ŎS-tē-ō-sīts

10–27   Bone is living tissue composed of oste/o/cytes, blood vessels, and nerves. Determine the medical term for bone cells.

_____/_____/_____

oste/itis
ŏs-tē-Ī-tĭs

oste/o/pathy
ŏs-tē-ŎP-ă-thē

oste/o/tomy
ŏs-tē-ŎT-ō-mē

oste/o/rrhaphy
ŏs-tē-OR-ă-fē

oste/o/scler/osis
ŏs-tē-ō-sklĕ-RŌ-sĭs

10–28   Practice developing medical words that mean

inflammation of bone: _____/_____.

disease of bone: _____/_____/_____.

incision of bone: ___ _____/_____/_____.

suture of bone (wiring of bone fragments):

_____/_____/_____.

abnormal condition of bone hardening:

_____/_____/_____/_____.

dist/o

10–29   Dist/al is a directional word that means pertaining to *(a structure) farthest from the point of attachment to the trunk, or far from the beginning of a structure.*

From dist/al, build the CF that means far or farthest.

_____/_____

proxim/o

10–30   Proxim/al is a directional word that means pertaining to *(a structure) near the point of attachment to the trunk, or near the beginning of a structure.*

From *proxim/al,* build the CF that means *near or nearest.*

_____/_____

Pink indicates a prefix. Blue indicates a suffix. Boldface indicates a word root or combining form.

oste/o/malacia ŏs-tē-ō-mă-LĀ-shē-ă **oste/o/genesis** ŏs-tē-ō-JĔN-ĕ-sĭs	**10–31** Milk is a good source of calcium and vitamin D. Deficiency of calcium and vitamin D results in softening and weakening of the skeleton, causing pain and bowing of the bones. Construct medical terms that mean *softening of bones:* _____/_____/_____. *producing or forming bone:* _____/_____/_____.
oste/o/malacia ŏs-tē-ō-mă-LĀ-shē-ă	**10–32** A form of oste/o/malacia known as *rickets* is seen in infants and children in many underdeveloped countries. It is a result of vitamin D deficiency. Symptoms of rickets include soft, pliable bones that cause deformities, such as bowlegs and knock-knees. Rickets is another name for _____/_____/_____.
rickets RĬK-ĕts	**10–33** Calcium provides bone strength needed for its supportive functions. Rickets occurs in many children in underdeveloped countries because of inadequate availability of milk. When oste/o/malacia occurs in children, it is called ___*Rickets*___.
bone(s)	**10–34** Oste/o/porosis is a condition in which there is a decrease in bone density (mass) that results in a thinning and weakening of bone(s). (See Figure 10-5.) To prevent osteoporosis, it is important to maintain a balanced diet rich in calcium and vitamin D. When you see the term oste/o/porosis in a medical report, you will know it refers to porous _____.
oste/o/porosis ŏs-tē-ō-por-ō-sis	**10–35** Oste/o/porosis commonly occurs in older women as a consequence of estrogen deficiency with menopause. Prevention and treatment of oste/o/porosis is crucial in preserving strong bones and avoiding fractures such as those of the hip and spine. (See Figure 10-5.) Loss of bone mass that occurs throughout the skeleton, predisposing patients to fractures is a condition known as _____/_/_____.

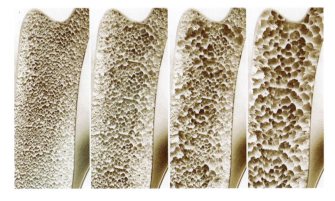

Figure 10-5 Stages of osteoporosis. Healthy bone at far left begins to lose density as shown by porous areas of the bone becoming greater.

calc/emia kăl-SĒ-mē-ă	**10–36** Combine *calc/o* and *-emia* to form a word that means *calcium in blood*. _____/_____
hyper/calc/emia hī-pĕr-kăl-SĒ-mē-ă	**10–37** Hypo/calc/emia is a deficiency of calcium in blood. The term that means *excessive amount of calcium in blood* is _____/_____/_____.
radi/o/logist rā-dē-ŎL-ō-jĭst	**10–38** Radi/o/logy, initially widely called *roentgen/o/logy,* was developed after discovery of an unknown ray in 1895 by Wilhelm Roentgen, who called his discovery a *roentgen* (x-ray). Occasionally you still may see words with **roentgen/o,** but **radi/o** is the preferred element used in the context of medical imaging today. Radi/o/logy is the branch of medicine concerned with the use of radioactive substances to diagnose path/o/log/ical conditions of the skeletal system. A physician who specializes in the study and interpretation of x-ray images is called a _____/_____/_____.
radi/o/therapy rā-dē-ō-THĔR-ă-pē	**10–39** Radiation is used for diagnostic and therapeutic purposes. Radiation therapy, also called *radi/o/therapy,* is treatment of diseases by using an external source of high-energy rays or internally implanted radioactive substances. These rays and substances are effective in destroying cancer cells and halting their growth. Treatment of disease using radiation is called _____/_____/_____.
muscle, bone marrow, spinal cord	**10–40** Although *my/o* and *myel/o* sound alike, they have different meanings. *My/o* refers to _____. *Myel/o* refers to _____ _____ or the _____ _____.
myel/o	**10–41** A myel/o/gram is a radi/o/graph of the spin/al cord after injection of a contrast medium. The CF for *bone marrow and spinal cord* is _____/_____.
myel/o/genesis mī-ĕ-lō-JĔN-ĕ-sĭs	**10–42** Use *-genesis* to build a word that means *formation of bone marrow*. _____/_____/_____
myel/o/malacia mī-ĕl-ō-mă-LĀ-shē-ă **myel/o/gram** MĪ-ĕl-ō-grăm	**10–43** Develop medical words that mean *softening of the spinal cord:* _____/_____/_____. *record of the spinal cord:* _____/_____/_____.

Pink indicates a prefix. Blue indicates a suffix. Boldface indicates a word root or combining form.

myel/o/gram MĪ-ĕl-ō-grăm	**10–44** A myel/o/gram, a radiograph of the spinal canal after injection of a contrast medium, is used to identify and study spinal lesions caused by trauma or disease. To identify any distortions of the spinal cord, the physician may order a radiograph called a _____/_____/_____.
oste/o/myel/itis *Inflammation or* ŏs-tē-ō-mī-ĕ-LĪ-tĭs	**10–45** Oste/o/myel/itis is an inflammation of bone and bone marrow, most commonly caused by infection. (See Figure 10-6.) Localized or generalized infection of bone and bone marrow is charted as _____/_____/_____/_____.
bone **bone marrow, spinal cord** **inflammation**	**10–46** Oste/o/myel/itis is usually caused by bacteria introduced through trauma or surgery, by direct extension from a nearby infection, or via the bloodstream. Staphylococci are the most common causative agents. Analyze the elements of the term *oste/o/myelitis.* *oste/o:* _bone_ *myel:* _Spinal_ _Cord_ ; _bone_ _marrow._ *-itis:* _Inflammation_

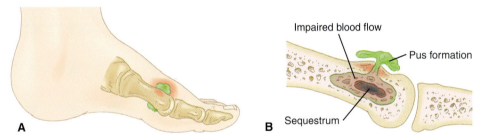

Figure 10-6   Osteomyelitis. (A) Bone infection in the toe. (B) Blocked blood flow in the area of infection with sequestrum (bone death) and pus formation at the infection site.

SECTION REVIEW 10-4

Using the following table, write the CF, suffix, or prefix that matches its definition in the space provided to the left of the definition. There may be more than one word element that matches a definition.

Combining Forms

calc/o	radi/o
chondr/o	scler/o
dist/o	
my/o	
myel/o	
oste/o	
proxim/o	

Suffixes

-algia	-graphy
-cele	-itis
-cyte	-logist
-dynia	-malacia
-emia	-oma
-genesis	-rrhaphy
-gram	-tomy

Prefixes

hyper-
hypo-
peri-

1. _____ excessive, above normal

2. _____ around

3. _____ blood condition

4. _____ bone

5. _____ cartilage

6. _____ calcium

7. _____ cell

8. _____ far, farthest

9. _____ hardening; sclera (white of eye)

10. _____ hernia; swelling

11. _____ incision

12. _____ inflammation

13. _____ near, nearest

14. _____ muscle

15. _____ pain

16. _____ process of recording

17. _____ forming, producing; origin

18. _____ record, writing

19. _____ softening

20. _____ specialist in study of

21. _____ bone marrow; spinal cord

22. _____ suture

23. _____ tumor

24. _____ under, below; deficient

25. _____ radiation, x-ray; radius (lower arm bone on thumb side)

Competency Verification: Check your answers in Appendix B: Answer Key, page 614. If you are not satisfied with your level of comprehension, go back to Frame 10–17, and rework the frames.

Correct Answers _____ x 4 = _____ % Score

Pink indicates a prefix. Blue indicates a suffix. Boldface indicates a word root or combining form.

Joints

synarthroses sĭn-ăr-THRŌ-sēz **diarthroses** dī-ăr-THRŌ-sēz **amphiarthroses** ăm-fē-ăr-THRŌ-sēz	**10-47** For body movements to function, <u>bones must</u> have points where they meet (articulate). These articulating points form joints that have various degrees of mobility. Some are freely movable (diarthroses); others are only slightly movable (amphiarthroses), and the remaining are totally immovable (synarthroses). All three types are necessary for smooth, coordinated body movements. Use the information above to identify the term that means *totally immovable joints:* _____. *freely movable joints:* _____. *slightly movable joints:* _____.

arthr/o/pathy ăr-THRŎP-ă-thē **arthr/itis** ăr-THRĪ-tĭs **arthr/o/centesis** ăr-thrō-sĕn-TĒ-sĭs	**10-48** Use *arthr/o* (joint) to develop medical words that mean *disease of a joint:* _____ / ____ / _____. *inflammation of a joint:* _arthr_ / _itis_ . *surgical puncture of a joint:* _____ / ____ / _____.

arthr/o/scope ĂR-thrō-skōp	**10-49** Arthr/o/scopy is the visual examination of the interior of a joint performed by inserting an endo/scope through a small incision. Arthr/o/scopy is performed to repair and remove joint tissue, especially of the knee, ankle, and shoulder. (See Figure 10-7.) The endo/scope used to perform arthr/o/scopy is called an _____ / ____ / _____.

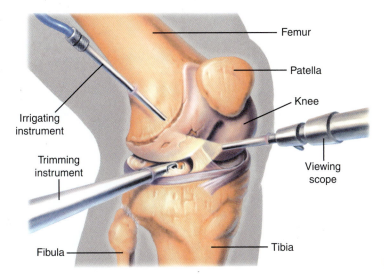

Figure 10-7 Arthroscopy.

arthr/o/plasty
ĂR-thrō-plăs-tē

10–50 Total hip replacement (THR), or total hip arthr/o/plasty, is a surgical procedure that replaces the upper end of the thighbone (femur) with a metal ball and resurfaces the hip socket (acetabulum) with a metal shell and plastic liner. The acetabulum is plastic coated to avoid metal-to-metal articulating surfaces. (See Figure 10-8.)

Use *arthr/o* to build a term that means surgical *repair of a joint.*

_____ / _____ / _____

THR

10–51 The surgical procedure to replace a hip joint that has been destroyed by disease or osteoarthritis is known as *total hip arthroplasty,* or _____ (abbreviation).

---

joints

10–52 Just as a piece of machinery is lubricated by oil, joints are lubricated by synovial fluid. The fluid is secreted within the synovial membranes.

Synovial fluid enables free movement of the _____.

---

arthr/itis
ăr-THRĪ-tĭs

oste/o/arthr/itis
ŏs-tē-ō-ăr-THRĪ-tĭs

10–53 Although there are various forms of arthr/itis, all types result in inflammation of the joints, usually accompanied by pain and swelling.

Form medical words that mean

inflammation of joints: _____ / _____.

inflammation of bones and joints:

_____ / _____ / _____ / _____.

---

oste/o/arthr/o/pathy
ŏs-tē-ō-ăr-THRŎP-ă-thē

10–54 A disease of the bones and joints is called

_____ / _____ / _____ / _____ / _____.

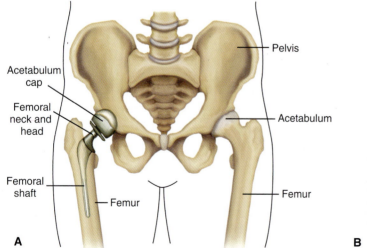 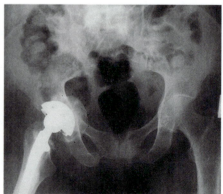

Figure 10-8   Total hip replacement. (A) Right total hip replacement. (B) Radiograph showing total hip replacement of an arthritic hip.

Pink indicates a prefix. Blue indicates a suffix. Boldface indicates a word root or combining form.

Combining Forms Related to Specific Bones

10–55 The word roots (WRs) for bones are derived from the specific anatomical names of the bones. Use the following information to learn the CFs of the bones as you label them in Figure 10-9.

- *Crani/o* refers to the (1) **cranium** (skull).
- *Stern/o* refers to the (2) **sternum** (breastbone).
- *Cost/o* refers to the (3) **ribs,** which are attached to the sternum.
- *Vertebr/o* refers to the (4) **vertebra** (backbone). The vertebral column, also called the spinal column, is composed of 26 bones called *vertebr/ae.*
- *Humer/o* refers to the (5) **humerus** (upper arm bone). The humerus articulates with the scapula at the shoulder and with the radius and ulna at the elbow.
- *Carp/o* refers to the (6) **carpus** (wrist bones). There are eight wrist bones.
- *Metacarp/o* refers to the (7) **metacarpus** (hand bone). The metacarpals (plural) radiate from the wristlike spokes and form the palm of the hand.
- *Phalang/o* refers to the (8) **phalanges** (bones of the fingers and toes).

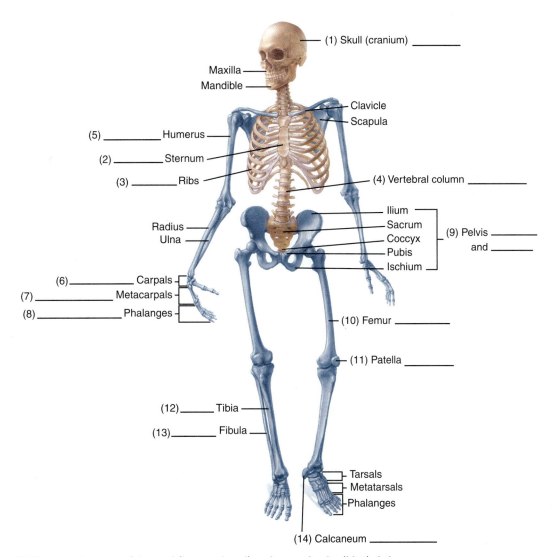

Figure 10-9   Anterior view of the axial (bone-colored) and appendicular (blue) skeleton.

- *Pelv/i* and *pelv/o* refer to the (9) **pelvis.** The pelvis, also called the *pelvic girdle,* is composed of three pairs of fused bones (the ilium, pubis, and ischium), the sacrum, and the coccyx. The pelvis provides attachment for the legs and supports the soft organs of the abdominal cavity.
- *Femor/o* refers to the (10) **femur** (thigh bone). The femur is the longest and strongest bone in the body. It articulates with the hip bone and the bones of the lower leg.
- *Patell/o* refers to the (11) **patella** (kneecap). The patella articulates with the femur but is, essentially, a floating bone. The main function of this bone is to protect the knee joint, but its exposed position makes it susceptible to dislocation and fracture.
- *Tibi/o* refers to the (12) **tibiav** (larger bone of the lower leg). The tibia is the weight-bearing bone of the lower leg.
- *Fibul/o* refers to the (13) **fibula** (smaller bone of the lower leg). The fibula is not a weight-bearing bone but is important because muscles are attached and anchored to it.
- *Calcane/o* refers to the (14) **calcaneum** (heel bone).

Competency Verification: Check your labeling of Figure 10-9 with Appendix B: Answer Key, page 614.

 You are not expected to know the CFs and the names of bones from memory. If needed, you can always refer to Appendix A: Glossary of Medical Word Elements, or a medical dictionary to obtain information about a bone or its CF.

pain, head	**10–56** Words that contain *cephal/o* refer to the head. *Cephal/o/dynia* is a _____ in the _____.
cephal/algia sĕf-ă-LĂL-gē-ă	**10–57** *Cephal/o/dynia* is the medical term for a headache. Construct another word that means *pain in the head.* _____ / _____
head **-meter**	**10–58** A meter is a metric unit of length equal to 39.37 inches. However, when used as a suffix *-meter* means *instrument for measuring.* Thus, a *cephal/o/meter is an* instrument for measuring the _____. In *cephal/o/meter,* the element that means *instrument for measuring* is _____.
encephal/o	**10–59** The prefix *en-* means in, within. Combine *en-* + *cephal/o* to create a new CF that refers to the brain. _____ / _____
encephal/oma ĕn-sĕf-ă-LŌ-mă **encephal/itis** ĕn-sĕf-ă-LĪ-tĭs **encephal/o/malacia** ĕn-sĕf-ă-lō-mă-LĀ-sē-ă	**10–60** Use *encephal/o* to build words that mean *tumor of the brain:* _____ / _____. *inflammation of the brain:* _____ / _____. *softening of the brain (tissue):* _____ / _____ / _____.

Pink indicates a prefix. Blue indicates a suffix. Boldface indicates a word root or combining form.

encephal/itis ĕn-sĕf-ă-LĪ-tĭs	**10–61** Encephal/itis is usually caused by viruses (e.g., arbovirus and herpes virus). Less commonly, it may occur as a component of rabies and acquired immune deficiency syndrome (AIDS). It may also occur as a result of systemic viral diseases, such as influenza, rubella, and chickenpox. The medical term for an inflammatory condition of the brain is _____ / _____.
disease, brain	**10–62** Encephal/o/pathy is a _____ of the _____.
brain	**10–63** An encephal/o/cele is a protrusion of _____ substance through an opening of the skull.
inter- **cost** **-al**	**10–64** Inter/cost/al muscles, located between the ribs, move the ribs during the breathing process. Write the elements in this frame that mean *between:* _____. *ribs:* _____. *pertaining to:* _____.
under *or* below, ribs	**10–65** *Sub/cost/al* refers to the area _____ the _____.

Fractures and Repairs

10–66 A fracture is a break or crack in the bone. Fractures are defined according to the type and extent of the break. (See Figure 10-10.) A (1) **closed fracture** means the bone is broken without causing an open wound, and surrounding tissue damage is minimal. An (2) **open fracture,** also called a *compound fracture,* means the broken end of a bone pierces the skin, creating an open wound. In such a fracture, there may be extensive damage to surrounding blood vessels, nerves, and muscles. An (3) **incomplete fracture** occurs when the line of fracture does not completely go through the bone. Whereas, a **complete fracture** occurs when the fracture goes completely through the bone, separating it in two. (See Figure10-11.) Label the closed, open, and incomplete fractures in Figure 10-10.

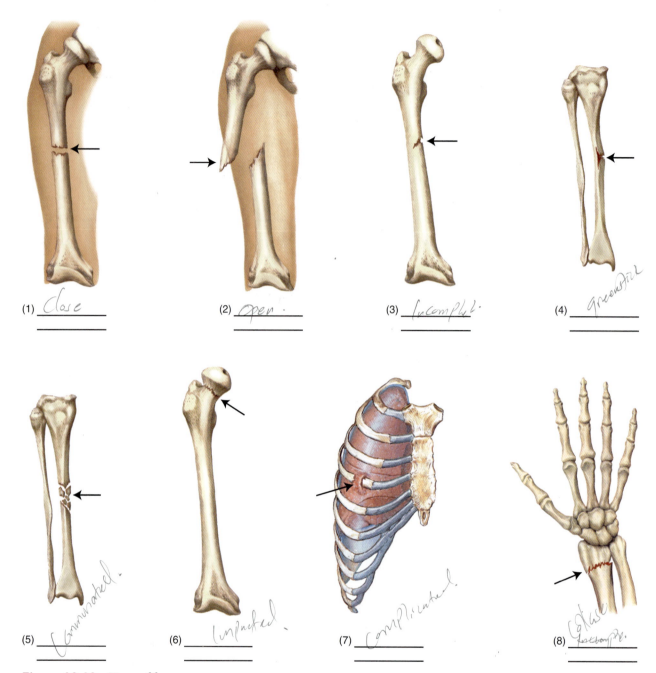

(1) _Close_ _____

(2) _Open._ _____

(3) _Incomplet._ _____

(4) _Greenstick_ _____

(5) _Comminuated._ _____

(6) _Impacted._ _____

(7) _Complicated._ _____

(8) _Colles_ _____ _lockway PF._

Figure 10-10   Types of fractures.

10-67 In addition to determining the extent of a break in a fracture, there are many different types of fractures, some of which are discussed here. A (4) **greenstick fracture** is an incomplete break of a soft bone and means that the bone is partially bent and partially broken. These fractures usually occur in children because their growing bones are soft and tend to splinter, rather than break completely. A (5) **comminuted fracture** occurs when the bone is broken into pieces. In an (6) **impacted fracture**, the broken ends of a bone are forced into one another; many bone fragments may be created by such a fracture. A (7) **complicated fracture** involves extensive soft tissue injury, such as when a broken rib pierces a lung. A (8) **Colles fracture** is a break of the lower end of the radius, which occurs just above the wrist. It causes displacement of the hand and usually occurs as a result of flexing a hand to cushion a fall. Label and study the different types of fractures in Figure 10-10.

Competency Verification: Check your labeling of Figure 10-10 in Appendix B: Answer Key, page 614.

open fracture

compound fracture

closed fracture

10-68 Identify the fractures that describe the following statements. (Refer to Figure 10–10.)

A bone pierces the skin and causes extensive damage to surrounding blood vessels:

_____ _____, also called

_____ _____.

A bone is broken with no external wound present:

_____ _____.

greenstick fracture

impacted fracture

10-69 Identify the fractures that describe the following statements. (Refer to Figure 10-10.)

A bone is partially bent and partially broken (found more commonly in children):

_____ _____.

The broken ends of bone segments are wedged into one another:

_____ _____.

10-70 Recall, a complete fracture occurs when a break goes completely through the bone, separating it in two portions. These types of fractures are based on the way the bone breaks and are categorized as: (1) **spiral**, (2) **oblique**, (3) **longitudinal**, and (4) **transverse**. (See Figure 10-11.) A **spiral fracture** occurs when a strong rotational or twisting force is applied along the axis of a bone. Spiral fractures often occur when the body is in motion while one extremity is planted. Label the spiral fracture in Figure 10-11.

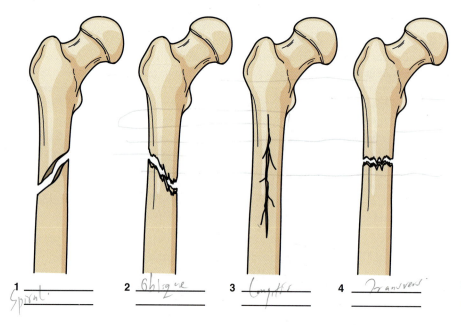

1 _Spiral_   2 _Oblique_   3 _Longitu_   4 _Transvers_

Figure 10-11   Complete fractures.

10-71   A _____ fracture results from a twisting force along the axis of a bone when the body is in motion with one extremity planted, and breaks in two. A spiral fracture is often slower to heal than other types of fractures. Figure 10-12 is an x-ray of a spiral fracture in the tibia of a 6-year-old boy. He was getting off a bike when he was hit by a bicyclist traveling downhill at a high speed.

spiral

10-72   Identify the fractures that describe the following statements, and then label them on Figure 10-11.

A fracture in which the break is diagonal (oblique to the long axis of the bone):

_____ .

The fracture runs nearly parallel to the long axis of the bone:

Longitudinal .

The fracture is across the bone (right angle to the long axis of the bone):

transverse .

oblique

longitudinal

transverse

Competency Verification: Check your labeling of Figure 10-11 in Appendix B: Answer Key, page 614.

Vertebral Column

10–73   The vertebr/al or spin/al column supports the body and provides a protective bony canal for the spinal cord.

Another name for the vertebr/al column is

_____ / _____ _____ .

From the word _spin/al_, construct the CF for _spine_.

_____ / _____

spin/al column
SPĪ-năl

spin/o

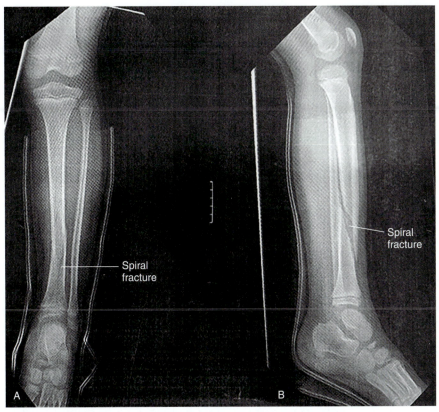

Figure 10-12   X-ray showing spiral fracture in the left distal tibia. (A) Anteroposterior view of lower leg. (B) Lateral view of lower leg.

---

vertebra VĔR-tĕ-bră	**10-74** *Spondyl/o* and *vertebr/o* are CFs that refer to the vertebrae (backbone). The singular form of vertebrae is _____.
vertebra VĔR-tĕ-bră **vertebra** VĔR-tĕ-bră	**10-75** Vertebr/ectomy is excision of a _____. Spondyl/o/dynia is a painful condition of a _____.
vertebrae VĔR-tĕ-brē **bursae** BĔR-sē **pleurae** PLOO-rē	**10-76** Change the following words from singular to plural form by retaining the *a* and adding an *e*. **Singular** **Plural** vertebra _____ bursa _____ pleura _____

spondyl/itis spŏn-dĭl-Ī-tĭs **spondyl/o/pathy** spŏn-dĭl-ŎP-ă-thē **spondyl/o/malacia** spŏn-dĭl-ō-mă-LĀ-shē-ă	**10–77** *Vertebr/o* is used to form words that describe the vertebra (backbone), and *spondyl/o* is used to form words about the condition of the vertebra. Build medical words that mean *inflammation of vertebrae:* _____ / _____ . *disease of vertebrae:* _____ / _____ / _____ . *softening of vertebrae:* _____ / _____ / _____ .
vertebra, vertebra VĔR-tĕ-bră	**10–78** As discussed previously, *vertebr/o* is used to form words that describe the vertebral structure. For example, *vertebr/o/cost/al* means *pertaining to a* _____ *and a rib. Vertebr/o/stern/al means pertaining to a* _____ *and the sternum, or chest plate.*
	10–79 Label Figure 10-13 as you learn about the vertebr/al or spin/al column. Vertebrae are separated and cushioned from each other by (1) **intervertebral disks** composed of cartilage.
inter- **vertebr/o** **-al**	**10–80** Determine the elements in *inter/vertebr/al* that mean *between:* _____ . *vertebra (backbone):* _____ / _____ . *pertaining to:* _____ .
	10–81 The vertebr/al column, also called the *spin/al column* or *backbone,* is composed of 26 bones known as *vertebrae* (singular, *vertebra*). There are five regions of these bones in the vertebr/al column, each of which derives its name from its location along the length of the spin/al column. Seven (2) **cervical vertebrae** form the skeletal framework of the neck. The first cervic/al vertebra is called the (3) **atlas** and supports the skull. The second, the (4) **axis,** enables the skull to rotate on the neck. Label these structures in Figure 10-13.
neck	**10–82** The CF *cervic/o* means *neck; cervix uteri (neck of the uterus). Cervic/o/facial* refers to the face and _____ .
atlas ĂT-lăs **cervic/al** SĔR-vĭ-kăl	**10–83** The name of the first cervic/al vertebra is the _____ . A term that means pertaining to the neck is _____ / _____ .
C5	**10–84** In medical reports, the first cervical vertebra is designated as C1. The fifth cervical vertebra is designated as _____ .

Pink indicates a prefix. Blue indicates a suffix. Boldface indicates a word root or combining form.

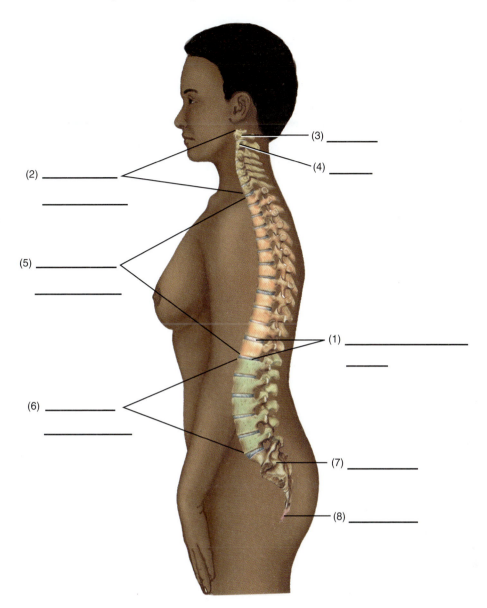

Figure 10-13   Vertebral column, lateral view, with regions of the spine shown with normal curves.

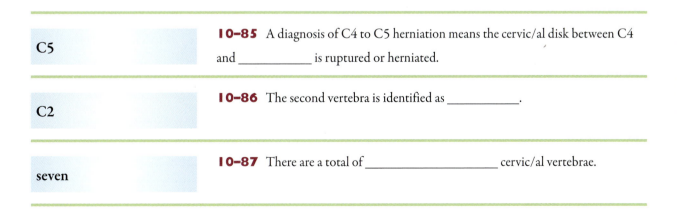

C5	**10–85** A diagnosis of C4 to C5 herniation means the cervic/al disk between C4 and _____ is ruptured or herniated.
C2	**10–86** The second vertebra is identified as _____.
seven	**10–87** There are a total of _____ cervic/al vertebrae.

10–88 Twelve (5) **thoracic vertebrae** support the chest and serve as a point of articulation (joining together to allow motion between parts) for the ribs. The next five vertebrae are the (6) **lumbar vertebrae.** These are situated in the lower back and carry most of the weight of the torso. Label these structures in Figure 10-13.

---

articulation
ăr-tĭk-ū-LĀ-shŭn

thorac/ic
thō-RĂS-ĭk

10–89 Identify the terms in Frame 10–88 that mean

a place where two bones meet: _____.

pertaining to the chest: _____ / _____.

---

pertaining to, back

10–90 The CF *lumb/o* refers to the *loins (lower back).*

Lumb/ar means _____ _____ *the loins or lower*

_____.

---

pain

10–91 Lumb/o/dynia is _____ in the lower back.

---

lumbar, five
LŬM-băr

10–92 Examine the position of the five lumbar vertebrae in Figure 10-13, designated as L1 to L5 in medical reports. An obese person with weak abdominal muscles tends to experience pain in the lower back area, or L1 to L5.

L5 refers to _____ vertebra _____.

10–93 Below the lumbar vertebrae are five sacral vertebrae that are fused into a single bone in the adult. The single bone is known as the (7) **sacrum** and the tail of the vertebral column, the (8) **coccyx.** Label the sacrum and coccyx in Figure 10-13.

---

pain

sacr/um, spine
SĀ-krŭm

10–94 The CF *sacr/o* means *sacr/um.* The suffix in the term *sacr/um* means *structure, thing.*

Sacr/o/dynia is _____ in the sacrum.

Sacr/o/spin/al refers to the _____ / _____ and

_____.

S5

10–95 Although the sacral vertebrae are fused into a single bone, to designate the exact position of abnormalities on the sacrum, the labels S1 to S5 are used. The first vertebra of the sacrum is designated as S1.

The fifth vertebra of the sacrum is designated as _____.

---

lumbar, sacrum
LŬM-băr, SĀ-krŭm

10–96 A ruptured disk can cause severe pain, muscle weakness, or numbness in either leg. The disk that commonly ruptures is the L5 to S1 disk. L5 refers to _____ *five.* S1 refers to _____ *one.*

Competency Verification: Check your labeling of Figure 10-13 in Appendix B: Answer Key, page 614.

Pink indicates a prefix. Blue indicates a suffix. Boldface indicates a word root or combining form.

SECTION REVIEW 10-5

Using the following table, write the CF or suffix that matches its definition in the space provided to the left of the definition. There may be more than one word element that matches a definition.

Combining Forms

arthr/o	oste/o
cephal/o	sacr/o
cervic/o	spondyl/o
cost/o	thorac/o
encephal/o	vertebr/o
lumb/o	

Suffixes

-centesis
-ectomy
-osis
-pathy
-um

1. _____ abnormal condition; increase (used primarily with blood cells)

2. _____ bone

3. _____ brain

4. _____ chest

5. _____ disease

6. _____ excision, removal

7. _____ head

8. _____ joint

9. _____ loins (lower back)

10. _____ neck; cervix uteri (neck of the uterus)

11. _____ structure, thing

12. _____ ribs

13. _____ sacrum

14. _____ surgical puncture

15. _____ vertebra (backbone)

Competency Verification: Check your answers in Appendix B: Answer Key, page 614. If you are not satisfied with your level of comprehension, go back to Frame 10–47, and rework the frames.

Correct Answers _____ x 6.67 = _____% Score

Abbreviations

This section introduces musculoskeletal system–related abbreviations and their meanings.

Abbreviation	Meaning	Abbreviation	Meaning
AIDS	acquired immune deficiency syndrome	HNP	herniated nucleus pulposus (herniated disk)
AP	anteroposterior	L1, L2 to L5	first lumbar vertebra, second lumbar vertebra, and so on
C1, C2 to C7	first cervical vertebra, second cervical vertebra, and so on	MG	myasthenia gravis
D.O., DO	Doctor of Osteopathy	RA	rheumatoid arthritis
CT	computed tomography	S1, S2 to S5	first sacral vertebra, second sacral vertebra, and so on
CTS	carpal tunnel syndrome	THR	total hip replacement
Fx	fracture	T1, T2 to T12	first thoracic vertebra, second thoracic vertebra, and so on

Additional Medical Terms

The following are additional terms related to the musculoskeletal system. Recognizing and learning these terms will help you understand the connections among a pathological condition, its diagnosis, and the rationale behind the method of treatment selected for a particular disorder.

Diseases and Conditions

Muscular Disorders

muscular dystrophy
MŬS-kū-lăr DĬS-trō-fē
muscul: muscle
   -ar: pertaining to
dys-: bad; painful; difficult
-trophy: development, nourishment

Group of hereditary diseases characterized by gradual atrophy and weakness of muscle tissue; also called *muscular dystrophy Duchenne type*

There is no cure for muscular dystrophy. Duchenne dystrophy is the most common form, and patients with this disease form have an average life span of 20 years.

myasthenia gravis (MG)
mī-ăs-THĒ-nē-ă GRĂV-ĭs

Autoimmune neuromuscular disorder characterized by severe muscular weakness and progressive fatigue

sprain

Trauma to a joint that causes injury to the surrounding ligament, accompanied by pain and disability

strain	Trauma to a muscle or tendon (stretch or tear) from overuse or excessive forcible stretch
torticollis tōr-tĭ-KŎL-ĭs	Spasmodic contraction of the neck muscles, causing stiffness and twisting of the neck; also called *wryneck* *Torticollis may be congenital or acquired.*

Bone and Joint Disorders

bunion BŬN-yŭn	Deformity characterized by lateral deviation of the great toe as it turns in toward the second toe (angulation), which may cause the tissues surrounding the metatarsophalangeal joint to become swollen and tender; also called *hallux valgus* (See Figure 10-14.) *Bunion is associated with rheumatoid arthritis, chronic irritation and pressure from tight-fitting shoes, or heredity. Treatment includes proper footwear, wearing padding around the toes to relieve pressure, medication for pain and swelling, or bunionectomy and arthroplasty.*

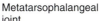
Metatarsophalangeal joint

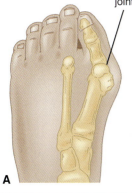
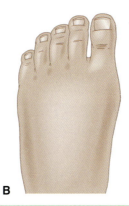

A   B

Figure 10-14   Bunion. (A) Preoperative. (B) Postoperative.

carpal tunnel syndrome (CTS) KĂR-păl TŬN-ĕl SĬN-drōm	Pain or numbness resulting from compression of the median nerve within the carpal tunnel (wrist canal through which the flexor tendons and median nerve pass)
contracture kŏn-TRĂK-chŭr	Fibrosis of connective tissue in skin, fascia, muscle, or joint capsule preventing normal mobility of the related tissue or joint
crepitation krĕp-ĭ-TĀ-shŭn	Grating sound made by movement of bone ends rubbing together, indicating a fracture or joint destruction
Ewing sarcoma Ū-ĭng săr-KŌ-mă	Malignant tumor that develops from bone marrow, usually in the long bones or the pelvis; also called *malignant neoplasm of bone by site* *Ewing sarcoma occurs most commonly in adolescent boys.*

ganglion cyst
GĂNG-lē-ŏn SĬST

Fluid-filled tumor that most commonly develops along the tendons or joint of the wrists or hands but may also occur in the ankles and feet

In most instances, ganglion cysts cause no pain, require no treatment, and go away on their own. Reasons for treatment are cosmetic or when the cyst causes pain (presses on a nearby nerve) or interferes with joint movement. Treatment involves removing the fluid or excising the cyst. (See Figure 10-15.)

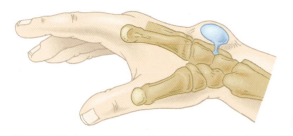

Figure 10-15   Ganglion cyst of the wrist.

gout
GOWT

Hereditary metabolic disease that is a form of acute arthritis, characterized by excessive uric acid in blood and around the joints

herniated disk
HĔR-nē-āt-ĕd

Herniation or rupture of the nucleus pulposus (center gelatinous material within an intervertebral disk) between two vertebrae; also called prolapsed disk (See Figure 10-16.)

A herniated disk places pressure on a spinal root nerve or the spinal cord. Displacement of the disk irritates the spinal nerves, causing muscle spasms and pain. It occurs most commonly in the lower spine.

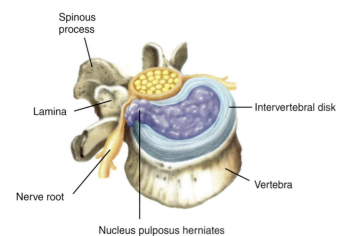

Spinous process

Lamina

Nerve root

Nucleus pulposus herniates and compresses nerve root

Intervertebral disk

Vertebra

Figure 10-16   Herniated disk.

Paget disease
PĂJ-ĕt

Skeletal disease that affects older people and causes chronic inflammation of bones, resulting in thickening and softening of bones and bowing of the long bones; also called *osteitis deformans*

rheumatoid arthritis (RA) ROO-mă-toyd ăr-THRĪ-tĭs *arthr*: joint *-itis*: inflammation	Chronic, systemic, inflammatory, autoimmune disease affecting the synovial membranes of multiple joints, eventually resulting in crippling deformities (See Figure 10-17.) *As RA develops, congestion and edema of the synovial membrane and joint occur, causing formation of a thick layer of granulation tissue. This tissue invades cartilage, destroying the joint and bone. Eventually, a fibrous immobility of joints (ankylosis) occurs, causing visible deformities and total immobility.*

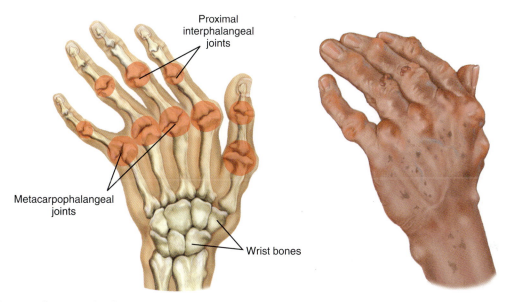

Proximal interphalangeal joints

Metacarpophalangeal joints

Wrist bones

Figure 10-17   Rheumatoid arthritis.

rotator cuff injury	Trauma to the capsule of the shoulder joint, which is reinforced by muscles and tendons; also called *musculotendinous rotator cuff injury* *Rotator cuff injuries occur in sports and in which there is a complete abduction of the shoulder, followed by a rapid and forceful rotation and flexion of the shoulder. This type of injury occurs most commonly in baseball when the player throws the ball.*
subluxation sŭb-lŭk-SĀ-shŭn	Partial or complete dislocation
sequestrum sē-KWĔS-trŭm	Fragment of a necrosed bone that has become separated from surrounding tissue
talipes equinovarus TĂL-ĭ-pēz ē-kwī-nō-VĀR-ŭs	Congenital deformity of the foot; also called *clubfoot* (See Figure 10-18.) *In talipes, the heel never rests on the ground. Treatment consists of applying casts to progressively straighten the foot and surgical correction for severe cases.*

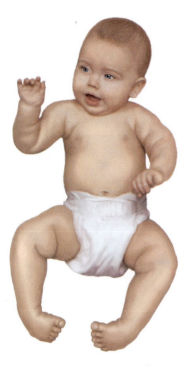

Figure 10-18   Talipes equinovarus.

Spinal Disorders

ankylosing spondylitis
ĂNG-kĭ-lōs-ĭng
spŏn-dĭl-Ī-tĭs
  spondyl/o: vertebra
    (backbone)
  -itis: inflamma-
    tion
	Chronic inflammatory disease of unknown origin that first affects the spine and is characterized by fusion and loss of mobility of two or more vertebrae; also called *rheumatoid spondylitis*
	
	Treatment includes nonsteroidal anti-inflammatory drugs (NSAIDs) and, in advanced cases of a badly deformed spine, surgery.

kyphosis
kī-FŌ-sĭs
  kyph: humpback
  -osis: abnormal
  condition; increase
  (used primarily with
  blood cells)
	Increased curvature of the thoracic region of the vertebral column, leading to a humpback posture; also called *hunchback*
	
	Kyphosis may be caused by poor posture, arthritis, or osteomalacia. (See Figure 10-19.)

lordosis
lōr-DŌ-sĭs
  lord: curve, swayback
  -osis: abnormal
  condition; increase
  (used primarily with
  blood cells)
	Forward curvature of the lumbar region of the vertebral column, leading to a swayback posture
	
	Lordosis may be caused by increased weight in the abdomen, such as during pregnancy. (See Figure 10-19.)

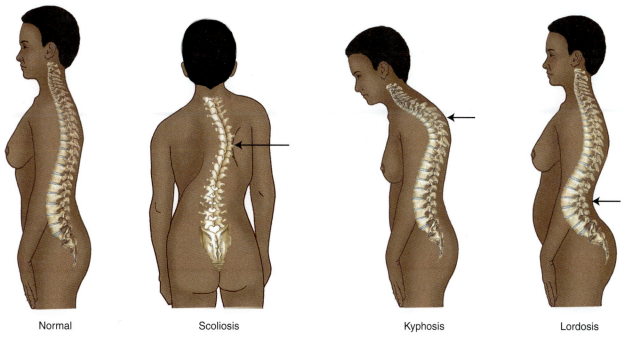

| Normal | Scoliosis | Kyphosis | Lordosis |

Figure 10-19   Spinal curvatures.

scoliosis
skō-lē-Ō-sĭs
    scoli: crooked, bent
    -osis: abnormal
            condition;
            increase (used
            primarily with
            blood cells)
	Abnormal sideward curvature of the spine to the left or right
	
	Scoliosis eventually causes back pain, disk disease, or arthritis. It is commonly a congenital disease but may result from poor posture. (See Figure 10-19.)

spinal stenosis
SPĪ-năl stĕ-NŌ-sĭs
    spin: spine
     -al: pertaining to
    sten: narrowing
    *-osis: abnormal
            condition; increase
            (used primarily
            with blood cells)*
	Narrowing of one or more spaces within the spine that results in the nerves becoming compressed or pinched, which leads to back pain; commonly occurs in the cervical or lumbar area (See Figure 10-20.)
	
	Spinal stenosis usually develops slowly over time and is commonly caused by osteoarthritis or wear and tear due to the aging process.

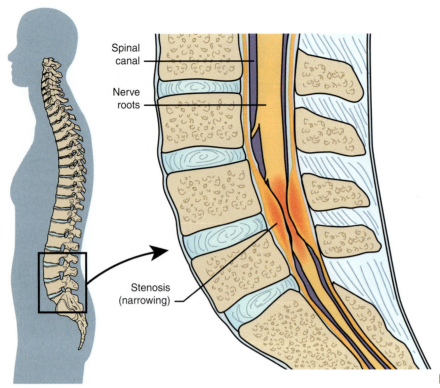

Spinal canal

Nerve roots

Stenosis (narrowing)

Figure 10-20   Spinal stenosis.

spondylolisthesis spŏn-dĭ-lō-lĭs-THĒ-sĭs *spondyl/o:* vertebra (backbone) *-listhesis:* slipping	Partial forward dislocation of one vertebra over the one below it, most commonly the fifth lumbar vertebra over the first sacral vertebra; also called *spinal cord compression*

Diagnostic Procedures

arthrocentesis ăr-thrō-sĕn-TĒ-sĭs *arthr/o:* joint *-centesis:* surgical puncture	Puncture of a joint space with a needle to remove fluid *Arthrocentesis is performed to obtain samples of synovial fluid for diagnostic purposes. It may also be used to instill medications and remove accumulated fluid from joints to relieve pain.*
bone density test (bone densitometry)	Low-energy x-ray absorption of the wrist, pelvis, and spinal column to measure bone density for purposes of diagnosis and management of osteoporosis; also called *dual-energy x-ray absorptiometry (DEXA)*

bone scan	Nuclear medicine procedure that visualizes bone(s) after the intravenous injection of a radiopharmaceutical
	A special scanning device detects areas of increased uptake of the radiopharmaceutical to indicate abnormalities of bone, such as infection, inflammation, fractures, and tumors.
rheumatoid factor ROO-mă-toyd	Blood test to detect the presence of rheumatoid factor, a substance present in patients with RA

Medical and Surgical Procedures

arthroplasty ĂR-thrō-plăs-tē *arthr/o:* joint *-plasty:* surgical repair	Surgical reconstruction or replacement of a painful, degenerated joint to restore mobility in RA or osteoarthritis or to correct a congenital deformity
bone immobilization	Process of holding a bone(s) in place to prevent the fracture from moving while it heals
casting	Protective shell of fiberglass, plaster, or plastic, that is molded to protect and facilitate alignment of bone as the fracture heals
splinting	Use of a rigid material, such as a thin piece of wood or metal, to maintain the injured body part in a fixed position to facilitate alignment of bone as the fracture heals
traction	Use of devices such as ropes, pulleys, and weights to apply tension and facilitate alignment of bone as the fracture heals
	Traction is also used to relieve back pain caused from a herniated disc by alleviating nerve pressure and stress on the vertebral discs
sequestrectomy sē-kwĕs-TRĔK-tō-mē *sequestr:* separation *-ectomy:* excision, removal	Excision of a sequestrum (segment of necrosed bone)

Pharmacology

The following table lists common drug categories used to treat musculoskeletal disorders, as well as their therapeutic actions.

Drug Category	Action
bone resorption inhibitors	Reduce resorption of bone; used in the treatment of weak and fragile bones, as seen in osteoporosis and Paget disease
calcium supplements	Treat and prevent hypocalcemia *Calcium supplements help to prevent osteoporosis when the diet is lacking in calcium and usually contain vitamin D, which is needed for calcium to be absorbed by the body.*
gold salts	Treat rheumatoid arthritis by inhibiting activity within the immune system to prevent further disease progression
muscle relaxants	Relieve muscle spasm and stiffness
nonsteroidal anti-inflammatory drugs (NSAIDs) nŏn-stĕr-OYD-ăl ăn-tē-ĭn-FLĂM-ă-tō-rē	Relieve mild to moderate pain and reduce inflammation in the treatment of musculoskeletal conditions, such as sprains and strains, and inflammatory disorders, such as RA, osteoarthritis, bursitis, gout, and tendinitis

Pronunciation Help	Long Sound	ā in rāte	ē in rēbirth	ī in īsle	ō in ōver	ū in ūnite
	Short Sound	ă in ăpple	ĕ in ĕver	ĭ in ĭt	ŏ in nŏt	ŭ in cŭt

Word Elements Review

This review provides a verification of your knowledge of the word elements covered in this chapter. First, use a slash to break the term into its component parts and identify each element by labeling it P for prefix, WR for word root, CF for combining form, or S for suffix. Then, provide the meaning of the medical term. Remember to define the suffix first, define the beginning of the word next, and define the middle part of the term last. The first word is a sample completed for you.

Term	Meaning
arthr/o/centesis CF S	*Surgical puncture of a joint*
1. chondr/o/malacia	
2. patell/ectomy	
3. hemi/plegia	
4. spondyl/it is	
5. lord/osis	

Matching the following medical terms with the definitions in the numbered list.

arthritis   fascioplasty   myoma   osteomalacia
arthrocentesis   kyphosis   myorrhaphy   osteoporosis
calcaneodynia   leiomyoma   myorrhexis   sequestrectomy
craniotomy   myelocele   osteochondritis

6. _____ inflammation of the joint(s)

7. _____ porous bones

8. _____ abnormal condition of a humpback

9. _____ surgical puncture of a joint

10. _____ excision, removal of a sequestrum (segment of necrosed bone)

11. _____ surgical repair of fascia

12. _____ rupture of a muscle

13. _____ tumor of smooth muscle

14. _____ herniation of the spinal cord

15. _____ inflammation of bone and cartilage

16. _____ softening of bone(s)

17. _____ tumor of muscle

18. _____ suture of muscle

19. _____ incision of the skull

20. _____ pain in the heel bone

Competency Verification: Check your answers in Appendix B: Answer Key, page 615. If you are not satisfied with your level of comprehension, review the vocabulary, and retake the review.

Correct Answers _____ x 6.67 = _____ % Score

Additional Medical Terms Review

Match the following medical terms with the definitions in the numbered list.

ankylosis	gout	NSAIDs	sequestrum
arthroplasty	herniated disk	Paget disease	sprain
arthroscopy	kyphosis	RA	strain
bunion	lordosis	rheumatoid factor	talipes
crepitation	muscular dystrophy	scoliosis	tendinitis
CTS	myasthenia gravis	sequestrectomy	torticollis
Ewing sarcoma			

1. _____ is a deformity characterized by lateral deviation of the great toe.

2. _____ is inflammation of a tendon.

3. _____ refers to trauma to a joint, causing injury to the surrounding ligament.

4. _____ refers to trauma to a muscle that results from overuse or excessive, forcible stretch.

5. _____ refers to a hunchback or humpback.

6. _____ is a malignant tumor that develops from bone marrow, usually in long bones or the pelvis, and occurs most commonly in adolescent boys.

7. _____ is characterized by spasmodic contraction of the neck muscles and is also called *wryneck*.

8. _____ is a disease characterized by excessive uric acid in blood and around the joints.

9. _____ is a disease characterized by inflammatory changes in joints and related structures that result in crippling deformities.

10. _____ is a skeletal disease of older adults causing chronic inflammation of bones, thickening and softening of bones, and bowing of the long bones, and is also called *osteitis deformans*.

11. _____ is a fragment of necrosed bone that has become separated from surrounding tissue.

12. _____ is the replacement of a joint.

13. _____ is a grating sound made by the ends of bone rubbing together.

14. _____ is a neuromuscular disorder characterized by muscular weakness and progressive fatigue.

15. _____ refers to a forward curvature of the lumbar spine, also called *swayback*.

16. _____ refers to a group of hereditary diseases characterized by gradual atrophy and weakness of muscle, with the most common form being *Duchenne*.

17. _____ are drugs that relieve mild to moderate pain and reduce inflammation in treatment of musculoskeletal disorders, such as sprains and strains.

18. _____ is immobility of a joint.

19. _____ refers to rupture of the nucleus pulposus between two vertebrae.

20. _____ is pain or numbness resulting from compression of the median nerve within the carpal tunnel.

21. _____ is excision of a necrosed piece of bone.

22. _____ is a blood test to detect a substance present in the blood of patients with rheumatoid arthritis.

23. _____ is a congenital foot deformity that is also called clubfoot.

24. _____ is the visual examination of a joint.

25. _____ is an abnormal sideward curvature of the spine to the left or right.

Competency Verification: Check your answers in Appendix B: Answer Key, page 615. If you are not satisfied with your level of comprehension, review the additional medical terms, and retake the review.

Correct Answers _____ x 4 = _____ % Score

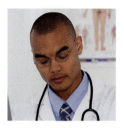

Medical Record Activities

To develop a working vocabulary of medical terms and to understand how those terms are used in the health-care industry, it is important that you complete the following activities.

MEDICAL RECORD ACTIVITY 10-1

RADIOLOGY REPORT: DEGENERATIVE INTERVERTEBRAL DISK DISEASE

This activity contains a radiology report in which a patient is diagnosed with degenerative intervertebral disk disease. Read the radiology report that follows, and underline the medical terms. Then complete the terminology and critical thinking exercises.

RADIOLOGY REPORT

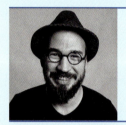

PATIENT NAME: Rexon, Arthur
MEDICAL RECORD ID: 24-58-73
DATE: October 19, 20xx

Anteroposterior (AP) and lateral views of the lumbar spine and AP view of the sacrum show a displacement of L5 on S1. The L5–S1 intervertebral disk space contains a slight shadow of decreased density. There is now slight narrowing of the L3–L4 and L4–L5. Bilateral laminectomies appear to have been done at L5–S1. Slight hypertrophic lipping of the upper lumbar vertebral bodies is now seen, as is slight lipping of the upper margin of the body of L4. The sacroiliac joint spaces are well preserved. Lateral views of the lumbosacral spine taken with the spine in flexion and extension show slight motion at all of the lumbar and lumbosacral levels.

IMPRESSION: 1. Degenerative, intervertebral disk disease at L5–S1, now also accompanied by slight narrowing of the L3–L4 and L4–L5.
2. Slight motion at all of the lumbar and lumbosacral levels.

Geoff Meyerson, M.D.

Geoff Meyerson, M.D.

GM:rsd

D: 10/19/20xx: T: 10/19/20xx

Terminology 10-1

*Terms listed in the following table come from the previous Radiology Report: Degenerative Intervertebral Disk
Disease. Use a medical dictionary, such as Taber's Cyclopedic Medical Dictionary; the appendices of this book; or
other resources to define each term. Then, pronounce the term, and place a checkmark (✓) in the box after you do so.*

Term	Definition
bilateral bī-LĂT-ĕr-ăl ☐	
degenerative dĕ-JĔN-ĕr-ă-tĭv ☐	
hypertrophic hī-pĕr-TRŌF-ĭk ☐	
intervertebral ĭn-tĕr-VĔRT-ĕ-brăl ☐	
L5	
laminectomies lăm-ĭ-NĔK-tō-mēz ☐	
lipping LĬP-ĭng ☐	
lumbar LŬM-băr ☐	
S1	
sacroiliac sā-krō-ĬL-ē-ăk ☐	
sacrum SĀ-krŭm ☐	

 Visit the *Medical Terminology Simplified* online resource center at FADavis.com to hear pronunciation and meanings
of selected terms in this medical report.

Critical Thinking 10-1

Review the previous Radiology Report: Intervertebral Disk Disease to answer the following questions. Use a medical dictionary, such as Taber's Cyclopedic Medical Dictionary, *and other resources, if needed.*

1. Why does the radiograph show decreased density at L5–S1?

_____

_____

2. What is the most common cause of degenerative intervertebral disk disease?

_____

_____

3. What happens to the gelatinous material of the disk as aging occurs?

_____

_____

4. What is the probable cause of the narrowing of the L3–L4 and L4–L5?

_____

_____

MEDICAL RECORD ACTIVITY 10-2

OPERATIVE REPORT: ROTATOR CUFF TEAR, RIGHT SHOULDER

This activity contains an operative report in which a patient receives treatment for a rotator cuff tear in the right shoulder. Read the operative report that follows, and underline the medical terms. Then, complete the terminology and critical thinking exercises.

OPERATIVE REPORT

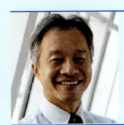

PATIENT NAME: Zang, Chen
MEDICAL RECORD ID: 33-1845-75
DATE: April 3, 20xx

PREOPERATIVE DIAGNOSIS: Rotator cuff tear, right shoulder. Degenerative arthritis, right acromioclavicular joint. Calcific tendinitis at the level of the superior glenoid tuberosity, right shoulder. Early degenerative osteoarthritis of the right shoulder. History of gouty arthritis.

ANESTHESIA: Xylocaine 1% local anesthetic with IV sedation.

OPERATION: Open repair of rotator cuff, open incision outer end of clavicle, anterior acromioplasty, glenohumeral and subacromial arthroscopy with arthroscopic bursectomy.

FINDINGS: Glenohumeral arthroscopy revealed that the superior, anterior, inferior, and posterior glenoid labra were intact. There was some fraying of the anterior glenoid labrum. The long head of the biceps was intact. We were unable to visualize any intra-articular calcification. We observed the takeoff of the long head of the biceps from the posterosuperior edge of the glenoid labrum and the glenoid tuberosity. There was an osteophyte inferiorly on the humeral head. There was a deep surface tear of the rotator cuff at the posterosuperior corner of the greater tuberosity of the humerus at the infraspinatus insertion. There was an extremely dense subacromial bursal scar. There was prominence of the inferior edge of the AC joint, with inferior AC joint and anterior acromial spurs.

Andrew Anderson, M.D.

Andrew Anderson, M.D.

AA: srr

D: 4/3/20xx; T: 4/3/20xx

Terminology 10-2

Terms listed in the following table come from the previous Operative Report: Rotator Cuff Tear, Right Shoulder. Use a medical dictionary, such as Taber's Cyclopedic Medical Dictionary; *the appendices of this book; or other resources to define each term. Then, pronounce the term and place a ✓ in the box after you do so.*

Term	Definition
AC joint	
acromial ăk-RŌ-mē-ăl ☐	
acromioclavicular ă-krō-mē-ō-klă-VĬK-ū-lăr ☐	
arthroscopy ăr-THRŎS-kō-pē ☐	
biceps BĪ-sĕps ☐	
bursectomy bŭr-SĔK-tō-mē ☐	
calcification kăl-sĭ-fĭ-KĀ-shŭn ☐	
degenerative dĕ-JĔN-ĕr-ă-tĭv ☐	
glenohumeral glē-nō-HŪ-mĕr-ăl ☐	
glenoid GLĒ-noyd ☐	
gouty GOW-tē ☐	

Term	Definition
intra-articular ĭn-tră-ăr-TĬK-ū-lăr ☐	
labra (singular, *labrum*) LĂ-bră ☐	
osteophyte ŎS-tē-ō-fīt ☐	
spur SPĔR ☐	
tuberosity tū-bĕr-ŎS-ĭ-tē ☐	

Visit the *Medical Terminology Simplified* online resource center at FADavis.com to hear pronunciation and meanings of selected terms in this medical report.

Critical Thinking 10-2

Review the previous Operative Report: Rotator Cuff Tear, Right Shoulder to answer the following questions. Use a medical dictionary, such as Taber's Cyclopedic Medical Dictionary, *and other resources, if needed.*

1. What type of arthritis did the patient have?

   _____

   _____

2. Did the patient have calcium deposits in the right shoulder?

   _____

   _____

3. What type of instrument did the physician use to visualize the glenoid labra?

   _____

   _____

4. What are labra?

   _____

   _____

5. Did the patient have any outgrowths of bone? If so, where?

   _____

   _____

MEDICAL RECORD ACTIVITY 10-3

CLINICAL APPLICATION

This activity is a clinical application that will help you integrate and reinforce your understanding of how the following medical terms are used in the clinical environment.

arthrocentesis	gouty arthritis	scoliosis
arthroplasty	myasthenia gravis	sprain
carpal tunnel syndrome	osteoarthritis	strain
costochondritis	rickets	torticollis

1. Jason sees the orthopedist for a follow-up visit for chronic pain in his left knee. He states that physical therapy and medications are not working and his pain is getting worse. The physician suggests surgical reconstruction of the knee. The medical term for surgical repair of a joint is known as _____.

2. This 33-year-old male presents with a complaint of rib pain when he takes a deep breath or when he coughs. The physician suspects the patient has inflammation of one or more costal cartilages and charts the diagnosis as _____.

3. This 62-year-old female is seen in the emergency department with complaints of left ankle pain and swelling after tripping on a curb. Radiographs are taken, and the radiologist notes there are no fractures. However, the surrounding ligament of the joint is damaged. This condition is known as a(n) _____.

4. Joyce, a 26-year-old administrative assistant, presents with a complaint of chronic pain in her left hand that extends to the forearm. She states that the pain started as a tingling in her fingers and has gradually worsened. The physician diagnoses compression of the median nerve. This condition is called _____.

5. Melanie, a 17-year-old female, is accompanied by her mother to the clinic. Her mother states that Melanie always seems to lean to the left when she stands and that she complains of chronic back pain. The physician orders radiographs, which reveal a sideward curvature of the spine. This is a condition known as _____.

6. A 5-year-old female child is brought to the pediatrician by her parents. The child's short stature and her continuous complaints of back and leg pain are of concern to the parents. After performing a physical examination and several tests, the pediatrician diagnoses softening of bones. The doctor notes that it is caused by vitamin D deficiency, a condition known as _____.

7. Mr. Y., a 38-year-old male, complains of recurrent pain in the joint of his big toe. Microscopic examination of fluid withdrawn from the joint capsule shows high uric acid levels. The physician diagnoses this condition as _____.

8. A 58-year-old male complains of a chronic stiff neck. He also experiences pain when trying to turn his head forward and is most comfortable when keeping his head tilted to the side. The physician explains this condition is caused by spasmodic contraction of the neck muscles and charts a diagnosis of _____.

9. Mr. E. complains of a swollen left elbow that began after being tackled while playing football. The physician orders radiography, and the result is negative for a fracture of the left elbow. He informs the patient that he will puncture the joint space with a needle to remove accumulated fluid, a surgical procedure called _____.

10. Dan, a 66-year-old male, is seen today with complaints of muscle weakness and fatigue. During the examination, the physician notes drooping of the eyelids. He suspects the patient suffers from an autoimmune neuromuscular disorder known as _____.

Competency Verification: Check your answers in Appendix B: Answer Key, page 616. If you are not satisfied with your level of comprehension, review the material in this chapter, and retake the review.

Correct Answers _____ x 10 = _____ % Score

MUSCULOSKELETAL SYSTEM CHAPTER REVIEW

WORD ELEMENTS SUMMARY

The following table summarizes CFs, suffixes, and prefixes related to the musculoskeletal system. Study the word elements and their meanings before completing the Vocabulary Review that follows.

Word Element	Meaning	Word Element	Meaning
Combining Forms			
arthr/o	joint	**metacarp/o**	metacarpus (hand bones)
calc/o	calcium	**myel/o**	bone marrow; spinal cord
calcane/o	calcaneum (heel bone)	**my/o**	muscle
carp/o	carpus (wrist bones)	**oste/o**	bone
cephal/o	head	**patell/o**	patella (kneecap)
cervic/o	neck; cervix uteri (neck of the uterus)	**proxim/o**	near
chondr/o	cartilage	**radi/o**	radiation, x-ray; radius (lower arm bone on the thumb side)
cost/o	ribs	**roentgen/o**	x-ray
crani/o	cranium (skull)	**sacr/o**	sacrum
cyt/o	cell	**scler/o**	hardening; sclera (white of the eye)
dist/o	far, farthest	**spin/o**	spine
encephal/o	brain	**spondyl/o, vertebr/o**	vertebra (backbone)
femor/o	femur (thigh bone)	**stern/o**	sternum (breastbone)
humer/o	humerus (upper arm bone)	**tend/o**	tendon
lumb/o	loin (lower back)	**tibi/o**	tibia (larger inner bone of the lower leg)
Suffixes			
-algia, -dynia	pain	**-logist**	specialist in the study of
-cele	hernia, swelling	**-malacia**	softening
-centesis	surgical puncture	**-meter**	instrument for measuring
-cyte	cell	**-oma**	tumor
-ectomy	excision, removal	**-osis**	abnormal condition
-emia	blood condition	**-pathy**	disease
-genesis	forming, producing; origin	**-plasty**	surgical repair
-gram	record, writing	**-plegia**	paralysis
-graphy	process of recording	**-rrhaphy**	suture
-ist	specialist	**-rrhexis**	rupture
-itis	inflammation	**-tomy**	incision

Word Element	Meaning	Word Element	Meaning
Prefixes			
en-	in, within	inter-	between
hemi-	one half	peri-	around
hypo-	under, below; deficient	quadri-	four

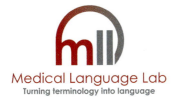

Medical Language Lab
Turning terminology into language

Visit the *Medical Language Lab* at *medicallanguagelab.com.* Use the flash-card–word elements exercise to reinforce your study of word elements. We recommend you complete the flash-card activity before starting the Vocabulary Review that follows.

Vocabulary Review

Match the following medical terms with the definitions in the numbered list.

AP	*bone marrow*	*distal*	*proximal*
arthrocentesis	*cephalometer*	*intervertebral*	*quadriplegia*
articulation	*cervical vertebrae*	*myelogram*	*radiologist*
atlas	*closed fracture*	*myorrhexis*	*radiology*
bilateral	*diaphysis*	*open fracture*	*spondylomalacia*

1. _____ is the study of x-rays and radioactive substances used for diagnosing and treating diseases.

2. _____ is the shaft, or main part, of a bone.

3. _____ refers to passing from the front to the rear.

4. _____ is a fracture in which the bone is broken, but there is no external wound and surrounding tissue damage is minimal.

5. _____ means *pertaining to or affecting two sides.*

6. _____ means *near the point of attachment to the trunk.*

7. _____ is the place of union between two or more bones and is also called a joint.

8. _____ is a fracture in which the broken end of a bone has moved so that it pierces the skin, with possibly extensive damage to surrounding blood vessels, nerves, and muscles.

9. _____ is the first cervical vertebra, which supports the skull.

10. _____ is a surgical puncture of a joint to remove fluid.

11. _____ is soft tissue that fills the medullary cavities of long bones.

12. _____ is an instrument used to measure the head.

13. _____ refers to a radiograph of the spinal canal after injection of a contrast medium.

14. _____ means *rupture of a muscle.*

15. _____ means *softening of vertebrae.*

16. _____ is a directional term that means *farthest from the point of attachment* to the trunk.

17. _____ is a physician who specializes in the use of x-rays for the diagnosis and treatment of disease.

18. _____ are bones that form the skeletal framework of the neck.

19. _____ is situated between two adjacent vertebrae.

20. _____ means *paralysis of all four extremities.*

Competency Verification: Check your answers in Appendix B: Answer Key, page 616. If you are not satisfied with your level of comprehension, review the chapter vocabulary, and retake the review.

Correct Answers: _____ x 5 = _____ % Score

Special Senses: Eyes and Ears

OBJECTIVES

Upon completion of this chapter, you will be able to:

- Describe the type of medical treatment the ophthalmologist and otolaryngologist provide.
- Identify the structures of the eye and ear by labeling them on the anatomical illustrations.
- Describe the primary functions of the eye and the ear.
- Describe diseases, conditions, and procedures related to the eye and the ear.
- Apply your word-building skills by constructing medical terms related to the eye and the ear.
- Describe common abbreviations and symbols related to the eye and the ear diseases.
- Recognize, define, pronounce, and spell terms correctly.
- Demonstrate your knowledge of this chapter by successfully completing the frames, reviews, and activities.

MEDICAL SPECIALTIES: OPHTHALMOLOGY AND OTOLARYNGOLOGY

Ophthalmology

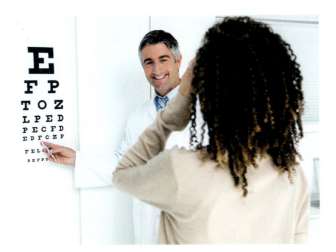

Ophthalmology is the branch of medicine concerned with diagnosis and treatment of eye disorders. The medical specialist in ophthalmology is called an **ophthalmologist.** Although ophthalmologists specialize in the treatment of the eyes only, it is important for them to be cognizant of other abnormalities that may be revealed during an eye examination. The importance of an eye examination cannot be overestimated because it commonly reveals the first signs of systemic illnesses (e.g., diabetes) that may be occurring in other parts of the body. The medical practice of ophthalmology includes prescribing corrective lenses and performing various types of corrective eye surgeries. Specialized surgeries involve techniques that are as delicate and precise as that of neurosurgery and are commonly performed by using magnifying glasses and laser beams. Corrective eye surgeries include cornea transplantation, cataract removal, repair of ocular muscle dysfunction, glaucoma treatment, lens removal, and radial keratotomy.

Two other providers involved in ophthalmology, the **optometrist** and the **optician,** specialize in providing corrective lenses for the eyes. They are not medical doctors but are licensed to examine and test the eyes. They also diagnose and treat visual defects by prescribing corrective lenses.

Otolaryngology

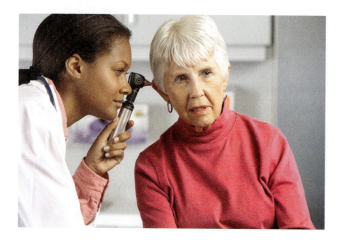

Otolaryngology is the medical and surgical management of patients with disorders of the ear, nose, and throat (ENT) and related structures of the head and neck. **Otolaryngologists,** also known as **ENT physicians,** commonly treat disorders related to the sinuses, including allergies and disorders of the sense of smell. Their diagnostic techniques help detect the causes of such symptoms as hoarseness, hearing and breathing difficulty, and swelling around the head or neck. Another important part of the ENT physician's practice is treatment of sleep disorders, most commonly sleep apnea. Various types of procedures, including but not limited to surgery, may be performed to treat sleep apnea or snoring disorders. ENT physicians are also involved in introducing rehabilitative programs for children and adults who have suffered hearing loss. Such programs commonly include collaborations with community agencies to identify individuals with hearing impairment (through public screenings) and provide them with needed medical treatment. Another provider involved in otolaryngology, the **audiologist** (not a medical doctor), detects, evaluates, and treats hearing loss.

Anatomy and Physiology Overview

The major senses of the body are sight, hearing, smell, taste, and touch. These sensations are identified with specific body organs. Senses of smell, taste, and touch were discussed in previous chapters. This chapter focuses on the eyes and ears, which include the senses of sight and hearing as well as balance.

Eyes

The eyes and their accessory structures are receptor organs that provide vision. As one of the most important sense organs of the body, the eyes provide most of the information not only about what we see but also from what we learn from reading printed material. Similar to other sensory organs, the eyes are constructed to detect stimuli in the environment to transmit those observations to the brain for interpretation.

WORD ELEMENTS

This section introduces word elements related to the eye. Review the word elements and their meanings in the following table, then pronounce each term in the word analysis column, and place a ✓ in the box after you do so.

Word Element	Meaning	Word Analysis
Combining Forms		
blephar/o	eyelid	**blephar/o/spasm** (BLĔF-ă-rō-spăzm ☐): involuntary contraction of eyelid muscles -*spasm:* involuntary contraction, twitching *Blepharospasm may be caused by eye strain or nervous irritability.*
conjunctiv/o	conjunctiva	**conjunctiv/itis** (kŏn-jŭnk-tĭ-VĪ-tĭs ☐): inflammation of the conjunctiva; also called pinkeye -*itis:* inflammation *Conjunctivitis can be caused by bacteria, allergy, irritation, or a foreign body.*
choroid/o	choroid	**choroid/o/pathy** (kō-roy-DŎP-ă-thē ☐): noninflammatory degeneration of the choroid -*pathy:* disease *The choroid is a thin, highly vascular layer of the eye between the retina and sclera.*
corne/o	cornea	**corne/itis** (kŏr-nē-Ī-tĭs ☐): inflammation of the cornea; also called *keratitis* -*itis:* inflammation

cor/o	pupil	**aniso/cor/ia** (ăn-ī-sō-KŌ-rē-ă ☐): inequality of pupil size
		  aniso-: *unequal, dissimilar*
		    -ia: *condition*
		Anisocoria may be congenital or associated with a neurological injury or disease.

core/o		**core/o/meter** (kō-rē-ŎM-ĕ-tĕr ☐): instrument for measuring the pupil -meter: instrument for measuring
pupill/o		**pupill/ary** (PŪ-pĭ-lăr-ē ☐): pertaining to the pupil -*ary:* pertaining to
dacry/o	tear; lacrimal apparatus (duct, sac, or gland)	**dacry/o/rrhea** (dăk-rē-ō-RĒ-ă ☐): excessive secretion of tears -*rrhea:* discharge, flow
lacrim/o		**lacrim/ation** (lăk-rĭ-MĀ-shŭn ☐): secretion and discharge of tears -*ation:* process (of)
dipl/o	double	**dipl/opia** (dĭp-LŌ-pē-ă ☐): two images of an object seen at the same time; also called *double vision* -*opia:* vision
irid/o	iris	**irid/o/plegia** (ĭr-ĭd-ō-PLĒ-jē-ă ☐): paralysis of the sphincter of the iris -*plegia:* paralysis
kerat/o	horny tissue; hard; cornea	**kerat/o/plasty** (KĔR-ă-tō-plăs-tē ☐): replacement of a cloudy cornea with a transparent one, typically derived from an organ donor; also called *corneal transplantation* -*plasty:* surgical repair

ocul/o	eye	**intra/ocul/ar** (ĭn-tră-ŎK-ū-lăr ☐): within the eyeball
		  intra-: in, within
		    -ar: pertaining to

ophthalm/o		**ophthalm/o/scope** (ŏf-THĂL-mō-skōp ☐): instrument for examining the interior of the eye, especially the retina -*scope:* instrument for examining

Continued

Word Element	Meaning	Word Analysis
opt/o	eye, vision	**opt**/ic (ŎP-tĭk ☐): pertaining to the eye or vision *-ic:* pertaining to
retin/o	retina	**retin/o**/pathy (rĕt-ĭn-ŎP-ă-thē ☐): disease of the retina *-pathy:* disease
scler/o	hardening; sclera (white of the eye)	**scler**/itis (sklĕ-RĪ-tĭs ☐): inflammation of the sclera *-itis:* inflammation

Suffixes

Word Element	Meaning	Word Analysis
-opia	vision	ambly/**opia** (ăm-blē-Ō-pē-ă ☐): reduction or dimness of vision, usually in one eye, with no apparent pathological condition; also called *lazy eye* *ambly:* dull, dim
-opsia		heter/**opsia** (hĕt-ĕr-ŎP-sē-ă ☐): inequality of vision in the two eyes *heter-:* different
-ptosis	prolapse, downward displacement	blephar/o/**ptosis** (blĕf-ă-rō-TŌ-sĭs ☐): drooping of the upper eyelid *blephar/o:* eyelid
-tropia	Turning	hyper/**tropia** (hī-pĕr-TRŌ-pē-ă ☐): ocular deviation (strabismus), with one eye located higher than the other *hyper-:* excessive, above normal *Upward deviation of the eye is usually caused by paresis of one of the muscles that either elevate or depress the eye. This condition is congenital or acquired.*

Pronunciation Help	*Long Sound*	ā in rāte	ē in rēbirth	ī in īsle	ō in ōver	ū in ūnite
	Short Sound	ă in ăpple	ĕ in ĕver	ĭ in ĭt	ŏ in nŏt	ŭ in cŭt

 Visit the *Medical Terminology Simplified* online resource center at FADavis.com for an audio exercise of the terms in this table to help master pronunciations and meanings of the selected medical terms.

SECTION REVIEW 11-1

For the following medical terms, first, write the suffix and its meaning. Then, translate the meaning of the remaining elements starting with the first part of the word. The first word is completed for you.

Term	Meaning
1. conjunctiv/it is	–itis: inflammation; conjunctiva
2. blephar/o/ptosis	
3. ambly/opia	
4. retin/o/pathy	
5. scler/itis	
6. ophthalm/o/scope	
7. intra/ocul/ar	
8. dacry/o/rrhea	
9. dipl/opia	
10. blephar/o/spasm	

Competency Verification: Check your answers in Appendix B: Answer Key, page 616. If you are not satisfied with your level of comprehension, review the vocabulary, and retake the review.

Correct Answers _____ x 10 = _____ % Score

Fibrous Tunic

eye

11-1 The eye is a globe-shaped, hollow structure set within a bony cavity. The bony cavity, or *orbit*, houses the eyeball and associated structures, such as the eye muscles, nerves, and blood vessels. Most of the eyeball is protected from trauma by the orbit's bony cavity. The eyeball consists of three basic layers: the fibrous tunic, the vascular tunic, and the sensory tunic, or *retina*. (See Figure 11-1.)

The CFs *ocul/o* and *ophthalm/o* refer to the _____.

11-2 The fibrous tunic is the outer layer of the eyeball. It consists of the posterior opaque (1) **sclera** and the anterior transparent (2) **cornea.** The sclera is the white part of the eyeball. It is composed of tightly bound elastic and collagenous fibers, which give shape to the eyeball and protect its inner structures. The sclera is avascular but does contain sensory receptors for pain. At the junction of the sclera and cornea is an opening known as the *canal of Schlemm.* A fluid called *aqueous humor* drains into this sinus. The cornea is transparent and convex permitting passage and causing refraction (bending) of incoming lightwaves. The optic nerve exits through the sclera at the posterior portion of the eyeball.

Observe the location of the outer layer of the eyeball (fibrous tunic) as you label the sclera and cornea in Figure 11-1.

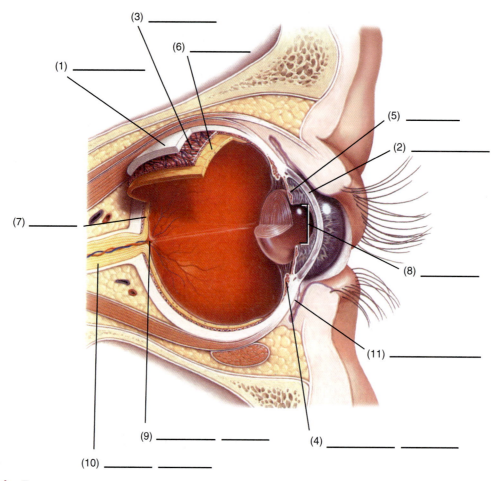

(3) _____

(6) _____

(1) _____

(5) _____

(2) _____

(7) _____

(8) _____

(11) _____

(9) _____ _____

(4) _____ _____

(10) _____ _____

Figure 11-1 Eye structures.

Vascular Tunic

11-3 The vascular tunic, or uvea, is the middle layer of the eyeball. It is composed of the choroid, ciliary body, and iris. The (3) **choroid** layer lies below the sclera and contains blood vessels. It also contains a dark, pigmented tissue that prevents glare within the eyeball because of its ability to absorb light. The anterior portion of the choroid is modified and forms the (4) **ciliary body** (or muscle) and the (5) **iris,** the colored portion of the eye. Observe the location of the middle layer of the eyeball (vascular tunic) as you label the choroid, ciliary body, and iris in Figure 11-1.

Sensory Tunic

11-4 The innermost layer, the **sensory tunic,** is the delicate, double-layered (6) **retina.** This structure lines the posterior two thirds of the eyeball and is the beginning of the visual pathway. It contains rods and cones, the sensory receptors for vision and image formation. Rods perceive the presence of light only, whereas cones perceive different wavelengths of light as colors. Cones are concentrated in the depression near the center of the retina called the (7) **fovea,** which is the area of sharpest vision. Surrounding the fovea is the yellowish macula, which also has an abundance of cones. In addition, the retina is the only place in the body where blood vessels can be seen directly. Label Figure 11-1 as you observe the location of the structures responsible for image formation.

scler/itis sklĕ-RĪ-tĭs **choroid/itis** kō-royd-Ī-tĭs **retin/itis** rĕt-ĭ-NĪ-tĭs	**11–5** The CF *scler/o* refers to hardening; sclera (*white of the eye*); *choroid/o* refers to the choroid; and *retin/o* refers to the retina. Use these CFs to build medical terms that mean *inflammation of the sclera:* _____/_____. *inflammation of the choroid:* _____/_____. *inflammation of the retina:* _____/_____.
choroid/o/pathy kō-roy-DŎP-ă-thē **retin/o/pathy** rĕt-ĭn-ŎP-ă-thē	**11–6** Practice building medical words that mean *disease of the choroid:* _____/_____/_____. *disease of the retina:* _____/_____/_____.
kerat/o/rrhexis kĕr-ă-tō-RĔK-sĭs **irid/o/cele** ĭ-RĬD-ō-sēl	**11–7** The CF *kerat/o* refers to horny tissue; hard; cornea. The CF *irid/o* refers to the iris. Use these CFs to build medical terms that mean *rupture of the cornea:* _____/_____/_____. *herniation of the iris:* _____/_____/_____.
kerat/o	**11–8** Kerat/itis, a vision-threatening infection, can occur if contact lenses are not cleaned and disinfected properly. From *kerat/itis,* construct the CF for cornea. _____/_____
scler/itis sklĕ-RĪ-tĭs **scler/o/malacia** sklĕ-rō-mă-LĀ-shē-ă	**11–9** Form medical words that mean *inflammation of the sclera:* _____/_____. *softening of the sclera:* _____/_____/_____.
kerat/o/tomy kĕr-ă-TŎT-ō-mē	**11–10** In some cases, laser kerat/o/tomy can be used to correct vision. Doing so eliminates the need for contact lenses or glasses. Shallow, bloodless, hairline, radial incisions are made with a laser in the outer portion of the cornea, where they will not interfere with vision. This allows the cornea to flatten and helps correct near-sightedness. About two thirds of patients are able to eliminate the use of glasses or contact lenses by undergoing the surgical procedure called laser _____/_____/_____.

11-11 The opening in the center of the iris is called the (8) **pupil.** The amount of light entering the eye is controlled by contractions and dilations of the pupil. Constriction of the pupil permits a sharper near vision. It is also a reflex that protects the retina from intense light. Label the pupil in Figure 11-1.

11-12 Nerve fibers unite at the (9) **optic disk** and form the (10) **optic nerve.** Because the optic disk has no rods or cones for vision, it is known as the *blind spot.* The optic nerve transmits impulses to the brain for processing visual information. Label the two structures in Figure 11-1.

ŏf-THĂL-mō

11-13 Words with *ophthalm/o* (eye) may be difficult to pronounce when you first encounter them. To avoid confusion, copy the pronunciation ŏf-THĂL-mō below, and practice saying it aloud.

_____

eye(s)

11-14 An ophthalm/o/logist is a physician who specializes in disorders and treatment of the _____. (See Figure 11-2.)

instrument

11-15 An ophthalm/o/scope is an _____ for examining the interior of the eye. (See Figure 11-2.)

ophthalm/o/scopy
ŏf-thăl-MŎS-kō-pē

11-16 The diagnostic term that describes visual examination of the eye is Ophthalm / o / scopy .

ophthalm/ectomy
ŏf-thăl-MĔK-tō-mē

ophthalm/o/malacia
ŏf-thăl-mō-mă-LĀ-shē-ă

ophthalm/o/plegia
ŏf-thăl-mō-PLĒ-jē-ă

11-17 Use *ophthalm/o* to build words that mean

surgical excision of the eye: _____ / _____.

softening of the eye: _____ / _____ / _____.

paralysis of the eye: _____ / _____ / _____.

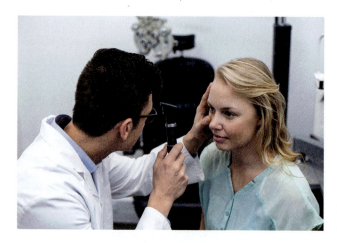

Figure 11-2 An ophthalmologist examining the eye with an ophthalmoscope.

Pink indicates a prefix. Blue indicates a suffix. Boldface indicates a word root or combining form.

ophthalm/o/plegia ŏf-thăl-mō-PLĒ-jē-ă	**11–18** A stroke can prevent eye movement and cause paralysis of eye muscles. A person with paralysis of eye (muscles) has a condition called _____/_____/_____.
conjuctiv/itis kŏn-jŭnk-tĭ-VĪ-tĭs	**11–19** The (11) **conjunctiva** is a thin, mucus-secreting membrane that lines the interior surface of the eyelids and the exposed anterior surface of the eyeballs. Conjuctiv/itis is commonly caused by an allergy and manifests as itchy, watery, red eyes. The medical term for *inflammation of the conjunctiva is* _____/_____.

Competency Verification: Check your labeling of Figure 11-1 in Appendix B: Answer Key, page 617.

blephar/o/plasty BLĔF-ă-rō-plăs-tē	**11–20** The surgical procedure to remove wrinkles from the eyelids is known as *blephar/o/plasty.* This procedure is performed for functional and cosmetic reasons. Surgical repair of the eyelid(s) is known as _____/_____/_____.
blephar/o/plasty BLĔF-ă-rō-plăs-tē	**11–21** Excessive skin around the upper eyelids may cause a decrease or lack of peripheral vision. To improve vision, the surgical procedure to remove the excessive skin is performed. This procedure is known as _____/_____/_____.
blephar/ectomy blĕf-ă-RĔK-tō-mē **blephar/o/tomy** blĕf-ă-RŎT-ō-mē **blephar/o/spasm** BLĔF-ă-rō-spăzm **blephar/o/plegia** blĕf-ă-rō-PLĒ-jē-ă	**11–22** Form medical words that mean *excision of part or all of the eyelid:* _____/_____. *surgical incision of eyelid:* _____/_____/_____. *twitching or spasm of eyelid:* _____/_____/_____. *paralysis of an eyelid:* _____/_____/_____. *blephar*
red **yellow**	**11–23** The suffix *-opia* is used in words to mean *vision.* Erythr/opia is a condition in which objects that are not red appear to be _____. Xanth/opia is a condition in which objects that are not yellow appear to be _____.
dipl/opia dĭp-LŌ-pē-ă	**11–24** Elements *dipl-* and **dipl/o** mean *double.* Dipl/opia occurs when both eyes are used but are not in focus. A person with double vision has a condition called _____/_____.

dipl/opia dĭp-LŌ-pē-ă	**11–25** Dipl/opia can occur with brain tumors, strokes, head trauma, and migraine headaches. Write the word in this frame that means *double vision.* _____/_____
hyper- **-opia** **my/o**	**11–26** Two common vision defects are my/opia (nearsightedness) and hyper/opia (farsightedness). See Figure 11-3 to compare a normal eye (emmetropia) with my/opia and hyper/opia. Write the elements in this frame that mean *excessive, above normal:* _____. *vision:* _____. *muscle:* _____/_____.
hyper/opia hī-pĕr-Ō-pē-ă	**11–27** In normal vision, the lens focuses the visual image on the retina. Hyper/opia, also called *farsightedness,* occurs when the lens focuses the visual image beyond the retina (see Figure 11-3), causing difficulty in seeing objects that are close. This is a condition common in people over 40 years old but can be corrected with "reading" glasses. The medical term for farsightedness is _____/_____.
close	**11–28** People with hyper/opia (farsightedness) have difficulty seeing objects that are _____.

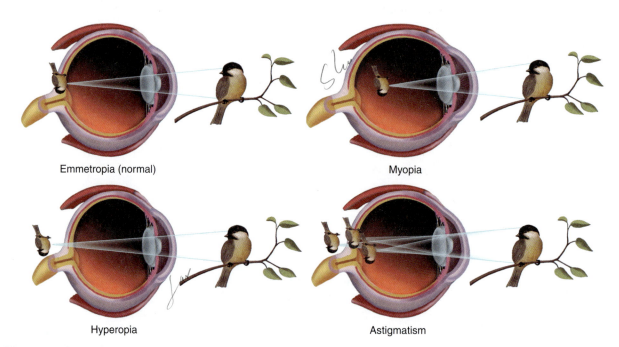

Emmetropia (normal)   Myopia

Hyperopia   Astigmatism

Figure 11-3   Refraction of the eye.

my/opia mī-Ō-pē-ă	**11–29** If the eyeball is too long, the visual image falls in front of the retina (see Figure 11-3), causing difficulty seeing objects that are far away. The medical term for *nearsightedness* is _____/_____.
hyper/opia hī-pĕr-Ō-pē-ă	**11–30** The opposite of my/opia, or *nearsightedness,* is _____/_____, or *farsightedness.*
blephar/o/plasty BLĔF-ă-rō-plăs-tē **blephar/o/spasm** BLĔF-ă-rō-spăzm **blephar/o/ptosis** blĕf-ă-rō-TŌ-sĭs	**11–31** Eyelids shade the eyes during sleep, protect them from excessive light and foreign objects, and spread lubricating secretions over the eyeballs. Use *blephar/o* (eyelid) to construct medical words that mean *surgical repair of eyelid:* _____/_____/_____. *twitching of an eyelid:* _____/_____/_____. *prolapse of an eyelid:* _____/_____/_____.
blephar/o **-ptosis**	**11–32** Blephar/o/ptosis is commonly seen after a stroke because the muscles leading to the eyelids become paralyzed. Indicate the elements in this frame that mean *eyelid:* _____/_____. *prolapse, downward displacement:* _____.
tears	**11–33** The lacrimal apparatus (see Figure 11-4) includes the (1) **lacrimal gland,** (2) **lacrimal sac,** and (3) **nasolacrimal duct.** The lacrimal gland is located above the outer corner of each eye. These glands produce tears, which keep the eyeballs moist. The lacrimal sac collects and drains tears into the nasolacrimal duct. Label the lacrimal structures in Figure 11-4.
tears	**11–34** The CF *dacry/o* is used in words to mean *tear; lacrimal sac.* Dacry/o/rrhea is an excessive flow of _____.
pain	**11–35** Dacry/aden/algia is _____ in a tear gland.
tear gland	**11–36** Dacry/aden/itis is inflammation of a _____ _____.

Competency Verification: Check your labeling of Figure 11-4 in Appendix B: Answer Key, page 617.

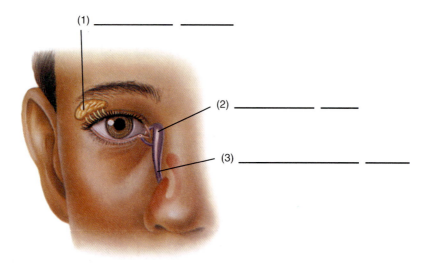

(1) _____ _____

(2) _____ _____

(3) _____ _____

Figure 11-4   Lacrimal apparatus.

Ears

The ears and their accessory structures are receptor organs that enable us to hear and maintain balance. Each ear consists of three divisions: external ear, middle ear, and inner ear. The external ear and the middle ear conduct sound waves through the ear. The inner ear contains auditory structures that receive sound waves and transmit them to the brain for interpretation. The inner ear also contains specialized receptors that maintain balance and equilibrium in response to fluctuations in body position and motion.

WORD ELEMENTS

This section introduces word elements related to the ear. Review the word elements and their meanings in the following table, then pronounce each term in the word analysis column, and place a ✓ in the box after you do so.

Word Elements	Meaning	Word Analysis
Combining Forms		
acous/o	hearing	**acous/tic** (ă-KOOS-tĭk ☐): pertaining to sound or the sense of hearing *-tic:* pertaining to
audi/o		**audi/o/meter** (aw-dē-ŎM-ĕ-tĕr ☐): instrument for testing hearing *-meter:* instrument for measuring
audit/o		**audit/ory** (AW-dĭ-tō-rē ☐): pertaining to the sense of hearing *-ory:* pertaining to
myring/o	tympanic membrane (eardrum)	**myring/o/tomy** (mĭr-ĭn-GŎT-ō-mē ☐): incision of the tympanic membrane *-tomy:* incision
tympan/o		**tympan/o/plasty** (tĭm-păn-ō-PLĂS-tē ☐): surgical repair of the tympanic membrane; also called myringoplasty *-plasty:* surgical repair *Tympanoplasty is any of several surgical procedures designed to cure a chronic inflammatory process in the middle ear or to restore function to the sound-transmitting mechanism of the middle ear.*
ot/o	ear	**ot/o/rrhea** (ō-tō-RĒ-ă ☐): inflammation of the ear with purulent discharge *-rrhea:* discharge, flow

salping/o	tube (usually fallopian or eustachian [auditory] tubes)	**salping/o/pharyng/eal** (săl-pĭng-gō-fă-RĬN-jē-ăl ☐): concerning the eustachian tube and pharynx
		   pharyng: pharynx (throat)
		      -eal: pertaining to

Suffix		
-acusis	hearing	**an/acusis** (ăn-ă-KŪ-sĭs ☐): total deafness *an-:* without, not

Pronunciation Help	*Long Sound* *Short Sound*	ā in rāte ă in ăpple	ē in rēbirth ĕ in ĕver	ī in īsle ĭ in ĭt	ō in ōver ŏ in nŏt	ū in ūnite ŭ in cŭt

 Visit the *Medical Terminology Simplified* online resource center at FADavis.com for an audio exercise of the terms in this table. It will help you master pronunciations and meanings of the selected medical terms.

SECTION REVIEW 11-2

For the following medical terms, first, write the suffix and its meaning. Then, translate the meaning of the remaining elements starting with the first part of the word. The first word is completed for you.

Term	Meaning
1. tympan/o/centesis	–centesis: surgical puncture; tympanic membrane (eardrum)
2. acous/tic	
3. hyper/tropia	
4. ot/o/rrhea	
5. an/acusis	
6. myring/o/tomy	
7. tympan/o/plasty	
8. audi/o/meter	
9. ot/o/scope	
10. salping/o/pharyng/eal	

Competency Verification: Check your answers in Appendix B: Answer Key, page 617. If you are not satisfied with your level of comprehension, review the vocabulary, and retake the review.

Correct Answers _____ x 10 = _____ % Score

11–37 The ear can be divided into three anatomical sections: external, middle, and inner. (See Figure 11-5.) The external ear includes the (1) **auricle,** which directs sound waves to the (2) **ear canal.** Eventually, the sound waves hit the (3) **tympanic membrane** (eardrum) and make the eardrum vibrate. Transmission of sound waves ultimately generates impulses that are transmitted to and interpreted by the brain as sound. Label Figure 11-5 as you learn about the ear.

ot/o/scopy
ō-TŎS-kŏ-pē

ot/o/scope
Ō-tō-skōp

11–38 The CF *ot/o* refers to the ear.

Ear infections can be diagnosed with an ot/o/scope as shown in Figure 11-6. Visual examination of the ear is known as _____/_____/_____.

The instrument to examine the ear is known as an

_____/_____/_____.

ot/algia
ō-TĂL-jē-ă

11–39 Swimmer's ear, resulting from an infection transmitted in the water of a swimming pool, may cause severe ot/o/dynia or _____/_____.

Pink indicates a prefix. Blue indicates a suffix. Boldface indicates a word root or combining form.

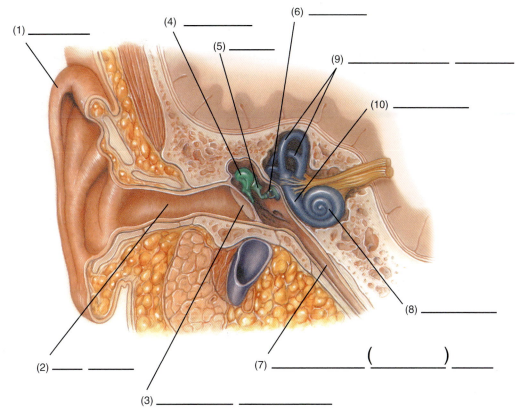

(1) _____ _____

(4) _____ _____

(5) _____

(6) _____

(9) _____ _____

(10) _____

(8) _____

(2) ____ _____

(7) _____ (_____) _____

(3) _____ _____

Figure 11-5 Ear structures.

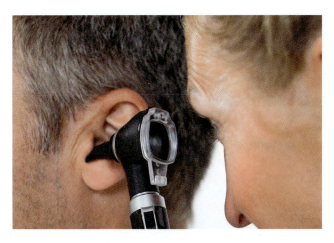

Figure 11-6 Examination with an otoscope.

ot/o/plasty Ō-tō-plăs-tē	**11–40** Surgical repair, or *plastic surgery,* of the ear (to correct defects and deformities) is a procedure known as _____/_____/_____.
URI	**11–41** Ot/itis media, infection of the middle ear, usually occurs after upper respiratory infection (URI). During ot/o/scopy, redness and stiffness of the tympanic membrane are observed, indicating inflammation. The abbreviation for upper respiratory infection is _____.

myring/o/tomy mĭr-ĭn-GŎT-ō-mē	**11-42** Ot/itis media caused by bacteria is commonly treated with antibiotics. When the condition persists and becomes chronic, a myring/o/tomy may be required. During this surgical procedure, a pressure-equalizing (PE) tube is inserted into the eardrum to relieve pressure and promote drainage. (See Figure 11-7.) Build the medical word that means *incision into the eardrum.* _____/_____/_____
eardrum	**11-43** The CFs *tympan/o* and *myring/o* refer to the tympanic membrane (eardrum). Tympan/itis is an inflammation of the tympanic membrane, or _____.
tympan/o, myring/o	**11-44** The tympan/ic membrane is stretched across the end of the ear canal and vibrates when sound waves strike it. The CFs for the tympanic membrane (eardrum) are _____/_____ and _____/_____.

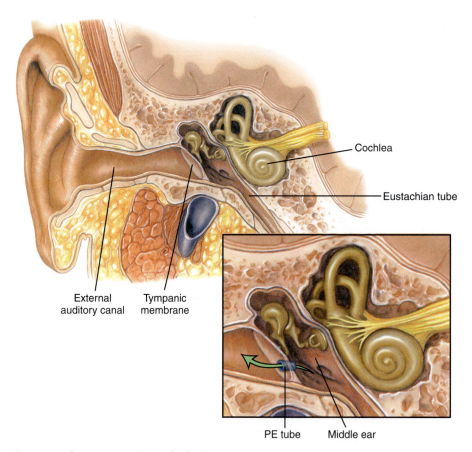

Figure 11-7   Placement of pressure-equalizing (PE) tubes.

11–45 Vibrations of the tympanic membrane are transmitted to the three auditory bones in the middle ear: the (4) **malleus,** the (5) **incus,** and the (6) **stapes.** The (7) **eustachian (auditory) tube** leads from the middle ear to the nasopharynx and permits air to enter or leave the middle ear cavity. Label and review the position of the middle ear structures in Figure 11-5.

---

salping/itis
săl-pĭn-JĪ-tĭs

11–46 The CF *salping/o* means tube (*usually fallopian or eustachian [auditory] tubes*). Inflammation of the eustachian tube would be diagnosed as _____/_____.

---

salping/o/scope
săl-PĬNG-gō-skōp

salping/o/scopy
săl-pĭng-GŎS-kō-pē

salping/o/stenosis
săl-pĭng-gō-stĕn-NŌ-sĭs

11–47 The eustachian tube equalizes air pressure in the middle ear with that of the outside atmosphere. Air pressure must be equalized for the eardrum to vibrate properly.

Build medical words that mean

instrument for examining the eustachian tube: _____/_____/_____.

visual examination of the eustachian tube: _____/_____/_____.

narrowing or stricture of the eustachian tube: _____/_____/_____.

11–48 Components of the inner ear include the (8) **cochlea** for hearing, the (9) **semicircular canals** for equilibrium, and the (10) **vestibule,** which is a chamber that joins the cochlea and semicircular canals. The inner surface of the cochlea is lined with highly sensitive nerve structures for hearing called the *organ of Corti.* Label inner ear structures in Figure 11-5.

11–49 The inner ear, also called the *labyrinth,* consists of a circular, mazelike structure, all of which contain the functional organs for hearing and equilibrium. The structures that make up the labyrinth are illustrated in Figure 11-8.

Use your medical dictionary to define labyrinth and list two types of inner ear labyrinths.

_____

_____

---

ot/o

11–50 The CF *ot/o* refers to the ear. From *ot/o/sclero/sis,* determine the CF for ear.

_____/_____

---

ot/o/sclerosis
ō-tō-sklĕ-RŌ-sĭs

11–51 Ot/o/sclerosis is a hereditary condition of unknown cause in which irregular ossification occurs in the ossicles of the middle ear, especially of the stapes, causing hearing loss.

Chronic progressive deafness, especially for low tones, may be caused by a hereditary condition called _____/_____/_____.

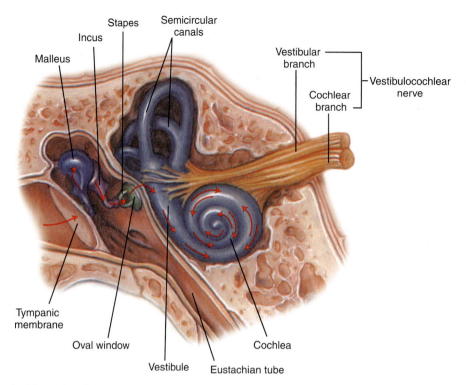

Malleus
Incus
Stapes
Semicircular canals
Vestibular branch
Cochlear branch
Vestibulocochlear nerve
Tympanic membrane
Oval window
Vestibule
Eustachian tube
Cochlea

Figure 11-8 The labyrinths of the inner ear, with arrows in the cochlea that indicate the *path of vibrations*.

staped/ectomy stā-pē-DĔK-tō-mē	**11-52** A patient diagnosed with ot/o/scler/osis may have hearing restored with a surgical procedure called *staped/ectomy*. To improve hearing, especially in cases of ot/o/scler/osis, the surgeon may excise the stapes using a surgical procedure called _____/_____.
staped/ectomy stā-pē-DĔK-tō-mē	**11-53** Staped/ectomy involves removal of the stapes and placement of a prosthesis to restore hearing. When the surgeon excises the stapes, the surgery performed is called _____/_____.
hearing	**11-54** Recall that the inner ear contains the receptors for two senses: hearing and equilibrium. The anterior portion, called the *cochlea,* is the part of the inner ear involved in hearing. The posterior portion, called the vestibular apparatus, is the part of the inner ear involved in maintenance of equilibrium and balance. The CFs *acous/o, audi/o,* and *audit/o* refer to _____.
audi/o/logist aw-dē-ŎL-ō-jĭst	**11-55** The branch of science that studies hearing, balance, and related disorders is known as *audi/o/logy*. It encompasses rehabilitation of persons with hearing impairments. The specialist in the study of hearing is called an _____/_____/_____.

Competency Verification: Check your labeling of Figure 11-5 in Appendix B: Answer Key, page 617.

Pink indicates a prefix. Blue indicates a suffix. Boldface indicates a word root or combining form.

SECTION REVIEW 11-3

Using the following table, write the CF, suffix, or prefix that matches its definition in the space provided to the left of the definition. There may be more than one word element that matches a definition.

Combining Forms

aden/o	myring/o
audi/o	ophthalm/o
blephar/o	ot/o
choroid/o	retin/o
corne/o	salping/o
dacry/o	scler/o
dipl/o	tympan/o
irid/o	xanth/o
kerat/o	

Suffixes

-acusis	-spasm
-edema	-stenosis
-logist	
-malacia	
-opia	
-opsia	
-ptosis	
-rrhexis	
-salpinx	

Prefixes

dipl-
hyper-

1. _____ excessive, above normal

2. _____ choroid

3. _____ horny tissue; hard; cornea

4. _____ double

5. _____ ear

6. _____ tube (usually fallopian or eustachian [auditory] tubes)

7. _____ eye

8. _____ eyelid

9. _____ gland

10. _____ hardening; sclera (white of the eye)

11. _____ involuntary contraction, twitching

12. _____ iris

13. _____ prolapse, downward displacement

14. _____ specialist in the study of

15. _____ retina

16. _____ rupture

17. _____ softening

18. _____ hearing

19. _____ narrowing, stricture

20. _____ swelling

21. _____ tear; lacrimal apparatus (duct, sac, or gland)

22. _____ tympanic membrane (eardrum)

23. _____ cornea

24. _____ vision

25. _____ yellow

Competency Verification: Check your answers in Appendix B: Answer Key, page 617. If you are not satisfied with your level of comprehension, go back to Frame 11–1, and rework the frames.

Correct Answers _____ x 4 = _____ % Score

Abbreviations

This section introduces abbreviations related to the eyes and ears and their meanings.

Abbreviation	Meaning	Abbreviation	Meaning
Eyes			
ARMD, AMD	age-related macular degeneration	LASIK	laser-assisted in situ keratomileusis
Ast	astigmatism	MD	muscular dystrophy, macular degeneration
ECCE	extracapsular cataract extraction	O.D.	doctor of optometry
IOL	intraocular lens	PERRLA	pupils equal, round, and reactive to light and accommodation
IOP	intraocular pressure	RK	radial keratotomy
IVFA	intravenous fluorescein angiography	VA	visual acuity
Ears			
AC	air conduction	OM	otitis media
BC	bone conduction	PE	physical examination; pulmonary embolism; pressure-equalizing (tube)
ENT	ear, nose, and throat	URI	upper respiratory infection
NIHL	noise-induced hearing loss		

Additional Medical Terms

The following are additional terms related to the eyes and ears. Recognizing and learning these terms will help you understand the connections among a pathological condition, its diagnosis, and the rationale behind the method of treatment selected for a particular disorder.

Diseases and Conditions

Eye

achromatopsia
ă-krō-mă-TŎP-sē-ă
 	
     a-: without, not
chromat: color
  -opsia: vision
	Congenital deficiency in color perception; also called color blindness
	
	Achromatopsia is more common in men.

astigmatism (Ast)
ă-STĬG-mă-tĭzm
 	
     a-: without, not
stigmat: point, mark
   -ism: condition
	Defective curvature of the cornea and lens, which causes light rays to focus unevenly over the retina, rather than being focused on a single point, resulting in a distorted image (See Figure 11-3.)

cataract KĂT-ă-răkt	Degenerative disease in which the lens of the eye becomes progressively cloudy, causing decreased vision (see Figure 11-9). *Cataracts are usually a result of the aging process and are caused by protein deposits on the surface of the lens that slowly build up until vision is lost. Treatment includes surgical intervention to remove the cataract.*

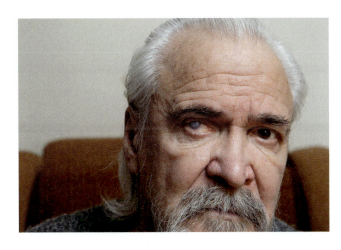

Figure 11-9 Cataract. This man has a cataract in the right eye. Left eye is normal.

diabetic retinopathy dī-ă-BĔT-ĭk rĕt-ĭn-ŎP-ă-thē *retin/o:* retina *-pathy:* disease	Retinal damage marked by aneurysmal dilation and bleeding of blood vessels or the formation of new blood vessels, causing visual changes *Diabetic retinopathy occurs in people with diabetes, manifested by small hemorrhages, edema, and formation of new vessels leading to scarring and eventual loss of vision.*
glaucoma glaw-KŌ-mă *glauc:* gray *-oma:* tumor	Condition in which aqueous humor fails to drain properly and accumulates in the anterior chamber of the eye, causing elevated intraocular pressure (IOP) (See Figure 11-10.) *Glaucoma eventually leads to loss of vision and, commonly, blindness. Treatment for glaucoma includes miotics (eye drops), which cause the pupils to constrict, permitting aqueous humor to escape from the eye, thereby relieving pressure. If miotics are ineffective, surgery may be necessary.*
open-angle	Most common form of glaucoma that results from degenerative changes that cause congestion and reduce flow of aqueous humor through the canal of Schlemm. *Open-angle glaucoma is painless but destroys peripheral vision, causing tunnel vision.*
closed-angle	Type of glaucoma caused by an anatomically narrow angle between the iris and the cornea, which prevents outflow of aqueous humor from the eye into the lymphatic system, causing a sudden increase in IOP *Closed-angle glaucoma constitutes an emergency situation. Symptoms include severe pain, blurred vision, and photophobia.*
hordeolum hor-DĒ-ō-lŭm	Small, purulent inflammatory infection of a sebaceous gland of the eyelid; also called *sty* (See Figure 11-11.)

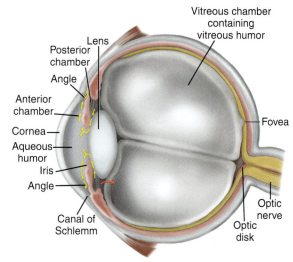

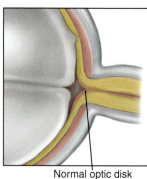

Figure 11-10   Glaucoma.

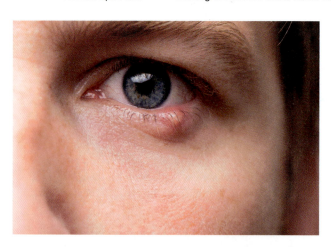

Figure 11-11   Hordeolum.

macular degeneration (MD) MĂK-ū-lăr	Breakdown of the tissues in the macula, resulting in loss of central vision *Macular degeneration is the most common cause of visual impairment in persons over age 50 years. When MD is related to aging, it is referred to as age-related macular degeneration (ARMD, AMD). (See Figure 11-12.)*
photophobia fō-tō-FŌ-bē-ă *phot/o:* light *-phobia:* fear	Unusual intolerance and sensitivity to light *Photophobia occurs in such disorders as meningitis, eye inflammation, measles, and rubella.*

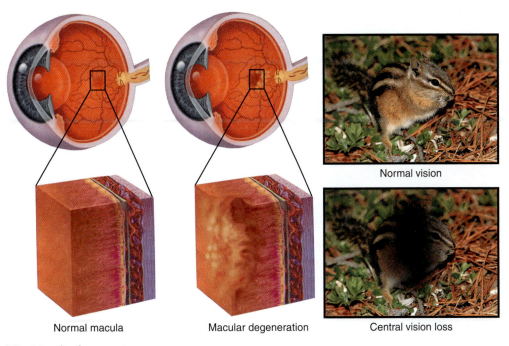

Normal macula   Macular degeneration   Central vision loss

Normal vision

Figure II-I2   Macular degeneration.

retinal detachment
RĔT-ĭ-năl
 	
   retin: retina
     -al: pertaining to
	Separation of the retina from the choroid, which disrupts vision and results in blindness if not repaired
	
	Retinal detachment may follow trauma, choroidal hemorrhages, or tumors and may be associated with diabetes mellitus.

strabismus stră-BĬZ-mŭs	Muscular eye disorder in which the eyes turn from the normal position so that they deviate in different directions *Various forms of strabismus are referred to as* tropias, *their direction being indicated by the appropriate prefix, such as* esotropia *and* exotropia. *(See Figure 11-13.)*

esotropia
    ĕs-ō-TRŌ-pē-ă
 	
       eso-: inward
     -tropia: turning
	Strabismus in which there is deviation of the visual axis of one eye toward that of the other eye, resulting in diplopia; also called cross-eye and convergent strabismus

exotropia
    ĕks-ō-TRŌ-pē-ă
 	
       exo-: outside,
             outward
     -tropia: turning
	Strabismus in which there is deviation of the visual axis of one eye away from that of the other eye, resulting in diplopia; also called wall-eye and divergent strabismus

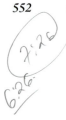

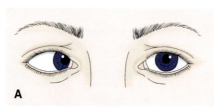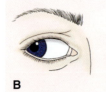

A   B

Figure 11-13   Types of strabismus. (A) Esotropia. (B) Exotropia.

Ear

acoustic neuroma a-KOOS-tĭk nū-RŌ-mă *acous:* hearing *-tic:* pertaining to *neur:* nerve *-oma:* tumor	Benign tumor that develops from the eighth cranial (vestibulocochlear) nerve and grows within the auditory canal *Depending on the location and size of the tumor, progressive hearing loss, headache, facial numbness, dizziness, and an unsteady gait may result.*
hearing loss	Decreased ability to perceive sounds compared with what the individual or examiner would regard as normal
anacusis ăn-ă-KŪ-sĭs *an-:* without, not *-acusis:* hearing	Total deafness (complete hearing loss)
conductive kŏn-DŬK-tĭv	Hearing loss resulting from any condition that prevents sound waves from being transmitted to the auditory receptors *Conductive hearing loss may result from wax obstructing the external auditory canal, inflammation of the middle ear, ankylosis of the ear bones, or fixation of the footplate of the stirrup.*
noise-induced	Hearing loss that results from exposure to very loud sounds *Working with noisy machinery; listening to loud music; or discharging rifles, guns, or explosives may cause noise-induced hearing loss (NIHL).*
sensorineural sĕn-sō-rē-NŪ-răl *sensori:* to feel *neur:* nerve *-al:* pertaining to	Hearing loss caused by permanent or temporary damage to the sensory cells or nerve fibers of the inner ear
Ménière disease mĕn-ē-ĀR	Rare disorder of unknown etiology within the labyrinth of the inner ear that can lead to a progressive loss of hearing; also called *endolymphatic/labyrinthine hydrops* *Symptoms of Ménière disease include vertigo, hearing loss, tinnitus, and a sensation of pressure in the ear.*

otitis externa
ō-TĪ-tĭs
 	
    ot: ear
    -itis: inflammation
	Infection of the external auditory canal
	
	Otitis externa can develop when water remains in the outer ear canal, most commonly after swimming (swimmer's ear). Other causes include allergies, eczema, and a foreign object lodged in the ear.

otitis media (OM)
ō-TĪ-tĭs MĒ-dē-ă
 	
    ot: ear
    -itis: inflammation
    med: middle
    -ia: condition
	Inflammation of the middle ear, which is commonly the result of an upper respiratory infection (URI)

serous	Noninfectious inflammation of the middle ear with accumulation of serum (clear fluid) *Treatment for serous OM may include myringotomy to aspirate fluid and the surgical insertion of pressure-equalizing (PE) tubes. (See Figure 11-7.)*
suppurative	Inflammation of the middle ear with pus formation *Suppurative OM is a common affliction in infants and young children caused by the horizontal orientation and small diameter of the eustachian tube in such patients, which predisposes them to infection. If left untreated, complications include ruptured tympanic membrane, mastoiditis, labyrinthitis, hearing loss, and meningitis.*

presbycusis
prĕz-bĭ-KŪ-sĭs
 	
    presby: old age
    -cusis: hearing
	Impairment of hearing that results from the aging process

tinnitus tĭn-Ī-tĭs	Ringing or tinkling noise heard constantly or intermittently in one or both ears, even in a quiet environment *Tinnitus may be a sign of injury to the ear, some disease process, or toxic levels of some medications (e.g., aspirin).*
vertigo VĔR-tĭ-gō	Sensation of moving around in space or a feeling of spinning or dizziness *Vertigo usually results from damage to the inner ear structure that is associated with balance and equilibrium.*

Diagnostic Procedures

Eye

slit-lamp examination	Eye evaluation that provides a stereoscopic (three-dimensional) view of the eye's interior with use of a binocular microscope (slit lamp) of a high-intensity light source to accentuate the anatomical structure of the eye, allowing close inspection *The slit lamp provides greater magnification (10–25 times) and illumination than most handheld devices. (See Figure 11-14.)*

tonometry
tōn-ŎM-ĕ-trē
  ton/o: tension
  -metry: act of measuring
	Test to measure increased intraocular pressure (IOP) to detect glaucoma
	
	Tonometry is performed with the slit lamp, but also uses a sensor to depress the cornea or a short burst of air directed at the cornea to measure IOP. (See Figure 11-14.)

intravenous fluorescein angiography (IVFA)
  intra-: in, within
  ven: vein
  -ous: pertaining to
  angi/o: vessel (usually blood or lymph)
  -graphy: process of recording
	Imaging technique used to study retinal blood vessels and circulation of blood in the retina using photographs of the retina after injection of a fluorescent dye
	
	IVFA produces images that show retinal blood flow and an angiogram that helps detect vascular changes in diabetic retinopathy, macular degeneration, and retinal vascular disease, as well as other types of macular disease.

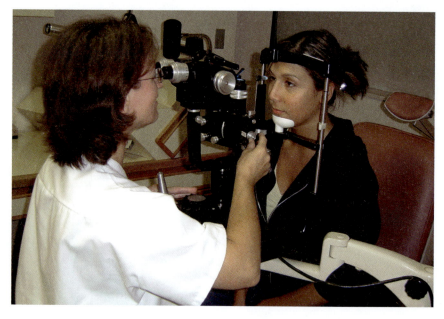

Figure 11-14 Slit-lamp examination measuring intraocular pressure by tonometry.

visual acuity (VA) test ă-KŪ-ĭ-tē	Examination that identifies the smallest letters that can be correctly read on a standardized Snellen vision chart from a distance of 20 feet. *VA is expressed as a ratio. The first number is the distance at which a person reads the chart, and the second number is the distance at which a person with normal vision can read the same chart. For example, 20/20 indicates that the person correctly reads at 20 feet letters that can be read by a person with normal vision at 20 feet. Normal vision is 20/20. (See Figure 11-15.)*

Ear

audiometry ăw-dē-ŎM-ĕ-trē *audi/o:* hearing *-metry:* act of measuring	Test that measures hearing acuity at various sound frequencies *In audiometry, an instrument called an audiometer delivers acoustic stimuli at different frequencies, and results are plotted on a graph called an* audiogram.

otoscopy ō-TŎS-kŏ-pē *ot/o:* ear *-scopy:* visual examination	Visual examination of the external auditory canal and the tympanic membrane by using an otoscope
pneumatic nū-MĂT-ĭk	Otoscopic procedure that assesses the ability of the tympanic membrane to move in response to a change in air pressure *In pneumatic otoscopy, the increase and decrease in pressure cause the healthy tympanic membrane to move in and out. Lack of movement indicates increased impedance or eardrum perforation.*

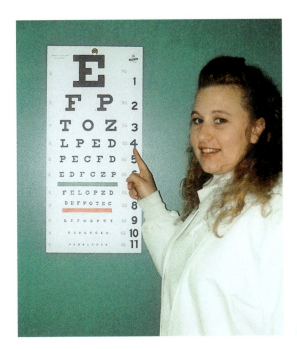

Figure 11-15   Snellen chart with letters.

tuning fork test	Hearing test that uses a turning fork (instrument that produces constant pitch when struck) that is struck and then placed against or near the bones on the side of the head to assess nerve and bone conduction of sound
	There are two types of tuning fork tests: the Rinne test and the Weber test.
Rinne RĬN-nē	Tuning fork test that evaluates bone conduction of sound in one ear at a time; also called air and bone conduction hearing test (See Figure 11-16.)
	The Rinne test is useful for differentiating between conductive hearing loss and sensorineural hearing loss.
Weber	Tuning fork test that evaluates bone conduction of sound in both ears at the same time; also called conductive and sensorineural hearing loss test
	During the Weber test, hearing sound equally in both ears indicates normal hearing.

Medical and Surgical Procedures

Eye

cataract surgery KĂT-ă-răkt	Excision of a lens affected by a cataract
	Extracapsular cataract extraction (ECCE) and phacoemulsification are the two primary ways to remove a cataract. In both surgeries, the central part of the lens is removed and replaced with an artificial intraocular lens (IOL) implant.
extracapsular cataract extraction (ECCE) ĕks-tră-KĂP-sū-lăr KĂT-ă-răkt	Excision of the anterior segment of the lens capsule along with the lens, allowing for the insertion of an IOL implant
phacoemulsification făk-ō-ē-mŭl-sĭ-fĭ-KĀ-shŭn	Excision of the lens by inserting an ultrasonic probe whose sound waves break the lens into tiny particles which are suctioned out of the eye and the IOL is implanted (See Figure 11-17.)

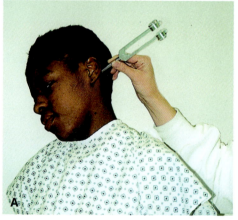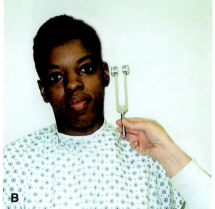

Figure 11-16   Rinne test. (A) Bone conduction. (B) Air conduction.

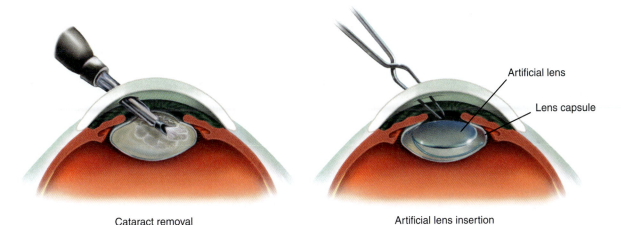

Cataract removal

Artificial lens insertion

Artificial lens

Lens capsule

Figure 11-17   Phacoemulsification.

corneal transplant KŎR-nē-ăl *corne:* cornea *-al:* pertaining to	Surgical transplantation of a donor cornea (from a cadaver) into the eye of a recipient; also called keratoplasty
iridectomy ĭr-ĭ-DĔK-tŏ-mē *irid:* iris *-ectomy:* excision, removal	Excision of a portion of the iris used to relieve intraocular pressure in patients with glaucoma *Iridectomy is usually performed to create an opening through which aqueous humor can drain.*
laser photocoagulation	Use of an argon laser to treat diabetic retinopathy by sealing leaking blood vessels in the retina; also called retinal photocoagulation *The laser uses the gas argon to produce blue-green wavelengths that are absorbed by the cells that lie under the retina and the red hemoglobin in blood but pass through fluid in the eye without damaging structures. Laser photocoagulation is also used to treat macular degeneration and to repair a detached retina. (See Figure 11-18.)*
laser-assisted in situ keratomileusis (LASIK)	Use of an excimer laser to correct errors of refraction, such as myopia, hyperopia, and astigmatism, by reshaping the cornea and improving visual acuity *LASIK provides a permanent alternative to wearing corrective lenses or contact lenses. Many patients who are treated with LASIK find an improvement of up to 20/20 vision. (See Figure 11-19.)*
vitrectomy vĭ-TRĔK-tō-mē	Removal of the vitreous gel from the middle of the eye and replacement of the gel with a clear artificial fluid *Vitrectomy may be performed in cases of retinal detachment, failure of blood to clear from the vitreous gel, scar tissue on the retina (complication of diabetic retinopathy), or tears or holes in the macula. (See Figure 11-20.)*

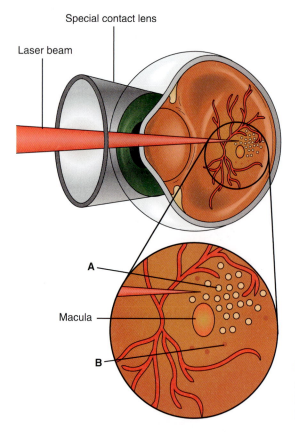

Laser beam

Special contact lens

A

Macula

B

Figure 11-18 Photocoagulation of the retina in diabetic retinopathy. (A) Retinal scars after laser treatment. (B) Untreated blood vessels that continue to bleed and cause visual distortion or blindness.

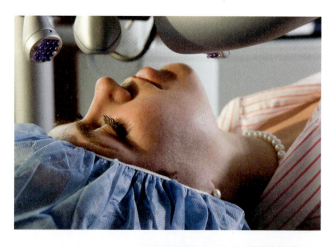

Figure 11-19 Lasik surgery.

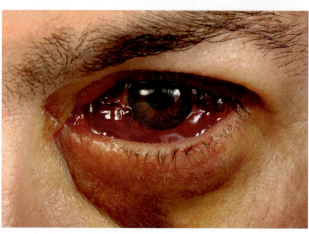

Figure 11-20 Vitrectomy.

Ear

cochlear implant KŎK-lē-ăr *cochle:* cochlea *-ar:* pertaining to	Electronic transmitter surgically implanted into the cochlea of a deaf person to restore hearing
ear irrigation	Process of flushing the external ear canal with sterile water or sterile saline solution to treat patients who complain of foreign body or cerumen (ear wax) impaction (See Figure 11-21.)

myringotomy
mĭr-ĭn-GŎT-ō-mē
myring/o: tympanic
        membrane
        (eardrum)
   -tomy: incision
	Incision of the eardrum to relieve pressure and release pus or serous fluid from the middle ear or to insert PE tubes (tympanostomy tubes) in the eardrum via surgery
	
	PE tubes provide ventilation and drainage of the middle ear when recurring ear infections do not respond to antibiotic treatment. They are used when persistent, severely negative middle ear pressure is present. (See Figure 11-7.)

Ear irrigation

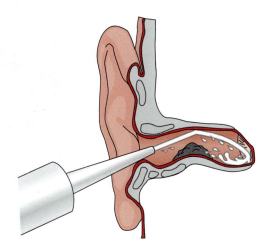

Figure 11-21   Ear irrigation.

Pharmacology

The following table lists common drug categories used to treat ophthalmology and otolaryngology disorders and their therapeutic actions.

Drug Category	Action
antiglaucoma agents ăn-tĭ-glaw-KŌ-mă	Reduce intraocular pressure by lowering the amount of aqueous humor in the eyeball, reducing its production or increasing its outflow
miotics mī-ŎT-ĭks	Cause the pupil to constrict *Miotics are used to treat glaucoma.*
mydriatics mĭd-rē-ĂT-ĭks	Cause the pupil to dilate and prepare the eye for an internal examination *Mydriatics provide accurate measurements for prescribing corrective lenses.*
vertigo and motion sickness drugs VĔR-tĭ-gō	Decrease sensitivity of the inner ear to motion and prevent nerve impulses from the inner ear from reaching the vomiting center of the brain
wax emulsifiers ē-MŬL-sĭ-fĭ-ĕrs	Loosen and help remove impacted cerumen (ear wax)

Pronunciation Help   *Long Sound*   ā in rāte   ē in rēbirth   ī in īsle   ō in ōver   ū in ūnite
Short Sound   ă in ăpple   ĕ in ĕver   ĭ in ĭt   ŏ in nŏt   ŭ in cŭt

Word Elements Review

This review provides a verification of word elements covered in this chapter. First, use a slash to break the term into its component parts, and identify each element by labeling it P for prefix, WR for word root, CF for combining form, and S for suffix. Then, provide the meaning of the medical term. Remember to define the suffix first, define the beginning of the word next, and define the middle part of the term last. The first word is a sample completed for you.

Term	Meaning
scler/itis WR S	*inflammation of the sclera (white of the eye)*
1. intra/ocul/ar	
2. myring/o/tomy	
3. ophthalm/o/scope	
4. tympan/o/plasty	
5. blephr/o/ptosis	

Match the following medical terms with the definitions in the numbered list.

anacusis   coreometer   iridocele   otalgia
anisocoria   conjunctivitis   keratoplasty   retinopathy
audiologist   dacryorrhea   optic   salpingostenosis

6. _____ specialist in the study of hearing

7. _____ inflammation of the conjunctiva

8. _____ without hearing; total deafness

9. _____ pertaining to the eye or vision

10. _____ flow or discharge of tears

11. _____ narrowing or stricture of the eustachian tube

12. _____ disease of the retina

13. _____ pain in the ear

14. _____ instrument for measuring the pupil

15. _____ condition of unequal or dissimilar pupil size

Competency Verification: Check your answers in Appendix B: Answer Key, page 618. If you are not satisfied with your level of comprehension, review the vocabulary, and retake the review.

Correct Answers _____ × 6.67 = _____ % Score

Additional Medical Terms Review

Match the following medical terms with the definitions in the numbered list.

achromatopsia	diabetic retinopathy	myringotomy	retinal detachment
acoustic neuroma	glaucoma	otitis media	Rinne test
anacusis	hordeolum	otosclerosis	strabismus
astigmatism	macular degeneration	phacoemulsification	tinnitus
cataract	Ménière disease	photophobia	tonometry
conductive hearing loss	mydriatics	presbycusis	vertigo
conjunctivitis			

1. _____ means *ringing in the ears.*

2. _____ is progressive deafness caused by ossification in the bony labyrinth of the inner ear.

3. _____ means *color blindness.*

4. _____ is a rare disorder characterized by progressive deafness, vertigo, and tinnitus.

5. _____ is a disorder in which both eyes cannot focus on the same point, resulting in looking in different directions at the same time.

6. _____ means *total deafness.*

7. _____ refers to middle ear infection that is most commonly seen in young children.

8. _____ refers to pinkeye.

9. _____ means *intolerance or unusual sensitivity to light.*

10. _____ is hearing loss resulting from aging.

11. _____ refers to intraocular pressure caused by the failure of the aqueous humor to drain.

12. _____ refers to a feeling of spinning or dizziness.

13. _____ refers to separation of the retina from the choroid.

14. _____ is another term for sty.

15. _____ is abnormal curvature of the cornea, which causes light rays to focus unevenly over the retina, resulting in a distorted image.

16. _____ is a benign tumor of the eighth cranial nerve.

17. _____ measures intraocular pressure and is used to diagnose glaucoma.

18. _____ cause dilation of the pupil to enable internal examination of the eye.

19. _____ is caused by an impairment in sound transmission because of damage to the eardrum or ossicles or by ear canal obstruction.

20. _____ refers to opacity (cloudiness) of the lens as a result of protein deposits on its surface.

21. _____ is a type of cataract surgery.

22. _____ is a hearing acuity test that is performed with a vibrating tuning fork.

23. _____ refers to retinal damage marked by aneurysmal dilation of blood vessels.

24. _____ is loss of central vision due to the aging process.

25. _____ is an incision of the eardrum to relieve pressure and release pus or serous fluid from the middle ear.

Competency Verification: Check your answers in Appendix B: Answer Key, page 618. If you are not satisfied with your level of comprehension, review the additional medical terms, and retake the review.

Correct Answers _____ × 4 = _____ % Score

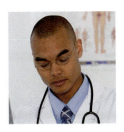

Medical Record Activities

To develop a working vocabulary of medical terms and to understand how those terms are used in the health-care industry, it is important that you complete the following activities.

MEDICAL RECORD ACTIVITY 11-1

OPERATIVE REPORT: RETINAL DETACHMENT REPAIR

This activity contains an operative report for repair of a retinal detachment. Read the report that follows and underline the medical terms. Then complete the terminology and critical thinking exercises.

OPERATIVE REPORT

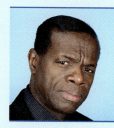

PATIENT NAME: Holler, Henry
MEDICAL RECORD ID: 41-99083
DATE: May 25, 20xx

PREOPERATIVE DIAGNOSIS: Total retinal detachment, left eye, secondary to complications of retinitis.

POSTOPERATIVE DIAGNOSIS: Total retinal detachment, left eye, secondary to complications of retinitis.

PROCEDURE: Retinal detachment repair

DESCRIPTION OF PROCEDURE: Patient was taken to the operating room, placed on the operating table, IV infusion started, electrocardiography (ECG) lead monitor attached, and retrobulbar anesthetic given, resulting in good anesthesia and akinesia. The patient was scrubbed, prepped, and draped in a standard sterile fashion for retinal surgery. A 360-degree conjunctival opening was made, and 2-0 silk sutures were placed around each rectus muscle. Four millimeters from the limbus, a mark was made in the sclera, and preplaced 5-0 Mersilene suture was passed. A mitrovitreoretinal stab incision was made, and a 4-mm infusion cannula was slipped into position and visualized inside the eye. Similar sclerotomy sites were made superior nasally and superior temporally. Trans pars plana vitrectomy was undertaken. Dense vitreous hemorrhage and debris were found and removed. There was incomplete posterior vitreous attachment. The retina was almost totally detached, and a small amount of nasal retina was still attached. A linear retinal break was seen just above the disk along a vessel. Gradually, all of the peripheral vitreous was removed.

Air–fluid exchange was performed, but with some difficulty because some vitreous was found anteriorly, loculating the bubble. It gave a peculiar view, but slowly the retina became totally flat, and we treated the retinal break with the diode laser. A 240 band was wrapped around the eye and fixed with the Watke sleeve superior temporally. The sclerotomies were all sewn closed. Before the last sclerotomy was closed, the air was exchanged for silicone. The eye was left soft because the patient had poor perfusion. The patient left the operating room in satisfactory condition.

Cathy Cannan, M.D.
_____
Cathy Cannan, M.D.

CC:sr
D: 5/25/20xx; T: 5/25/20xx

Terminology 11-1

Terms listed in the following table come from the previous Operative Report: Retinal Detachment Repair. Use a medical dictionary, such as Taber's Cyclopedic Medical Dictionary; *the appendices of this book; or other resources to define each term. Then, pronounce the term, and place a checkmark (✓) in the box after you do so.*

Term	Definition
akinesia ă-kĭ-NĒ-zē-ă ☐	
cannula KĂN-ū-lă ☐	
conjunctival kŏn-jŭnk-TĪ-văl ☐	
limbus LĬM-bŭs ☐	
mm	
retinal detachment| RĔT-ĭ-năl ☐	
retrobulbar rĕt-rō-BŬL-băr ☐	
sclerotomy sklĕ-RŎT-ō-mē ☐	
vitrectomy vĭ-TRĔK-tō-mē ☐	

 Visit the *Medical Terminology Simplified* online resource center at FADavis.com to hear pronunciation and meanings of the selected terms in this medical report listed in the previous table.

Critical Thinking 11-1

Review the Operative Report: Retinal Detachment Repair above to answer the following questions. Use a medical dictionary, such as Taber's Cyclopedic Medical Dictionary, *and other resources, if needed.*

1. Where is the retina located?

_____

_____

2. Was the anesthetic administered behind or in front of the eyeball?

_____

_____

3. How much movement remained in the eye after anesthesia?

_____

_____

4. Where was the hemorrhage located?

_____

_____

5. What type of vitrectomy was undertaken?

_____

_____

6. Why was the eye left soft?

_____

_____

MEDICAL RECORD ACTIVITY 11-2

SOAP NOTE: OTITIS MEDIA

This activity is based on an office visit for a child accompanied by her mother and is diagnosed with otitis media in the left ear. Read the SOAP note that follows, and underline the medical terms. Then, complete the terminology and critical thinking exercises.

SOAP NOTE

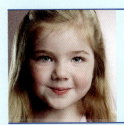

PATIENT NAME: Strew, Mary
MEDICAL RECORD ID: 34-27887
DATE: December 1, 20xx

SUBJECTIVE: The patient, accompanied by her mother, presents with fever and irritability that had lasted for the last couple of days. According to the mother, the patient had some upper respiratory symptoms, including a runny nose and clear discharge, for about 8 days. The patient had a little bit of a cough but no shortness of breath or noticeable difficulty breathing. The patient was seen in our office last week and her lungs had been clear at the time. She was diagnosed with a viral infection and advised to return if her condition got worse. Yesterday, she developed a temperature of 104°F, and this morning, it was again 104°F. The patient had been eating well until about 2 days ago and now is not eating so well, but she is drinking lots of juice, according to her mother.

OBJECTIVE: Vital signs revealed a temperature of 102.2°F axillary. In general, this is a minimally to mildly ill-appearing 4-year-old girl, who is crying and appears agitated during the examination, but she is in no acute distress. **HEENT:** The pupils were equal, round, and reactive to light. Extraocular movements were intact. The left tympanic membrane was red. Right tympanic membrane was pink. The oropharynx was red, especially the left tonsil. No exudates and no petechiae were noted. The mucous membranes were moist. The neck was supple and had full range of motion. No significant lymphadenopathy was present. **PULMONARY:** Lungs were clear, with good aeration throughout. **CARDIAC:** Heart rate and rhythm were regular. No murmurs were appreciated. The skin revealed no significant rash upon examination.

LABORATORY DATA: Rapid strep was negative.

ASSESSMENT: Left otitis media.

PLAN:
1. Prescription for amoxicillin 200 mg per 5 mL, 1 teaspoon b.i.d. 10 days.
2. Alternate with Tylenol and ibuprofen throughout the day to keep the fever down.
3. Patient to come for follow-up appointment in two weeks to ensure resolution of the ear infection, but sooner if any of her symptoms persist or worsen.

Robert S. Dukota, M.D.

Robert S. Dukota, M.D.

RD:ks
D: 11/19/20xx; T: 11/19/20xx

Terminology 11-2

Terms listed in the following table come from the previous SOAP Note: Otitis Media. Use a medical dictionary, such as Taber's Cyclopedic Medical Dictionary; the appendices of this book; or other resources to define each term. Then, pronounce the term, and place a checkmark (✓) in the box after you do so.

Term	Definition
amoxicillin ă-mŏk-sĭ-SĬL-ĭn ☐	
axillary ĂK-sĭ-lăr-ē ☐	
extraocular ĕks-tră-ŎK-yū-lăr ☐	
exudates ĔKS-ū-dāts ☐	
lymphadenopathy lĭm-făd-ĕ-NŎP-ă-thē ☐	
oropharynx or-ō-FĂR-ĭnks ☐	
otitis media ō-TĪ-tĭs MĒ-dē-ă ☐	
petechiae pē-TĒ-kē-ă ☐	
rapid strep	
tympanic membrane tĭm-PĂN-ĭk MĔM-brān ☐	

 Visit the *Medical Terminology Simplified* online resource center at FADavis.com to hear pronunciation and meanings of terms in this medical report.

Critical Thinking 11-2

Review the SOAP Note: Otitis Media above to answer the following questions. Use a medical dictionary, such as Taber's Cyclopedic Medical Dictionary, *and other resources, if needed.*

1. What was the chief complaint that brought the child to the clinic?

   _____

   _____

2. What laboratory test(s) were performed in the clinic?

   _____

   _____

3. Where was the patient's infection located?

   _____

   _____

4. What medication(s) was prescribed for the patient's infection?

   _____

   _____

5. What medication(s) was prescribed for the patient's fever?

   _____

   _____

MEDICAL RECORD ACTIVITY 11-3

CLINICAL APPLICATION

This activity is a clinical application that will help you integrate and reinforce your understanding of how the following medical terms are used in the clinical environment. Complete the following clinically related sentences by selecting an appropriate term from the list.

achromatopsia	conjunctivitis	mydriatics	presbycusis
audiometry	esotropia	myringotomy	tonometry
cochlear implant	iridectomy	photophobia	wax emulsifiers

1. A 66-year-old male complains of bilateral hearing loss that has worsened over the last year. The physician performs a series of hearing tests and diagnoses him with a type of hearing deficit that is related to the aging process. This condition is known as _____.

2. Denise, a 6-year-old female, complains of red, itchy eyes. Upon examination, the physician diagnoses her with inflammation of the eye, commonly caused by a bacterium or virus. This condition is commonly called *pinkeye* or _____.

3. Mr. B. complains of recurrent migraine headaches with eye pain and a sensitivity to light. His physician tells him that sensitivity to light will commonly accompany a migraine and is a condition called _____.

4. Lori is a 68-year-old female who presents with complaints of progressive vision loss and eye pain. The physician performs a test to measure the pressure of the intraocular fluid and diagnoses her with glaucoma. The diagnostic test used to detect glaucoma is _____.

5. A 29-year-old male presents for a Department of Transportation physical examination. During the Ishihara color plate test, he is unable to distinguish many of the numbers. The physician diagnoses him with color blindness, also known as _____.

6. Bobbie is a 4-year-old female who is diagnosed with bilateral nerve deafness. The physician explains there is a device that can be placed within the inner ear to help restore her hearing. This type of electronic transmitter is known as a(n) _____.

7. A 38-year-old female complains of chronic blurry vision. The ophthalmologist administers eye drops to dilate the pupils to see the internal structures of the eye and detect abnormalities. Medications that dilate the pupil for an internal examination of the eye are known as _____.

8. Mitzy, a 7-year-old girl accompanied by her parents, presents to the pediatrician with complaints of vision problems and an abnormal inward turning of her right eye. After a series of examinations, the physician diagnoses her with a type of strabismus known as _____.

9. This 28-year-old male complains of diminished hearing in both ears. Otoscopic examination of the external auditory canal reveals impacted cerumen bilaterally. The practitioner administers drops of medication to loosen and help remove the cerumen. Agents that perform this action are known as _____.

10. An 8-year-old female is diagnosed with acute otitis media. A procedure is recommended in which an incision is made in the eardrum to allow the build-up of fluids in the middle ear to drain into the ear canal. This surgical procedure to incise the tympanic membrane (eardrum) is called a(n) _____.

Correct Answers: _____ × 10 = _____ % Score

Competency Verification: Check your answers in Appendix B: Answer Key, page 619. If you are not satisfied with your level of comprehension, review the material in this chapter, and retake the review.

SPECIAL SENSES: EYES AND EARS CHAPTER REVIEW

WORD ELEMENTS SUMMARY

The following table summarizes CFs, suffixes, and prefixes related to the special senses. Study the word elements and their meanings before completing the Vocabulary Review that follows.

Word Element	Meaning	Word Element	Meaning
Combining Forms			
acous/o, audi/o, audit/o	hearing	**my/o**	muscle
blephar/o	eyelid	**myring/o, tympan/o**	tympanic membrane (eardrum)
choroid/o	choroid	**neur/o**	nerve
chromat/o	color	**ocul/o, ophthalm/o**	eye
cochle/o	cochlea	**ot/o**	ear
corne/o	cornea	**presby/o**	old age
dacry/o, lacrim/o	tear; lacrimal apparatus (duct, sac, or gland)	**retin/o**	retina
dipl/o	double	**salping/o**	tube (usually fallopian or eustachian [auditory] tubes)
erythr/o	red	**scler/o**	hardening; sclera (white of the eye)
irid/o	iris	**ton/o**	tension
kerat/o	horny tissue; hard; cornea	**xanth/o**	yellow
Suffixes			
-acusis	hearing	**-pathy**	disease
-algia, -dynia	pain	**-plasty**	surgical repair
-ectomy	excision, removal	**-ptosis**	prolapse, downward displacement
-edema	swelling	**-rrhexis**	rupture
-logist	specialist in the study of	**-salpinx**	tube (usually fallopian or eustachian [auditory] tubes)
-logy	study of	**-scope**	instrument for examining
-malacia	softening	**-scopy**	visual examination
-metry	act of measuring	**-spasm**	involuntary contraction, twitching
-oma	tumor	**-stenosis**	narrowing, stricture
-opia, -opsia	vision	**-tomy**	incision
-osis	abnormal condition; increase (used primarily with blood cells)	**-tropia**	turning

Continued

Word Element	Meaning	Word Element	Meaning
Prefixes			
a-	without; not	**eso-**	inward
ana-	against; up; back	**exo-**	outside, outward
dipl-	Double	**hyper-**	excessive, above normal

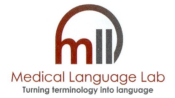

Medical Language Lab
Turning terminology into language

Visit the *Medical Language Lab* at *medicallanguagelab.com*. Use the flash-card activity to reinforce your study of word elements. We recommend you complete the flash-card activity before starting the following Vocabulary Chapter Review.

Vocabulary Review

Match the following medical terms with the definitions in the numbered list.

blepharoptosis	*diplopia*	*mastoid surgery*	*otitis media*
cholesteatoma	*general anesthetic*	*miotics*	*postoperatively*
chronic	*hyperopia*	*mucoserous*	*salpingostenosis*
dacryorrhea	*keratitis*	*myopia*	*sclera*
diagnosis	*labyrinth*	*ophthalmologist*	*tympanic membrane*

1. _____ means *double vision*.

2. _____ refers to the white of the eye.

3. _____ is the eardrum; it vibrates when soundwaves strike it.

4. _____ means *excessive flow of tears*.

5. _____ cause the pupil to constrict.

6. _____ refers to inflammation of the cornea caused by a vision-threatening infection and sometimes occurs when contact lenses are not disinfected properly.

7. _____ is a process of determining the cause and nature of a pathological condition.

8. _____ means *composed of mucus and serum*.

9. _____ is inflammation of the middle ear.

10. _____ is a tumorlike sac filled with keratin debris most commonly found in the middle ear.

11. _____ is an operation on the mastoid process of the temporal bone.

12. _____ is anesthesia that affects the entire body with loss of consciousness.

13. _____ is a physician who specializes in the treatment of eye disorders.

14. _____ means *of long duration,* designating a disease showing little change or slow progression.

15. _____ means *farsightedness*.

16. _____ means *occurring after surgery*.

17. _____ is a system of intercommunicating canals, especially of the inner ear.

18. _____ is prolapse of an eyelid.

19. _____ is narrowing or stricture of the eustachian tube.

20. _____ means *nearsightedness*.

Competency Verification: Check your answers in Appendix B: Answer Key, page 619. If you are not satisfied with your level of comprehension, review the chapter vocabulary, and retake the review.

Correct Answers: _____ × 5 = _____ % Score

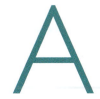
Glossary of Medical Word Elements

The following glossary contains an alphabetical list of medical word elements with corresponding meanings.

Medical Word Element	Meaning	Medical Word Element	Meaning
A		-algia	pain
a-	without; not	allo-	other, differing from the normal
ab-	from; away from	alveol/o	alveolus; air sac
abdomin/o	abdomen	ambly/o	dull, dim
abort/o	to miscarry	amni/o	amnion (amniotic sac)
-ac	pertaining to	an-	without; not
acid/o	acid	an/o	anus
acous/o	hearing	ana-	against; up; back
acr/o	extremity	andr/o	male
acromi/o	acromion (projection of the scapula)	aneurysm/o	widened blood vessel
		angi/o	vessel (usually blood or lymph)
-acusis	hearing	aniso-	unequal; dissimilar
ad-	toward	ankyl/o	stiffness; bent, crooked
-ad	toward	ante-	before, in front of
aden/o	gland	anter/o	anterior, front
adenoid/o	adenoids	anthrac/o	coal, coal dust
adip/o	fat	anti-	against
adren/o	adrenal glands	aort/o	aorta
adrenal/o	adrenal glands	append/o	appendix
aer/o	air	appendic/o	appendix
af-	toward	aque/o	water
agglutin/o	clumping, gluing	-ar	pertaining to
agora-	marketplace	-arche	beginning
-al	pertaining to	arteri/o	artery
albin/o	white	arteriol/o	arteriole
albumin/o	albumin (protein)	arthr/o	joint
-algesia	pain		

Continued

Medical Word Element	Meaning	Medical Word Element	Meaning
-ary	pertaining to	cauter/o	heat, burn
asbest/o	asbestos	cec/o	cecum
-asthenia	weakness, debility	-cele	hernia; swelling
astr/o	star	-centesis	surgical puncture
-ate	having the form of; possessing	cephal/o	head
atel/o	incomplete; imperfect	-ceps	head
ather/o	fatty plaque	-ception	conceiving
-ation	process (of)	cerebell/o	cerebellum
atri/o	atrium	cerebr/o	cerebrum
audi/o	hearing	cervic/o	neck; cervix uteri (neck of the uterus)
audit/o	hearing		
aur/o	ear	chalic/o	limestone
auricul/o	ear	cheil/o	lip
auto-	self, own	chem/o	chemical; drug
ax/o	axis; axon	chlor/o	green
azot/o	nitrogenous compounds	chol/e	bile, gall
		cholangi/o	bile vessel
B		cholecyst/o	gallbladder
bacteri/o	bacteria (singular, *bacterium*)	choledoch/o	bile duct
balan/o	glans penis	chondr/o	cartilage
bas/o	base (alkaline, opposite of acid)	chori/o	chorion
bi-	two	choroid/o	choroid
bi/o	life	chrom/o	color
bil/i	bile, gall	chromat/o	color
-blast	embryonic cell	-cide	killing
blast/o	embryonic cell	cine-	movement
blephar/o	eyelid	circum-	around
brachi/o	arm	cirrh/o	yellow
brachy-	short	-cision	a cutting
brady-	slow	-clasia	to break; surgical fracture
bronch/o	bronchus (plural, *bronchi*)	-clasis	to break; surgical fracture
bronchi/o	bronchus (plural, *bronchi*)	-clast	to break; surgical fracture
bronchiol/o	bronchiole	clavicul/o	clavicle (collar bone)
bucc/o	cheek	-cleisis	closure
		clon/o	clonus (turmoil)
C		-clysis	irrigation, washing
calc/o	calcium	coccyg/o	coccyx (tailbone)
calcane/o	calcaneum (heel bone)	cochle/o	cochlea
-capnia	carbon dioxide (CO_2)	col/o	colon
carcin/o	cancer	colon/o	colon
cardi/o	heart	colp/o	vagina
-cardia	heart condition	condyl/o	condyle
carp/o	carpus (wrist bones)	coni/o	dust
cata-	down		
caud/o	tail		

Medical Word Element	Meaning	Medical Word Element	Meaning
conjunctiv/o	conjunctiva	dipl/o	double
-continence	to hold back	dips/o	thirst
contra-	against; opposite	-dipsia	thirst
cor/o	pupil	dist/o	far, farthest
core/o	pupil	dors/o	back (of the body)
corne/o	cornea	duct/o	to lead; carry
coron/o	heart	-duction	act of leading, bringing, conducting
corp/o	body	duoden/o	duodenum (first part of the small intestine)
corpor/o	body		
cortic/o	cortex	dur/o	dura mater; hard
cost/o	ribs	-dynia	pain
crani/o	cranium (skull)	dys-	bad; painful; difficult
crin/o	secrete	**E**	
-crine	secrete	-eal	pertaining to
cruci/o	cross	ec-	out; out from
cry/o	cold	echo-	a repeated sound
crypt/o	hidden	-ectasis	dilation, expansion
culd/o	cul-de-sac	ecto-	outside; outward
-cusia	hearing	-ectomy	excision, removal
-cusis	hearing	-edema	swelling
cutane/o	skin	ef-	away from
cyan/o	blue	electr/o	electricity
cycl/o	ciliary body of the eye; circular; cycle	-ema	state of; condition
		embol/o	embolus (plug)
-cyesis	pregnancy	-emesis	vomiting
cyst/o	bladder	-emia	blood condition
cyt/o	cell	emphys/o	to inflate
-cyte	cell	en-	in, within
D		encephal/o	brain
dacry/o	tear; lacrimal apparatus (duct, sac, or gland)	end-	in, within
		endo-	in, within
dacryocyst/o	lacrimal sac	enter/o	intestine (usually small intestine)
dactyl/o	fingers; toes	eosin/o	dawn (rose-colored)
de-	cessation	epi-	above; upon
dendr/o	tree	epididym/o	epididymis
dent/o	teeth	epiglott/o	epiglottis
derm/o	skin	episi/o	vulva
-derma	skin	erythem/o	red
dermat/o	skin	erythemat/o	red
-desis	binding, fixation (of a bone or joint)	erythr/o	red
		eschar/o	scab
di-	double	-esis	condition
dia-	through; across		
dipl-	double		

Continued

Medical Word Element	Meaning	Medical Word Element	Meaning
eso-	inward	-grade	to go
esophag/o	esophagus	-graft	transplantation
esthes/o	feeling	-gram	record, writing
-esthesia	feeling	granul/o	granule
eti/o	cause	-graph	instrument for recording
eu-	good; normal	-graphy	process of recording
ex-	out; out from	-gravida	pregnant woman
exo-	outside; outward	gyn/o	woman, female
extra-	outside	gynec/o	woman, female
F		**H**	
faci/o	face	hallucin/o	hallucination
fasci/o	band, fascia (fibrous membrane supporting and separating muscles)	hedon/o	pleasure
		hem/o	blood
femor/o	femur (thigh bone)	hemangi/o	blood vessel
-ferent	to carry	hemat/o	blood
fibr/o	fiber, fibrous tissue	hemi-	one half
fibul/o	fibula (smaller bone of the lower leg)	hepat/o	liver
		hetero-	different
fluor/o	luminous, fluorescent	hidr/o	sweat
G		hist/o	tissue
galact/o	milk	histi/o	tissue
gangli/o	ganglion (knot or knotlike mass)	home/o	same, alike
gastr/o	stomach	homeo-	same, alike
-gen	forming, producing; origin	homo-	same
gen/o	forming, producing; origin	humer/o	humerus (upper arm bone)
-genesis	forming, producing; origin	hydr/o	water
genit/o	genitalia	hyp-	under, below; deficient
gest/o	pregnancy	hyp/o	under, below; deficient
gingiv/o	gum(s)	hyper-	excessive; above normal
glauc/o	gray	hypn/o	sleep
gli/o	glue; neuroglial tissue	hypo-	under, below; deficient
-glia	glue; neuroglial tissue	hyster/o	uterus (womb)
-globin	protein	**I**	
glomerul/o	glomerulus	-ia	condition
gloss/o	tongue	-iac	pertaining to
glott/o	glottis	-iasis	abnormal condition (produced by something specified)
gluc/o	sugar, sweetness		
glucos/o	sugar, sweetness	iatr/o	physician; medicine; treatment
glyc/o	sugar, sweetness	-iatry	medicine; treatment
glycos/o	sugar, sweetness	-ic	pertaining to
gnos/o	knowing	-ical	pertaining to
-gnosis	knowing	-ice	noun ending
gon/o	seed (ovum or spermatozoon)	ichthy/o	dry; scaly
gonad/o	gonads, sex glands	-ician	specialist

Medical Word Element	Meaning	Medical Word Element	Meaning
-icle	small, minute	kinesi/o	movement
-icterus	jaundice	-kinesia	movement
idi/o	unknown; peculiar	kinet/o	movement
-ile	pertaining to	kyph/o	humpback
ile/o	ileum (third part of the small intestine)	**L**	
ili/o	ilium (lateral, flaring portion of the hip bone)	labi/o	lip
		labyrinth/o	labyrinth (inner ear)
im-	not	lacrim/o	tear; lacrimal apparatus (duct, sac, or gland)
immun/o	immune, immunity, safe		
in-	in; not	lact/o	milk
-ine	pertaining to	-lalia	speech, babble
infer/o	lower, below	lamin/o	lamina (part of vertebral arch)
infra-	below, under	lapar/o	abdomen
inguin/o	groin	laryng/o	larynx (voice box)
insulin/o	insulin	later/o	side; to one side
inter-	between	lei/o	smooth
intestin/o	intestine	leiomy/o	smooth muscle (visceral)
intra-	in, within	-lepsy	seizure
-ion	the act of	lept/o	thin, slender
-ior	pertaining to	leuk/o	white
irid/o	iris	lingu/o	tongue
-is	noun ending	lip/o	fat
isch/o	to hold back; block	lipid/o	fat
ischi/o	ischium (lower portion of the hip bone)	-listhesis	slipping
		-lith	stone, calculus
-ism	condition	lith/o	stone, calculus
iso-	same; equal	lob/o	lobe
-ist	specialist	log/o	study of
-isy	state of; condition	-logist	specialist in the study of
-itic	pertaining to	-logy	study of
-itis	inflammation	lord/o	curve, swayback
-ive	pertaining to	-lucent	to shine; clear
-ization	process (of)	lumb/o	loins (lower back)
		lymph/o	lymph
J		lymphaden/o	lymph gland (node)
jaund/o	yellow	lymphangi/o	lymph vessel
jejun/o	jejunum (second part of the small intestine)	-lysis	separation; destruction; loosening
K		**M**	
kal/i	potassium (an electrolyte)	macro-	large
kary/o	nucleus	mal-	bad
kel/o	crab	-malacia	softening
kerat/o	horny tissue; hard; cornea	mamm/o	breast
ket/o	ketone bodies (acids and acetones)	-mania	state of mental disorder, frenzy
keton/o	ketone bodies (acids and acetones)	mast/o	breast

Continued

Medical Word Element	Meaning	Medical Word Element	Meaning
mastoid/o	mastoid process	nat/o	birth
maxill/o	maxilla (upper jaw bone)	natr/o	sodium (an electrolyte)
meat/o	opening, meatus	necr/o	death, necrosis
medi-	middle	neo-	new
medi/o	middle	nephr/o	kidney
mediastin/o	mediastinum	neur/o	nerve
medull/o	medulla	neutr/o	neutral; neither
mega-	enlargement	nid/o	nest
megal/o	enlargement	noct/o	night
-megaly	enlargement	nucle/o	nucleus
melan/o	black	nulli-	none
men/o	menses, menstruation	nyctal/o	night
mening/o	meninges (membranes covering the brain and spinal cord)	*O*	
meningi/o	meninges (membranes covering the brain and spinal cord)	obstetr/o	midwife
ment/o	mind	ocul/o	eye
meso-	middle	odont/o	teeth
meta-	change; beyond	-oid	resembling
metacarp/o	metacarpus (hand bones)	-ole	small, minute
metatars/o	metatarsus (foot bones)	olig/o	scanty
-meter	instrument for measuring	-oma	tumor
metr/o	uterus (womb); measure	omphal/o	navel (umbilicus)
metri/o	uterus (womb)	onc/o	tumor
-metry	act of measuring	onych/o	nail
mi/o	smaller; less	oophor/o	ovary
micr/o	small	-opaque	obscure
micro-	small	ophthalm/o	eye
mono-	one	-opia	vision
morph/o	form, shape; structure	-opsia	vision
muc/o	mucus	-opsy	view of
multi-	many, much	opt/o	eye, vision
muscul/o	muscle	optic/o	eye, vision
mut/a	genetic change	or/o	mouth
my/o	muscle	orch/o	testis (plural, *testes*)
myc/o	fungus (plural, *fungi*)	orchi/o	testis (plural, *testes*)
mydr/o	widen, enlarge	orchid/o	testis (plural, *testes*)
myel/o	bone marrow; spinal cord	-orexia	appetite
myos/o	muscle	orth/o	straight
myring/o	tympanic membrane (eardrum)	-ory	pertaining to
myx/o	mucus	-ose	pertaining to; sugar
N		-osis	abnormal condition; increase (used primarily with blood cells)
narc/o	stupor; numbness; sleep	-osmia	smell
nas/o	nose	oste/o	bone

Medical Word Element	Meaning	Medical Word Element	Meaning
ot/o	ear	phleb/o	vein
-ous	pertaining to	-phobia	fear
ovari/o	ovary	-phonia	voice
ox/i	oxygen	-phoresis	carrying; transmission
ox/o	oxygen	-phoria	feeling (mental state)
-oxia	oxygen	phot/o	light
P		phren/o	diaphragm; mind
palat/o	palate (roof of mouth)	-phylaxis	protection
pan-	all	-physis	growth
pancreat/o	pancreas	pil/o	hair
para-	near, beside; beyond	pituitar/o	pituitary gland
-para	to bear (offspring)	-plakia	plaque
parathyroid/o	parathyroid glands	plas/o	formation; growth
-paresis	partial paralysis	-plasia	formation; growth
patell/o	patella (kneecap)	-plasm	formation; growth
path/o	disease	-plasty	surgical repair
-pathy	disease	-plegia	paralysis
pector/o	chest	pleur/o	pleura
ped/i	foot; child	-plexy	stroke
ped/o	foot; child	-pnea	breathing
pedicul/o	lice	pneum/o	air; lung
pelv/i	pelvis	pneumon/o	air; lung
pelv/o	pelvis	pod/o	foot
pen/o	penis	-poiesis	formation; production
-penia	decrease; deficiency	poikil/o	varied; irregular
-pepsia	digestion	poli/o	gray; gray matter (of the brain or spinal cord)
peri-	around	poly-	many, much
perine/o	perineum (area between the scrotum [or vulva in the female] and anus)	polyp/o	small growth
		-porosis	porous
peritone/o	peritoneum	post-	after; behind
-pexy	fixation (of an organ)	poster/o	back (of the body), behind, posterior
phac/o	lens	-potence	power
phag/o	swallowing, eating	-prandial	meal
-phage	swallowing, eating	pre-	before, in front of
-phagia	swallowing, eating	presby/o	old age
phalang/o	phalanges (bones of the fingers and toes)	primi-	first
pharmaceutic/o	drug, medicine	pro-	before, in front of
pharyng/o	pharynx (throat)	proct/o	anus, rectum
-phasia	speech	prostat/o	prostate gland
-phil	attraction for	proxim/o	near, nearest
phil/o	attraction for	pseudo-	false
-philia	attraction for		

Continued

Medical Word Element	Meaning	Medical Word Element	Meaning
psych/o	mind	scapul/o	scapula (shoulder blade)
-ptosis	prolapse, downward displacement	-schisis	a splitting
ptyal/o	saliva	schiz/o	split
-ptysis	spitting	scler/o	hardening; sclera (white of the eye)
pub/o	pelvis bone (anterior part of the pelvic bone)	scoli/o	crooked, bent
pulmon/o	lung	-scope	instrument for examining
pupill/o	pupil	-scopy	visual examination
py/o	pus	scot/o	darkness
pyel/o	renal pelvis	seb/o	sebum, sebaceous
pylor/o	pylorus	semi-	one half
pyr/o	fire	semin/i	semen; seed
Q, R		semin/o	semen; seed
quadri-	four	sept/o	septum
rachi/o	spine	septic/o	infection
radi/o	radiation, x-ray; radius (lower arm bone on the thumb side)	sequestr/o	separation
radicul/o	nerve root	ser/o	serum
rect/o	rectum	sial/o	saliva, salivary gland
ren/o	kidney	sider/o	iron
reticul/o	net, mesh	sigmoid/o	sigmoid colon
retin/o	retina	sin/o	sinus, cavity
retro-	backward; behind	sinus/o	sinus, cavity
rhabd/o	rod-shaped (striated)	-sis	state of; condition
rhabdomy/o	rod-shaped (striated) muscle	somat/o	body
rhin/o	nose	somn/o	sleep
rhytid/o	wrinkle	son/o	sound
roentgen/o	x-ray	-spadias	slit, fissure
-rrhage	bursting forth (of)	-spasm	involuntary contraction, twitching
-rrhagia	bursting forth (of)	sperm/i	spermatozoa, sperm cells
-rrhaphy	suture	sperm/o	spermatozoa, sperm cells
-rrhea	discharge, flow	spermat/o	spermatozoa, sperm cells
-rrhexis	rupture	sphygm/o	pulse
-rrhythm/o	rhythm	-sphyxia	pulse
rube/o	red	spin/o	spine
S		spir/o	breathe
sacr/o	sacrum	splen/o	spleen
salping/o	tube (usually fallopian or eustachian [auditory] tubes)	spondyl/o	vertebra (backbone)
-salpinx	tube (usually fallopian or eustachian [auditory] tubes)	squam/o	scale
sarc/o	flesh (connective tissue)	staped/o	stapes
-sarcoma	malignant tumor of connective tissue	-stasis	standing still
		steat/o	fat
		sten/o	narrowing, stricture

Medical Word Element	Meaning	Medical Word Element	Meaning
-stenosis	narrowing, stricture	-tome	instrument to cut
stern/o	sternum (breastbone)	-tomy	incision
steth/o	chest	ton/o	tension
sthen/o	strength	tonsill/o	tonsils
stigmat/o	point, mark	tox/o	poison
stomat/o	mouth	-toxic	pertaining to poison
-stomy	forming an opening (mouth)	toxic/o	poison
sub-	under, below	trabecul/o	trabecula (supporting bundles of fibers)
sudor/o	sweat		
super-	upper, above	trache/o	trachea (windpipe)
super/o	upper, above	trans-	across; through
supra-	above; excessive; superior	tri-	three
sym-	union, together, joined	trich/o	hair
syn-	union, together, joined	trigon/o	trigone (triangular region at the base of the bladder)
synapt/o	synapsis, point of contact		
synov/o	synovial membrane, synovial fluid	-tripsy	crushing
T		-trophy	development; nourishment
tachy-	rapid	-tropia	turning
tax/o	order; coordination	-tropin	stimulate
-taxia	order; coordination	tubercul/o	a little swelling
ten/o	tendon	tympan/o	tympanic membrane (eardrum)
tend/o	tendon	**U**	
tendin/o	tendon	-ula	small, minute
-tension	to stretch	-ule	small, minute
test/o	testis (plural, *testes*)	uln/o	ulna (lower arm bone on the opposite side of the thumb)
thalam/o	thalamus		
thalass/o	sea	ultra-	excess; beyond
thec/o	sheath (usually referring to the meninges)	-um	structure; thing
		umbilic/o	umbilicus, navel
thel/o, theli/o	nipple	ungu/o	nail
therapeut/o	treatment	uni-	one
-therapy	treatment	ur/o	urine, urinary tract
therm/o	heat	ureter/o	ureter
thorac/o	chest	urethr/o	urethra
-thorax	chest	-uria	urine
thromb/o	blood clot	urin/o	urine, urinary tract
thym/o	thymus gland	-us	condition; structure
-thymia	mind; emotion	uter/o	uterus (womb)
thyr/o	thyroid gland	uvul/o	uvula
thyroid/o	thyroid gland	**V, W**	
tibi/o	tibia (larger bone of the lower leg)	vagin/o	vagina
-tic	pertaining to	valv/o	valve
-tocia	childbirth, labor	varic/o	dilated vein
tom/o	to cut, slice	vas/o	vessel; vas deferens; duct

Continued

Medical Word Element	Meaning	Medical Word Element	Meaning
vascul/o	vessel (usually blood or lymph)	vitr/o	vitreous body (of the eye)
ven/o	vein	vitre/o	glassy
ventr/o	belly, belly side	vol/o	volume
ventricul/o	ventricle (of the heart or brain)	vulv/o	vulva
-version	turning	**X, Y, Z**	
vertebr/o	vertebra (backbone)	xanth/o	yellow
vesic/o	bladder	xen/o	foreign, strange
vesicul/o	seminal vesicle	xer/o	dry
vest/o	clothes	xiph/o	sword
viscer/o	internal organs	-y	condition; process

Answer Key

CHAPTER 1: INTRODUCTION TO PROGRAMMED LEARNING AND MEDICAL WORD BUILDING

Frame 1-49

Medical Term	Combining Form (Root + o)	Word Root	Suffix
arthr/o/scop/ic ăr-thrōs-KŎP-ĭk	*arthr/o*	*scop*	*-ic*
erythr/o/cyt/osis ĕ-rĭth-rō-sī-TŌ-sĭs	erythr/o	cyt	-osis
dermat/itis dĕr-mă-TĪ-tĭs		dermat	-itis
gastr/o/enter/itis găs-trō-ĕn-tĕr-Ī-tĭs	gastr/o	enter	-itis
orth/o/ped/ic or-thō-PĒ-dĭk	orth/o	ped	-ic
oste/o/arthr/itis ŏs-tē-ō-ăr-THRĪ-tĭs	oste/o	arthr	-itis

Section Review 1-1

1. breve
2. macron
3. long
4. short
5. pn
6. hard
7. n
8. eye
9. second
10. separate

Surgical Suffixes

Term	Meaning
arthr/o/**centesis** ăr-thrō-sĕn-TĒ-sĭs	*surgical puncture of a joint*
arthr/o/**desis** ăr-thrō-DĒ-sĭs	binding or fixation of a joint
append/**ectomy** ăp-ĕn-DĔK-tō-mē	excision or removal of the appendix
thromb/o/**lysis** thrŏm-BŎL-ĭ-sĭs	separation, destruction, or loosening of a blood clot
mast/o/**pexy** MĂS-tō-pĕks-ē	fixation of the breast(s)
rhin/o/**plasty** RĬ-nō-plăs-tē	surgical repair of the nose (to change the shape or size)
my/o/**rrhaphy** mī-OR-ă-fē	suture of a muscle
trache/o/**stomy** trā-kē-ŎS-tō-mē	forming an opening (mouth) into the trachea
oste/o/**tome** ŎS-tē-ō-tōm	instrument to cut bone
trache/o/**tomy** trā-kē–ŎT-ō–mē	incision into the trachea
lith/o/**tripsy** LĬTH-ō-trĭp-sē	crushing a stone or calculus

Diagnostic Suffixes

Term	Meaning
electr/o/cardi/o/**gram** ē-lĕk-trō-KĂR-dē-ō-grăm	record of electrical activity of the heart
electr/o/cardi/o/**graph** ē-lĕk-trō-KĂR-dē-ōg-răf	instrument to record electrical activity of the heart
electr/ocardi/o/**graphy** ē-lĕk-trō-kăr-dē-ŌG-ră-fē	process of recording electrical activity of the heart
pelv/i/**meter** pĕl-VĬM-ĕ-tĕr	instrument for measuring the pelvis
pelv/i/**metry** pĕl-VĬM-ĕ-trē	act of measuring the pelvis
endo/**scope** ĔN-dō-skōp	instrument for examining within (or inside a hollow organ or cavity)
endo/**scopy** ĕn-DŎS-kō-pē	visual examination within (a cavity or canal using a specialized lighted instrument called an endoscope)

Pathologic Suffixes

Term	Meaning
neur/**algia** nū-RĂL-jē-ă	pain of a nerve (or pain along the path of a nerve)
ot/o/**dynia** ō-tō-DĬN-ē-ă	pain in the ear (earache)
hepat/o/**cele** hĕ-PĂT-ō-sēl	hernia or swelling of the liver
bronchi/**ectasis** brŏng-kē-ĔK-tă-sĭs	abnormal dilation or expansion of a bronchus or bronchi
lymph/**edema** lĭmf-ĕ-DĒ-mă	swelling of lymph tissue (swelling resulting from accumulation of tissue fluid)
hyper/**emesis** hī-pĕr-ĔM-ĕ-sĭs	excessive or above normal vomiting
an/**emia** ă-NĒ-mē-ă	literally means without blood (blood condition caused by iron deficiency or a decrease in red blood cells)
chol/e/**lith/iasis** kō-lē-lĭ-THĪ-ă-sĭs	presence or formation of gallstones (in the gallbladder or common bile duct)
gastr/**itis** găs-TRĪ-tĭs	inflammation of the stomach
chol/e/**lith** KŌ-lē-lĭth	gallstone
chondr/o/**malacia** kŏn-drō-mă-LĀ-shē-ă	softening of cartilage
cardi/o/**megaly** kăr-dē-ō-MĔG-ă–lē	enlargement of the heart
neur/**oma** nū-RŌ-mă	tumor composed of nerve cells
cyan/**osis** sī-ă-NŌ-sĭs	abnormal condition of dark blue coloration (bluish or purple discoloration of the skin and mucous membrane)
my/o/**pathy** mī-ŎP-ă-thē	any disease of muscle
erythr/o/**penia** ĕ-rĭth-rō-PĒ-nē-ă	abnormal decrease in or deficiency of red blood cells
hem/o/**phobia** hĕ-mō-FŌ-bē-ă	fear of blood
hemi/**plegia** hĕm-ē-PLĒ-jē-ă *hemi-:* one half	paralysis of one half (paralysis of one side of the body)
hem/o/**rrhage** HĔM-ĕ-rĭj	bursting forth of blood (loss of large amounts of blood within a short period, externally or internally)
men/o/**rrhagia** mĕn-ō-RĀ-jē-ă	bursting forth of menses (profuse discharge of blood during menstruation)

Continued

Term	Meaning
dia/rrhea dī-ă-RĒ-ă	discharge or flow through (abnormally frequent discharge or flow of fluid fecal matter from the bowel)
arteri/o/rrhexis ăr-tē-rē-ō-RĔK-sĭs	rupture of an artery
arteri/o/stenosis ăr-tē-rē-ō-stĕ-NŌ-sĭs	narrowing or stricture of an artery
hepat/o/toxic HĔP-ă-tō-tŏk-sĭk	potentially destructive to the liver
dys/trophy DĬS-trō-fē	bad state of development or nourishment (abnormal condition caused by defective nutrition or metabolism)

Section Review 1-2

Singular	Plural	Rule
sarcoma	*sarcomata*	*Retain the ma and add ta.*
thrombus	thrombi	Drop *us* and add *i.*
appendix	appendices	Drop *ix* and add *ices.*
diverticulum	diverticula	Drop *um* and add *a.*
ovary	ovaries	Drop *y* and add *ies.*
diagnosis	diagnoses	Drop *is* and add *es.*
lumen	lumina	Drop *en* and add *ina.*
vertebra	vertebrae	Retain the *a* and add *e.*
thorax	thoraces	Drop the *x* and add *ces.*
spermatozoon	spermatozoa	Drop *on* and add *a.*

Common Prefixes

Term	Meaning
a/mast/ia ă-MĂS-tē-ă	without a breast
an/esthesia ăn-ĕs-THĒ-zē-ă	without feeling (partial or complete loss of sensation with or without loss of consciousness)
auto/graft AW-tō-grăft	transplantation to self
circum/duction sĕr-kŭm-DŬK-shŭn	act of leading around (movement of a part, such as an extremity, in a circular direction)
peri/odont/al pĕr-ē-ō-DŎN-tăl	pertaining to "around a tooth"

Term	Meaning
dia/rrhea dī-ă-RĒ-ă	flow through
trans/vagin/al trăns-VĂJ-ĭn-ăl	pertaining to "across the vagina"
dipl/opia dĭp-LŌ-pē-ă	double vision
diplo/bacteri/al dĭp-lō-băk-TĔR-ē-ăl	pertaining to bacteria linked together in pairs
endo/crine ĔN-dō-krīn	secrete within
intra/muscul/ar ĭn-tră-MŬS-kū-lăr	pertaining to "within the muscle"
hetero/graft HĔT-ĕ-rō-grăft	different transplantation
homo/graft HŌ-mō-grăft	literally means transplantation of same (transplantation of tissue between the same species)
homeo/plasia hō-mē-ō-PLĀ-zē-ă	formation or growth of new tissue similar to that already existing in a part
hypo/derm/ic hī-pō-DĔR-mĭk	pertaining to "under the skin" (under or inserted under the skin, as in a hypodermic injection)
macro/cyte MĂK-rō-sīt	abnormally large cell (usually erythrocyte), such as those found in pernicious anemia
micro/scope MĪ-krō-skōp	instrument for examining minute objects
mono/cyte MŎN-ō-sīt	large mononuclear leukocyte
uni/nucle/ar ū-nĭ-NŪ-klē-ăr	pertaining to a single nucleus
post/nat/al pōst-NĀ-tăl	pertaining to (the period) after birth
pre/nat/al prē-NĀ-tăl	pertaining to (the period) before birth
pro/gnosis prŏg-NŌ-sĭs	before knowing; knowing beforehand (prediction of the course and end of a disease, and the estimated chance of recovery)
primi/gravida prī-mĭ-GRĂV-ĭ-dă	woman during her first pregnancy
retro/version rĕt-rō-VĔR-shŭn	literally means turning backward (tipping backward of an organ, such as the uterus, from its normal position)
super/ior soo-PĒ-rē-or	pertaining to upper or above (toward the head or upper portion of a structure)

CHAPTER 2: BODY STRUCTURE

Section Review 2-1

Term	Meaning
1. dist/al	*-al: pertaining to; far, farthest*
2. poster/ior	-ior: pertaining to; back (of body), behind, posterior
3. hist/o/logist	-logist: specialist in study of; tissue
4. dors/al	-al: pertaining to; back (of body)
5. anter/ior	-ior: pertaining to; anterior, front
6. later/al	-al: pertaining to; side; to one side
7. medi/ad	-ad: toward; middle
8. chondr/oma	-oma: tumor
9. proxim/al	-al: pertaining to; near, nearest
10. ventr/al	-al: pertaining to; belly, belly side

Section Review 2-2

1. hist/o	4. proxim/o	7. ventr/o	10. caud/o	13. infer/o
2. -al, -ior	5. -logy	8. -toxic	11. -logist	14. -lysis
3. medi/o	6. cyt/o	9. -ad	12. dist/o	15. later/o

Section Review 2-3

Term	Meaning
1. ili/ac	*-ac: pertaining to; ilium (lateral, flaring portion of hip bone)*
2. abdomin/al	-al: pertaining to; abdomen
3. inguin/al	-al: pertaining to; groin
4. spin/al	-al: pertaining to; spine
5. peri/umbilic/al	-al: pertaining to; around; umbilicus, navel
6. cephal/ad	-ad: toward; head
7. gastr/ic	-ic: pertaining to; stomach
8. thorac/ic	-ic: pertaining to; chest
9. cervic/al	-al: pertaining to; neck, cervix uteri (neck of the uterus)
10. lumb/ar	-ar: pertaining to; loins (lower back)

Section Review 2-4

1. -ad	4. pelv/o	7. -ac, -al, -ic, -ior	10. hypo-	13. umbilic/o
2. inguin/o	5. chondr/o	8. lumb/o	11. crani/o	14. poster/o
3. gastr/o	6. epi-	9. thorac/o	12. spin/o	15. abdomin/o

Word Elements Review

Medical Term	Meaning
1. **cephal/ad** 　　WR S	toward the head
2. **crani/o/meter** 　　CF　　S	instrument for measuring the cranium (skull)
3. **epi/gastr/ic** 　P　WR S	PT above the stomach
4. **peri/umbilic/al** 　P　　WR　　S	PT around the umbilicus or navel
5. **poster/o/later/al** 　　CF WR S	PT to the back side (of the body)

6. endoscopy	8. cytology	10. septic	12. cephalad	14. superior
7. hypogastric	9. lateral	11. toxic	13. radiology	15. transverse

Additional Medical Terms Review

1. CT	5. C&S	9. tomography	13. adhesion
2. fluoroscopy	6. endoscope	10. radiopharmaceutical	14. radiography
3. US	7. anastomosis	11. endoscopy	15. septicemia
4. MRI	8. inflammation	12. cauterize	

CHAPTER 3: INTEGUMENTARY SYSTEM

Section Review 3-1

Term	Meaning
1. hypo/derm/ic	-ic: pertaining to; under, below; deficient; skin
2. melan/oma	-oma: tumor; black
3. kerat/osis	-osis: abnormal condition, increase (used primarily with blood cells); horny tissue; hard; cornea
4. cutane/ous	-ous: pertaining to; skin
5. lip/o/cyte	-cyte: cell; fat
6. onych/o/malacia	-malacia: softening; nail
7. scler/o/derma	-derma: skin; hardening; sclera (white of the eye)
8. dia/phoresis	-phoresis: carrying; transmission; through; across
9. dermat/o/myc/osis	-osis: abnormal condition, increase (used primarily with blood cells); skin; fungus
10. cry/o/therapy	-therapy: treatment; cold

Labeling Review—Figure 3-2: Identifying Integumentary Structures

Check your labeling of Figure 3-2 on page 70.

1. epidermis
2. dermis
3. stratum corneum
4. basal layer

5. hair follicle
6. sebaceous (oil) gland
7. sudoriferous (sweat) gland
8. subcutaneous tissue

Labeling Review—Figure 3-5: Structure of a Fingernail

Check your labeling of Figure 3-5 on page 79.

1. nail root
2. matrix
3. cuticle

4. nail bed
5. nail body
6. lunula

Section Review 3-2

1. -pathy
2. xer/o
3. lip/o, adip/o, steat/o

4. -rrhea
5. trich/o, pil/o
6. scler/o
7. -cele

8. onych/o
9. derm/o, dermat/o, cutane/o, -derma

10. -malacia
11. -logist
12. epi-
13. -osis

14. hidr/o
15. hypo-

Section Review 3-3

1. melan/o
2. cyan/o
3. -emia

4. cyt/o, -cyte
5. -penia
6. -pathy

7. -rrhea
8. erythr/o
9. auto-

10. -derma
11. -oma
12. leuk/o

13. xanth/o
14. necr/o
15. -osis

Word Elements Review

Medical Term	Meaning
1. an/hidr/osis P WR S	abnormal condition of being without sweat
2. dermat/o/plasty CF S	surgical repair of skin
3. sub/cutane/ous P WR S	pertaining to "under the skin"
4. onych/o/malacia CF S	softening of a nail
5. lip/ectomy WR S	excision of fat

6. lipocyte
7. melanoma
8. trichopathy

9. squamous
10. xeroderma
11. melanocyte

12. diaphoresis
13. lipocele
14. carcinoma

15. leukocytopenia

Additional Medical Terms Review

1. verruca	4. furuncle	7. corticosteroids	10. cryosurgery	13. alopecia
2. vitiligo	5. eczema	8. dermabrasion	11. débridement	14. comedo
3. tinea	6. urticaria	9. fulguration	12. scabies	15. petechia

Critical Thinking 3-1: Consultation Letter

1. What was the predisposing factor causing the patient's present condition?

   Exposing her skin to the sun

2. What did the physician recommend to the patient to prevent future problems with solar keratosis?

   Protect her skin from the sun (photoprotection)

3. What treatment did the physician perform on the precancerous lesions?

   Freezing the lesions with liquid nitrogen on an applicator

4. When does the physician want to see the patient again?

   Only as required

Critical Thinking 3-2: Progress Note

1. What causes psoriasis?

   The etiology is unknown, but heredity is a significant determining factor.

2. On what parts of the body does psoriasis typically occur?

   Scalp; elbows; knees; sacrum; and around the nails, arms, legs, and abdomen

3. How is psoriasis treated?

   Treatment for mild to moderate psoriasis includes corticosteroids and phototherapy.

4. What is a histiocytoma?

   A tumor containing histiocytes, which are macrophages present in all loose connective tissue

Medical Record Activity 3-3

1. antipruritics	3. biopsy	5. I&D	7. alopecia	9. abscess
2. hirsutism	4. débridement	6. scabies	8. vitiligo	10. petechia

Vocabulary Review

1. subcutaneous	5. Kaposi sarcoma	9. leukemia	13. pustule	17. melanoma
2. diaphoresis	6. suction lipectomy	10. ecchymosis	14. papules	18. lipocele
3. trichopathy	7. onychomycosis	11. onychoma	15. erythrocyte	19. xanthoma
4. autograft	8. pressure ulcers	12. hirsutism	16. xeroderma	20. onychomalacia

CHAPTER 4: RESPIRATORY SYSTEM

Section Review 4-1

Term	Meaning
1. laryng/o/scope	-scope: instrument for examining; larynx (voice box)
2. py/o/thorax	-thorax: chest; pus
3. hyp/oxia	-oxia: oxygen; under, below; deficient
4. trache/o/stomy	-stomy: forming an opening (mouth); trachea (windpipe)
5. a/pnea	-pnea: breathing; without; not
6. pulmon/o/logist	-logist: specialist in the study of; lung
7. pneumon/ia	-ia: condition; air; lung
8. rhin/o/rrhea	-rrhea: discharge, flow; nose
9. an/osmia	-osmia: smell; without; not
10. pneum/ectomy	-ectomy: excision, removal; air; lung

Section Review 4-2

1. aer/o	5. -stomy	9. -cele	13. pharyng/o	17. -therapy
2. para-	6. -tomy	10. neo-	14. -stenosis	18. a-, an-
3. myc/o	7. -tome	11. nas/o, rhin/o	15. -phagia	19. -scopy
4. -ectasis	8. laryng/o	12. -plegia	16. trache/o	20. hydr/o

Labeling Review—Figure 4-3: Identifying Upper and Lower Respiratory Tracts

Check your labeling of Figure 4-3 on page 120.

1. nasal cavity	5. trachea	7. bronchioles	10. pulmonary
2. pharynx (throat)	(windpipe)	8. left lung	capillaries
3. larynx (voice box)	6. right and left	9. alveoli	11. pleura
4. epiglottis	primary bronchi		12. diaphragm

Section Review 4-3

1. -osis	8. thorac/o	15. -spasm	22. -stenosis
2. brady-	9. -ectasis	16. macro-	23. -centesis
3. dys-	10. -phobia	17. tachy-	24. a-
4. melan/o	11. myc/o	18. pneum/o, pneumon/o	25. chondr/o
5. -pnea	12. eu-	19. pleur/o	
6. bronch/o, bronchi/o	13. -cele	20. micro-	
7. hem/o	14. -scope	21. orth/o	

Word Elements Review

Medical Term	Meaning
1. a/pnea P S	without breathing
2. pleur/o/dynia CF S	pain in the pleura
3. trache/o/stomy CF S	creation of an opening (mouth) into the trachea
4. bronchi/ectasis WR S	dilation of the bronchi
5. pneumon/ectomy WR S	excision of a lung

6. erythrocyte
7. rhinorrhea
8. thoracotomy

9. pneumonocentesis
10. emphysema
11. tracheostenosis

12. laryngectomy
13. anosmia
14. intercostal

15. hemophobia

Additional Medical Terms Review

1. stridor
2. epistaxis
3. influenza
4. acidosis

5. coryza
6. cystic fibrosis
7. lung cancer
8. pleural effusion

9. pneumothorax
10. rales
11. bronchodilators
12. ARDS

13. COVID-19
14. atelectasis
15. epiglottitis
16. pertussis

17. hypoxemia
18. SIDS
19. hypoxia
20. rhonchi

Critical Thinking 4-1: Referral Letter

1. What surgeries did the patient have last year?

   Septoplasty and turbinate reduction

2. What was the outcome of last year's surgery?

   Significant improvement in airway passage

3. What seasonal symptoms are currently noted by the patient?

   Sneezing and watery rhinorrhea, tickling of the palate, and burning of the eyes

4. How is the nasal mucosa described?

   Somewhat pale and edematous, with a serous discharge

5. What was the recommendation of the physician?

   Double-strength Vancenase AQ and Allegra and referral to an allergist to undergo definitive allergy testing

Critical Thinking 4-2: Pulmonary Function Report

1. Did this patient have any difficulty breathing?

    Yes

2. What was the presenting diagnosis?

    Shortness of breath

3. What was the hydrogen ion concentration?

    7.38

4. What was the level of bicarbonate radical?

    22

5. What was the partial pressure of carbon dioxide? (*Clue:* This patient is retaining carbon dioxide.)

    78

Medical Record Activity 4-3

1. laryngoscope	3. bronchorrhagia	5. thoracocentesis	7. tracheotomy	9. rales
2. influenza	4. pneumonia	6. bronchodilator	8. PFT	10. acidosis

Vocabulary Review

1. pyothorax	5. tracheostomy	9. aspirate	13. pharyngoplegia	17. rhinoplasty
2. thoracentesis	6. corticosteroids	10. mucolytics	14. pleurisy	18. TB
3. asthma	7. apnea	11. atelectasis	15. *Pneumocystis*	19. COPD
4. croup	8. aerophagia	12. anosmia	16. catheter	20. pneumothorax

CHAPTER 5: CARDIOVASCULAR AND LYMPHATIC SYSTEMS

Section Review 5-1

Term	Meaning
1. endo/cardi/um	-um: structure, thing; in, within; heart
2. cardi/o/megaly	-megaly: enlargement; heart
3. aort/o/stenosis	-stenosis: narrowing, stricture; aorta
4. tachy/cardia	-cardia: heart condition; rapid
5. phleb/itis	-itis: inflammation; vein
6. thromb/o/lysis	-lysis: separation; destruction; loosening; blood clot
7. vas/o/spasm	-spasm: involuntary contraction, twitching; vessel; vas deferens; duct
8. ather/oma	-oma: tumor; fatty plaque
9. electr/o/cardi/o/graphy	-graphy: process of recording; electricity; heart
10. atri/o/ventricul/ar	-ar: pertaining to; atrium; ventricle (of the heart or brain)

Labeling Review—Figure 5-2: Heart Structures

Check your labeling of Figure 5-2 on page 168.

1. endocardium
2. myocardium
3. pericardium
4. aorta
5. right atrium

6. superior vena cava
7. inferior vena cava
8. pulmonary trunk
9. right lung
10. left lung

11. left atrium
12. right pulmonary veins
13. left pulmonary veins

Labeling Review—Figure 5-4: Internal Structures of the Heart

Check your labeling of Figure 5-4 on page 172.

1. right atrium (RA)
2. left atrium (LA)
3. right ventricle (RV)
4. left ventricle (LV)
5. interventricular septum (IVS)
6. superior vena cava (SVC)

7. inferior vena cava (IVC)
8. tricuspid valve
9. pulmonary valve
10. right pulmonary artery
11. left pulmonary artery
12. right pulmonary veins

13. left pulmonary veins
14. mitral valve
15. aortic valve
16. aorta
17. branches of the aorta
18. descending aorta

Labeling Review—Figure 5-6: Heart Structures With Valves and Cusps

Check your labeling of Figure 5-6 on page 180.

1. tricuspid valve
2. mitral valve

3. chordae tendineae
4. pulmonary valve

5. aortic valve
6. three cusps

7. two cusps

Section Review 5-2

1. -osis
2. epi-
3. aort/o
4. peri-
5. arteri/o
6. atri/o
7. hem/o, hemat/o

8. -pnea
9. -pathy
10. -ectasis
11. scler/o
12. cardi/o
13. -spasm
14. my/o

15. tachy-
16. -rrhexis
17. brady-
18. -ole, -ule
19. -rrhaphy
20. -stenosis
21. -phagia

22. tri-
23. bi-
24. phleb/o, ven/o
25. ventricul/o

Labeling Review—Figure 5-7: Anterior View of the Conduction Pathway of the Heart

Check your labeling of Figure 5-7 on page 183.

1. sinoatrial (SA) node
2. right atrium (RA)
3. atrioventricular (AV) node

4. bundle of His
5. bundle branches
6. Purkinje fibers

Section Review 5-3

Term	Meaning
1. agglutin/ation	*-ation: process (of); clumping, gluing*
2. thym/oma	-oma: tumor; thymus gland
3. phag/o/cyte	-cyte: cell; swallowing, eating
4. lymphaden/itis	-itis: inflammation; lymph gland (node)
5. splen/o/megaly	-megaly: enlargement; spleen
6. aden/o/pathy	-pathy: disease; gland
7. ana/phylaxis	-phylaxis: protection; against; up; back
8. lymphangi/oma	oma: tumor; lymph vessel
9. lymph/o/poiesis	-poiesis: formation, production; lymph
10. immun/o/gen	-gen: forming, producing; origin; immune, immunity, safe

Labeling Review—Figure 5-11: Lymphatic System

Check your labeling of Figure 5-11 on page 192.

1. lymph capillaries
2. lymph vessels
3. thoracic duct
4. right lymphatic duct
5. cervical nodes
6. axillary nodes
7. inguinal nodes
8. tonsil
9. spleen
10. thymus

Section Review 5-4

1. aort/o
2. hem/o
3. thromb/o
4. -cyte
5. cerebr/o
6. necr/o
7. -pathy
8. electr/o
9. -megaly
10. cardi/o
11. lymph/o
12. my/o
13. -graphy
14. -gram
15. -al, -ic
16. -rrhexis
17. -lysis
18. -stenosis
19. -plasty
20. angi/o

Word Elements Review

Medical Term	Meaning
1. lymphangi/oma WR S	tumor composed of lymph vessels
2. hemat/o/poiesis CF S	formation or production of blood
3. phleb/o/stenosis CF S	stricture or narrowing of a vein
4. thromb/ectomy WR S	excision or removal of a blood clot
5. peri/cardi/o/centesis P CF S	surgical puncture around the heart

6. agglutination
7. tachycardia
8. arteriosclerosis

9. aneurysmorrhaphy
10. vasospasm
11. electrocardiograph

12. intraventricular
13. atherectomy
14. arrhythmia

15. immunogen

Additional Medical Terms Review

1. mononucleosis
2. thrombolytics
3. embolus
4. DVT
5. statins

6. bruit
7. Doppler US
8. rheumatic heart disease
9. Holter monitor
10. Raynaud disease

11. ischemia
12. Hodgkin lymphoma
13. AIDS
14. HF
15. fibrillation

16. valvuloplasty
17. lymphangiography
18. tissue typing
19. troponin I
20. CABG

Critical Thinking 5-1: Emergency Department Report

1. What symptoms did the patient experience before admission to the hospital?

   A burning midsternal pain that lasted several seconds

2. What was found during clinical examination?

   No abnormalities were found.

3. What was the cause of the patient's prior myocardial infarctions?

   Cocaine use

4. Did the patient have a prior history of heart problems? If so, describe them.

   Yes, a history of two previous myocardial infarctions related to his use of cocaine

5. How was the chest pain treated?

   The patient received 45 cc of Mylanta and 10 cc of viscous lidocaine.

Critical Thinking 5-2: Operative Report

1. Which coronary arteries were under examination?

   The left and right coronary arteries

2. Which surgical procedure was used to clear the stenosis?

   Balloon angioplasty

3. What symptoms did the patient exhibit before balloon inflation?

   The patient had significant ST elevations in the inferior leads and severe throat tightness and shortness of breath.

4. Why was the patient put on heparin?

   To prevent formation of postsurgical clots

Medical Record Activity 5-3

1. angina pectoris
2. Kaposi sarcoma
3. mononucleosis

4. AIDS
5. beta blocker
6. statin

7. Holter monitor
8. Hodgkin disease
9. cardiac catheterization

10. lymphangiography

Vocabulary Review

1. myocardium
2. tachypnea
3. arteriosclerosis
4. phagocyte

5. systole
6. diastole
7. ECG
8. malaise

9. desiccated
10. cardiomegaly
11. aneurysm
12. angina pectoris

13. MI
14. agglutination
15. statins
16. anaphylaxis

17. capillaries
18. hemangioma
19. arterioles
20. pacemaker

CHAPTER 6: DIGESTIVE SYSTEM

Section Review 6-1

Term	Meaning
1. gingiv/itis	*-itis: inflammation; gum(s)*
2. dys/pepsia	-pepsia: digestion; bad; painful; difficult
3. pylor/o/my/o/tomy	-tomy: incision; pylorus; muscle
4. dent/ist	-ist: specialist; teeth
5. esophag/o/scope	-scope: instrument for examining; esophagus
6. gastr/o/scopy	-scopy: visual examination; stomach
7. dia/rrhea	-rrhea: discharge, flow; through; across
8. hyper/emesis	-emesis: vomiting; excessive; above normal
9. an/orexia	-orexia: appetite; without; not
10. sub/lingu/al	-al: pertaining to; under, below; tongue

Labeling Review—Figure 6-2: Oral Cavity, Esophagus, Pharynx, and Stomach

Check your labeling of Figure 6-2 on page 234.

1. oral cavity
2. sublingual gland
3. submandibular gland
4. parotid gland
5. bolus
6. pharynx (throat)
7. esophagus
8. stomach

Section Review 6-2

1. -oma
2. -al, -ary, -ic
3. peri-
4. hypo-
5. -rrhea
6. myc/o
7. gingiv/o
8. pylor/o
9. dys-
10. hyper-
11. sial/o
12. gastr/o
13. -ist
14. orth/o
15. dent/o, odont/o
16. dia-
17. lingu/o, gloss/o
18. -scope
19. -tomy
20. -orexia
21. stomat/o, or/o
22. -algia, -dynia
23. -phagia
24. an-
25. -pepsia

Section Review 6-3

Term	Meaning
1. duoden/o/scopy	*-scopy: visual examination; duodenum (first part of the small intestine)*
2. appendic/itis	-itis: inflammation; appendix
3. enter/o/pathy	-pathy: disease; intestine (usually small intestine)
4. col/o/stomy	-stomy: forming an opening (mouth); colon
5. rect/o/cele	-cele: hernia; swelling; rectum
6. sigmoid/o/tomy	-tomy: incision; sigmoid colon
7. proct/o/logist	-logist: specialist in the study of; anus, rectum
8. jejun/o/rrhaphy	-rrhaphy: suture; jejunum (second part of the small intestine)
9. append/ectomy	-ectomy: excision, removal; appendix
10. ile/o/stomy	-stomy: forming an opening (mouth); ileum (third part of the small intestine)

Labeling Review—Figure 6-4: Small Intestine and Colon

Check your labeling of Figure 6-4 on page 247.

1. duodenum
2. jejunum
3. ileum

4. ascending colon
5. transverse colon
6. descending colon

7. sigmoid colon
8. rectum
9. anus

Section Review 6-4

1. enter/o
2. -tome
3. rect/o

4. -spasm
5. ile/o
6. -scopy

7. jejun/o
8. col/o, colon/o
9. duoden/o

10. -stomy
11. proct/o
12. -stenosis

13. -rrhaphy
14. -tomy
15. sigmoid/o

Section Review 6-5

Term	Meaning
1. hepat/itis	*-itis: inflammation; liver*
2. hepat/o/megaly	-megaly: enlargement; liver
3. chol/e/lith	-lith: stone, calculus; bile, gall
4. cholangi/ole	-ole: small, minute; bile vessel
5. cholecyst/ectomy	-ectomy: excision, removal; gallbladder
6. post/prandial	-prandial: meal; after; behind
7. chol/e/lith/iasis	-iasis: abnormal condition (produced by something specified); bile, gall; stone, calculus
8. choledoch/o/tomy	-tomy: incision; bile duct
9. pancreat/o/lith	-lith: stone, calculus; pancreas
10. pancreat/itis	-itis: inflammation; pancreas

Labeling Review—Figure 6-10: Liver, Gallbladder, Pancreas, and Duodenum With Associated Ducts and Blood Vessels

Check your labeling of Figure 6-10 on page 259.

1. liver
2. gallbladder
3. pancreas
4. duodenum

5. common bile duct
6. right hepatic duct
7. left hepatic duct
8. hepatic duct

9. cystic duct
10. pancreatic duct

Section Review 6-6

1. -oma
2. -iasis
3. choledoch/o
4. chol/e
5. cyst/o

6. -megaly
7. -ectomy
8. -stomy
9. cholecyst/o
10. therm/o

11. hepat/o
12. -algia, -dynia
13. pancreat/o
14. toxic/o, tox/o, -toxic
15. -graphy

16. -gram
17. -lith
18. -plasty
19. -rrhaphy
20. -emesis

Word Elements Review

Medical Term	Meaning
1. hepat/o/megaly CF S	enlargement of the liver
2. lith/iasis WR S	abnormal condition of stones
3. chol/e/cyst/ectomy CF WR S	excision or removal of the gallbladder
4. cholangi/oma WR S	tumor of the bile vessel
5. lapar/o/scop/ic CF WR S	pertaining to visual examination of the abdomen

6. choledochoplasty
7. toxicology
8. postprandial

9. sigmoidoscopy
10. gastroenterologist
11. colonoscope

12. pancreatectomy
13. biliary
14. pylorotomy

15. sublingual

Additional Medical Terms Review

1. hemoccult
2. antiemetics
3. polyp
4. ascites

5. Crohn disease
6. lithotripsy
7. fistula
8. jaundice

9. barium enema
10. IBD
11. hematochezia
12. volvulus

13. cirrhosis
14. barium swallow
15. IBS

Critical Thinking 6-1: Progress Note

1. What symptom made the patient seek medical help?

    Weight loss of 40 pounds since his last examination

2. What surgical procedures were performed on the patient for regional enteritis?

    Ileostomy and appendectomy

3. What abnormality was found with the sigmoidoscopy?

    Dark blood and rectal bleeding

4. What is causing the rectal bleeding?

    The bleeding could be caused by a polyp, bleeding diverticulum, or rectal carcinoma.

5. Write the plural form of diverticulum.

    Diverticula

Critical Thinking 6-2: Operative Report

1. What surgery was performed on this patient?

    Resection of the esophagus with anastomosis of the stomach; mediastinal lymph node excision

2. What diagnostic testing confirmed malignancy?

    Pathology tests on the biopsy specimen from esophagoscopy

3. Where was the carcinoma located?

    Middle third of the esophagus

4. Why was the adjacent lymph node excised?

    Metastasis was suspected.

Medical Record Activity 6-3

1. volvulus	4. ascites	7. antiemetic	10. hernioplasty
2. dysentery	5. polypectomy	8. jaundice	
3. GERD	6. cholangiography	9. diverticulitis	

Vocabulary Review

1. gastroscopy	6. celiac disease	11. cholecystectomy	16. ileostomy
2. dyspepsia	7. stomatalgia	12. anastomosis	17. cholelithiasis
3. hematemesis	8. duodenotomy	13. sigmoidotomy	18. friable
4. ultrasound	9. hepatomegaly	14. rectoplasty	19. peritonitis
5. H$_2$ blockers	10. dysphagia	15. GERD	20. bariatric

CHAPTER 7: URINARY SYSTEM

Section Review 7-1

Term	Meaning
1. glomerul/o/scler/osis	-osis: abnormal condition, increase (used primarily with blood cells); glomerulus; hardening; sclera (white of the eye)
2. cyst/o/scopy	-scopy: visual examination; bladder
3. poly/uria	-uria: urine; many, much
4. lith/o/tripsy	-tripsy: crushing; stone, calculus
5. dia/lysis	-lysis: separation; destruction; loosening; through; across
6. ureter/o/stenosis	-stenosis: narrowing, stricture; ureter
7. meat/us	-us: condition, structure; opening, meatus
8. ur/emia	-emia: blood condition; urine
9. nephr/oma	-oma: tumor; kidney
10. azot/emia	-emia: blood; nitrogenous compounds

Section Review 7-2

1. -osis	5. -megaly	9. -tome	13. lith/o
2. -iasis	6. dia-	10. -tomy	14. -rrhaphy
3. supra-	7. -pexy	11. nephr/o, ren/o	15. poly-
4. -pathy	8. scler/o	12. -ptosis	

Labeling Review—Figure 7-2: Urinary Structures

Check your labeling of Figure 7-2 on page 297.

1. right kidney	3. renal medulla	5. renal vein	7. ureters	9. urethra
2. renal cortex	4. renal artery	6. nephron	8. urinary bladder	10. urinary meatus

Section Review 7-3

1. -iasis
2. cyst/o, vesic/o
3. carcin/o
4. -pathy
5. -megaly
6. -ectomy
7. -ectasis
8. aden/o
9. -tomy
10. -itis
11. -scope
12. enter/o
13. pyel/o
14. rect/o
15. -lith
16. -plasty
17. -rrhaphy
18. -oma
19. ureter/o
20. urethr/o

Labeling Review—Figure 7-9: Structure of a Nephron

Check your labeling of Figure 7-9 on page 312.

1. renal cortex
2. renal medulla
3. glomerular capsule
4. glomerulus
5. renal tubule
6. collecting tubule

Section Review 7-4

1. cyst/o, vesic/o
2. hemat/o
3. -logist
4. glomerul/o
5. scler/o
6. -ist
7. nephr/o, ren/o
8. py/o
9. azot/o
10. pyel/o
11. olig/o
12. ureter/o
13. urethr/o
14. ur/o
15. noct/o
16. -cele
17. poly-
18. -ptosis
19. intra-
20. a-, an-

Word Elements Review

Medical Term	Meaning
1. lith/o/tripsy CF S	crushing of a stone or calculus
2. nephr/o/megaly CF S	enlargement of the kidney(s)
3. ur/emia WR S	blood in urine
4. ureter/o/stenosis CF S	narrowing or stricture of a ureter
5. vesic/o/cele CF S	hernia of the bladder

6. pyuria
7. nephralgia
8. cystocele
9. nephrosclerosis
10. pyeloplasty
11. adenocarcinoma
12. pyelography
13. benign
14. glomerulonephritis
15. nephroptosis

Additional Medical Terms Review

1. diuretics
2. Wilms tumor
3. azoturia
4. antibiotics
5. diuresis
6. retrograde pyelography
7. hemodialysis
8. interstitial nephritis
9. BUN
10. enuresis
11. catheterization
12. VCUG
13. uremia
14. renal hypertension
15. dialysis

Critical Thinking 7-1: Hospital Admission

1. What prompted the consultation with the urologist, Dr. Moriati?

   Preoperative catheterization was not possible.

2. What abnormality did the urologist discover?

   Mild to moderate benign prostatic hypertrophy

3. Did the patient have any previous surgery on his prostate?

   No

4. Where was the patient's hernia?

   In the groin and scrotum (hydrocele)

5. What in the patient's past medical history contributed to his present urological problem?

   Nothing in his past history contributed to his benign prostatic hypertrophy; he had a previous colon resection for carcinoma of the colon.

Critical Thinking 7-2: Progress Note

1. What was found when the patient had a cystoscopy?

   Cystitis

2. What are the symptoms of cystitis?

   Nocturia, urinary frequency, pelvic pain, and, in this case, hematuria

3. What is the patient's past surgical history?

   Cholecystectomy, choledocholithotomy, and incidental appendectomy

4. What is the treatment for cystitis?

   Antibiotics and consumption of a lot of fluids

5. What are the dangers of untreated cystitis?

   Spreading of infection to the kidneys or to the bloodstream (sepsis)

6. What instrument is used to perform a cystoscopy?

   A cystoscope

Medical Record Activity 7-3

1. cystoscopy
2. enuresis
3. BUN
4. catheterization
5. uremia
6. nephrolithiasis
7. hypertension
8. Wilms tumor
9. dialysis
10. cystourethrography

Vocabulary Review

1. malignant
2. nephrons
3. cholelithiasis
4. renal pelvis
5. IVP
6. diuretics
7. edema
8. benign
9. nephrolithotomy
10. acute renal failure
11. nephroptosis
12. ureteropyeloplasty
13. bilateral
14. nocturia
15. urinary incontinence
16. hematuria
17. polyuria
18. oliguria
19. anuria
20. cystocele

CHAPTER 8: REPRODUCTIVE SYSTEMS

Section Review 8-1

Term	Definition
1. primi/gravida	-gravida: pregnant woman; first
2. colp/o/scopy	-scopy: visual examination; vagina
3. gynec/o/logist	-logist: specialist in the study of; woman, female
4. perine/o/rrhaphy	-rrhaphy: suture; perineum
5. hyster/ectomy	-ectomy: excision, removal; uterus (womb)
6. oophor/oma	-oma: tumor; ovary
7. dys/tocia	-tocia: childbirth, labor; bad; painful; difficult
8. endo/metr/itis	-itis: inflammation; in, within; uterus (womb); measure
9. mamm/o/gram	-gram: record, writing; breast
10. amni/o/centesis	-centesis: surgical puncture; amnion (amniotic sac)

Section Review 8-2

1. cyst/o
2. hemat/o, hem/o
3. -rrhage, -rrhagia
4. hyster/o, uter/o, metr/o
5. -cele
6. -tomy
7. -tome

8. -scope
9. salping/o, -salpinx
10. -pexy
11. muc/o
12. oophor/o, ovari/o
13. -arche
14. metr/o

15. -ptosis
16. -oid
17. -logist
18. -logy
19. -plasty
20. colp/o, vagin/o

Labeling Review—Figures 8-2 and 8-3: Lateral View of the Female Reproductive System

Check your labeling of Figures 8-2 and 8-3 on pages 347 and 348.

Figure 8-2

1. ovary (singular)
2. fallopian tube (singular)
3. uterus

4. vagina
5. labia majora
6. labia minora

7. clitoris
8. Bartholin gland
9. cervix

Figure 8-3

1. ovary (singular)
2. fallopian tube (singular)
3. uterus
4. vagina
5. labia majora (shown in lateral view only)

6. labia minora (shown in lateral view only)
7. clitoris (shown in lateral view only)
8. Bartholin gland
9. cervix

Labeling Review—Figure 8-7: Structure of Mammary Glands

Check your labeling of Figure 8-7 on page 359.

1. adipose tissue
2. glandular tissue
3. lobe
4. lactiferous duct
5. nipple
6. areola

Section Review 8-3

1. post-
2. gynec/o
3. pre-
4. mamm/o, mast/o
5. -pathy
6. -ectomy
7. -rrhea
8. -itis
9. -tome
10. -scope
11. -scopy
12. men/o
13. cervic/o
14. -algia, -dynia
15. -ary, -ous
16. -logist
17. salping/o
18. colp/o, vagin/o
19. vulv/o, episi/o
20. dys-

Section Review 8-4

Term	Meaning
1. vas/ectomy	-ectomy: excision, removal; vessel; vas deferens; duct
2. balan/itis	-itis: inflammation; glans penis
3. spermi/cide	-cide: killing; spermatozoa, sperm cells
4. gonad/o/tropin	-tropin: stimulate; gonads, sex glands
5. orchi/o/pexy	-pexy: fixation (of an organ); testis (plural, testes)
6. a/sperm/ia	-ia: condition; without; not; spermatozoa, sperm cells
7. vesicul/itis	-itis: inflammation; seminal vesicle
8. orchid/ectomy	-ectomy: excision, removal; testis (plural, testes)
9. andr/o/gen	-gen: forming, producing; origin; male
10. crypt/orch/ism	-ism: condition; hidden; testis (plural, testes)

Labeling Review—Figure 8-10: Lateral View of the Male Reproductive System

Check your labeling of Figure 8-10 on page 367.

1. testis (singular) or testicle (singular)
2. scrotum
3. epididymis
4. vas deferens
5. seminal vesicle
6. prostate gland
7. bulbourethral gland
8. penis
9. glans penis
10. foreskin

Section Review 8-5

1. -rrhaphy
2. dys-
3. cyst/o
4. carcin/o
5. -cyte
6. -pathy
7. -megaly
8. -cele
9. -itis
10. -tome
11. vas/o
12. muc/o
13. neo-
14. -genesis
15. prostat/o
16. test/o, orchi/o, orchid/o
17. olig/o
18. spermat/o, sperm/o
19. -pexy
20. hyper-

Word Elements Review

Medical Term	Meaning
1. vas/ectomy WR S	excision or removal of a vessel or the vas deferens duct
2. amni/o/centesis CF S	surgical puncture of the amnion (amniotic sac)
3. mast/o/plasty CF S	surgical repair of the breast(s)
4. oophor/oma WR S	tumor of the ovary
5. crypt/orchid/ism WR WR S	condition of hidden testis (testes)

6. prostatocystitis
7. mastopexy
8. colposcopy

9. oligospermia
10. hysterectomy
11. balanitis

12. testopathy
13. galactorrhea
14. perineorrhaphy

15. primigravida

Additional Medical Terms Review

1. cryptorchidism
2. fibroid
3. sterility
4. anorchism
5. candidiasis

6. chlamydia
7. circumcision
8. cerclage
9. leukorrhea
10. endometriosis

11. mammography
12. gonorrhea
13. syphilis
14. toxic shock
15. trichomoniasis

16. D&C
17. phimosis
18. impotence
19. oligomenorrhea
20. gonadotropins

Critical Thinking 8-1: Emergency Department

1. What conditions are treated with the over-the-counter medication Monistat?

   An antifungal used to treat fungal and vaginal yeast infections

2. Place a "1" in the space provided for positive findings and a "−" for negative findings. A positive finding indicates the patient had these symptoms; a negative finding indicates the patient did not have the symptoms.

hematuria	−	*skin rash*	−
vaginal irritation	+	vaginal drainage	+
fever	−	foul-smelling drainage	+

3. What were the diagnoses in this patient?

   Probable pelvic inflammatory disease (PID), trichomoniasis, possible gonorrhea exposure

4. What is trichomoniasis and how is it treated?

   Most common sexually transmitted infection (STI) that is asymptomatic; treated with a single oral dose of a combined antibacterial and antiprotozoal medication

5. What are the possible complications if the patient does not treat her sexually transmitted infection (STI)?

   In the female, the prolonged presence of an untreated STI may result in infertility. In addition, the presence of an STI during pregnancy and childbirth could have potential negative effects on the health of the fetus and baby; the patient may also spread the STI to her sexual partner(s).

Critical Thinking 8-2: Operative Report

1. What is the end result of a bilateral vasectomy?

   Sterilization

2. Was the patient awake during the surgery? What type of anesthesia was used?

   Yes; 1% xylocaine

3. What was used to prevent bleeding?

   Hemostats, cautery, and sutures

4. What type of suture material was used to close the incision?

   2-0 chromic

5. What was the patient given for pain relief at home?

   Darvocet-N 100

6. Why is it important for the patient to go for a follow-up visit?

   To analyze his semen and confirm sterilization

Medical Record Activity 8-3

1. TURP	5. herpes genitalis	9. orchidoplasty
2. preeclampsia	6. ectopic pregnancy	10. lumpectomy
3. candidiasis	7. colposcopy	
4. cryptorchidism	8. endometriosis	

Vocabulary Review

1. prostatomegaly	6. oophoritis	11. epididymis	16. dysmenorrhea
2. testopathy	7. aspermatism	12. hydrocele	17. postmenopausal
3. testosterone	8. gravida 4	13. vas deferens	18. oxytocics
4. amenorrhea	9. uterus	14. para 4	19. vasectomy
5. estrogen	10. prostatic cancer	15. cervix uteri	20. PID

CHAPTER 9: ENDOCRINE AND NERVOUS SYSTEMS

Section Review 9-1

Term	Definition
1. toxic/o/logist	-logist: specialist in the study of; poison
2. pancreat/itis	-itis: inflammation; pancreas
3. thyr/o/megaly	-megaly: enlargement; thyroid gland
4. hyper/trophy	-trophy: development, nourishment; excessive, above normal
5. gluc/o/genesis	-genesis: forming, producing; origin; sugar, sweetness
6. hypo/calc/emia	-emia: blood condition; under, below; deficient; calcium
7. adrenal/ectomy	-ectomy: excision, removal; adrenal glands
8. poly/dipsia	-dipsia: thirst; many, much
9. aden/oma	-oma: tumor; gland
10. thyroid/ectomy	-ectomy: excision, removal; thyroid gland

Section Review 9-2

1. -osis	6. calc/o	11. aden/o	16. radi/o
2. hyper-	7. -pathy	12. -tomy	17. -logist
3. poster/o	8. -megaly	13. -tome	18. poly-
4. dys-	9. acr/o	14. neur/o	19. thyroid/o, thyr/o
5. -emia	10. anter/o	15. toxic/o	20. hypo

Labeling Review—Figure 9-3: Locations of Major Endocrine Glands

Check your labeling of Figure 9-3 on page 413.

1. pituitary gland	4. adrenal glands	7. thymus gland
2. thyroid gland	5. pancreas	8. ovaries
3. parathyroid glands	6. pineal gland	9. testes

Section Review 9-3

1. -iasis	8. para-	15. orch/o, orchi/o, orchid/o
2. supra-	9. pancreat/o	16. -dipsia
3. adrenal/o, adren/o	10. -gen, -genesis	17. thym/o
4. -pathy	11. -lysis	18. hypo-
5. -pexy	12. -lith	19. -uria
6. -rrhea	13. gluc/o, glyc/o	20. toxic/o
7. poly-	14. -phagia	

Section Review 9-4

Term	Meaning
1. meningi/oma	-oma: tumor; meninges
2. neur/o/lysis	-lysis: separation; destruction; loosening; nerve
3. hemi/paresis	-paresis: partial paralysis; one half
4. myel/algia	-algia: pain; bone marrow; spinal cord
5. cerebr/o/spin/al	-al: pertaining to; cerebrum; spine
6. a/phasia	-phasia: speech; without; not
7. mening/o/cele	-cele: hernia; swelling; meninges
8. encephal/itis	-itis: inflammation; brain
9. gli/oma	-oma: tumor; glue; neuroglial tissue
10. quadri/plegia	-plegia: paralysis; four

Labeling Review—Figure 9-10: Structures of the Brain

Check your labeling of Figure 9-10 on page 433.

1. cerebrum	3. pons
2. midbrain	4. medulla

Labeling Review—Figure 9-11: Spinal Nerves

Check your labeling of Figure 9-11 on page 435.

1. cervical nerves
2. thoracic nerves
3. lumbar nerves

4. sacral nerves
5. coccygeal nerves

Section Review 9-5

1. -osis
2. dys-
3. thromb/o
4. vascul/o

5. encephal/o
6. -rhage, -rrhagia
7. gli/o, -glia
8. scler/o

9. mening/o, meningi/o
10. neur/o
11. cerebr/o
12. -malacia

13. -phasia
14. myel/o
15. a-

Word Elements Review

Medical Term	Meaning
1. hemi/paresis P S	partial paralysis of one half of the body (right half or left half)
2. hyper/glyc/emia P WR S	condition of excessive glucose (sugar) in blood
3. hypo/pituitar/ism P WR S	condition of deficient (inadequate levels of) pituitary hormones in the body
4. meningi/oma WR S	tumor composed of meninges
5. poly/dipsia PR S	much (excessive) thirst
6. quadri/plegia PR S	paralysis of the four extremities
7. thyr/o/megaly CF S	enlargement of the thyroid gland
8. toxic/o/logist CF S	specialist in the study of poisons (toxins)

9. glioma
10. acromegaly
11. thrombogenesis
12. thymoma
13. thyropathy

14. neuralgia
15. aphasia
16. meningocele
17. adrenalectomy
18. neurolysis

19. hemiparesis
20. thalamotomy
21. myelitis
22. hypocalcemia
23. pancreatolithiasis

24. encephalitis
25. hypertrophy

Additional Medical Terms Review

1. Bell palsy
2. TIA
3. antipsychotics
4. exophthalmos
5. Graves disease
6. hypophysectomy
7. myxedema

8. pheochromocytoma
9. Parkinson disease
10. poliomyelitis
11. sciatica
12. spina bifida
13. EEG
14. neuroblastoma

15. Alzheimer disease
16. MRI
17. type 1 diabetes
18. shingles
19. quadriplegia
20. panhypopituitarism
21. Huntington chorea

22. lumbar puncture
23. epilepsy
24. thalamotomy
25. PET

Critical Thinking 9-1: Discharge Summary

1. What symptoms of diabetes mellitus (DM) did the patient experience before his office visit?

   Glycosuria, elevated blood glucose of 400, polydipsia, and increased appetite

2. What confirmed the patient's new diagnosis of DM?

   Elevated blood glucose and glycosuria

3. What conditions had to be met before the patient could be discharged from the hospital?

   He had to be able to draw up and give his own insulin and perform fingersticks.

4. How many times a day does the patient have to take insulin?

   Two times, once in the morning and once in the afternoon

5. Why does the patient have to perform fingersticks four times a day?

   To monitor his blood glucose levels closely and ensure they are within the normal range

6. What is an ADA 2,000-calorie diet? Why is it important?

   A 2,000-calorie diet designed by American Diabetic Association (ADA), which is important for maintaining the same number of calories each day to help control blood glucose levels

Critical Thinking 9-2: Chart Note

1. What are the patient's presenting complaints?

   Prolonged pain and burning in her feet, especially in the left foot; diminished proprioception; difficulty walking, particularly in the dark; and intermittent low back pain

2. Are the patient's cranial nerves intact?

   Yes, but the patient experiences hearing loss, which might arise from a problem with cranial nerve VIII.

3. How was the motor system examination described?

   The patient has normal gait and station and generally good strength, coordination, and reflexes. She was able to touch her fingertips to her toes but unable to straighten up unless she bent her knees.

4. How extensive is the patient's sensory loss?

   Decreased position, vibratory, and pinprick sense in the lower extremities, much more in the right foot up to the upper third of the shin, and in just the foot and ankle on the left

5. What test(s) did the doctor order to further understand the extent of her peripheral neuropathy?

   EMG and nerve conduction studies of the lower extremities

Medical Record Activity 9-3

1. myxedema
2. epilepsy
3. Graves disease
4. glucose tolerance test
5. sciatica
6. Addison disease
7. shingles
8. TIA
9. Alzheimer disease
10. pheochromocytoma

Vocabulary Review

1. acromegaly
2. pancreatolysis
3. adenohypophysis
4. cerebral palsy
5. hypercalcemia
6. insulin
7. neurohypophysis
8. pancreatopathy
9. polyphagia
10. diabetes mellitus
11. hyperglycemia
12. pancreatolith
13. polydipsia
14. thyrotoxicosis
15. adrenalectomy
16. adrenaline
17. glycogenesis
18. meningocele
19. neuromalacia
20. pruritus
21. deglutition
22. vertigo
23. jaundice
24. metastasis
25. hormone

CHAPTER 10: MUSCULOSKELETAL SYSTEM

Section Review 10-1

Term	Meaning
1. chondr/itis	-itis: inflammation; cartilage
2. my/o/rrhaphy	*-rrhaphy:* suture; muscle
3. hemi/plegia	-plegia: paralysis; one half
4. ten/o/tomy	-tomy: incision; tendon
5. leiomy/oma	-oma: tumor; smooth muscle
6. tend/o/lysis	-lysis: separation; destruction; loosening; tendon
7. my/o/pathy	-pathy: disease; muscle
8. lumb/o/cost/al	-al: pertaining to; loins (lower back); ribs
9. tendin/itis	-itis: inflammation; tendon
10. my/algia	-algia: pain; muscle

Section Review 10-2

1. -osis
2. cyst/o
3. -cyte
4. quadri-
5. hemi-
6. scler/o
7. -tomy
8. enter/o
9. hepat/o
10. my/o
11. -plegia
12. -genesis
13. -rrhexis
14. -plasty
15. -rrhaphy
16. ten/o, tendin/o, tend/o
17. -tome
18. chondr/o
19. -sarcoma
20. -lysis

Section Review 10-3

Term	Meaning
1. dia/physis	*-physis: growth; through, across*
2. sub/cost/al	-al: pertaining to; under, below; ribs
3. oste/o/malacia	-malacia: softening; bone
4. lamin/ectomy	-ectomy: excision, removal; lamina (part of the vertebral arch)
5. pelv/i/metry	-metry: act of measuring; pelvis
6. myel/o/cele	-cele: hernia; swelling; bone marrow; spinal cord
7. oste/o/porosis	-porosis: porous; bone
8. ankyl/osis	-osis: abnormal condition, increase (used primarily with blood cells); stiffness; bent, crooked
9. carp/o/ptosis	-ptosis: prolapse, downward displacement; carpus (wrist bones)
10. crani/o/tomy	-tomy: incision; cranium (skull)

Labeling Review—Figure 10-4: Longitudinal Section of a Long Bone (Femur) and Interior Bone Structure

Check your labeling of Figure 10-4 on page 487.

1. diaphysis	3. compact bone	5. distal epiphysis	7. spongy bone
2. periosteum	4. medullary cavity	6. proximal epiphysis	

Section Review 10-4

1. hyper-	8. dist/o	15. -algia, -dynia	22. -rrhaphy
2. peri-	9. scler/o	16. -graphy	23. -oma
3. -emia	10. -cele	17. -genesis	24. hypo-
4. oste/o	11. -tomy	18. -gram	25. radi/o
5. chondr/o	12. -itis	19. -malacia	
6. calc/o	13. proxim/o	20. -logist	
7. -cyte	14. my/o	21. myel/o	

Labeling Review—Figure 10-9: Anterior View of the Skeleton

Check your labeling of Figure 10-9 on page 495.

1. crani/o	4. vertebr/o	7. metacarp/o	10. femor/o	13. fibul/o
2. stern/o	5. humer/o	8. phalang/o	11. patell/o	14. calcane/o
3. cost/o	6. carp/o	9. pelv/i, pelv/o	12. tibi/o	

Labeling Review—Figure 10-10: Types of Fractures

Check your labeling of Figure 10-10 on page 498.

1. closed fracture	3. incomplete fracture	5. comminuted fracture	7. complicated fracture
2. open fracture	4. Greenstick fracture	6. impacted fracture	8. Colles fracture

Labeling Review—Figure 10-11: Complete Fractures

Check your labeling of Figure 10-11 on page 500.

1. spiral fracture	2. oblique fracture	3. longitudinal fracture	4. transverse fracture

Labeling Review—Figure 10-13: Vertebral Column, Lateral View

Check your labeling of Figure 10-13 on page 503.

1. intervertebral disks	3. atlas	5. thoracic vertebrae	7. sacrum
2. cervical vertebrae	4. axis	6. lumbar vertebrae	8. coccyx

Section Review 10-5

1. -osis	5. -pathy	9. lumb/o	13. sacr/o
2. oste/o	6. -ectomy	10. cervic/o	14. -centesis
3. encephal/o	7. cephal/o	11. -um	15. spondyl/o, vertebr/o
4. thorac/o	8. arthr/o	12. cost/o	

Word Elements Review

Medical Term	Meaning
1. chondr/o/malacia 　　CF　　S	softening of cartilage
2. patell/ectomy 　　WR　　S	excision of the kneecap
3. hemi/plegia 　　P　　S	paralysis of one half (of the body)
4. spondyl/itis 　　WR　　S	inflammation of any of the vertebrae (plural)
5. lord/osis 　　WR　S	abnormal condition of a curved or swayback

6. arthritis
7. osteoporosis
8. kyphosis
9. arthrocentesis

10. sequestrectomy
11. fascioplasty
12. myorrhexis
13. leiomyoma

14. myelocele
15. osteochondritis
16. osteomalacia
17. myoma

18. myorrhaphy
19. craniotomy
20. calcaneodynia

Additional Medical Terms Review

1. bunion
2. tendinitis
3. sprain
4. strain
5. kyphosis
6. Ewing sarcoma
7. torticollis

8. gout
9. RA
10. Paget disease
11. sequestrum
12. arthroplasty
13. crepitation
14. myasthenia gravis

15. lordosis
16. muscular dystrophy
17. NSAIDs
18. ankylosis
19. herniated disk
20. CTS
21. sequestrectomy

22. rheumatoid factor
23. talipes
24. arthroscopy
25. scoliosis

Critical Thinking 10-1: Radiology Report

1. Why does the x-ray show a decreased density at L5–S1?

   Appears that a bilateral laminectomy had been done

2. What is the most common cause of degenerative intervertebral disk disease?

   Aging, with degenerative intervertebral disk disease being a common finding in individuals age 50 years or greater

3. What happens to the gelatinous material of the disk as aging occurs?

   The gelatinous material is replaced by harder fibrocartilage.

4. What is the probable cause of the narrowing of the L3–L4 and L4–L5?

   Narrowing commonly occurs as a result of degenerative intervertebral disk disease.

Critical Thinking 10-2: Operative Report

1. What type of arthritis did the patient have?

   Degenerative

2. Did the patient have calcium deposits in the right shoulder?

   No

3. What type of instrument did the physician use to visualize the glenoid labra?

   Arthroscope

4. What are labra?

   Liplike structures; in this case, edges or rims of bones

5. Did the patient have any outgrowths of bone? If so, where?

   Yes, spurs were found at the inferior and anterior acromioclavicular joint.

Medical Record 10-3

1. arthroplasty	5. scoliosis	9. arthrocentesis
2. costochondritis	6. rickets	10. myasthenia gravis
3. sprain	7. gouty arthritis	
4. carpal tunnel syndrome	8. torticollis	

Vocabulary Review

1. radiology	6. proximal	11. bone marrow	16. distal
2. diaphysis	7. articulation	12. cephalometer	17. radiologist
3. AP	8. open fracture	13. myelogram	18. cervical vertebrae
4. closed fracture	9. atlas	14. myorrhexis	19. intervertebral
5. bilateral	10. arthrocentesis	15. spondylomalacia	20. quadriplegia

CHAPTER 11: SPECIAL SENSES: EYES AND EARS

Section Review 11-1

Term	Meaning
1. conjunctiv/itis	*-itis; inflammation; conjunctiva*
2. blephar/o/ptosis	-ptosis: prolapse, downward displacement; eyelid
3. ambly/opia	-opia: vision; dull, dim
4. retin/o/pathy	-pathy: disease; retina
5. scler/itis	-itis: inflammation; hardening; sclera (white of the eye)
6. ophthalm/o/scope	-scope: instrument for examining; eye
7. intra/ocul/ar	-ar: pertaining to; within, in; eye
8. dacry/o/rrhea	-rrhea: discharge, flow; tear; lacrimal apparatus (duct, sac, or gland)
9. dipl/opia	-opia: vision; double
10. blephar/o/spasm	-spasm: involuntary contraction, twitching; eyelid

Labeling Review—Figure 11-1: Eye Structures

Check your labeling of Figure 11-1 on page 534.

1. sclera
2. cornea
3. choroid
4. ciliary body

5. iris
6. retina
7. fovea
8. pupil

9. optic disc
10. optic nerve
11. conjunctiva

Labeling Review—Figure 11-4: Lacrimal Apparatus

Check your labeling of Figure 11-4 on page 540.

1. lacrimal gland

2. lacrimal sac

3. nasolacrimal duct

Section Review 11-2

Term	Meaning
1. tympan/o/centesis	*-centesis: surgical puncture; tympanic membrane (eardrum)*
2. acous/tic	-tic: pertaining to; hearing
3. hyper/tropia	-tropia: turning; excessive; above normal
4. ot/o/rrhea	-rrhea: discharge, flow; ear
5. an/acusis	-acusis: hearing; without; not
6. myring/o/tomy	-tomy: incision; tympanic membrane (eardrum)
7. tympan/o/plasty	-plasty: surgical repair; tympanic membrane (eardrum)
8. audi/o/meter	-meter: instrument for measuring; hearing
9. ot/o/scope	-scope: instrument for examining; ear
10. salping/o/pharyng/eal	-eal: pertaining to; tube (usually fallopian or eustachian [auditory] tubes); pharynx (throat)

Labeling Review—Figure 11-5: Ear Structures

Check your labeling of Figure 11-5 on page 543.

1. auricle
2. ear canal
3. tympanic membrane
4. malleus

5. incus
6. stapes
7. eustachian (auditory) tube
8. cochlea

9. semicircular canals
10. vestibule

Section Review 11-3

1. hyper-
2. choroid/o
3. kerat/o
4. dipl/o, dipl-
5. ot/o
6. salping/o, -salpinx
7. ophthalm/o

8. blephar/o
9. aden/o
10. scler/o
11. -spasm
12. irid/o
13. -ptosis
14. -logist

15. retin/o
16. -rrhexis
17. -malacia
18. audi/o, -acusis
19. -stenosis
20. -edema
21. dacry/o

22. tympan/o, myring/o
23. corne/o
24. -opia, -opsia
25. xanth/o

Word Elements Review

Medical Term	Meaning
1. intra/ocul/ar P WR S	pertaining to "within the eye"
2. myring/o/tomy CF S	incision of the tympanic membrane (eardrum)
3. ophthalm/o/scope CF S	instrument for examining the eye
4. tympan/o/plasty CF S	surgical repair of the tympanic membrane (eardrum)
5. blephar/o/ptosis CF S	prolapse or downward displacement of the eyeball

6. audiologist	9. optic	12. retinopathy	15. anisocoria
7. conjunctivitis	10. dacryorrhea	13. otalgia	
8. anacusis	11. salpingostenosis	14. coreometer	

Additional Medical Terms Review

1. tinnitus	8. conjunctivitis	15. astigmatism	22. Rinne test
2. otosclerosis	9. photophobia	16. acoustic neuroma	23. diabetic retinopathy
3. achromatopsia	10. presbycusis	17. tonometry	24. macular degeneration
4. Ménière disease	11. glaucoma	18. mydriatics	25. myringotomy
5. strabismus	12. vertigo	19. conductive hearing loss	
6. anacusis	13. retinal detachment	20. cataract	
7. otitis media	14. hordeolum	21. phacoemulsification	

Critical Thinking 11-1: Operative Report

1. Where is the retina located?

   The retina is the innermost layer of the eye.

2. Was the anesthetic administered behind or in front of the eyeball?

   Behind the eyeball (retrobulbar)

3. How much movement remained in the eye following anesthesia?

   None; akinesia

4. Where was the hemorrhage located?

   In the orbit of the eye behind the lens, where the vitreous humor is located

5. What type of vitrectomy was undertaken?

   Trans pars plana vitrectomy

6. Why was the eye left soft?

   Because it had poor perfusion

Critical Thinking 11-2: SOAP Note

1. What was the chief complaint that brought the child into the office?

   She had been diagnosed with a virus last week and advised to follow up if anything got worse. Yesterday, she developed a temperature of 104°F; and this morning, it was 104°F, and she is not eating well.

2. What laboratory test(s) were performed in the office?

   Rapid strep test, which had a negative result

3. Where was the patient's infection located?

   The left ear

4. What medication was prescribed for the patient's infection?

   Amoxicillin 200 mg per 5 mL, 1 teaspoon twice a day for 10 days

5. What medication(s) was prescribed for the patient's fever?

   Alternating Tylenol and ibuprofen throughout the day to keep the fever down

Medical Record Activity 11-3

1. presbycusis
2. conjunctivitis
3. photophobia
4. tonometry
5. achromatopsia
6. cochlear implant
7. mydriatics
8. esotropia
9. wax emulsifiers
10. myringotomy

Vocabulary Review

1. diplopia
2. sclera
3. tympanic membrane
4. dacryorrhea
5. miotics
6. keratitis
7. diagnosis
8. mucoserous
9. otitis media
10. cholesteatoma
11. mastoid surgery
12. general anesthetic
13. ophthalmologist
14. chronic
15. hyperopia
16. postoperatively
17. labyrinth
18. blepharoptosis
19. salpingostenosis
20. myopia

Index of Diagnostic, Medical, and Surgical Procedures

This section provides a list of the diagnostic, medical, and surgical procedures covered in the textbook, along with page numbers. Diagnostic procedures help the physician assess a patient's health status, evaluate the factors influencing that status, and determine a method of treatment. Medical and surgical procedures are performed to treat a specific disorder that is diagnosed by the physician.

Diagnostic Procedures

Amniocentesis, Chapter 8, Reproductive Systems, 381
Arterial blood gas (ABG), Chapter 4, Respiratory System, 143
Arthrocentesis, Chapter 10, Musculoskeletal System, 512
Audiometry, Chapter 11, Special Senses: Eyes and Ears, 555
Barium enema (BE), Chapter 6, Digestive System, 271
Barium swallow, Chapter 6, Digestive System, 272
Biopsy, Chapter 3, Integumentary System, 94
Blood urea nitrogen (BUN), Chapter 7, Urinary System, 321
Bone density test (bone densitometry), Chapter 10, Musculoskeletal System, 512
Bone scan, Chapter 10, Musculoskeletal System, 513
Bone marrow aspiration biopsy, Chapter 5, Cardiovascular and Lymphatic Systems, 207
Bronchoscopy, Chapter 4, Respiratory System, 143
Capsule endoscopy, Chapter 6, Digestive System, 272
Cardiac catheterization (CC), Chapter 5, Cardiovascular and Lymphatic Systems, 204
Cardiac enzyme studies, Chapter 5, Cardiovascular and Lymphatic Systems, 204
Cerebrospinal fluid (CSF) analysis, Chapter 9, Endocrine and Nervous Systems, 450
Colposcopy, Chapter 8, Reproductive Systems, 381
Computed tomography (CT), Chapter 2, Body Structure, 57
    Chapter 4, Respiratory System, 144
    Chapter 6, Digestive System, 272
    Chapter 7, Urinary System, 321
    Chapter 9, Endocrine and Nervous Systems, 451
COVID-19 test, antibody test, Chapter 4, Respiratory System, 144
COVID-19 test, nose swab, Chapter 4, Respiratory System, 144
Creatinine clearance, Chapter 7, Urinary System, 321
Culture and sensitivity (C&S), Chapter 2, Body Structure, 55
Digital rectal examination (DRE), Chapter 8, Reproductive Systems, 383

Doppler Ultrasonography (DUS), Chapter 5, Cardiovascular and Lymphatic Systems, 206

Echocardiography, Chapter 5, Cardiovascular and Lymphatic Systems, 204

Electrocardiography (ECG), Chapter 5, Cardiovascular and Lymphatic Systems, 204

Electroencephalography (EEG), Chapter 9, Endocrine and Nervous Systems, 450

Enzyme-linked immunosorbent assay (ELISA), Chapter 5, Cardiovascular and Lymphatic Systems, 207

Endoscopy, Chapter 2, Body Structure, 56
    Chapter 6, Digestive System, 272

Fasting blood glucose (FBG), Chapter 9, Endocrine and Nervous Systems, 449

Fluoroscopy, Chapter 2, Body Structure, 57

Glucose tolerance test (GTT), Chapter 9, Endocrine and Nervous Systems, 450

Holter monitor, Chapter 5, Cardiovascular and Lymphatic Systems, 205

Hysterosalpingo-oophorectomy, Chapter 8, Reproductive Systems, 385

Intravenous fluorescein angiography (IVFA), Chapter 11, Special Senses: Eyes and Ears, 554

Intravenous pyelography (IVP), Chapter 7, Urinary System, 322

Kidney, ureter, bladder (KUB), Chapter 7, Urinary System, 313

Laparoscopy, Chapter 8, Reproductive Systems, 382

Lipid panel, Chapter 5, Cardiovascular and Lymphatic Systems, 205

Lumbar puncture, Chapter 9, Endocrine and Nervous Systems, 450

Lymphangiography, Chapter 5, Cardiovascular and Lymphatic Systems, 207

Magnetic resonance imaging (MRI), Chapter 2, Body Structure, 57
    Chapter 4, Respiratory System, 144
    Chapter 6, Digestive System, 273
    Chapter 9, Endocrine and Nervous Systems, 451

Magnetoencephalography (MEG), Chapter 9, Endocrine and Nervous Systems, 451

Mammography, Chapter 8, Reproductive Systems, 382

Nuclear scan, Chapter 2, Body Structure, 57
    Chapter 7, Urinary System, 322

Nuclear stress test, Chapter 5, Cardiovascular and Lymphatic Systems, 205

Otoscopy, Chapter 11, Special Senses: Eyes and Ears, 555

Papanicolaou (Pap) test, Chapter 8, Reproductive Systems, 382

Polysomnography (PSG), Chapter 4, Respiratory System, 144

Spirometry, Chapter 4, Respiratory System, 145

Pneumatic otoscopy, Chapter 11, Special Senses: Eyes and Ears, 555

Positron emission tomography (PET), Chapter 9, Endocrine and Nervous Systems, 451

Prostate-specific antigen (PSA) test, Chapter 8, Reproductive Systems, 370

Pulmonary function tests (PFTs), Chapter 4, Respiratory System, 145

Pyelography, Chapter 7, Urinary System, 322

Radioactive iodine uptake (RAIU) test, Chapter 9, Endocrine and Nervous Systems, 450

Radiography, Chapter 2, Body Structure, 47

Radiopharmaceutical, Chapter 2, Body Structure, 57

Renal scan, Chapter 7, Urinary System, 322

Retrograde pyelography, Chapter 7, Urinary System, 322

Rheumatoid factor, Chapter 10, Musculoskeletal System, 513

Rinne test, Chapter 11, Special Senses: Eyes and Ears, 556

Spirometry, Chapter 4, Respiratory System, 145

Skin test, Chapter 3, Integumentary System, 94

Slit lamp examination, Chapter 11, Special Senses: Eyes and Ears, 554

Stool guaiac, Chapter 6, Digestive System, 273

Stress test, Chapter 5, Cardiovascular and Lymphatic Systems, 205

Tissue typing, Chapter 5, Cardiovascular and Lymphatic Systems, 207

Tomography, Chapter 2, Body Structure, 57

Tonometry, Chapter 11, Special Senses: Eyes and Ears, 554

Transrectal ultrasound (TRUS) and biopsy of the prostate, Chapter 8, Reproductive Systems, 384

Troponin I, Chapter 5, Cardiovascular and Lymphatic Systems, 206

Tuberculosis test, Mantoux, Chapter 4, Respiratory System, 146

Tuberculosis test, tine test, Chapter 4, Respiratory System, 146

Tuning fork test, Chapter 11, Special Senses: Eyes and Ears, 556

Ultrasonography (US), Chapter 2, Body Structure, 59
   Chapter 5, Cardiovascular and Lymphatic Systems, 206
   Chapter 6, Digestive System, 273
   Chapter 7, Urinary System, 322
   Chapter 8, Reproductive Systems, 383
Urinalysis, Chapter 7, Urinary System, 305
Visual acuity test, Chapter 11, Special Senses: Eyes and Ears, 555
Voiding cystourethrography (VCUG), Chapter 7, Urinary System, 323
Weber test, Chapter 11, Special Senses: Eyes and Ears, 556
X-ray, Chapter 2, Body Structure, 57

Medical and Surgical Procedures

Allograft, Chapter 3, Integumentary System, 96
Anastomosis, Chapter 2, Body Structure, 59
Angioplasty, Chapter 5, Cardiovascular and Lymphatic Systems, 208
Appendectomy, Chapter 6, Digestive System, 273
Arthroplasty, Chapter 10, Musculoskeletal System, 513
Autograft, Chapter 3, Integumentary System, 96
Automatic external defibrillator (AED), Chapter 5, Cardiovascular and Lymphatic Systems, 210
Automatic implantable cardioverter defibrillator (AICD), Chapter 5, Cardiovascular and Lymphatic Systems, 210
Bariatric surgery, Chapter 6, Digestive System, 274
Bone immobilization, casting, Chapter 10, Musculoskeletal System, 513
Bone immobilization, splinting, Chapter 10, Musculoskeletal System, 513
Bone immobilization, traction, Chapter 10, Musculoskeletal System, 513
Bone marrow transplantation, Chapter 5, Cardiovascular and Lymphatic Systems, 212
Brachytherapy, Chapter 8, Reproductive Systems, 388
Cardioversion, Chapter 5, Cardiovascular and Lymphatic Systems, 209
Cataract surgery, Chapter 11, Special Senses: Eyes and Ears, 556
Catheterization (Cath), Chapter 7, Urinary System, 323
Cauterization, Chapter 2, Body Structure, 60
Cauterize, Chapter 2, Body Structure, 60
Cerclage, Chapter 8, Reproductive Systems, 384
Chemical peel, Chapter 3, Integumentary System, 96
Circumcision, Chapter 8, Reproductive Systems, 388
Cochlear implantation, Chapter 11, Special Senses: Eyes and Ears, 559
Colonoscopy, Chapter 6, Digestive System, 272
Corneal transplantation, Chapter 11, Special Senses: Eyes and Ears, 557
Coronary artery bypass graft (CABG), Chapter 5, Cardiovascular and Lymphatic Systems, 210
Craniotomy, Chapter 9, Endocrine and Nervous Systems, 453
Cryosurgery, Chapter 3, Integumentary System, 95
Cutaneous laser, Chapter 3, Integumentary System, 96
Débridement, Chapter 3, Integumentary System, 95
Defibrillation, Chapter 5, Cardiovascular and Lymphatic Systems, 210
Dermabrasion, Chapter 3, Integumentary System, 96
Dialysis, Chapter 7, Urinary System, 324
Ear irrigation, Chapter 11, Special Senses: Eyes and Ears, 559
Endarterectomy, Chapter 5, Cardiovascular and Lymphatic Systems, 211
Endotracheal intubation, Chapter 4, Respiratory System, 146
Excimer laser, Chapter 3, Integumentary System, 95
Extracapsular cataract extraction (ECCE), Chapter 11, Special Senses: Eyes and Ears, 556
Extracorporeal shock-wave lithotripsy (ESWL), Chapter 6, Digestive System, 275
Fulguration, Chapter 3, Integumentary System, 95
Hemodialysis (HD), Chapter 7, Urinary System, 324
Hysterosalpingo-oophorectomy, Chapter 8, Reproductive Systems, 385
Incision and drainage (I&D), Chapter 3, Integumentary System, 95

Insulin pump therapy, Chapter 9, Endocrine and Nervous System, 452

Iridectomy, Chapter 11, Special Senses: Eyes and Ears, 557

Laser photocoagulation, Chapter 11, Special Senses: Eyes and Ears, 557

Laser-assisted in situ keratomileusis (LASIK), Chapter 11, Special Senses: Eyes and Ears, 557

Lithotripsy, Chapter 6, Digestive System, 275

Lumpectomy, Chapter 8, Reproductive Systems, 385

Lymphangiectomy, Chapter 5, Cardiovascular and Lymphatic Systems, 212

Mastectomy, Chapter 8, Reproductive Systems, 386

Modified radical mastectomy, Chapter 8, Reproductive Systems, 386

Mohs surgery, Chapter 3, Integumentary System, 95

Myringotomy, Chapter 11, Special Senses: Eyes and Ears, 559

Nasogastric intubation, Chapter 6, Digestive System, 275

Percutaneous transluminal coronary angioplasty (PTCA), Chapter 5, Cardiovascular and Lymphatic Systems, 208

Peritoneal dialysis, Chapter 7, Urinary System, 324

Phacoemulsification, Chapter 11, Special Senses: Eyes and Ears, 556

Pneumonectomy, Chapter 4, Respiratory System, 128

Postural drainage, Chapter 4, Respiratory System, 146

Radical mastectomy, Chapter 8, Reproductive Systems, 386

Reconstructive breast surgery, Chapter 8, Reproductive Systems, 386

Renal transplantation, Chapter 7, Urinary System, 320

Roux-en-Y gastric bypass (RGB), Chapter 6, Digestive System, 274

Sclerotherapy, Chapter 5, Cardiovascular and Lymphatic Systems, 212

Sequestrectomy, Chapter 10, Musculoskeletal System, 513

Skin graft, Chapter 3, Integumentary System, 96

Skin resurfacing, Chapter 3, Integumentary System, 96

Synthetic, Chapter 3, Integumentary System, 96

Thalamotomy, Chapter 9, Endocrine and Nervous Systems, 453

Tissue (skin) expansion, Chapter 8, Reproductive Systems, 386

Total mastectomy, Chapter 8, Reproductive Systems, 386

Transsphenoidal hypophysectomy, Chapter 9, Endocrine and Nervous Systems, 452

Transurethral resection of the prostate (TURP), Chapter 8, Reproductive Systems, 389

Transverse rectus abdominis muscle (TRAM) flap, Chapter 8, Reproductive Systems, 386

Trephination, Chapter 9, Endocrine and Nervous Systems, 453

Tubal ligation, Chapter 8, Reproductive Systems, 388

Ureteral stent, Chapter 7, Urinary System, 326

Valvuloplasty, Chapter 5, Cardiovascular and Lymphatic Systems, 212

Vertical banded gastroplasty, Chapter 6, Digestive System, 274

Vitrectomy, Chapter 11, Special Senses: Eyes and Ears, 557

Xenograft, Chapter 3, Integumentary System, 96

Drug Classifications

This section provides a quick reference of common drug categories. They include prescription and over-the-counter drugs that are used to treat signs, symptoms, and diseases of the various body systems.

Drug Classification	Description
A	
alkylawtes ĂL-kĭ-lāts	Treat certain types of malignancies *Alkylates break deoxyribonucleic acid (DNA) strands in the cancerous cell by substituting an alkyl group for a hydrogen molecule in DNA.*
analgesics ăn-ăl-JĒ-zĭks	Relieve minor to severe pain *Analgesics include nonprescription drugs, such as aspirin and other nonsteroidal anti-inflammatory agents, and those classified as controlled substances that are available only by prescription.*
androgens ĂN-drō-jĕnz	Increase testosterone levels *Hyposecretion of testosterone may be caused by surgical removal of the testes or decreased levels of luteinizing hormone (LH) from the anterior pituitary gland.*
anesthetics ăn-ĕs-THĔT-ĭks	Produce partial or complete loss of sensation with or without loss of consciousness *General anesthetics act on the brain to produce complete loss of feeling with loss of consciousness. Local anesthetics act on nerves or nerve tracts to affect a local area only without loss of consciousness.*
angiotensin-converting enzyme inhibitors ăn-jē-ō-TĔN-sĭn, ĔN-zīm	Lower blood pressure by inhibiting conversion of angiotensin I (an inactive enzyme) to angiotensin II (a potent vasoconstrictor)
antacids ănt-ĂS-ĭds	Neutralize excess acid in the stomach and help relieve gastritis and ulcer pain *Antacids are also used to relieve indigestion and reflux esophagitis (heartburn).*
antianginals ăn-tĭ-ĂN-jĭ-năls	Relieve angina pectoris by vasodilation
antianxiety drugs ăn-tē-ăng-ZĪ-ĕ-tē	Decrease anxiety and tension *Antianxiety drugs are classified as minor tranquilizers and anxiolytics.*
antiarrhythmics ăn-tē-ă-RĬTH-mĭks	Treat cardiac arrhythmias by stabilizing the electrical conduction of the heart

Continued

Drug Classification	Description
antibiotics ăn-tĭ-bī-ŎT-ĭks	Inhibit growth of or destroy microorganisms *Antibiotics are used extensively in treatment of infectious diseases.*
anticoagulants ăn-tĭ-kō-ĂG-ū-lănts	Prevent or delay blood coagulation *Anticoagulants prevent deep vein thrombosis (DVT) and postoperative clot formation and decrease the risk of stroke.*
anticonvulsants ăn-tĭ-kŏn-VŬL-sănts	Prevent or reduce the severity of epileptic or other convulsive seizures; also called *antiepileptics*
antidepressants ăn-tĭ-dē-PRĔS-săntz	Regulate mood and reduce symptoms of depression by affecting the amount of neurotransmitters in the brain
antidiabetics ăn-tĭ-dī-ă-BĔT-ĭks	Stimulate the pancreas to produce more insulin and decrease peripheral resistance to insulin *Oral antidiabetics help treat type 2 diabetes mellitus.*
antidiarrheals ăn-tĭ-dī-ă-RĒ-ăls	Control loose stools and relieve diarrhea by absorbing excess water in the bowel or slowing peristalsis in the intestinal tract
antidiuretics ăn-tĭ-dī-ū-RĔT-ĭks	Reduce the production of urine
antiemetics ăn-tĭ-ē-MĔT-ĭks	Prevent or suppress vomiting *Antiemetics also help treat vertigo, motion sickness, and nausea.*
antifungals ăn-tĭ-FŬNG-ăls	Alter the cell wall of fungi or disrupt enzyme activity, resulting in cellular death
antiglaucoma agents ăn-tĭ-glaw-KŌ-mă	Reduce intraocular pressure by lowering the amount of aqueous humor in the eyeball, reducing its production, or increasing its outflow
antihistamines ăn-tĭ-HĬS-tă-mēns	Counteract the effects of a histamine *Antihistamines inhibit allergic reactions of inflammation, redness, and itching, especially hay fever and other allergic disorders of the nasal passages.*
antihyperlipidemics ăn-tĭ-hī-pĕr-lĭp-ĭ-DĒ-mĭcs	Lower lipid levels in the bloodstream *Antihyperlipidemics reduce the risk of heart attack by lowering lipid levels.*
antihypertensives ăn-tĭ-hī-pĕr-TĔN-sĭvs	Lower blood pressure
anti-impotence agents	Treat erectile dysfunction (impotence) by increasing blood flow to the penis, resulting in an erection
anti-infectives, **antibacterials, antifungals** ăn-tĭ-ĭn-FĔK-tĭvs, ăn-tĭ-băk-TĒ-rē-ăls, ăn-tĭ-FŬNG-ăls	Eliminate or inhibit bacterial or fungal infections *Anti-infectives, antibacterials, and antifungals can be administered topically or systemically.*
anti-inflammatories ăn-tĭ-ĭn-FLĂM-ă-tō-rēz	Relieve the swelling, tenderness, redness, and pain of inflammation *Anti-inflammatories may be classified as steroidal (corticosteroids) or nonsteroidal.*
antimetabolites ăn-tĭ-mĕ-TĂB-ō-līts	Interfere with the use of enzymes required for cell division *Antimetabolites block folic acid, a B vitamin required for synthesis of some amino acids in the DNA of cancerous cells.*

Drug Classification	Description
antimicrobials ăn-tĭ-mī-KRŌ-bē-ălz	Destroy or inhibit the growth of bacteria, fungi, and protozoa, depending on the particular drug, generally by interfering with the functions of their cell membrane or their reproductive cycle
antiparkinsonians ăn-tĭ-păr-kĭn-SŌN-ē-ănz	Control tremors and muscle rigidity associated with Parkinson disease by increasing dopamine levels in the brain
antipruritics ăn-tĭ-proo-RĬT-ĭks	Prevent or relieve itching
antipsychotics ăn-tĭ-sī-KŎT-ĭks	Treat psychosis, paranoia, and schizophrenia by altering the chemicals in the brain, including the limbic system (group of brain structures), which controls emotions
antiseptics ăn-tĭ-SĔP-tĭks	Topically applied agent that destroys or inhibits the growth of bacteria, preventing infection in cuts, scratches, and surgical incisions
antispasmodics ăn-tĭ-spăz-MŎD-ĭks	Act on the autonomic nervous system to reduce spasms in the bladder or gastrointestinal (GI) tract
antithyroids ăn-tĭ-THĪ-royds	Treat hyperthyroidism by impeding the formation of triiodothyronine (T_3) and thyroxine (T_4) hormones
antituberculars ăn-tĭ-too-BĔR-kū-lărs	Treat tuberculosis *Several antituberculars are used in combination for effective treatment.*
antitussives ăn-tĭ-TŬS-ĭvz	Relieve or suppress coughing by blocking the cough reflex in the medulla of the brain
antivirals ăn-tĭ-VĪ-rălz	Prevent replication of viruses within host cells *Antivirals treat HIV infection and AIDS, as well as other viral diseases.*
astringents ă-STRĬN-jĕnts	Shrink the blood vessels locally, dry up secretions from seeping lesions, and lessen skin sensitivity
B	
beta blockers BĀ-tă	Decrease heart rate and dilate arteries by blocking beta receptors *Beta blockers are used to treat angina pectoris, arrhythmias, and hypertension.*
birth control	Delivers two synthetic hormones, progestin and estrogen, through a transdermal patch, injectable, or oral pill, impeding pregnancy by preventing the ovaries from releasing eggs (ovulation) and thickening the cervical mucus; also called contraceptives
bone reabsorption inhibitors	Inhibit breakdown of bone *Bone resorption inhibitors treat osteoporosis.*
bronchodilators brŏng-kō-DĪ-lă-tors	Stimulate bronchial muscles to relax, thereby expanding air passages and resulting in increased airflow to the lungs
C	
calcium channel blockers KĂL-sē-ŭm	Selectively block movement of calcium (required for blood vessel contraction) into myocardial cells and arterial walls, causing heart rate and blood pressure to decrease *Calcium channel blockers treat angina pectoris, arrhythmias, heart failure, and hypertension.*
calcium supplements KĂL-sē-ŭm	Treat and prevent hypocalcemia *Calcium supplements help prevent osteoporosis when the normal diet is lacking adequate amounts of calcium.*

Continued

Drug Classification	Description
contraceptives kŏn-tră-SĔP-tĭvz	Prevent conception or ovulation; also called birth control
corticosteroids (glucocorticoids) kor-tĭ-kō-STĒR-oydz	Relieve inflammation and replace hormones for adrenal insufficiency (Addison disease) *Corticosteroids are widely used to suppress the immune system's inflammatory response to tissue damage, control allergic reactions, reduce the rejection process in tissue and organ transplantation, and treat some cancers.*
cycloplegics sī-klō-PLĒ-jĭks	Paralyze the ciliary muscles, resulting in pupil dilation *Cycloplegics dilate the pupils to facilitate certain eye examinations and surgical procedures.*
cytotoxics sī-tō-TŎKS-ĭks	Disrupt nucleic acid and protein synthesis, causing immunosuppression and cancer cell death *Cytotoxics treat cancer and autoimmune diseases, such as inflammatory bowel disease and systemic vasculitis. They also help prevent rejection of transplants.*
D	
decongestants	Decrease congestion of mucous membranes of the sinuses and nose *Decongestants are used for temporary relief of nasal congestion associated with the common cold, hay fever, other upper respiratory allergies, and sinusitis.*
diuretics dī-ū-RĔT-ĭks	Act on the kidney to promote the excretion of sodium and water *Diuretics treat edema and hypertension.*
E	
emetics ĕ-MĔT-ĭks	Induce vomiting, especially in cases of poisoning
erectile agents ĕ-RĔK-tīl	Treat erectile dysfunction (impotence) by increasing blood flow to the penis, resulting in an erection
estrogens ĔS-trō-jĕnz	Treat symptoms of menopause (hot flashes, vaginal dryness) through hormone replacement therapy (HRT)
estrogen hormone ĔS-trō-jĕn HOR-mōn	Used in estrogen replacement therapy (ERT) during menopause to correct estrogen deficiency and as chemotherapy for some types of cancer, including tumors of the prostate
expectorants ĕk-SPĔK-tō-rănts	Liquefy respiratory secretions so that they are more easily expelled during coughing episodes
F, G	
fibrinolytics	Trigger the body to produce plasmin, an enzyme that dissolves clots *Fibrinolytics treat acute pulmonary embolism and, occasionally, DVT.*
gold compound drugs, gold salts	Treat rheumatoid arthritis by inhibiting activity within the immune system to prevent further disease progression *Gold compound drugs actually contain gold.*
gonadotropins gŏn-ă-dō-TRŌ-pĭnz	Raise sperm count in infertility cases
growth hormone replacements	Increase skeletal growth in children and growth hormone deficiencies in adults
H	
H₂ blockers	Block histamine 2 (H_2) receptors in the stomach to prevent the release of acid to treat heartburn, peptic ulcers, and gastroesophageal reflux disease (GERD)

Drug Classification	Description
hemostatics hē-mō-STĂT-ĭks	Prevent or control bleeding *Hemostatics treat blood disorders and certain bleeding problems associated with surgery.*
hormone replacement therapy (HRT) HOR-mōn	Correct deficiency of such hormones as estrogen, testosterone, or thyroid hormone *HRT may include oral administration or injection of synthetic hormones.*
hypnotics hĭp-NŎT-ĭks	Depress the central nervous system (CNS) to induce or maintain sleep
I	
inotropics, cardiotonics ĭn-ō-TRŎP-ĭks, kăr-dē-ō-TŎN-ĭks	Increase the efficiency of heart muscle contractions *Inotropics treat cardiac arrhythmias and cardiac failure.*
insulins ĬN-sŭ-lĭns	Lower glucose (sugar) level in blood *Insulins are synthetic forms of the insulin hormone used to treat diabetes and are administered by injection.*
K, L, M	
keratolytics kĕr-ă-tō-LĬT-ĭks	Destroy and soften the outer layer of skin so that it is sloughed off or shed *Strong keratolytics are effective for removing warts and corns. Milder preparations promote the shedding of scales and crusts in eczema, psoriasis, and seborrheic dermatitis. Weak keratolytics irritate inflamed skin, acting as tonics that speed up the healing process.*
laxatives (cathartics, purgatives) LĂK-să-tĭvz, kă-THĂR-tĭks, PŬR-gă-tĭvs	Induce bowel movements or loosen stool *When used in smaller doses, laxatives relieve constipation. When used in larger doses, they evacuate the entire GI tract—for example, as preparation for surgery or intestinal radiological examinations.*
miotics mī-ŎT-ĭks	Constrict the pupil of the eye *Miotics help treat glaucoma.*
mucolytics	Liquefy sputum or reduce its viscosity so that it can be coughed up more easily
muscle relaxants	Relieve muscle spasms and stiffness
mydriatics mĭd-rē-ĂT-ĭks	Dilate the pupil and paralyze the muscles of accommodation of the iris *Mydriatics help prepare the eye for internal examination and treat inflammatory conditions of the iris.*
N	
nitrates NĪ-trāts	Dilate arteries and increase blood flow to the myocardium *Nitrates treat angina pectoris.*
nonsteroidal anti-inflammatory drugs (NSAIDs) nŏn-STĔR-oyd-ăl ăn-tĭ-ĭn-FLĂM-ă-tō-rē	Relieve mild to moderate pain and reduce inflammation in the treatment of musculoskeletal conditions, such as sprains and strains, and inflammatory disorders, such as rheumatoid arthritis, osteoarthritis, bursitis, gout, and tendinitis
O	
opiates Ō-pē-ĭts	Relieve pain *Opiates contain opium or its derivative. They are commonly prescribed on a short-term basis because of their strong addictive property.*

Continued

Drug Classification	Description
oral hypoglycemics hī-pō-glī-SĒ-mĭcs	Stimulate insulin secretion from pancreatic cells in patients with non–insulin-dependent diabetes with some pancreatic function
oxytocics ŏk-sē-TŌ-sĭks	Induce labor at term by increasing the strength and frequency of uterine contractions
P	
parasiticides păr-ă-SĬT-ĭ-sīds	Destroy systemic parasites, such as pinworm or tapeworm, in oral form or insect parasites, such as mites and lice, in topical form
potassium supplements pō-TĂS-ē-ŭm	Increase the potassium level in blood *Potassium can be administered orally or intravenously when dangerously low levels occur. It is used as a replacement for potassium loss caused by diuretics.*
prostaglandins prŏs-tă-GLĂN-dĭns	Used to induce labor, terminate pregnancy, or treat erectile dysfunction, patent ductus arteriosus, or pulmonary hypertension
protectives prŏk-TĔK-tĭvs	Function by covering, cooling, drying, or soothing inflamed skin *Protectives do not penetrate or soften the skin but form a long-lasting film that protects the skin from air, water, and clothing during the natural healing process.*
proton pump inhibitors PRŌ-tŏn	Block the final stage of hydrochloric acid production in the stomach *Proton pump inhibitors treat peptic ulcers and GERD.*
psychotropics sī-kō-TRŎP-ĭks	Alter chemical balance in the brain, causing changes in perception, mood, and behavior *Psychotropics are commonly employed in the management of psychiatric disorders.*
Q, R, S	
relaxants rē-LĂK-sănts	Reduce tension, causing relaxation of muscles or bowel
salicylates săl-ĬS-ĭl-āts	Relieve mild to moderate pain and reduce inflammation and fever
sedatives SĔD-ă-tĭvs	Exert a calming or tranquilizing effect
skeletal muscle relaxants SKĔL-ĕ-tăl rē-LĂK-sănts	Relieve muscle spasms and stiffness
spermicides SPĔR-mĭ-sīdz	Chemically destroy sperm *Spermicidals are available as jellies, creams, and foams and do not require a prescription. They are commonly placed within the woman's vagina for contraceptive purposes.*
statins STĂ-tĭnz	Lower cholesterol in the blood and reduce its production in the liver by blocking the enzyme that produces it
T	
thrombolytics thrŏm-bō-LĬT-ĭks	Dissolve blood clots by destroying their fibrin strands *Thrombolytics are used to break apart, or lyse, thrombi.*
thyroid supplements THĪ-royd	Replace or supplement thyroid hormones

Drug Classification	Description
topical anesthetics ăn-ĕs-THĔT-ĭks	Block sensation of pain by numbing the skin layers and mucous membranes *Topical anesthetics are applied directly in sprays, creams, gargles, suppositories, and other preparations. They are also used to numb skin to make the injection of medication more comfortable.*
tranquilizers TRĂNG-kwĭ-lī-zĕrz	Reduce anxiety, agitation, and tension; used for sedation.
U	
uricosurics Ū-rĭ-kō-soo-rĭks	Increase urinary excretion of uric acid, reducing the concentration of uric acid in blood *Uricosurics are used to treat gout.*
uterine stimulants Ū-tĕr-ĭn	Induce labor at term, control postpartum hemorrhage, and induce therapeutic abortion; also called *oxytocic agents* *Oxytocin is a pharmaceutically prepared chemical that is similar to the pituitary hormone oxytocin. Uterine stimulants are also used to treat infertility in females.*
V	
vasoconstrictors vă-sō-kŏn-STRĬK-tĕrs	Narrow or constrict the diameter of blood vessels *Vasoconstrictors decrease blood flow and increase blood pressure.*
vasodilators văs-ō-dī-LĀ-torz	Dilate the diameter of blood vessels *Vasodilators help treat angina pectoris and hypertension.*
vitamin B$_{12}$	Treats pernicious anemia *Vitamin B$_{12}$ is delivered by nasal spray or intramuscular injection.*
vertigo and motion sickness agents VĔR-tĭ-gō	Decrease sensitivity of the inner ear to motion and prevent nerve impulses in the inner ear from reaching the vomiting center of the brain
W, X, Y, Z	
wax emulsifiers ē-MŬL-sĭ-fĭ-ĕrz	Loosen and help remove impacted cerumen (ear wax)

Abbreviations, Discontinued Abbreviations, and Common Symbols

Abbreviations

The table below lists common abbreviations used in health care and related fields along with their meanings.

Abbreviation	Meaning	Abbreviation	Meaning
A		AED	automatic external defibrillator
A&P	anatomy and physiology; auscultation and percussion	AF	atrial fibrillation
		AFB	acid-fast bacillus (TB organism)
A, B, AB, O	blood types in ABO blood group	AGN	acute glomerulonephritis
AAA	abdominal aortic aneurysm	AI	artificial insemination
AB, Ab, ab	antibody; abortion	AICD	automatic implantable cardioverter-defibrillator
ABC	aspiration, biopsy, cytology		
ABG	arterial blood gas	AIDS	acquired immune deficiency syndrome
a.c.*	before meals		
ACE	angiotensin-converting enzyme (inhibitor)	AK	above the knee
		ALL	acute lymphocytic leukemia
ACL	anterior cruciate ligament	ALS	amyotrophic lateral sclerosis (also called *Lou Gehrig disease*)
ACTH	adrenocorticotropic hormone		
AD*	right ear	ALT	alanine aminotransferase
ad lib	as desired	AM, a.m.	in the morning or before noon
ADH	antidiuretic hormone (vasopressin)	AML	acute myelogenous leukemia
		ANS	autonomic nervous system
ADHD	attention-deficit hyperactivity disorder	ant	anterior
		AOM	acute otitis media
ADLs	activities of daily living	AP	anteroposterior
AE	above the elbow		

Continued

Abbreviation	Meaning	Abbreviation	Meaning
ARDS	acute respiratory distress syndrome	CAT	computed axial tomography
ARF	acute renal failure	Cath	catheterization; catheter
ARMD, AMD	age-related macular degeneration	CBC	complete blood count
AS	aortic stenosis	CC	cardiac catheterization; chief complaint
AS*	left ear		
ASD	atrial septal defect	cc*	cubic centimeters; same as milliliters (1/1,000 of a liter)
ASHD	arteriosclerotic heart disease		
AST	angiotensin sensitivity test	CCU	coronary care unit
Ast	astigmatism	CDH	congenital dislocation of the hip
AU*	both ears	CF	cystic fibrosis
AV	atrioventricular; arteriovenous	CHB	complete heart block
B		CHD	coronary heart disease
Ba	barium	chemo	chemotherapy
baso	basophil (type of white blood cell)	CHF	congestive heart failure
BBB	bundle branch block	Chol	cholesterol
BC	bone conduction	CLL	chronic lymphocytic leukemia
BCC	basal cell carcinoma	CK	creatine kinase (cardiac enzyme); conductive keratoplasty
BE	barium enema; below the elbow		
BG	blood glucose	cm	centimeter (1/100 of a meter)
b.i.d.*	twice a day	CML	chronic myelogenous leukemia
BK	below the knee	CNS	central nervous system
BKA	below-knee amputation	c/o	complains of, complaints
BM	bowel movement	CO	cardiac output
BMI	body mass index	CO₂	carbon dioxide
BMR	basal metabolic rate	COPD	chronic obstructive pulmonary disease
BMT	bone marrow transplant		
BNO	bladder neck obstruction	COVID-19	coronavirus disease 2019
BP, B/P	blood pressure	CP	cerebral palsy
BPH	benign prostatic hyperplasia; benign prostatic hypertrophy	CPAP	continuous positive airway pressure
BS	blood sugar	CPD	cephalopelvic disproportion
BSE	breast self-examination	CPK	creatine phosphokinase (enzyme released into the bloodstream after a heart attack)
BSO	bilateral salpingo-oophorectomy		
BUN	blood urea nitrogen	CPR	cardiopulmonary resuscitation
Bx, bx	biopsy	CRF	chronic renal failure
C		CRRT	continuous renal replacement therapy
C1, C2, and so on	first cervical vertebra, second cervical vertebra, and so on	C&S	culture and sensitivity
CA	cancer; chronological age; cardiac arrest	CS, C-section	cesarean section
		CSF	cerebrospinal fluid
Ca	calcium; cancer	CT	computed tomography
CABG	coronary artery bypass graft	CTL	cytotoxic T lymphocytes
CAD	coronary artery disease	CTS	carpal tunnel syndrome
CAH	chronic active hepatitis; congenital adrenal hyperplasia	CV	cardiovascular
		CVA	cerebrovascular accident

CO_2 carbon dioxide

Abbreviation	Meaning	Abbreviation	Meaning
CVD	cardiovascular disease	ED	erectile dysfunction; emergency department
CVS	chorionic villus sampling	EEG	electroencephalography; electroencephalogram
CWP	childbirth without pain		
CXR	chest x-ray, chest radiography	EF	ejection fraction
cysto	cystoscopy	EGD	esophagogastroduodenoscopy
D		ELISA	enzyme-linked immunosorbent assay
D	diopter (lens strength)		
dc, DC, D/C*	discharge; discontinue	ELT	endovenous laser ablation; endoluminal laser ablation
D&C	dilation and curettage		
Decub	decubitus (lying down)	Em	emmetropia
derm	dermatology	EMG	electromyography
DES	diffuse esophageal spasm; drug-eluting stent	ENT	ears, nose, and throat
		EOM	extraocular movement
DEXA, DXA	dual energy x-ray absorptiometry	eos	eosinophil (type of white blood cell)
DI	diabetes insipidus; diagnostic imaging		
		ERCP	endoscopic retrograde cholangiopancreatography
diff	differential count (white blood cells)		
		ESR	erythrocyte sedimentation rate
DJD	degenerative joint disease	ESRD	end-stage renal disease
DKA	diabetic ketoacidosis	ESWL	extracorporeal shock-wave lithotripsy
DMARDs	disease-modifying antirheumatic drugs		
		ETT	exercise tolerance test; endotracheal tube
DM	diabetes mellitus		
DNA	deoxyribonucleic acid	**F**	
D.O., DO	Doctor of Osteopathy	FBS	fasting blood sugar
DOE	dyspnea on exertion	FECG, FEKG	fetal electrocardiogram; fetal electrocardiography
DPI	dry powder inhaler		
D.P.M.	Doctor of Podiatric Medicine	FH	family history
DPT	diphtheria, pertussis, tetanus	FHR	fetal heart rate
DRE	digital rectal examination	FHT	fetal heart tone
DSA	digital subtraction angiography	FS	frozen section
DSM-V	Diagnostic and Statistic Manual of Mental Disorders (5th edition)	FSH	follicle-stimulating hormone
		FTND	full-term normal delivery
		FVC	forced vital capacity
DUB	dysfunctional uterine bleeding	Fx	fracture
DVT	deep vein thrombosis; deep venous thrombosis	**G**	
		G	gravida (pregnant)
Dx	diagnosis	g, gm	gram
E		GB	gallbladder
EBV	Epstein-Barr virus	GBS	gallbladder series (x-ray studies)
ECCE	extracapsular cataract extraction	GC	gonococcus (*Neisseria gonorrhoeae*)
ECG, EKG	electrocardiogram; electrocardiography		
		G-CSF	granulocyte colony-stimulating factor
ECHO	echocardiogram; echocardiography; echoencephalogram; echoencephalography		
		GER	gastroesophageal reflux

Continued

Abbreviation	Meaning	Abbreviation	Meaning
GERD	gastroesophageal reflux disease	ICD	implantable cardioverter-defibrillator
GFR	glomerular filtration rate	ICP	intracranial pressure
GH	growth hormone	ICU	intensive care unit
GI	gastrointestinal	ID	intradermal
GTT	glucose tolerance test	IDDM	insulin-dependent diabetes mellitus
GU	genitourinary	Ig	immunoglobulin
GVHD	graft-versus-host disease	IM	intramuscular; infectious mononucleosis
GVHR	graft-versus-host reaction		
GYN	gynecology	IMP	impression (synonymous with diagnosis)
H		IOL	intraocular lens
HAV	hepatitis A virus	IT	intensive therapy
Hb, Hgb, hgb	hemoglobin	IVP	intravenous pyelogram; intravenous pyelography
HBV	hepatitis B virus		
HCG	human chorionic gonadotropin	IOP	intraocular pressure
HCl	hydrochloric acid	IPPB	intermittent positive-pressure breathing
HCO^3	bicarbonate		
HCT, Hct	hematocrit	IRDS	infant respiratory distress syndrome
HCV	hepatitis C virus		
HD	hemodialysis; hip disarticulation; hearing distance	IT	intensive therapy
		IUD	intrauterine device
HDL	high-density lipoprotein	IUGR	intrauterine growth rate; intrauterine growth retardation
HDN	hemolytic disease of the newborn		
HDV	hepatitis D virus	IV	intravenous
HEV	hepatitis E virus	IVC	intravenous cholangiogram; intravenous cholangiography
HF	heart failure		
HIV	human immunodeficiency virus	IVF	in vitro fertilization
HMD	hyaline membrane disease	IVFA	intravenous fluorescein angiography
HNP	herniated nucleus pulposus (herniated disk)		
		IVF-ET	in vitro fertilization and embryo transfer
H$_2$O	water		
HP	hemipelvectomy	IVP	intravenous pyelogram, intravenous pyelography
HPV	human papillomavirus		
HRT	hormone replacement therapy	IVS	interventricular septum
h.s.*	at bedtime	**K**	
hs*	half strength	K	potassium (an electrolyte)
HSG	hysterosalpingography	KD	knee disarticulation
HSV	herpes simplex virus	KUB	kidney, ureter, bladder
HTN	hypertension	**L**	
Hx	history	L	liter
I, J		L1, L2, and so on	first lumbar vertebra, second lumbar vertebra, and so on
IAS	interatrial septum		
I&D	incision and drainage; irrigation and débridement	LA	left atrium
		LASIK	laser-assisted in situ keratomileusis
IBD	inflammatory bowel disease	LAT, lat	lateral
IBS	irritable bowel syndrome		

Abbreviation	Meaning	Abbreviation	Meaning
LBBB	left bundle branch block	MSH	melanocyte-stimulating hormone
LD	lactate dehydrogenase; lactic acid dehydrogenase (cardiac enzyme)	MUGA	multiple-gated acquisition (scan)
		MVP	mitral valve prolapse
LDL	low-density lipoprotein	MVR	mitral valve replacement; massive vitreous retraction (blade); microvitreoretinal
LES	lower esophageal sphincter		
LFT	liver function test		
LH	luteinizing hormone	Myop	myopia (nearsightedness)
LLQ	left lower quadrant	*N*	
LMP	last menstrual period	Na	sodium (an electrolyte)
LOC	loss of consciousness	NB	newborn
LP	lumbar puncture	NCV	nerve conduction velocity
LPR	laryngopharyngeal reflux	NG	nasogastric
LS	lumbosacral spine	NIDDM	non–insulin-dependent diabetes mellitus
LSO	left salpingo-oophorectomy		
lt	left	NIHL	noise-induced hearing loss
LUQ	left upper quadrant	NK	natural killer cell
LV	left ventricle	NMT	nebulized mist treatment
lymphos	lymphocytes	NPO, n.p.o.*	nothing by mouth
M		NSAID	nonsteroidal anti-inflammatory drug
MCH	mean cell hemoglobin (average amount of hemoglobin per red blood cell)		
		NSR	normal sinus rhythm
		O	
MCHC	mean cell hemoglobin concentration (average concentration of hemoglobin per red blood cell)	O₂	oxygen
		OB	obstetrics
		OB/GYN	obstetrics and gynecology
		OCP	oral contraceptive pill
MCV	mean cell volume (average volume or size per red blood cell)	O.D.	Doctor of Optometry
		OD	overdose
M.D., MD	doctor of medicine; macular degeneration; muscular dystrophy	OD*	right eye
		OM	otitis media
MDI	metered-dose inhaler	OP	outpatient; operative procedure
MEG	magnetoencephalography	OR	operating room
MG	myasthenia gravis	ORTH, ortho	orthopedics
mg	milligram (1/1,000 of a gram)	OS*	left eye; by mouth (pharmacology)
mg/dl, mg/dL	milligram per deciliter	OSA	obstructive sleep apnea
MI	myocardial infarction	OU*	both eyes
mix astig	mixed astigmatism	*P*	
ml, mL	milliliter (1/1,000 of a liter)	P	phosphorus; pulse
mm	millimeter (1/1,000 of a meter)	PA	posteroanterior; pernicious anemia; pulmonary artery; physician assistant
mm Hg	millimeters of mercury		
MR	mitral regurgitation		
MRA	magnetic resonance angiogram; magnetic resonance angiography	PAC	premature atrial contraction
		Pap	Papanicolaou (test)
MRI	magnetic resonance imaging	para 1, 2, 3, and so on	unipara, bipara, tripara, and so on (according to number of viable births)
MS	mitral stenosis; musculoskeletal; multiple sclerosis; mental status; magnesium sulfate		

Continued

Abbreviation	Meaning	Abbreviation	Meaning
PAT	paroxysmal atrial tachycardia	PTH	parathyroid hormone (also called *parathormone*)
PBI	protein-bound iodine		
pc, p.c.*	after meals	PTHC	percutaneous transhepatic cholangiography
PCI	percutaneous coronary intervention	PTT	partial thromboplastin time
PCL	posterior cruciate ligament	PUD	peptic ulcer disease
PCNL	percutaneous nephrolithotomy	PVC	premature ventricular contraction
PCO_2, $PaCO^2$, pCO^2	partial pressure of carbon dioxide	*Q*	
PCP	*Pneumocystis* pneumonia; primary care physician	q.2h.*	every 2 hours
		qAM*	every morning
PE	physical examination; pulmonary embolism; pressure-equalizing (tube)	q.d.*	every day
		q.h.*	every hour
		q.i.d.*	four times a day
PERRLA	pupils equal, round, and reactive to light and accommodation	q.o.d.*	every other day
		qPM*	every evening
PET	positron emission tomography	*R*	
PFT	pulmonary function test		
PGH	pituitary growth hormone	RA	right atrium; rheumatoid arthritis
pH	symbol for degree of acidity or alkalinity	RAI	radioactive iodine
		RAIU	radioactive iodine uptake
PID	pelvic inflammatory disease	RBC, rbc	red blood cell
PIH	pregnancy-induced hypertension	RD	respiratory distress
PKD	polycystic kidney disease	RDS	respiratory distress syndrome
PMH	past medical history	RF	rheumatoid factor; radiofrequency
PMI	point of maximal impulse		
PMN, PMNL	polymorphonuclear leukocyte	RGB	Roux-en-Y gastric bypass
PMP	previous menstrual period	RK	radial keratotomy
PMS	premenstrual syndrome	RLQ	right lower quadrant
PND	paroxysmal nocturnal dyspnea	R/O	rule out
PNS	peripheral nervous system	ROM	range of motion
p.o.*	by mouth	RP	retrograde pyelogram; retrograde pyelography
PO_2	partial pressure of oxygen		
poly	polymorphonuclear leukocyte	RSO	right salpingo-oophorectomy
post	posterior	rt	right
PPD	purified protein derivative (substance used in a tuberculosis test)	RUQ	right upper quadrant
		RV	residual volume; right ventricle
		S	
p.r.n.*	as required	S1, S2, and so on	first sacral vertebra, second sacral vertebra, and so on
PSA	prostate-specific antigen		
PSG	polysomnography	SA, S-A	sinoatrial
pt	patient	SaO_2	arterial oxygen saturation
PT	prothrombin time; physical therapy	SARS	severe acute respiratory syndrome
		SAT	saturation
PTCA	percutaneous transluminal coronary angioplasty	SD	shoulder disarticulation

Abbreviation	Meaning	Abbreviation	Meaning
SIADH	syndrome of inappropriate antidiuretic hormone	TRAM	transverse rectus abdominis muscle
SICS	small incision cataract surgery	TRUS	transrectal ultrasonography
SIDS	sudden infant death syndrome	TSE	testicular self-examination
SLE	systemic lupus erythematosus; slit lamp examination	TSH	thyroid-stimulating hormone
		TSS	toxic shock syndrome
SMAS	superficial musculoaponeurotic system (flap)	TURP	transurethral resection of the prostate
SNS	sympathetic nervous system	TVH	total vaginal hysterectomy
SOB	shortness of breath	TVH-BSO	total vaginal hysterectomy–bilateral salpingo-oophorectomy
sono	sonogram; sonography		
SPECT	single-photon emission computed tomography	Tx	treatment
		U	
sp. gr.	specific gravity	UA	urinalysis
ST	esotropia	UC	uterine contractions
stat., STAT	immediately	UGI	upper gastrointestinal
STD	sexually transmitted disease	UGIS	upper gastrointestinal series
STI	sexually transmitted infection	U&L, U/L	upper and lower
subcu, Sub-Q, subQ*	subcutaneous (injection)	ung	ointment
SVC	superior vena cava	UPP	uvulopalatopharyngoplasty
Sx	symptom	URI	upper respiratory infection
T		US	ultrasound; ultrasonography
T1, T2, and so on	first thoracic vertebra, second thoracic vertebra, and so on	UTI	urinary tract infection
		V	
T_3	triiodothyronine (thyroid hormone)	VA	visual acuity
		VC	vital capacity
T_4	thyroxine (thyroid hormone)	VCUG	voiding cystourethrography
T&A	tonsillectomy and adenoidectomy	VD	venereal disease
TAH	total abdominal hysterectomy	VF	visual field
TB	tuberculosis	VSD	ventricular septal defect
TFT	thyroid function test	VT	ventricular tachycardia
THA	total hip arthroplasty	VUR	vesicoureteral reflux
ther	therapy	**W**	
THR	total hip replacement	WBC, wbc	white blood cell
TIA	transient ischemic attack	WD	well-developed
t.i.d.*	three times a day	WN	well-nourished
TKA	total knee arthroplasty	WNL	within normal limits
TKR	total knee replacement	**X, Y, Z**	
TPPV	trans pars plana vitrectomy	XP, XDP	xeroderma pigmentosum
TPR	temperature, pulse, and respiration	XT	exotropia

*Although these abbreviations are currently found in medical records and clinical notes, they are easily misinterpreted. Thus, the Joint Commission (formerly Joint Commission on Accreditation of Healthcare Organizations [JCAHO]) has recommended that they be discontinued. Instead, it recommends writing out the full forms. For a summary of these abbreviations, see the table that follows.

Common Symbols

The table below lists some common symbols used in the health care and related fields.

Abbreviation	Meaning	Abbreviation	Meaning
@	at	+	plus, positive
āā	of each	–	minus, negative
′	foot	±	plus or minus; either positive or negative; indefinite
″	inch	#	number; following a number; pounds
c̄	with	÷	divided by
p̄	after	×	multiplied by; magnification
pH	degree of acidity or alkalinity	=	equals
℞	prescription, treatment, therapy	°	degree
→	to, in the direction of	%	percent
↑	increase(d), up	♀	female
↓	decrease(d), down	♂	male

Discontinued Abbreviations

The Joint Commission (JC) and the Institute for Safe Medication Practices (ISMP) report that the following abbreviations are commonly misinterpreted and have resulted in harmful medical errors. Both organizations have compiled a comprehensive "Do Not Use" list (available on their websites) for health-care providers.

To prevent harmful medical errors, both organizations recommend discontinuance of use of these abbreviations. Instead, the abbreviations should be written out. Nevertheless, some of the abbreviations on the "Do Not Use" list are still used by health-care providers. A selected number are listed below.

Abbreviation	Meaning
Medication and Therapy Time Schedule	
a.c.	before meals
b.i.d.	twice a day
hs	half strength
h.s.	at bedtime
NPO, n.p.o.	nothing by mouth
p.c.	after meals
p.o.	by mouth (orally)
p.r.n.	as required
qAM	every morning
q.d.	every day
q.h.	every hour
q.2h.	every 2 hours
q.i.d.	four times a day
q.o.d.	every other day
qPM	every evening
t.i.d.	three times a day
Other Related Abbreviations	
AD	right ear
AS	left ear
AU	both ears
cc	cubic centimeter; same as milliliter (1/1,000 of a liter)
	Use mL *for milliliters, or write out the meaning.*
dc, DC, D/C	discharge; discontinue
OD	right eye
OS	left eye
OU	both eyes
subcu, Sub-Q, subQ	subcutaneous (injection)
U	unit

Medical Specialties

This index provides a summary and description of medical specialties.

Medical Specialty	Medical Specialist	Description of Medical Specialty
Allergy	Allergist	Diagnosis and treatment of allergic disorders caused by hypersensitivity to foods, pollens, dusts, and medicines
Anesthesiology	Anesthesiologist	Administration of agents capable of bringing about loss of sensation with or without loss of consciousness
Cardiology	Cardiologist	Diagnosis and treatment of heart and vascular disorders
Dermatology	Dermatologist	Diagnosis and treatment of skin disorders
Emergency medicine	Emergency physician	Diagnosis and treatment of acute illness and injury that require sudden and immediate action in a hospital setting
Endocrinology	Endocrinologist	Diagnosis and treatment of endocrine gland disorders
Gastroenterology (sub-specialty of Internal Medicine)	Gastroenterologist	Treatment of stomach and intestinal disorders
General practice (GP), family medicine	General practitioner (GP)	Coordination of total health-care delivery, including counseling, to all members of the family, regardless of sex *GP encompasses several branches of medicine, including internal medicine, preventive medicine, pediatrics, surgery, obstetrics, and gynecology.*
Geriatrics, gerontology	Gerontologist, Geriatrician	Understanding of the physiological characteristics of aging and the diagnosis and treatment of diseases affecting older patients
Gynecology	Gynecologist	Diagnosis and treatment of diseases of the female reproductive organs
Hematology	Hematologist	Diagnosis and treatment of diseases of the blood and blood-forming tissues
Immunology	Immunologist	Study of various elements of the immune system and their functions *Immunology includes treatment of immune deficiency diseases, such as acquired immunodeficiency syndrome (AIDS); autoimmune diseases, such as systemic lupus erythematosus; allergies; and various types of cancer related to the immune system.*
Internal medicine	Internist	Study of the physiological and pathological characteristics of internal organs and the diagnosis and treatment of these organs
Neonatology	Neonatologist	Care and treatment of newborns
Nephrology	Nephrologist	Diagnosis and management of kidney disease, kidney transplantation, and dialysis therapies
Neurosurgery	Neurosurgeon	Surgery of the brain, spinal cord, and peripheral nerves

Continued

Medical Specialty	Medical Specialist	Description of Medical Specialty
Obstetrics	Obstetrician	Care of women during pregnancy, childbirth, and postnatal period
Oncology	Oncologist	Diagnosis, treatment, and prevention of cancer
		Oncologists are internal medicine physicians who specialize in the treatment of solid tumors (e.g., carcinomas and sarcomas) and liquid tumors (including hematological malignancies, such as leukemias).
Ophthalmology	Ophthalmologist	Diagnosis and treatment of eye diseases, including prescribing corrective lenses
Optometry	Optometrist	Primary eye care, including testing the eyes for visual acuity, diagnosing and managing eye health, prescribing corrective lenses, and recommending eye exercises
		An optometrist, licensed by the state, is not a medical doctor but is known as a Doctor of Optometry (D.O.).
Orthopedics	Orthopedist	Prevention, diagnosis, care, and treatment of musculoskeletal disorders
		Musculoskeletal disorders include injury to or disease of bones, joints, ligaments, muscles, and tendons.
Otolaryngology	Otolaryngologist	Medical and surgical management of disorders of the ear, nose, and throat (ENT) and related structures of the head and neck
Pathology	Pathologist	Identification of diseases and conditions by studying abnormal cells and tissues
		A pathologist is a physician who is an expert in the study of diseases and specializes in performing autopsy.
Pediatrics	Pediatrician	Diagnosis and treatment of disease in infants, children, and adolescents
Plastic surgery	Plastic surgeon	Surgery to alter, replace, or restore a body structure to treat a defect or injury or for cosmetic reasons
Physiatry, physical medicine	Physiatrist	Prevention, diagnosis, and treatment of disease or injury and the rehabilitation from resultant impairment and disability
		Physiatrists are physicians who use physical agents, such as light, heat, cold water, therapeutic exercise, mechanical apparatus, and, sometimes, pharmaceutical agents.
Pulmonology, pulmonary medicine	Pulmonologist	Diagnosis and treatment of diseases involving the lungs, their airways and blood vessels, and the chest wall (thoracic cage)
Psychiatry	Psychiatrist	Diagnosis, treatment, and prevention of mental, emotional, and behavioral disorders
		A psychiatrist is a medical doctor (an M.D. or D.O.) who specializes in mental health, including substance abuse disorders.
Radiology	Radiologist	Diagnosis using radiography and other diagnostic procedures, such as ultrasonography (US), computed tomography (CT), and magnetic resonance imaging (MRI)
		Radiology also employs various radiation techniques to treat disease through other subspecialties of radiology, such as interventional radiology and nuclear medicine.
Rheumatology	Rheumatologist	Diagnosis and treatment of inflammatory and degenerative diseases of the joints
Surgery	Surgeon	Use of operative procedures to treat deformity, injury, and disease
Thoracic surgery	Thoracic surgeon	Use of operative procedures to treat disease or injury of the thoracic area
Urology	Urologist	Diagnosis and treatment of the male urinary and reproductive systems and the female urinary system

Glossary of English-to-Spanish Translations

This appendix provides guidelines to help health-care practitioners communicate with their Spanish-speaking patients. The following information includes selected terms commonly used in various medical specialties.

Spanish Sounds

Although the spellings of some Spanish terms resemble English terms, the terms are still pronounced with a Spanish accent. Because of these spelling similarities, the practitioner should take care to learn the meaning and pronunciations of certain Spanish words. The first step in communicating with Spanish-speaking patients is to learn the Spanish sound system. This section provides Spanish pronunciations of vowels and consonants. The table below lists vowels and their Spanish pronunciations. Practice the pronunciations before continuing with the other information in this appendix.

Letter	Spanish Pronunciation Sounds Like
Vowels	
a	*ah* as in *father*
e	*eh* as in *net*
i	*ee* as in *keep*
o	*oh* as in *no*
u	*oo* as in *spoon;* silent following *q* or *g*
y	*ee* as in *bee*
Consonants	
c	*k* as in *kitten* (before *a, o, u,* and any consonant except *h*); s as in sit (before *e* or *i*); *k* after *e* or *i*
g	*h* as in *hit* (when followed by *e* or *i*); otherwise, like *g* as in *gold*
h	silent; never pronounced unless preceded by *c*
j	*h* as in *hot*
ll	*y* as in *yellow*

Continued

Letter	Spanish Pronunciation Sounds Like
ñ	*ni* as in *onion*
qu*	*k* as in *kite*
r	trilled *r*
rr*	strongly trilled *r*
v	*b* as in *boy*
z	*s* as in *sun*

*Note: *qu* and *rr* are not consonants but, rather, sounds. As such, they are not part of the Spanish alphabet. We include them here
      purely as an aid in pronunciation for non–Spanish-speaking health-care providers.

Emphasis in Spanish

In the tables that follow, capitalization is used to indicate primary emphasis of Spanish words. The capital letters in the Spanish pronunciation column indicate that emphasis is placed on the capitalized syllable. You will note that some Spanish terms, such as *perspiración* and *úlcera*, have a diacritical mark above the vowel. This mark indicates emphasis that falls on a syllable other than the one predicted by the rules of Spanish pronunciation.

Although there are some exceptions to these rules, the suggested guidelines here will help you learn Spanish terms and pronunciations of selected key terms in each chapter. Start by reviewing the English and Spanish terms, and then practice the Spanish pronunciations by applying the English system of phonetics.

Adjective Endings

Many Spanish adjectives change the last letter of the word to denote the gender of the noun being modified. If the noun is feminine, the letter will be *a;* for a masculine noun, the letter used is *o*. For example, the adjective *lenta* (slow) modifies a feminine noun. The same adjective when modifying a masculine noun ends with the letter *o*, so it would be *lento*. To change the gender of an adjective to correspond with the noun it modifies, change the ending vowel. For example, if the noun is masculine, change the ending vowel to *o*. The table below clearly identifies Spanish adjectives that should receive a specific gender.

English-to-Spanish Translations

The following selected terms are used in the medical environment to denote anatomical structures and their functions; signs, symptoms, and diseases; and other related terms.

English	Spanish	Spanish Pronunciation
abdomen	abdomen	ab-DOH-men
adrenal gland	glándula adrenal	GLAN-doo-lah ah-dreh-NAHL
adrenaline	adrenalina	ah-dreh-nah-LEE-nah
allergy	alergia	ah-LEHR-hee-ah
alveolus	alvéolo	ahl-VEH-oh-loh
aneurysm	aneurisma	a-neh-oo-REES-mah
ankle	tobillo	toh-BEE-yoh
antacid	antiácido	ahn-tee-AH-see-doh
appendix	apéndice	ah-PEHN-dee-seh
appetite	apetito	ah-peh-TEE-toh

English	Spanish	Spanish Pronunciation
arm	brazo	BRAH-soh
artery	arteria	ahr-TEH-ree-ah
arthritis	artritis	ahr-TREE-tees
asphyxia	asfixia	ahs-FEEK-see-ah
asthma	asma	AHS-mah
belch	eructar	eh-rook-TAHR
belly	barriga	bahr-REE-gah
benign	benigno	beh-NEEG-noh
birth	nacimiento	nah-see-mee-EHN-toh
black	negra (feminine)	NEH-grah
	negro (masculine)	NEH-groh
bladder	vejiga	beh-HEE-gah
blepharospasm	blefaroespasmo	bleh-fah-roh-ehs-PAHS-moh
blister	ampolla	am-PO-yah
blood	sangre	SAHN-greh
blood clot	coágulo de sangre	koh-AH-goo-loh deh SAHN-greh
blood pressure	presión sanguínea	preh-see-OHN san-GEE-neh-ah
blue	azul	ah-SOOL
bones	huesos	oo-EH-sohs
brain	cerebro	seh-REH-broh
breast	pecho	PEH-cho
breathe	respirar	rehs-pee-RAHR
breathing	respiración	rehs-pee-rah-see-OHN
bronchus	bronquios	BROHN-kee-ohs
brown	marrón	mahr-ROHN
	OR	
	café	cah-FAY
burn	quemar	keh-MAHR
calcium	calcio	KAHL-see-oh
calculus	cálculo	KAHL-coo-loh
capillary	capilar	kah-pee-LAHR
cartilage	cartílago	kahr-TEE-lah-goh
catheter	catéter	kah-TEH-tehr
catheterization	cateterización	kah-teh-teh-ree-sah-see-OHN
cerumen	cera de los oídos	CEH-rah deh lohs oh-EE-dohs
cervix	cervix	SERH-beex
cesarean section	cesárea	seh-SAH-reh-ah

Continued

English	Spanish	Spanish Pronunciation
chew	masticar	mahs-tee-KAHR
choroidopathy	coroidopatía	coh-roh-ee-doh-pah-TEE-ah
circumcision	circuncisión	seer-koon-see-see-OHN
clear	clara (feminine)	KLAH-rah
	claro (masculine)	KLAH-roh
cloudy	nublado	noo-BLAH-doh
collarbone	clavícula	klah-BEE-coo-lah
colon	colon	KOH-lohn
colonoscopy	colonoscopia	koh-loh-nohs-koh-PEE-ah
conception	concepción	khon-sehp-see-OHN
concussion	concusión	kohn-koo-see-OHN
condom	condón	kohn-DOHN
conscious	consciente	kohns-see-EHN-teh
constipation	estreñimiento	ehs-treh-nyee-mee-EHN-toh
cough	toser	toh-SEHR
cystoscopy	cistoscopia	sees-toh-SCOH-pee-ah
dark	obscuro	obs-COO-roh
deafness	sordera	sohr-DEH-rah
defecate	defecar	deh-feh-KAHR
dermatology	dermatologia	der-mah-toh-loh-HEE-ah
diabetes	diabetes	dee-ah-BEH-tehs
dialysis	diálisis	dee-AH-lee-sees
diaphragm	diafragma	dee-ah-FRAHG-mah
diarrhea	diarrea	dee-ah-RREH-ah
digestion	digestión	dee-hes-tee-OHN
diplopia	diplopia	dee-PLOH-pee-ah
diuretic	diurético	dee-oo-REH-tee-coh
dizzy	mareado	mah-reh-AH-doh
dyspepsia	dispepsia	dees-PEHP-see-ah
dysphagia	disfagia	dees-FAH-hee-ah
dysuria	disuria	dee-SOO-ree-ah
eardrum	tímpano del oído	TEEM-pah-noh dehl oh-EE-doh
ears	oídos	oh-EE-dohs
encephalopathy	encefalopatía	ehn-ceh-fah-loh-pah-TEE-ah
endometriosis	endometriosis	ehn-doh-meh-tree-OH-sees
epiglottis	epiglotis	eh-pee-GLOH-tees
epilepsy	epilepsia	eh-pee-LEHP-see-ah

English	Spanish	Spanish Pronunciation
erection	erección	eh-rek-see-OHN
esophagus	esófago	eh-SOH-fah-goh
excretion	excreción	ex-kreh-see-OHN
eyelid	párpado	PAHR-pah-doh
eyes	ojos	OH-hohs
fainting	desmayo	dehs-MAH-yoh
fracture	fractura	frahk-TOO-rah
gallbladder	vesícula biliar	beh-SEE-koo-lah bee-lee-AHR
gallstone	cálculo biliar	KAHL-koo-loh bee-lee-AHR
genitalia	genitalia	heh-nee-TAH-lee-ah
glucose	glucosa	gloo-KO-sah
goiter	bocio	BOH-see-oh
gums	encia	ehn-SEE-ah
hair	pelo	PEH-loh
hardening	endurecimiento	en-doo-reh-see-mee-EHN-toh
heart	corazón	koh-rah-SOHN
heart attack	ataque al corazón	ah-TAH-keh ahl koh-rah-SOHN
	OR	
	ataque cardíaco	ah-TAH-keh kar-DEE-ah-koh
heart rate	ritmo cardíaco	REET-moh kar-DEE-ah-koh
hematuria	hematuria	eh-mah-TOO-ree-ah
hernia	hernia	EHR-nee-ah
herniated disk	disco herniado	DEES-coh ehr-nee-AH-doh
hip	cadera	kah-DEH-rah
hormone replacement	reemplazo de hormonas	reh-ehm-PLAH-soh deh or-MOH-nahs
hyperopia	hiperopía	ee-pehr-oh-PEE-ah
hysterectomy	histerectomía	ees-teh-rek-toh-MEE-ah
impotency	impotencia	eem-poh-TEHN-see-ah
influenza	influenza	een-floo-EHN-sah
inner ear	oído interior	oh-EE-doh een-teh-ree-OHR
insulin	insulina	in-soo-LEE-nah
intestine	intestino	een-tehs-TEE-noh
iodine	yodo	YOH-doh
iris	iris	EE-rees
jaundice	ictericia	eek-teh-REE-see-ah
joint	coyunturas	ko-yoon-TOO-rahs
kidney	riñón	ree-NYOHN

Continued

English	Spanish	Spanish Pronunciation
knee	rodilla	roh-DEE-yah
kneecap	rótula	ROH-too-lah
laparoscopy	laparoscopía	lah-pah-rohs-KOH-pee-ah
larynx	laringe	lah-REEN-heh
leukorrhea	leucorrea	leh-oo-koh-RREH-ah
ligament	ligamento	lee-gah-MEHN-toh
light	luz	loos
liver	hígado	EE-gah-doh
lobe	lóbulo	LOH-boo-loh
lungs	pulmones	pool-MOH-nehs
lymph	linfa	LEEN-fah
lymph node	nódulo linfático	NOH-doo-loh leen-FAH-tee-coh
lymphatic	linfático	leen-FAH-tee-coh
macular degeneration	degeneración macular	deh-heh-neh-rah-see-OHN mah-coo-LAHR
malignant	maligno	mah-LEEG-noh
mammogram	mamografía	mah-moh-grah-FEE-ah
masculine	masculino	mahs-koo-LEE-noh
menopause	menopausia	meh-noh-PAH-oo-see-ah
menstruation	menstruación	mehns-troo-ah-see-OHN
mouth	boca	BOH-kah
movement	movimiento	moh-bee-mee-EHN-toh
muscle	músculo	MOOS-koo-loh
myopia	miopía	mee-o-PEE-ah
nails	sarpullidos	sar-pooh-YEE-dohs
nerve	nervio	NER-bee-oh
newborn	recién nacida (feminine)	reh-see-EHN nah-SEE-dah
	recién nacido (masculine)	reh-see-EHN nah-SEE-doh
nocturia	nocturia	nok-TOO-ree-ah
nose	nariz	nah-REES
nostril	orificio de la nariz	o-ree-FEE-see-oh deh lah nah-REES
obstruction	obstrucción	obs-trook-see-OHN
oliguria	oliguria	oh-lee-GOO-ree-ah
ophthalmoscopy	oftalmoscopía	ohf-tahl-mohs-coh-PEE-ah
otalgia	otalgía	oh-tahl-HEE-ah
otitis media	otitis media	oh-TEE-tees MEH-dee-ah
otoscope	otoscopio	oh-tohs-COH-pee-oh
otoscopy	otoscopía	oh-tohs-coh-PEE-ah

English	Spanish	Spanish Pronunciation
ovary	ovario	oh-BAH-ree-oh
pain	dolor	doh-LOHR
pancreas	páncreas	PAHN-kreh-ahs
paralysis	parálisis	pah-RAH-lee-sees
penis	pene	PEH-neh
perspiration	perspiración	pehr-spee-rah-see-OHN
pink	rosada (female)	roh-SAH-dah
	rosado (male)	roh-SAH-doh
pituitary	pituitaria	pee-too-ee-TAH-ree-ah
pneumonia	pulmonía	pool-moh-NEE-ah
pregnant	embarazada	ehm-bah-rah-SAH-dah
prostate	próstata	PROHS-tah-tah
protein	proteína	proh-teh-EE-nah
pulse	pulso	POOL-soh
rapid	rápida (feminine)	RAH-pee-dah
	rápido (masculine)	RAH-pee-doh
rectum	recto	REHK-toh
reduction	reducción	reh-dook-see-OHN
renal pelvis	pelvis renal	PEHL-bees reh-NAHL
retina	retina	reh-TEE-nah
retinitis	retinitis	reh-tee-NEE-tees
rhythm	ritmo	REET-moh
rib	costilla	coh-STEE-yah
sacrum	sacro	SAH-croh
sclera	esclera	ehs-KLEH-rah
seizure	convulsion	con-buhl-see-OHN
	OR	
	ataque de apoplejía	ah-TAH-keh deh ah-pohp-leh-HEE-ah
sensation	sensación	sen-sah-see-OHN
sexual intercourse	coito	KOH-ee-toh
shoulder	hombro	OHM-broh
sigmoidoscopy	sigmoidoscopia	seeg-moh-ee-doh-SKOH-pee-ah
sinus	seno	SEH-noh
skin	piel	pee-EHL
slow	lenta (feminine)	LEHN-tah
	lento (masculine)	LEHN-toh

Continued

English	Spanish	Spanish Pronunciation
sore	llaga	YAH-gah
	OR	
	úlcera	OOL-seh-rah
spinal column	espina dorsal	ehs-PEE-nah dohr-SAHL
sprain	torcer	tohr-SEHR
sputum	esputo	ehs-POO-toh
sternum	esternón	ehs-tehr-NOHN
stiff	dura (feminine)	DOO-rah
	duro (masculine)	DOO-roh
stomach	estómago	es-TOH-mah-goh
stroke	ataque	ah-TAH-keh
stroke	ataque cerebral	ah-TAH-keh seh-reh-BRAHL
support	soporte	soh-POHR-teh
swallow	tragar	trah-GAHR
symptom	síntoma	SEEN-toh-mah
syncope	síncope	SEEN-coh-peh
teeth	diente	dee-EHN-teh
tendon	tendón	tehn-DOHN
testicle	testículo	tehs-TEE-koo-loh
thigh	muslo	MOOS-loh
thyroid	tiroides	tee-ROH-ee-dehs
tinnitus	tinitus	tee-NEE-toos
tissue	tejido	teh-HEE-doh
toe, finger	dedo	DEH-doh
tonsil	amígdala	ah-MEEG-dah-lah
trachea	tráquea	TRAH-keh-ah
ulcer	úlcera	OOL-seh-rah
ultrasonography	ultrasonografía	ool-trah-soh-noh-grah-FEE-ah
unconscious	inconsciente	een-kons-see-EHN-teh
ureter	uréter	oo-REH-tehr
urethra	uretra	oo-REH-trah
urinalysis	urinálisis	oo-ree-NAH-lee-sees
urinary	urinario	oo-ree-NAH-ree-oh
urinary tract infection	infección del tracto urinario	een-fek-see-OHN dehl TRAK-toh oo-ree-NAH-ree-oh
urinate	orinar	oh-ree-NAHR
urine	orina	oh-REE-nah
urology	urología	ooh-roh-loh-HEE-ah

English	Spanish	Spanish Pronunciation
uterus	útero	OO-teh-roh
vagina	vagina	bah-HEE-nah
valve	válvula	BAHL-boo-lah
varicose vein	vena varicosa	BEH-nah bah-ree-KOH-sah
vein	vena	BEH-nah
ventricle	ventrículo	behn-TREE-koo-loh
vertebrae	vértebra	BEHR-teh-brah
vision	visión	bee-see-OHN
voice	voz	bohs
vomit	vómito	BOH-mee-toh
wound	herida	eh-REE-dah
wrist	muñeca	moo-NYEH-kah
x-ray	rayos equis *OR* radiografía	RAH-yohs EH-kees rah-dee-oh-grah-FEE-yah
yellow	amarilla (feminine) amarillo (masculine)	ah-mah-REE-yah ah-mah-REE-yoh

INDEX

Note: An "f" following a page number indicates a figure, a "t" following a page number indicates a table

Abbreviations, 633–639, 641
  body structure, 54
  cardiovascular system, 197
  digestive system, 267
  discontinued, 641
  ear, 548
  endocrine system, 443
  eye, 548
  female reproductive system, 375
  integumentary system, 87
  lymphatic system, 197
  male reproductive system, 375
  musculoskeletal system, 506
  nervous system, 443
  radiographic procedures, 443
  radiology, 54
  respiratory system, 136
  sexually transmitted infections, 375
  urinary system, 319
Abdominal, 44
Abdominal adhesions, 54f
Abdominal cavity, 48f, 49
Abdominopelvic cavity, 48, 48f, 49
Abdominopelvic quadrants, 49–50, 51f
Abdominopelvic regions, 50f, 51–52
Abduction, 42, 42f, 479f
Abrasion, 87
Abscess, 87, 87f
Absence seizure, 448
Acetabulum, 494, 494f
Achilles tendon, 473f, 478
Achromatopsia, 548
Acidosis, 138
Acne, 88, 88f
Acoustic, 541
Acoustic neuroma, 552
Acquired immune deficiency syndrome
    (AIDS), 85, 134, 202
Acromegaly, 417, 418f
Acute renal failure (ARF), 317
Acute respiratory distress syndrome (ARDS), 138
Addison disease, 444
Adduction, 42, 42f, 479f
Adenocarcinoma, 310
Adenodynia, 310
Adenohypophysis, 413, 414
Adenoidectomy, 115
Adenoids, 114f, 115
Adenoma, 72, 310, 408
Adenopathy, 190
Adhesion, 54, 54f
Adipectomy, 72
Adipocele, 67, 79
Adipoma, 73
Adipose tissue, 66f, 358
Adrenal, 408, 416
Adrenal cortex hormones, 425t
Adrenal glands, 293f, 407f, 424–425
Adrenal hormones, 425t
Adrenal medullary hormones, 425t
Adrenalectomy, 408, 424
Adrenaline, 425t

Adrenocorticotropic hormone (ACTH), 411f,
    415, 416t
Adrenomegaly, 424
Adventitious breath sounds, 138
Aerophagia, 116, 119, 242
Age-related macular degeneration (ARMD,
    AMD), 550
Agglutination, 190
AIDS, 85, 134, 202
Albinism, 72, 81
Albino, 72
Alcoholism, 4, 408
Aldosterone, 425t
Alimentary canal, 230
Allergic rhinitis, 150–153
Allogenic BMT, 212
Allograft, 28, 96
Alopecia, 88
Alveolar, 115
Alveolus (alveoli), 115, 126
Alzheimer disease, 445
Amastia, 26
Amblyopia, 532
Amniocentesis, 344, 381, 381f
Amphiarthroses, 493
Amyotrophic lateral sclerosis (ALS), 445
Anacusis, 552
Anal fistula, 269
Anaphylaxis, 190
Anastomosis, 59, 59f, 249
Anatomical position, 37
Ancusis, 541
Androgen, 364
Androsterone, 364
Anemia, 198
Anesthesia, 373
Anesthetics, 454
Aneurysm, 188, 188f, 189, 438
Aneurysmectomy, 438
Aneurysmorrhaphy, 165
Angina pectoris, 198
Angiocarditis, 193
Angiography, 165
Angioma, 177
Angioplasty, 193, 208
Angiorrhaphy, 193
Angiorrhexis, 193
Angiotensin-converting enzyme (ACE)
    inhibitors, 213
Anhidrosis, 77
Anisocoria, 531
Ankylosing spondylitis, 482, 510
Ankylosis, 483
Anorchism, 378
Anorexia, 232
Anorexia nervosa, 439, 439f
Anosmia, 116
Anoxia, 138
Antacids, 276
Anterior, 33, 38, 38f, 412, 414
Anterolateral, 40
Anteroposterior (AP), 39

Antiarrhythmics, 213
Antibiotics, 97, 326
Anticoagulants, 188, 199, 213
Antidiarrheals, 276
Antidiuretic, 326
Antidiuretic hormone (ADH), 411f, 417t
Antiemetics, 276
Antiepileptics, 454
Antifungals, 97, 389
Antigen, 170
Antiglaucoma agents, 560
Antihypertensives, 213
Antiparkinsonian agents, 454
Antipruritics, 97
Antipsychotics, 454
Antispasmodics, 326
Antituberculars, 147
Antivirals, 213
Anuria, 314
Anus, 230f, 244, 251, 254f, 343f, 364f
Aorta, 165, 189
Aortic, 189
Aortic aneurysm, 188
Aortic stenosis, 177
Aortic valve, 177, 179
Aortopathy, 177
Aortostenosis, 165
Aphasia, 431
Aplasia, 372
Apnea, 116, 130
Appendectomy, 12, 13f, 244, 273, 273f
Appendicitis, 244
Appendicular skeleton, 481, 481f, 495f
Appendix, 230f, 244
Aqueous humor, 533
Arachnoid membrane, 434, 435f, 436
Areola, 358
Arrhythmia, 173
Arterial bleeding, 175
Arterial blood gas (ABG), 143
Arterial circulation, 175
Arteriole, 165, 178
Arteriolith, 176
Arteriolitis, 165
Arteriosclerosis, 165, 185, 187
Arteriostenosis, 166
Arthritis, 21, 22f, 483, 493, 494
Arthrocentesis, 18, 19f, 512
Arthrodesis, 484
Arthropathy, 493
Arthroplasty, 513
Arthroscope, 493
Arthroscopy, 493, 493f
Articulations, 473, 504
Ascending aorta, 177
Ascending colon, 230f
Ascites, 267, 268f
Aspermatism, 368
Aspermia, 365
Aspiration biopsy, 94
Asthma, 135, 135f
Astigmatism, 538f, 548

Atelectasis, 116, 139
Atheroma, 165
Atherosclerosis, 186, 186f, 187
Athlete's foot, 93
Atlas, 502
Atrial, 171
Atrial flutter, 173
Atrioventricular (AV), 165, 172, 182
Atrium, 165, 171
Atrophy, 419
Atropine, 200
Audiogram, 555
Audiologist, 530, 546
Audiology, 546
Audiometer, 541, 555
Audiometry, 555
Auditory, 541
Auricle, 542
Autoexamination, 85
Autograft, 26, 26f, 85, 96
Autograph, 85
Autohypnosis, 85
Autologous BMT, 212
Automatic external defibrillator (AED), 210
Automatic implantable cardioverter
    defibrillator (AICD), 210, 211f
Axial skeleton, 481, 481f, 495f
Axillary lymph nodes, 189, 194
Axis, 502
Axon, 430, 430f
Axon terminal synapse, 430f
Azotemia, 294
Azoturia, 319

Backbone, 502
Bacteriuria, 305
Balanitis, 364, 378
Baldness, 88
Balloon valvuloplasty, 212
Bariatric surgery, 274, 275f
Barium enema (BE), 271, 271f
Barium swallow, 272
Bartholin glands, 343f, 356
Basal cell carcinoma (BCC), 84, 84f
Basal layer, 66f, 70
Bed-wetting at night, 320
Bedsore, 93
Bell palsy, 446
Belly button, 52
Benign prostatic hypertrophy (BPH),
    329–332, 369, 369f
Benign tumor, 309, 371
Beta blockers, 213
Biceps brachii, 473f, 477
Biceps femoris, 473f, 477
Bicuspid valve, 175
Bilateral, 373
Bilateral vasectomy, 397–399
Bile, 260
Bile duct, 257, 262, 262f
Biliary colic, 264
Biliary tract disease, 408
Biopsy, 94, 360, 384
Bladder, 293f, 305, 306, 343f, 354
Blepharectomy, 537
Blepharoplasty, 537, 539
Blepharoplegia, 537
Blepharoptosis, 532, 539
Blepharospasm, 531, 537, 539

Blepharotomy, 537
Blind spot, 536
Blood, 170f, 170t
Blood clot, 165, 188, 199, 438
Blood poisoning, 55
Blood pressure (BP), 184
Blood types, 170t
Blood urea nitrogen (BUN), 321
Body cavities, 48–49
Body planes, 45–46
Body structure, 31–64
    abbreviations, 54
    abdominopelvic quadrants, 49–50, 51f
    abdominopelvic regions, 50f, 51–52
    basic units of structure, 35–36
    body cavities, 48–49
    body planes, 45–46
    combining forms, 33–34, 44
    diagnostic procedures, 55–59
    directional terms, 33, 36–43
    diseases and conditions, 54–55
    levels of organization, 31, 32f
    medical and surgical procedures, 59
Boil, 87
Bolus, 230f, 238
Bone and joint disorders, 507–510
Bone density test (bone densitometry), 512
Bone immobilization, 513
Bone marrow aspiration biopsy, 207, 207f
Bone marrow transplant (BMT), 212
Bone resorption inhibitors, 514
Bone scan, 513
Bones, 473, 482–492
Borborygmus, 267
Bowel movement, 236
Bowman capsule, 312
Brachialis, 473f
Brachioradialis, 473f
Brachytherapy, 388, 388f
Brain, 432–434
Brainstem, 433
Breast reconstruction, 386
Breasts, 358–360
Bronchial, 133
Bronchial tree, 124
Bronchiectasis, 21, 115, 126
Bronchiole, 114f, 124
Bronchiolitis, 115
Bronchitis, 126, 133, 134
Bronchodilators, 147
Bronchopneumonia, 133, 134
Bronchoscope, 115
Bronchoscopy, 143, 143f
Bronchospasm, 125, 126
Bronchostenosis, 126
Bronchus (bronchi), 115, 124, 125
Bruise, 90
Bruit, 198
Bulbourethral gland, 364f, 368
Bulla (bullae), 88, 92f
Bundle branches, 182
Bundle of His, 182
Bunion, 507, 507f
Burn, 88, 89f
Bursa (bursae), 501

C-section, 362
Calcaneodynia, 482
Calcaneum, 495f, 496

Calcemia, 421, 490
Calcitonin, 419t
Calcium supplements, 514
Calculus (calculi), 176, 257, 261, 263, 295, 300
Calyces, 293f
Canal of Schlemm, 533
Cancer, 119, 241
Cancerous, 309
Candia albicans, 375
Candidiasis, 375
Capillaries, 178
Capsule endoscopy, 272
Carbuncle, 87, 87f
Carcinoma, 84, 241, 254
Carcinophobia, 440
Cardiac, 177, 187
Cardiac catheterization, 204, 204f, 221–223
Cardiac center, 434
Cardiac enzyme studies, 204
Cardiac muscle fibers, 476
Cardiac tamponade, 168
Cardiologist, 162
Cardiology, 162
Cardiomegaly, 165, 185
Cardiothoracic surgeon, 162
Cardiovascular and lymphatic systems, 161–227
    abbreviations, 197
    anatomy and physiology overview, 163
    clinical application activity, 224
    combining forms, 165–166, 225
    emergency department report (ruling out
        myocardial infarction), 216–220
    interrelationship between cardiovascular and
        lymphatic systems, 164f
    operative report (cardiac catheterization),
        221–223
    prefixes, 226
    suffixes, 166, 225–226
Cardiovascular surgeon, 162
Cardiovascular system, 167–189
    blood/blood types, 170f, 170t
    blood flow through the heart, 175–179
    cardiac cycle and heart sounds, 183–189
    circulation and heart structures, 169–174
    conduction pathway of heart, 182, 183f
    diagnostic procedures, 204–206
    diseases and conditions, 198–202
    heart valves, 179–180
    heart wall, 167–169
    medical and surgical procedures, 208–212
    pharmacology, 213
Cardioversion, 209, 209f
Carotid endarterectomy, 211, 211f
Carpal tunnel syndrome (CTS), 507
Carpals, 481f
Carpoptosis, 482
Carpus, 495
Cartilage, 124
Casting, 513
Cataract, 548, 549f
Cataract surgery, 556
Catheter, 117, 302, 323
Catheter ablation, 208
Catheterization, 323, 324f
Caudal, 33
Cauterize, 59
Cecum, 230f
Celiac disease, 268
Cell, 35

Cellular level, 31, 32f
Cellular necrosis, 85
Central nervous system (CNS), 429
Cephalad, 41, 44
Cephalodynia, 496
Cephalometer, 496
Cerclage, 384
Cerebellum, 433, 433f
Cerebral, 189, 433
Cerebral cortex, 432
Cerebral degeneration, 445
Cerebral palsy (CP), 446
Cerebrospinal, 431
Cerebrospinal fluid (CSF), 436
Cerebrotomy, 433
Cerebrovascular accident (CVA), 438
Cerebrum, 432
Cervical, 44, 356, 482
Cervical cancer, 376, 376f
Cervical dilator, 352f
Cervical lymph nodes, 189, 194
Cervical nerves, 434, 435f
Cervical vertebrae, 502, 503
Cervicitis, 344, 356
Cervicofacial, 502
Cervix, 343f, 356
Cervix uteri, 357
Cesarean section (CS), 362
Chart note, 462–465
Chemabrasion, 96
Chemical peel, 96
Chest radiograph, 57, 58f
Chest x-ray, 39f
Chiropractic medicine, 472
Chiropractor, 472
Chlamydia, 362, 380
Cholangiography, 262
Cholangiole, 257
Cholangioma, 262
Cholangitis, 262
Cholecyst, 263
Cholecystalgia, 264
Cholecystectomy, 257, 264
Cholecystitis, 12, 13f, 263, 264
Cholecystodynia, 264
Cholecystolith, 261
Cholecystolithiasis, 264
Choledocholith, 262
Choledocholithiasis, 262, 262f
Choledochorrhaphy, 262
Choledochotomy, 257, 262
Cholelith, 257, 261
Cholelithiasis, 257, 261, 262f, 263
Cholemesis, 260
Chondritis, 124
Chondroma, 33, 124
Chondropathy, 124
Chondroplasty, 124
Chordae tendineae, 168f, 179
Choroid, 531, 534
Choroiditis, 535
Choroidopathy, 531, 535
Chronic bronchitis, 133, 134, 135f
Chronic obstructive pulmonary disease
    (COPD), 134, 135f
Chronic renal failure (CRF), 320
Chyme, 238
Ciliary body, 534
Circulatory system, 163

Circumcision, 388
Cirrhosis, 267
Clavicle, 481f
Clitoris, 343f, 356
Closed-angle glaucoma, 549
Closed fracture, 497, 499
Clot, 438
Clot buster, 213
Clubfoot, 509
CO₂, 126
Coccygeal nerve, 434, 435f
Coccyx, 481f, 504
Cochlea, 544f, 545, 546, 546f
Cochlear implant, 559
Cold (disease), 139
Colectomy, 250
Colitis, 250
Collecting tubule, 312
Colles fracture, 499
Colon, 244, 254f
Colon cancer, 254, 255, 329–332
Colonoscopy, 12, 13f, 244, 253, 254f, 272
Color blindness, 548
Colorrhaphy, 250
Coloscopy, 253
Colostomy, 244, 250, 250f
Colotomy, 250
Colpalgia, 351
Colpitis, 351
Colpocele, 344
Colpocervical, 356
Colpohysterectomy, 354
Colpopexy, 352
Colpoptosis, 352
Colporrhagia, 354
Colposcope, 344, 356, 381, 381f
Colposcopy, 344, 356, 381, 381f
Colpospasm, 352
Combining form (CF), 5–7
Comedo, 76
Comminuted fracture, 499
Compact bone, 486
Competent, 178
Complete fracture, 497, 500f
Complete heart block (CHB), 200
Complicated fracture, 499
Compound fracture, 497, 499
Computed tomography (CT scan), 57, 58f,
    144, 272, 321
Conductive and sensorineural hearing
    loss test, 556
Conductive hearing loss, 552
Congenital syphilis (CS), 380
Congestive heart failure (CHF), 201
Conjunctiva, 537
Conjunctivitis, 531, 537
Consultation letter, 101–104
Continence, 316
Continuous positive airway pressure (CPAP)
    machine, 130, 131f
Contraceptives, 389
Contracture, 507
Contusion, 90
Convergent strabismus, 551
Convulsion, 448
Coreometer, 531
Cornea, 76, 533
Corneal transplant, 531, 557
Corneitis, 531

Coronal plane, 46f, 47
Coronary, 165
Coronary angioplasty, 208
Coronary artery bypass graft (CABG), 210, 210f
Coronary artery disease (CAD), 185, 186
Coronavirus, 139
Corticoadrenal insufficiency, 444
Corticosteroids, 97, 147
Cortisol, 416, 425t
Coryza, 139
Costochondritis, 483
COVID-19, 139, 139f, 144, 144f
Cowper glands, 368
Crackles, 138
Cranial, 44
Cranial bones, 485
Cranial cavity, 48, 48f
Craniotomy, 453, 482
Cranium, 495, 495f
Creatinine clearance, 321
Crepitation, 507
Crohn disease, 249, 269
Cross-eye, 551
Cross-sectional plane, 47
Croup, 139
Cryosurgery, 95
Cryotherapy, 68
Cryptorchism, 365, 379
CT scan, 57, 58f, 144, 272, 321
Culture and sensitivity (C&S), 55, 56f
Curet (curette), 351, 352f
Cushing syndrome, 415, 416, 417f
Cutaneous, 67
Cutaneous laser, 96
Cuticle, 78
Cyanoderma, 81, 83
Cyanosis, 83, 116
Cyst, 89
Cystic, 260
Cystic duct, 260, 262f
Cystic fibrosis (CF), 140
Cystitis, 305, 308, 317
Cystocele, 294, 306, 306f
Cystolithiasis, 305
Cystolithotomy, 305
Cystorrhaphy, 305
Cystoscope, 307, 307f
Cystoscopy, 294, 307, 307f
Cystourethroscopy, 307
Cytologist, 36
Cytology, 34, 35, 81
Cytolysis, 34
Cytometer, 33, 36
Cytotoxic T lymphocyte (CTL), 195

Dacryadenalgia, 539
Dacryadenitis, 539
Dacryorrhea, 531, 539
Debridement, 95
Decubitus ulcer, 93
Deep vein thrombosis (DVT), 199, 200f
Defibrillator, 209, 210
Degenerative intervertebral disk disease,
    518–520
Deltoid, 473f, 478
Dendrites, 430, 430f
Dentist, 231, 237
Dentistry, 237
Deoxygenated, 171

Depressed lesions, 92f
Dermabrasion, 87, 96
Dermal, 71
Dermatitis, 72, 74
Dermatologist, 65, 67, 71, 75
Dermatology, 65, 71, 75
Dermatoma, 75
Dermatomycosis, 67, 72, 77
Dermatopathy, 75, 78
Dermatoplasty, 68, 74, 88
Dermic, 71
Dermis, 66f, 69
Dermoid, 68
Dermopathy, 70, 72
Descending aorta, 177
Descending colon, 230f
Diabetes mellitus (DM), 320, 427, 444, 458–461
Diabetic retinopathy, 549
Diagnosis (Dx), 87, 236
Diagnostic procedures, 621–623
Diagnostic suffix, 19–20
Dialysis, 295, 324
Diaphoresis, 67, 68
Diaphragm, 48, 49f, 131, 133f
Diaphragmatic hernia, 270f
Diaphysis, 484, 486
Diarrhea, 27, 232, 252
Diarthroses, 493
Diastole, 183, 184
Digestive system, 229–289
    abbreviations, 267
    accessory organs of digestion, 258–265
    anatomy and physiology overview, 230
    clinical application activity, 286
    combining forms, 231–232, 244–245, 257, 287
    diagnostic procedures, 271–273
    diseases and conditions, 267–271
    esophagus, pharynx, and stomach, 238–242
    gallbladder, 260–264
    liver, 259–260
    lower GI tract, 246–256
    medical and surgical procedures, 273–275
    operative report (esophageal carcinoma), 283–285
    oral cavity, 233–237
    organs, 230f
    pancreas, 264–265
    pharmacology, 276
    prefixes, 288
    progress note (rectal bleeding), 279–282
    rectum and anus, 251–255
    small and large intestines, 246–251
    suffixes, 232, 257, 287–288
    upper GI tract, 233–242
Digital rectal examination (DRE), 383, 383f
Dilation and curettage (D&C), 351, 352f
Diplobacteria, 27
Diplopia, 531, 537, 538
Dipstick test, 314, 315f
Discharge summary, 458–461
Dissecting aneurysm, 188f
Distal, 33, 41, 42, 315, 488
Distal epiphysis, 486
Diuresis, 320
Diuretics, 213, 326
Divergent strabismus, 551

Diverticular disease, 268
Diverticulitis, 268
Doppler ultrasonography, 206, 206f
Dorsal, 33, 37, 38
Dorsal cavity, 48, 48f
Dorsal root, 437
Dorsiflexion, 479f
Double vision, 531, 538
Drug classifications, 625–631
Dual diagnosis, 439
Dual-energy x-ray absorptiometry (DEXA), 512
Duchenne dystrophy, 506
Ductus deferens, 364, 368
Duodenal ulcer, 238, 239f
Duodenectomy, 247, 248
Duodenorrhaphy, 248
Duodenoscopy, 244, 272
Duodenostomy, 248
Duodenum, 230f, 239f, 244, 247, 248
Dura mater, 434, 435f, 436
Dwarfism, 415, 415f
Dysentery, 269
Dysmenorrhea, 357
Dyspepsia, 232, 242
Dysphagia, 232, 242
Dysplasia, 372
Dyspnea, 130, 135
Dystocia, 345
Dysuria, 305, 308, 309

Ear, 540–547
    abbreviations, 548
    clinical application activity, 570
    combining forms, 541, 571
    diagnostic procedures, 555–556
    diseases and conditions, 552–553
    external, 542
    inner, 545–546, 545f
    medical and surgical procedures, 559
    middle, 543–545
    pharmacology, 560
    prefixes, 572
    SOAP note (otitis media), 567–569
    suffixes, 541, 571
Ear canal, 542
Ear irrigation, 559, 559f
Eardrum, 542, 544
Ecchymosis, 90, 90f
Echocardiography, 204
Echogram, 57
Echography, 273
Eclampsia, 378
Ectopic pregnancy, 376, 377f
Eczema, 89, 90f
Eczematous rash, 89
Edema, 55, 55f, 301, 313
EEG, 19, 166, 183f, 184, 185, 204
Ejaculatory duct, 364f
Electrocardiogram (ECG, EKG), 19, 166, 183f, 184, 185, 204
Electrocardiograph, 19, 166
Electrocardiography, 19, 20f, 166
Electrodesiccation, 95
Electroencephalography (EEG), 450, 450f
Electronic medical record (EMR), 62
Elevated lesions, 92f
Embolus, 199, 438

Emergency department report, 216–220, 392–396
Emesis, 241
Emmetropia, 538f
Emphysema, 134, 135f
Empyema, 140
Encephalitis, 431, 432, 496, 497
Encephalocele, 497
Encephaloma, 432, 496
Encephalomalacia, 496
Encephalopathy, 497
End-stage renal disease (ESRD), 292, 320
End-to-end anastomosis, 59, 59f
End-to-side anastomosis, 59, 59f
Endarterectomy, 211
Endocardium, 166, 167, 179
Endocrine, 27
Endocrine system, 406–428
    abbreviations, 443
    adrenal glands, 424, 425t
    clinical application activity, 466
    combining forms, 408, 467
    diagnostic procedures, 449–450
    discharge summary (diabetes mellitus), 458–461
    diseases and conditions, 444–445
    hormones, 410–412
    major endocrine glands, 407f
    medical and surgical procedures, 452, 453f
    ovaries, 428
    pancreas, 425–427
    parathyroid glands, 423
    pharmacology, 454
    pineal gland, 428
    pituitary gland, 412–417
    prefixes, 468
    suffixes, 409, 467–468
    testes, 428
    thymus gland, 428
    thyroid gland, 418–421
Endocrinologist, 405
Endocrinology, 405
Endolymphatic/labyrinthine hydrops, 552
Endometriosis, 377, 377f
Endometritis, 344
Endoscope, 240, 272
Endoscopy, 56, 56f, 229, 239, 253, 272
Endotracheal intubation, 146, 146f
ENT physician, 530
Enterectomy, 250
Enterologist, 236
Enteropathy, 244
Enterorrhaphy, 250
Enuresis, 320
Enzyme-linked immunosorbent assay (ELISA), 207
Epidermis, 66f, 69, 70
Epididymis, 364f, 368
Epidural nerve block, 436, 436f
Epidural space, 436
Epigastric, 51, 241
Epigastric region, 50f
Epiglottis, 114f, 122, 131f
Epiglottitis, 140
Epilepsy, 445, 448
Epinephrine, 425t
Episiotomy, 345, 384, 385f
Epispadias, 379

Epistaxis, 140
Epstein-Barr virus (EBV), 203
Erectile agents, 389
Erectile dysfunction (ED), 379
Erthropia, 537
Erythema, 88
Erythrocyte, 82, 126, 169, 170
Erythrocytosis, 84
Erythroderma, 81
Erythropoiesis, 488
Erythrosis, 83
Esophageal carcinoma, 283–285
Esophageal ulcer, 238, 239f
Esophagogastroduodenoscopy (EGD), 240
Esophagoplasty, 240
Esophagoscope, 231
Esophagoscopy, 240, 272
Esophagotome, 240
Esophagotomy, 240
Esophagus, 230f, 231, 238, 239f, 240
Esotropia, 551, 552f
Estrogen, 342, 350, 358, 389
Ethmoidal sinuses, 118f
Eupnea, 130
Eustachian tube, 544f, 545, 546f
Eversion, 479f
Ewing sarcoma, 507
Excimer laser, 95
Exciplex laser, 95
Excoriation, 92f
Exhalation, 132
Exophthalmos, 420
Exotropia, 551, 552f
Expiration, 132
Extension, 479f
External ear, 542
External respiration, 114, 127
Extracapsular cataract extraction (ECCE), 556
Extracorporeal shock wave lithotripsy (ESWL), 275, 299, 300f
Eye, 530–540
    abbreviations, 548
    clinical application activity, 570
    combining forms, 531–532, 571
    diagnostic procedures, 554–555
    diseases and conditions, 548–552
    fibrous tunic, 533
    medical and surgical procedures, 556–558
    operative report (retinal detachment repair), 563–566
    pharmacology, 560
    prefixes, 572
    refraction of, 538f
    sensory tunic, 534
    suffixes, 532, 571
    vascular tunic, 534

Fallopian tube, 343f, 346, 349
Farsightedness, 538, 539
Fascioplasty, 474
Fasting blood glucose (FBG), 449
Fasting blood sugar (FBS), 236, 449
Fat cells, 73
Feces, 251
Female reproductive system, 342–361
    abbreviations, 375
    breasts, 358–360
    combining forms, 344–345, 401

diagnostic procedures, 381–383
diseases and conditions, 375–378
external structures, 356–358
internal structures, 346–355
lateral view, 343f
medical and surgical procedures, 384–388
pharmacology, 389
suffixes, 345
Femoral, 482
Femur, 481f, 496
Fertilization, 348
Fibroid, 377
Fibroma, 474
Fibrous tunic, 533
Fibula, 481f, 496
Fibular, 483
Filtrate, 312
Fingernail, 78, 79f
First-degree burn, 88, 89f
First-degree heart block, 200
Fissure, 92f
Fistula, 269, 353, 353f
Flat bones, 485, 486
Flat lesions, 92f
Flexion, 479f
Floating kidney, 300
Flu, 141
Fluoroscopy, 57
Foley catheter, 323
Follicle-stimulating hormone (FSH), 411f, 416t
Foreskin, 370
Fovea, 534
Fracture, 497–500
Frame, 2
Friction rub, 138
Frontal plane, 46f, 47
Frontal sinuses, 118f
Frozen-section biopsy, 94
Fulguration, 95
Full thickness burn, 88
Fungus, 78
Furuncle, 87, 87f
Fusiform aneurysm, 188f

Galactorrhea, 344
Gall, 260
Gallbladder, 230f, 257, 258, 260–264, 261
Gallbladder attack, 264
Gallstone, 261, 263
Gametes, 342, 364
Ganglion cyst, 508, 508f
Gangrene, 85
Gastralgia, 232
Gastrectomy, 240
Gastric, 44
Gastric bypass with gastroenterostomy, 274
Gastric ulcer, 238, 239, 239f
Gastritis, 241
Gastrocnemius, 473f, 478
Gastroduodenostomy, 249
Gastrodynia, 232, 239
Gastroenteroanastomosis, 249
Gastroenterologist, 229, 236
Gastroenterology, 229
Gastroenterostomy, 249
Gastroesophageal reflux disease (GERD), 269
Gastroileostomy, 249
Gastrointestinal, 236

Gastrointestinal (GI) system, 229
Gastrointestinal (GI) tract, 230
Gastrologist, 236
Gastrology, 236
Gastromegaly, 12, 13f, 232, 239
Gastroplasty, 240
Gastroscopy, 231, 240, 272
Gastrotomy, 241
Genitalia, 342, 356
Gestational hypertension, 378
GI tract, 230
Gigantism, 415, 415f
Gingivitis, 231, 237
Glandular tissue, 358
Glans penis, 364f, 370
Glaucoma, 549, 550f, 554, 557
Glioma, 431
Glomerular, 294
Glomerular capsule, 312
Glomerulitis, 313
Glomerulonephritis, 301, 313
Glomerulosclerosis, 313
Glomerulus, 294, 312, 313
Glucagon, 427t
Glucocorticoids, 425t
Glucogenesis, 408, 426
Glucometer, 427, 427f
Glucose tolerance test (GTT), 450
Gluteus maximus, 473f
Glycogen, 426
Glycogenesis, 426
Gold salts, 514
Gonadotropin, 365, 389
Gonads, 364
Gonorrhea, 362, 380
Gout, 508
Graft, 85
Grand mal seizure, 448
Graves disease, 420, 420f
Gravida, 361
Gray matter, 430, 435f, 448
Greenstick fracture, 499
Growth hormone (GH), 411f, 414, 416t
Gynecologist, 342, 344, 357
Gynecology, 342, 357
Gynecopathy, 357

H₂ blockers, 276
Hair follicle, 66f, 72
Hallucinations, 441
Hallux valgus, 507
Hardening of the arteries, 185
Hearing loss, 552
Heart, 165
Heart attack, 202
Heart block, 200
Heart failure (HF), 201
Heart surgeon, 162
Heart valves, 179–180
Heart wall, 167–169
Hemangiectasis, 177
Hematemesis, 351
Hematochezia, 269
Hematologist, 177, 351
Hematology, 177, 351
Hematoma, 90
Hematomesis, 242
Hematopathy, 351

Hematopoietic stem cells, 171
Hematosalpinx, 345
Hematuria, 314, 316
Hemiparesis, 431
Hemiplegia, 23, 474, 478
Hemoccult test, 273
Hemodialysis (HD), 324, 325f
Hemorrhage, 90, 189, 195, 354, 438
Hemorrhagic stroke, 438
Hemorrhoid, 269
Hepatectomy, 260
Hepatic, 260
Hepatic duct, 260, 262f
Hepatitis, 12, 13f, 257, 259
Hepatocyte, 260
Hepatodynia, 260
Hepatolith, 261
Hepatoma, 259
Hepatomegaly, 257, 259
Hepatorrhaphy, 260
Hepatosis, 263
Hernia, 79, 269, 306
Herniated disk, 508, 508f
Herpes genitalis, 380
Herpes simplex virus (HSV), 380
Herpes zoster virus, 448
Heterograft, 28, 28f, 96
Heteropsia, 532
Hiatal hernia, 270f
Hiccups, 131
Hidradenitis, 67, 77
Hidrosis, 77
Hirsutism, 91
Histologist, 34, 36
Histolysis, 33
HIV, 85, 202
Hives, 93
Hodgkin lymphoma, 191, 202
Holter monitor, 205, 205f
Homeostasis, 292, 312
Homograft, 28, 96
Hordeolum, 549, 550f
Horizontal plane, 46f
Hormone replacement therapy (HRT), 350, 454
Hormones, 410–412
    adrenal, 425t
    key characteristics, 411
    pancreatic, 427t
    parathyroid, 423t
    pituitary, 416–417t
    target organs, 411f
    thyroid, 419t
Hospital admission, 329–332
Human immunodeficiency virus (HIV), 85, 202
Human papillomavirus (HPV), 380
Humeral, 482
Humerus, 481f, 495
Hunchback, 510
Huntington chorea, 445
Hydrocele, 371
Hydrocephal, 431
Hydronephrosis, 315, 315f
Hydroureter, 315, 315f
Hypercalcemia, 490
Hyperemesis, 232, 241
Hyperglycemia, 408

Hyperhidrosis, 67, 68, 77
Hyperopia, 538, 538f, 539
Hyperparathyroidism, 423
Hyperplasia, 372, 416
Hypersalivation, 235
Hypersecretion, 410, 412, 416
Hypertension, 201
    gestational, 378
    glomerulonephritis, 313
    kidneys, 302
    polycystic kidney disease (PKD), 317
    renal, 301
Hyperthyroidism, 420
Hypertrophy, 409
Hypertropia, 532
Hypocalcemia, 408, 421
Hypochondriac, 51
Hypodermic, 67
Hypodermic needle, 28, 29f, 71
Hypogastric, 50f, 51
Hypogastric region, 50f, 52
Hypoglossal, 231
Hypophysis, 412
Hypopituitarism, 408
Hyposecretion, 410, 412
Hypospadias, 321, 379
Hypothalamus, 407f
Hypothyroidism, 419
Hypoxemia, 140
Hypoxia, 116, 140
Hysteralgia, 349
Hysterectomy, 344, 349, 349f, 354
Hysterocele, 349
Hysterodynia, 349
Hysteropathy, 349
Hysteroptosis, 350
Hysterosalpingooophorectomy, 385
Hysteroscopy, 350
Hysterospasm, 349
Hysterotomy, 349, 362

Ichthyosis, 67
Ileectomy, 247
Ileitis, 249
Ileorrhaphy, 248, 249
Ileostomy, 244, 248
Ileotomy, 248
Ileum, 230f, 244, 246, 247, 248, 249, 287
Iliac, 44
Iliac lymph nodes, 189
Ilium, 481f
Immunogen, 190
Immunologist, 163
Immunology, 163
Immunosuppressants, 213
Impacted fracture, 499
Impetigo, 91
Impotence, 379
In situ, 84
Incision, 300
Incision and drainage (I&D), 59, 95
Incompetent, 179
Incomplete fracture, 497
Incontinence, 316
Incus, 545, 546f
Inferior, 33, 38f, 40, 41, 47, 478
Inferior vena cava (IVC), 169, 175, 293f

Inflammation, 55
Inflammatory bowel disease (IBD), 269
Influenza, 141
Inguinal, 44, 51
Inguinal hernia, 270f
Inguinal lymph nodes, 189, 194
Inhalation, 132
Inhaler with spacer, 147f
Inner ear, 545–546, 545f
Inspiration, 132
Insulin, 427t
Insulin pump therapy, 452, 452f
Integumentary system, 65–111
    abbreviations, 87
    anatomy and physiology overview, 66
    clinical application activity, 109
    color, 81–86
    combining forms, 67–68, 110
    consultation letter (skin cancer check), 101–104
    diagnostic procedures, 94
    diseases and conditions, 87–94
    medical and surgical procedures, 95–96
    pharmacology, 97
    prefixes, 110
    progress note (psoriasis vulgaris), 105–108
    skin and accessory organs, 69–80
    structure of skin and subcutaneous tissue, 66f
    suffixes, 68, 110
Interatrial septum (IAS), 173
Intercostal, 132
Intercostal muscles, 497
Internal respiration, 114, 127
Interstitial nephritis, 321
Interventricular septum (IVS), 173
Intervertebral disk, 502
Intradermal allergy test, 94, 94f
Intradermal injection, 29f
Intramuscular injection, 29f
Intraocular, 531
Intraocular lens (IOL), 556
Intravenous fluorescein angiography (IVFA), 554
Intravenous pyelography, 322
Intraventricular, 166
Inversion, 479f
Iridectomy, 557
Iridocele, 535
Iridoplegia, 531
Iris, 534
Iron deficiency anemia, 21, 22f
Irregular bones, 485, 486
Irritable bowel syndrome (IBS), 270
Ischemia, 201
Ischemic stroke, 438
Ischium, 481f
Islets of Langerhans, 425

Jaundice, 261
Jejunal feeding tube, 248
Jejunectomy, 247
Jejunorrhaphy, 244, 249
Jejunostomy, 248
Jejunotomy, 248
Jejunum, 230f, 244, 247, 248
Jock itch, 93

Joints, 473, 493–494
Juvenile wart, 93

Kaposi sarcoma, 85, 203
Keloid, 74, 75f
Keratin, 71
Keratitis, 535
Keratoma, 76
Keratoplasty, 531, 557
Keratorrhexis, 535
Keratosis, 67, 76
Keratotomy, 535
Kidney, 293f, 296, 297
Kidney stone, 298, 299f
Killer T cells, 195
Kleptomania, 441
Kyphosis, 510, 511f

Labia majora, 343f, 356
Labia minora, 343f, 356
Labyrinth, 545
Lacrimal apparatus, 539, 540f
Lacrimal gland, 539
Lacrimal sac, 539
Lacrimation, 531
Lactation, 358
Lactiferous duct, 358
Lactogen, 344
Laminectomy, 483
Laparoscopic appendectomy, 273, 273f, 274f
Laparoscopy, 382, 382f
Laparotomy, 274
Large intestine, 244–245, 246–251
Laryngectomy, 121
Laryngitis, 122
Laryngoscope, 115, 122
Laryngoscopy, 122
Laryngostenosis, 121, 122
Larynx, 114f, 115, 121
Laser-assisted in situ keratomileusis (LASIK) surgery, 557, 558f
Laser keratotomy, 535
Laser photocoagulation, 557
LASIK, 557, 558f
Lateral, 33, 37, 40
Laxatives, 276
Lazy eye, 532
Left atrium (LA), 171, 183f, 201f
Left hypochondriac region, 50f
Left inguinal region, 50f
Left lower quadrant (LLQ), 50, 50f
Left lumbar region, 50f
Left lung, 171
Left pulmonary artery, 175
Left pulmonary vein, 171, 176
Left upper quadrant (LUQ), 50, 50f
Left ventricle (LV), 171, 183f, 201f
Leiomyoma, 377, 474
Leucocyte, 171
Leukemia, 82
Leukocyte, 82, 169, 171
Leukocytopenia, 82
Leukocytosis, 84
Leukoderma, 81, 94
Leukopenia, 82
Leukopoiesis, 488
Leukorrhea, 378
Lipectomy, 72

Lipid panel, 205
Lipocele, 79
Lipocyte, 67, 73
Lipoma, 73
Liposuction, 73, 74f
Lithectomy, 298
Lithiasis, 263, 295, 298
Lithotripsy, 275, 295, 298
Liver, 230f, 247f, 251, 257, 258, 259–260, 262f
Lobectomy, 128, 128f
Lobitis, 128
Lobotomy, 128
Long bones, 485, 486
Longitudinal fracture, 499, 500
Lordosis, 510, 511f
Lou Gehrig disease, 445
Low blood oxygen, 140
Low sperm count, 368
Lower GI series, 271
Lower GI tract, 246–256
Lower respiratory tract, 124–135
Lumbar, 44, 51
Lumbar nerves, 434, 435f
Lumbar puncture (LP), 450, 451f
Lumbar region, 52
Lumbar vertebrae, 504
Lumbocostal, 474
Lumbodynia, 474
Lumen, 308
Lumpectomy, 360, 360f, 385
Lung cancer, 135, 141
Lungs, 114f, 116, 125, 171
Lunula, 78
Luteinizing hormone (LH), 411f, 416t
Lymbodynia, 504
Lymph capillaries, 189, 191
Lymph nodes, 189
Lymph vessels, 191
Lymphadenitis, 190
Lymphangiography, 207
Lymphangioma, 190
Lymphatic system, 189–195
    combining forms, 190
    diagnostic procedures, 207
    diseases and conditions, 202–203
    functions, 189
    lymphatic structures, 191–194
    medical and surgical procedures, 212
    pharmacology, 213
    suffix, 190
    tonsils, spleen, and thymus, 194–195
Lymphedema, 21, 193, 194f
Lymphocyte, 171
Lymphogioma, 193
Lymphoma, 191, 202
Lymphopoiesis, 190, 191

Macrophage, 195
Macular degeneration (MD), 550, 551f
Macule, 92f
Magnetic resonance imaging (MRI), 57, 58f, 144, 273, 451
Magnetic source imaging (MSI), 451
Magnetoencephalography, 451
Male reproductive system, 364–373
    abbreviations, 375
    combining forms, 364–365, 401
    diagnostic procedures, 383–384

diseases and conditions, 378–379
    lateral view, 364f
    medical and surgical procedures, 388–389
    organs of reproduction, 366–373
    pharmacology, 389
Malignant melanoma, 83, 83f
Malignant neoplasm of bone by site, 507
Malignant neoplasm of soft tissue, 203
Malignant tumor, 309, 371
Malleus, 545, 546f
Mammary glands, 358, 359f
Mammogram, 344
Mammography, 360, 382
Mammoplasty, 360
Mandible, 481f
Mantoux test, 146
Masculinization, 364
Masseter, 473f
Mastalgia, 358
Mastectomy, 358, 386, 386f
Mastodynia, 358
Mastopexy, 18, 344, 360
Mastoplasty, 360
Matrix, 78
Maxilla, 481f
Maxillary sinus, 118f
Meatorrhaphy, 309
Meatotomy, 309
Meatus, 294
Mediad, 34, 40
Medial, 33, 38f, 40
Median plane, 46f
Medical and surgical procedures, 623–624
Medical imaging, 56–57, 58f
Medical record, 62
Medical record activities, 62
    chart note, 462–465
    consultation letter, 101–104
    discharge summary, 458–461
    emergency department report, 216–220, 392–396
    hospital admission, 329–332
    operative report, 221–223, 283–285, 397–399, 521–524, 563–566
    progress note, 105–108, 279–282, 333–335
    radiology report, 518–520
    SOAP note, 567–569
Medical specialties, 643–644
    cardiology, 162
    chiropractic medicine, 472
    dermatology, 65
    endocrinology, 405
    gastroenterology, 229
    gynecology, 341–342
    immunology, 163
    nephrology, 292
    neurology, 406
    obstetrics, 341–342
    ophthalmology, 530
    orthopedics, 472
    otolaryngology, 530
    pulmonology, 113
    rheumatology, 472
    urology, 291, 342
Medical word elements, 3–15, 17–24, 26–30, 575–584
Medulla, 433, 434
Medullary cavity, 486

Megalocardia, 165, 185
Megalogastria, 239
Megalomania, 441
Melanin, 71, 72
Melanocyte, 71, 72, 82, 83
Melanoderma, 81
Melanoma, 67, 83, 83f, 84
Melanosis, 83
Menarche, 345
Ménière disease, 552
Meninges, 434
Meningioma, 431, 436
Meningitis, 436
Meningocele, 431, 436, 437
Menopause, 350, 357
Menorrhagia, 344
Menorrhea, 357, 358
Menses, 357
Menstruation, 357, 358
Mental disorders, 439–441
Metacarpals, 481f
Metacarpectomy, 482
Metacarpus, 495
Metastasis, 135
Metastasize, 135
Metatarsals, 481f
Metered-dose inhaler, 147f
Microcardia, 185
Micrographic survey, 95
Midbrain, 433
Middle ear, 543–545
Midsagittal plane, 46, 46f
Mineralocorticoids, 425t
Miotics, 560
Mitral valve, 176, 179, 201f
Mitral valve murmur, 179
Mitral valve prolapse, 201, 201f
Mixed nerve, 437
Modified radical mastectomy, 386, 386f
Mohs surgery, 95
Mononucleosis, 203
Morbid obesity, 270
Motion sickness drugs, 560
MRI, 54, 57, 58f, 144, 273, 451
Mucoid, 238
Mucolytics, 147
Mucous, 238, 356, 368
Mucus, 368
Multigravida, 361
Multipara, 345
Multiple sclerosis (MS), 445
Muscle relaxants, 514
Muscles, 473–481, 477
Muscosal, 119
Muscular, 474
Muscular disorders, 506–507
Muscular dystrophy, 506
Musculoskeletal system, 471–528
    abbreviations, 506
    anatomy and physiology overview, 473, 473f
    bone and joint disorders, 507–510
    bones, 473, 482–492
    clinical application activity, 525
    combining forms, 474, 495–496, 526
    diagnostic procedures, 512–513
    diseases and conditions, 506–512
    fractures, 497–500
    joints, 473, 493–494

medical and surgical procedures, 513
    muscles, 473–481
    muscular disorders, 506–507
    operative report (rotator cuff injury),
        521–524
    pharmacology, 514
    prefixes, 527
    radiology report (degenerative intervertebral
        disk disease), 518–520
    skeletal system, 481–484
    spinal disorders, 510–512
    suffixes, 526
    vertebral column, 500–504
Musculotendinous rotator cuff injury, 509
Myalgia, 474, 477
Myasthenia, 474
Myasthenia gravis (MG), 506
Mycosis, 77, 236
Mydriatics, 560
Myelalgia, 431
Myelin sheath, 430, 430f
Myelitis, 437
Myelocele, 483
Myelogenesis, 490
Myelogram, 490, 491
Myeloma, 437
Myelomalacia, 437, 490
Myelopathy, 437
Myelotome, 437
Myocardial infarction (MI), 187, 202,
        216–220
Myocardium, 167, 169, 173
Myopathy, 474, 477
Myopia, 538, 538f, 539
Myoplasty, 477
Myorrhaphy, 475, 477
Myorrhexis, 474, 477
Myosarcoma, 475
Myosclerosis, 477
Myringoplasty, 541
Myringotomy, 541, 544, 553, 559
Myxedema, 419

Nail body, 78
Nail root, 78
Nailbed, 78
Nares, 117
Nasal, 115
Nasal cavity, 114f, 119
Nasogastric (NG), 117
Nasogastric (NG) intubation, 275
Nasolacrimal duct, 539
Natal, 361
Navel, 52
Nearsightedness, 538, 539
Nebulized mist treatment (NMT), 147
Nebulizer, 147f
Necrectomy, 187
Necrophobia, 440
Necrosis, 85, 187
Necrotic, 85
Needle biopsy, 94
Neonatologist, 361
Neonatology, 361
Neoplasm, 371
Nephralgia, 298
Nephrectomy, 298
Nephritis, 297, 298

Nephroblastoma, 321
Nephrolith, 298, 302
Nephrolithiasis, 298, 302
Nephrolithotomy, 300, 302
Nephrologist, 292, 316
Nephrology, 292
Nephroma, 294
Nephromegaly, 302
Nephron, 294, 296, 297f, 311, 312, 312f
Nephropathy, 295
Nephropexy, 295, 300
Nephroptosis, 295, 300
Nephrorrhaphy, 302
Nephrosclerosis, 302
Nephrosis, 302
Nephrostomy tube, 302
Nephrotic syndrome, 301
Nephrotomy, 302
Nerve block, 436, 436f
Nervous system, 429–438
    abbreviations, 443
    brain, 432–434
    chart note (peripheral neuropathy),
        462–465
    CNS/PNS, 429–430
    combining forms, 431, 467
    diagnostic procedures, 450–451
    diseases and conditions, 445–449
    medical and surgical procedures, 453
    pharmacology, 454
    prefixes, 468
    spinal cord, 434–437
    suffixes, 431, 467–468
Neuralgia, 437
Neuritis, 437
Neuroblastoma, 446
Neurocyte, 438
Neurodegenerative genetic disorder, 445
Neuroglandular glands, 431
Neuroglia, 430, 438
Neurohypophysis, 413, 414
Neurologist, 406
Neurology, 406
Neurolysis, 431
Neuroma, 437
Neuromuscular glands, 431
Neuron, 430, 438
Neuropathy, 437
Neurosis (neuroses), 440
Neurosurgeon, 406
Neurosurgery, 406
Neurotransmitter, 430–431, 430f
Nipple, 358
Nocturia, 316
Nocturnal enuresis, 320
Nodule, 92f
Noise-indued hearing loss (NIHL), 552
Non-Hodgkin lymphoma, 191, 202
Nonsteroidal anti-inflammatory drugs
        (NSAIDs), 514
Norepinephrine, 425t
Nose, 114f, 115, 117
Nose swab test, 144, 144f
Nosebleed, 140
Nostrils, 117
NSAIDs, 514
Nuclear, 33
Nuclear scan, 57, 58f, 322

Nuclear stress test, 205
Nucleotoxic substance, 35
Nucleus, 35

O₂, 126, 170, 171
Obesity, 270
Oblique fracture, 499, 500
Obstetrician, 342
Obstetrician/gynecologist, 341
Obstetrics, 342
Obstetrics and gynecology (OB-GYN), 341
Obstructive sleep apnea (OSA), 130, 131f
Occlusion of arteries, 186f, 187
Oligomenorrhea, 358
Oligospermia, 368
Oliguria, 313, 316
Onychoma, 79
Onychomalacia, 67, 79
Onychomycosis, 79
Onychopathy, 79
Oophoritis, 362
Oophoroma, 345, 346, 362
Oophoropathy, 428
Oophoropexy, 348
Oophoroplasty, 348
Oophorotomy, 428
Oophropathy, 348
Open-angle glaucoma, 549
Open appendectomy, 273, 273f
Open fracture, 497, 499
Operative report, 221–223, 283–285,
    397–399, 521–524, 563–566
Ophthalmectomy, 536
Ophthalmologist, 530, 536, 536f
Ophthalmology, 530
Ophthalmomalacia, 536
Ophthalmoplegia, 536, 537
Ophthalmoscope, 531, 536, 536f
Ophthalmoscopy, 536
Optic, 532
Optic disk, 536
Optic nerve, 536
Optician, 530
Optometrist, 530
Oral, 231
Oral cavity, 231, 233–237
Oral glucose tolerance test (OGTT), 450
Oral hypoglycemics, 454
Orbicularis oculi, 473f
Orchidectomy, 365
Orchidopexy, 428
Orchiopexy, 365, 368
Orchioplasty, 368
Orchiorrhaphy, 368
Organ level, 31, 32f
Organ of Corti, 545
Organism level, 31, 32f
Orthodontist, 231, 237
Orthopedics, 472, 483
Orthopedist, 472
Orthopnea, 131
Osteitis, 483, 488
Osteitis deformans, 508
Osteoarthritis, 494
Osteoarthropathy, 494
Osteoblast, 486
Osteoclast, 484
Osteocyte, 484, 487, 488

Osteogenesis, 487, 489
Osteomalacia, 484, 489
Osteomyelitis, 491, 491f
Osteopathy, 488
Osteoporosis, 484, 489, 489f
Osteorrhaphy, 488
Osteosclerosis, 488
Osteotomy, 488
Otalgia, 542
Otitis externa, 553
Otitis media (OM), 543, 544, 553, 567–569
Otolaryngologist, 530
Otolaryngology, 530
Otoplasty, 543
Otorrhea, 541
Otosclerosis, 545
Otoscope, 542, 543f
Otoscopy, 542, 555
Oval window, 546f
Ovariorrhexis, 345
Ovary (ovaries), 343f, 346, 348, 407f, 428
Oviduct, 348, 349
Ovulation, 348
Ovum, 348
Oxytocin, 411f, 417t
Oxytoxics, 389

P wave, 184
Pacemaker, 189, 200
Paget disease, 508
Palsy, 446
Pancreas, 230f, 247f, 258, 262f, 264–265, 407f,
    425–427
Pancreatectomy, 264
Pancreatic, 260
Pancreatic cancer, 264
Pancreatic duct, 260, 262f, 263
Pancreatic hormones, 427t
Pancreatitis, 12, 13f, 257, 270, 408
Pancreatolith, 261, 263, 426
Pancreatolithiasis, 263, 426
Pancreatolysis, 426
Pancreatoma, 426
Pancreatopathy, 426
Panhypopituitarism, 444
Papanicolaou (Pap) test, 382, 383f
Papule, 92f
Para, 361
Paralysis, 446, 447, 478
Paranasal, 118
Paranasal sinuses, 118f
Paraplegia, 446, 447
Parathyroid, 408
Parathyroid glands, 407f, 423
Parathyroid hormone (PTH), 423, 423t
Parkinson disease, 446
Parotid gland, 230f, 235
Partial occlusion, 186f
Partial thickness burn, 88
Patch test, 94, 94f
Patella, 481f, 496
Patellectomy, 483
Patency, 373
Patent ductus arteriosus, 202
Pathogen, 195, 362
Pathological, 253
Pathological suffix, 21
Pectoralis major, 473f, 477

Pediatric cardiologist, 162
Pediatric urologist, 291
Pelvic cavity, 48f, 49
Pelvic girdle, 481f, 496
Pelvic inflammatory disease (PID), 361, 362,
    392–396
Pelvic US, 383
Pelvimeter, 44
Pelvis, 481f, 483, 494, 494f, 496
Penis, 364, 364f, 370
Peptic ulcer disease (PUD), 238, 239f
Percutaneous coronary intervention (PCI), 208
Percutaneous nephrostomy, 302, 303, 303f
Percutaneous transluminal coronary
    angioplasty (PTCA), 208, 208f
Pericardiectomy, 168
Pericardiocentesis, 168
Pericardiorrhaphy, 169
Pericarditis, 168
Pericardium, 167, 169
Perineorrhaphy, 345
Perineum, 343f
Periodontist, 237
Periodontitis, 237
Periosteum, 486
Peripheral nervous system (PNS), 429–430
Peripheral neuropathy, 462–465
Peristalsis, 238, 251
Peritoneal dialysis, 324, 325f
Peritonitis, 270
Peritonsillar, 115
Periumbilical, 44
Pertussis, 142
PET scan, 58f, 451
Petechia, 90
Petit mal seizure, 448
Peyer patches, 189, 192f
Phacoemulsification, 556, 557f
Phagocyte, 190
Phalanges, 481f, 482, 485, 495
Phalangitis, 482
Pharyngalgia, 238
Pharyngeal suction catheter, 117
Pharyngitis, 115, 121, 238
Pharyngocele, 121
Pharyngodynia, 238
Pharyngomycosis, 119
Pharyngoparalysis, 119
Pharyngoplasty, 121
Pharyngoplegia, 119
Pharyngospasm, 116, 121
Pharyngostenosis, 121
Pharyngotome, 121
Pharyngotomy, 121
Pharyngotonsillitis, 231
Pharynx, 115, 117, 119, 230f, 231, 238
Pheochromocytoma, 445
Phimosis, 379
Phlebitis, 165
Phleborrhaphy, 176
Phleborrhexis, 176
Phlebostenosis, 176
Phlebotomy, 176
Photophobia, 550
Phrenospasm, 131
Pia mater, 434, 435f, 436
Pilocystic, 78
Pilonidal, 68

Pilonidal cyst, 68
Pineal gland, 407f, 428
Pinkeye, 531
Pitting edema, 55, 55f
Pituitary gland, 407f, 412–417, 433f
Pituitary hormones, 416–417t
Plantar flexion, 479f
Plantar wart, 93
Plastic surgery, 543
Pleura (pleurae), 501
Pleural effusion, 142
Pleural mesothelioma, 141, 141f
Pleural rub, 138
Pleuralgia, 116, 129
Pleurisy, 129
Pleuritic, 115
Pleuritis, 129
Pleurocele, 129
Pleurodynia, 129
Pleuropneumonia, 129
Plural suffix, 24
Pneumatic otoscopy, 555
Pneumectomy, 115
Pneumoconiosis, 128
Pneumocystis pneumonia (PCP), 134
Pneumomelanosis, 128
Pneumonectomy, 127, 128f
Pneumonia, 115, 127
Pneumonitis, 127
Pneumonocele, 127
Pneumonopathy, 127
Pneumonosis, 127
Pneumothorax, 142, 142f
Poison, 264
Polio (poliomyelitis), 448
Polycystic kidney disease (PKD), 317, 317f
Polydipsia, 409, 427
Polyp, 271
Polypectomy, 271f
Polyphagia, 427
Polysomnography (PSG), 144, 145f
Polyuria, 295, 316, 427
Pons, 433
Positron emission tomography (PET) scan, 58f, 451
Posterior, 33, 38, 38f, 412, 414
Posteroanterior (PA), 39, 39f
Posterolateral, 40
Postmenopause, 350
Postprandial, 257
Postural drainage, 146
Potassium supplements, 326
P-R interval, 183f
Preeclampsia, 378
Prefix, 13–15, 26–30
Premenopause, 350
Prenatal, 344, 361
Prepuce, 364f, 370
Presbycusis, 553
Pressure-equalizing (PE) tubes, 544, 544f, 559
Pressure ulcer, 93, 93f
Prick skin test, 94f
Primary lesions, 91, 92f
Primigravida, 345, 361
Proctalgia, 251
Proctitis, 253
Proctocele, 245
Proctologist, 244

Proctoscopy, 272
Proctospasm, 253
Progesterone, 350, 358
Programmed learning, 2
Progress note, 105–108, 333–335
Prolactin, 411f, 416t
Prolapse of uterus, 350
Prolapsed kidney, 300
Pronation, 479f
Pronunciation guidelines, 16
Prostate cancer, 371
Prostate gland, 293f, 364f, 368, 369f
Prostate-specific antigen (PSA), 370
Prostatectomy, 371
Prostatitis, 365, 370, 371, 373
Prostatocystitis, 370
Prostatomegaly, 368, 369
Proteinuria, 301, 316
Proximal, 33, 41, 42, 315, 488
Proximal epiphysis, 486
Psoriasis, 91, 91f
Psoriasis vulgaris, 105–108
Psychiatric disorders, 439
Psychiatry, 440
Psychosis (psychoses), 440
Psychotherapy, 440
Ptyalism, 231, 235
Puberty, 358
Pubis, 343f, 481f
Pulmonary, 177
Pulmonary artery, 175
Pulmonary capillaries, 126
Pulmonary function report, 154–156
Pulmonary function tests (PFTs), 145
Pulmonary medicine, 113
Pulmonary trunk, 171
Pulmonary valve, 175, 179
Pulmonologist, 113, 116
Pulmonology, 113
Punch biopsy, 94
Pupil, 536
Pupillary, 531
Purkinje fibers, 182
Pustule, 76, 92f
Pyelitis, 314
Pyelogram, 314, 322
Pyelography, 322
Pyelonephritis, 314
Pyelopathy, 313
Pyeloplasty, 294, 314
Pyloric stenosis, 252, 252f
Pyloromyotomy, 231, 252
Pyoderma, 68
Pyonephrosis, 314
Pyorrhea, 314
Pyothorax, 116
Pyromania, 441
Pyuria, 305, 314, 316

Q-T interval, 183f
QRS complex, 183f, 184
QRS wave, 184
Quadriplegia, 431, 446, 447f, 478

Radiation therapy, 490
Radical mastectomy, 386
Radioactive iodine uptake (RAIU) test, 450
Radiofrequency ablation, 208

Radiograph, 57, 483
Radiographic procedures, 443
Radiography, 307
Radiologist, 490
Radiology, 47, 490
Radiology report, 518–520
Radionuclide imaging, 57
Radiotherapy, 490
Radius, 481f
Rales, 138
Raynaud disease, 202
Reabsorption, 292
Receptor sites, 430f, 431
Reconstructive breast surgery, 386
Rectal bleeding, 279–282
Rectalgia, 251
Rectocele, 245, 306, 306f
Rectoplasty, 251
Rectospasm, 253
Rectovaginal fistula, 353
Rectum, 245, 251, 306, 343f, 364f
Rectus abdominis, 473f
Red blood cell (RBC), 171
Referral letter, 150–153
Regional ileitis, 249
Renal, 294, 297, 298, 301, 317, 322
Renal artery, 293f, 296
Renal calculus, 298, 315
Renal cortex, 293f, 296, 312
Renal failure, 317
Renal filtrate, 312
Renal hypertension, 301
Renal medulla, 293f, 296, 312
Renal pelvis, 293f, 294, 312f, 313, 314
Renal pyramid, 293f
Renal transplantation, 320, 320f
Renal tubule, 312
Renal tumor, 310
Renal vein, 293f, 296
Reproductive system, 341–404
  anatomy and physiology overview, 342
  clinical application activity, 400
  diagnostic procedures, 381–384
  diseases and conditions, 375–379
  emergency department report (PID), 392–396
  females. *See* Female reproductive system
  gynecology, 341–342
  males. *See* Male reproductive system
  medical and surgical procedures, 384–389
  obstetrics, 341–342
  operative report (bilateral vasectomy), 397–399
  pharmacology, 389
  prefixes, 402
  sexually transmitted infections (STIs), 375, 380
  suffixes, 401–402
  urology, 342
Resectoscope, 370, 370f, 389
Respiration, 114, 127
Respiratory center, 434
Respiratory system, 113–160
  abbreviations, 136
  anatomy and physiology overview, 114
  clinical application activity, 157
  combining forms, 115–116, 158
  diagnostic procedures, 143–146

diseases and conditions, 138–142
lower respiratory tract, 124–135
medical and surgical procedures, 146
pharmacology, 147
prefixes, 159
pulmonary function report, 154–156
referral letter (allergic rhinitis), 150–153
schematic of upper and lower respiratory
    tracts, 114f
suffixes, 116, 158–159
upper respiratory tract, 117–123
Retina, 534
Retinal detachment, 551
Retinal detachment repair, 563–566
Retinal photocoagulation, 557, 558f
Retinitis, 535
Retinopathy, 532, 535
Retrograde pyelography (RP), 322
Retroversion, 345
Rheumatic heart disease, 202
Rheumatoid arthritis, 472, 509, 509f
Rheumatoid factor, 513
Rheumatoid spondylitis, 510
Rheumatologist, 472
Rheumatology, 472
Rhinoplasty, 118
Rhinorrhagia, 119
Rhinorrhea, 115, 118, 119
Rhinotomy, 118
Rhonchi, 138
Ribs, 481f, 495
Rickets, 489
Right atrium (RA), 169, 171, 182, 201f
Right hypochondriac region, 50f
Right inguinal region, 50f
Right lower quadrant (RLQ), 50, 50f
Right lumbar region, 50f
Right lung, 171
Right lymphatic duct, 193
Right pulmonary artery, 175
Right pulmonary vein, 171, 176
Right upper quadrant (RUQ), 50, 261
Right ventricle (RV), 171, 183f, 201f
Ringworm, 93
Rinne test, 556, 556f
Roentgen, Wilhelm, 490
Root, 4
Rotation, 479f
Rotator cuff injury, 509, 521–524
Roux-en-Y gastric bypass (RGB), 274, 275f
Ruptured disk, 504

Saccular aneurysm, 188f
Sacral nerves, 434, 435f
Sacrodynia, 504
Sacrospinal, 504
Sacrum, 343f, 364f, 481f, 504
Saliva, 231, 235
Salivary glands, 230f, 235
Salpingectomy, 345, 348, 362
Salpingitis, 545
Salpingocele, 349
Salpingopharyngeal, 541
Salpingoplasty, 348
Salpingoscope, 348, 545
Salpingoscopy, 545
Salpingostenosis, 545
Salpinoscopy, 348

Scabies, 91
Scapula, 481f
Schizophrenia, 441
Sciatica, 448
Sclera, 533
Scleritis, 532, 535
Scleroderma, 68, 75
Scleromalacia, 535
Sclerosis, 75, 301, 477
Sclerotherapy, 212
Scoliosis, 511, 511f
Scratch test, 94, 94f
Scrotum, 364f, 366
Sebaceous cyst, 89
Sebaceous glands, 66f, 72, 76, 77
Seborrhea, 68
Sebum, 76
Second-degree burn, 88, 89f
Second-degree heart block, 200
Secondary lesions, 91, 92f
Segmental resection, 128f
Seizure, 448
Semen, 365
Semicircular canals, 545, 546f
Seminal fluid, 368
Seminal vesicle, 364f, 368
Seminiferous tubules, 364f
Sensorineural, 552
Sensory tunic, 534
Sepsis, 55
Septicemia, 55
Septum, 173
Sequestrectomy, 513
Sequestrum, 509
Serous OM, 553
Serrated, 351
Serrated curette, 352f
Sex hormones, 407f, 425t
Sexually transmitted infections (STIs), 362,
    375, 380
Shave biopsy, 94
Shingles, 448, 448f
Short bones, 485, 486
Sialitis, 235
Sialorrhea, 231, 235
Sickle cell anemia, 198, 199f
Side-to-side anastomosis, 59, 59f
Sigmoid colon, 230f, 245, 251, 254
Sigmoidectomy, 251, 254
Sigmoiditis, 251
Sigmoidoscope, 255
Sigmoidoscopy, 253, 254f, 272
Sigmoidotomy, 245
Sinoatrial (SA) node, 182
Sinus rhythm, 184
Skeletal muscle fibers, 476
Skeletal system, 481–484
Skin cancer check, 101–104
Skin graft, 96
Skin lesion, 91, 92f
Skin resurfacing, 96
Skin test, 94, 94f
Skull, 481f, 495f
Sleep apnea, 130, 131f
Slit-lamp examination, 554, 554f
Small intestine, 244, 246–251, 254f
Smooth muscle fibers, 476
Snellen chart, 555

SOAP note, 567–569
Soleus, 473f
Somatotropin, 416t
Sonogram, 57
Spanish-speaking patients, 645–653
Sperm, 368
Spermatocyte, 365, 367
Spermatogenesis, 367
Spermatoid, 367
Spermatolith, 367
Spermatozoa, 365, 367, 401
Spermaturia, 368
Spermicide, 4, 365, 389
Sphenoidal sinus, 118f
Spina bifida, 449, 449f
Spina bifida cystica, 449
Spina bifida occulta, 449, 449f
Spinal, 44
Spinal cavity, 48, 48f
Spinal column, 495, 500, 502
Spinal cord, 433f, 434–437
Spinal cord compression, 512
Spinal curvatures, 511f
Spinal disorders, 510–512
Spinal nerves, 434, 435f
Spinal stenosis, 511, 512f
Spiral fracture, 499, 500, 501f
Spirometry, 145
Spleen, 194, 195, 230f, 247f, 251
Splenomegaly, 12, 13f, 190
Splinting, 513
Spondylitis, 482, 502
Spondylolisthesis, 512
Spondylomalacia, 502
Spondylopathy, 502
Spongy bone, 486
Sprain, 506
Squamous, 68
Squamous cell carcinoma, 84, 85f
Stapedectomy, 546
Stapes, 545, 546f
Staphylococcal infection, 87
Staphylococcus (staphylococci), 491
Staphylococcus aureus, 378
Steatitis, 67
Stenosis, 252, 301, 309
Sterility, 378
Sternocleidomastoid, 473f
Sternocostal, 482
Sternum, 481f, 495
Stomach, 230f, 231, 238, 239f, 247f
Stomatalgia, 234
Stomatodynia, 234
Stomatomycosis, 235
Stomatopathy, 231
Stomatosis, 235
Stone, 176, 257, 263, 298, 300
Stool, 251
Stool guaiac, 273
Strabismus, 551, 552f
Straight catheter, 323
Strain, 507
Strangulated hernia, 270f
Stratum corneum, 66f, 70
Stress test, 205, 206f
Stridor, 138
Stroke, 186, 438
Sty, 549

Subarachnoid space, 435f
Subcostal, 482, 497
Subcutaneous, 71
Subcutaneous injection, 29f, 71
Subcutaneous tissue, 66f, 73
Subdural space, 436
Sublingual, 231, 235
Sublingual gland, 230f, 235
Subluxation, 509
Submandibular gland, 230f, 235
Submaxillary, 235
Suction-assisted lipectomy, 73
Sudden infant death syndrome (SIDS), 142
Sudoresis, 67, 68
Sudoriferous glands, 66f, 72, 76, 77
Suffix, 7–10
    diagnostic, 19–20
    pathological, 21
    plural, 24
    surgical, 17–18, 300
Superior, 33, 38f, 41, 47, 424
Superior vena cava (SVC), 169, 175
Supination, 479f
Suppurative OM, 553
Suprarenal, 301, 424
Suprarenal glands, 424
Surgical suffix, 17–18, 300
Suture, 305
Swayback, 510
Swelling, 301
Swimmer's ear, 542, 553
Symbols, 640
Symphysis pubis, 364, 364f
Synapse, 430, 430f
Synarthroses, 493
Synovial fluid, 494
Synthetic skin test, 96
Syphilis, 380
System level, 31, 32f
Systemic lupus erythematosus (SLE), 203, 203f
Systemic scleroderma, 75
Systemic sclerosis, 76
Systole, 183, 184

T cells, 195
T wave, 184
Tachycardia, 166
Talipes equinovarus, 509, 510f
Target organs, 406
Target tissues, 406
Tarsals, 481f
TB, 135, 146
Tears, 539
Tendinitis, 474
Tendoplasty, 474, 478
Tendotome, 478
Tendotomy, 478
Tenotomy, 474
Testalgia, 365
Testectomy, 366
Testes (testis), 364, 364f, 366, 407f, 428
Testicle, 366
Testitis, 366
Testopathy, 366
Testosterone, 364
Thalamotomy, 453
Thalassemia, 198
Third-degree burn, 88, 89f

Third-degree heart block, 200
Thoracentesis, 131, 132f
Thoracic, 44, 193, 504
Thoracic cavity, 48f, 49
Thoracic duct, 193
Thoracic nerves, 434, 435f
Thoracic vertebrae, 504
Thoracocentesis, 131
Thoracodynia, 116
Thoracopathy, 116
Thoracotomy, 131
Thrombectomy, 187
Thrombocyte, 169, 171, 438
Thrombogenesis, 188, 438
Thrombolysis, 18, 165, 188, 438
Thrombolytics, 213
Thrombosis, 187
Thrombus, 187, 188, 438
Thymectomy, 428
Thymolysis, 428
Thymoma, 190, 408, 428
Thymopathy, 428
Thymosin, 195
Thymus, 163, 194, 195
Thymus gland, 407f, 428
Thyroid gland, 407f, 418–421
Thyroid hormones, 419t
Thyroid-stimulating hormone (TSH), 411f,
    416t
Thyroidectomy, 4, 418, 420
Thyroidotomy, 408
Thyromegaly, 408
Thyropathy, 418
Thyrotomy, 418
Thyroxine (T$_4$), 419t
Tibia, 481f, 496
Tibial, 483
Tine test, 146
Tinea, 93
Tinea barbae, 93
Tinea corporis, 93
Tinea cruris, 93
Tinea pedis, 93
Tinea versicolor, 93
Tinnitus, 553
Tissue expansion, 386, 387f
Tissue level, 31, 32f
Tissue typing, 207
Tomography, 57
Tongue, 230f, 231, 235
Tonic-clonic seizure, 448
Tonometry, 554
Tonsils, 115, 194
Torticollis, 507
Total hip arthroplasty, 494
Total hip replacement (THR), 494, 494f
Total mastectomy, 386
Total occlusion, 186f
Toxic shock syndrome (TSS), 378
Toxicologist, 408, 421
Toxicology, 264, 265
Toxicopathy, 421
Toxicosis, 265
Trachea, 114f, 115, 124, 131f
Tracheomalacia, 124
Tracheopathy, 125
Tracheoplasty, 125
Tracheostenosis, 125

Tracheostomy, 18, 115, 124, 125f
Tracheotomy, 18, 125
Traction, 513
Transdermal, 350
Transient ischemic attack (TIA), 449
Transrectal ultrasound (TRUS) and biopsy of
    prostate, 384, 384f
Transsphenoidal hypophysectomy, 452, 453f
Transurethral resection of prostate (TURP),
    369, 370, 370f, 389
Transvaginal US, 383
Transverse colon, 230f
Transverse fracture, 499, 500
Transverse plane, 46f, 47
Transverse rectus abdominis muscle (TRAM)
    flap, 386, 387f
Trapezius, 473f
Trephination, 453
Trephine, 453
Triceps brachii, 473f, 477
Trichomoniasis, 380
Trichomycosis, 78
Trichopathy, 68, 78
Trichosis, 78
Tricuspid valve, 175, 179
Triiodothyronine (T$_3$), 419t
Trocars, 274f
Troponin I test, 206
Tubal ligation, 388
Tubal pregnancy, 377f
Tube, 117
Tubercle, 135
Tuberculosis (TB), 135, 146
Tumor, 92f
Tuning fork test, 556
Tympanic membrane, 542, 544, 544f, 546f
Tympanoplasty, 541
Tympanostomy tubes, 559
Type 1 diabetes, 444
Type 2 diabetes, 444

Ulcer, 92f, 93
Ulcerative colitis, 269
Ulna, 481f
Ultrasonic-assisted liposuction, 73
Ultrasonogram, 58f, 59f
Ultrasonography (US), 57, 206, 273, 322, 323f,
    383
Ultrasonography using sound pitch, 206
Umbilical, 50f, 51
Umbilical hernia, 270f
Umbilical region, 50f, 52
Upper GI endoscopy, 240
Upper GI series, 272
Upper GI tract, 233–242
Upper respiratory infection (URI), 543
Upper respiratory tract, 117–123
Uremia, 294
Ureter, 293f, 294, 304, 315f
Ureteral orifice, 293f
Ureteral stent, 326, 326f
Ureterorrhaphy, 305
Ureterostenosis, 294
Ureterovaginal fistula, 353
Urethra, 293f, 305, 308, 343f, 364f
Urethral, 308
Urethral orifice, 364f
Urethral stenosis, 309

Urethral stricture, 308, 309
Urethralgia, 308
Urethrectomy, 308
Urethritis, 308
Urethrocele, 294
Urethrocystitis, 309
Urethrodynia, 308
Urethropexy, 308
Urethroplasty, 308, 309
Urethroscope, 309
Urethroscopy, 309
Urgency, 321
Urinalysis, 305, 314
Urinary, 294
Urinary bladder, 293f, 305, 306, 343f, 364f
Urinary incontinence, 316
Urinary meatus, 293f, 305, 309
Urinary system, 291–339
    abbreviations, 319
    anatomy and physiology overview, 292, 293f
    clinical application activity, 336
    combining forms, 294, 314, 337
    diagnostic procedures, 321–323
    diseases and conditions, 319–321
    hospital admission (BPH, colon cancer),
        329–332
    macroscopic structures, 296–304
    medical and surgical procedures, 323–326
    microscopic structures, 311–318
    pharmacology, 326
    prefixes, 338
    progress note, 333–335
    suffixes, 294–295, 300, 337
    ureters, bladder, and urethra, 304–311
Urinary tract infection (UTI), 308
Urinary tract tumor, 310
Urination, 316
Urine dipstick, 315f
Urogenital disorders, 342
Urogram, 322
Urogynecologist, 291
Urologist, 291, 316, 342
Urology, 291, 342
Urticaria, 93
Uterine fibroids, 377
Uterine tube, 349
Uteroscopy, 350
Uterovaginal, 344

Uterus, 343f, 346, 349, 350, 357
Uvea, 534

Vagina, 343f, 346, 351, 354
Vaginal, 354, 356
Vaginal hemorrhage, 354
Vaginal hysterectomy, 354
Vaginitis, 351
Vaginocele, 344
Vaginoplasty, 352
Vaginoscope, 352
Vaginotomy, 352
Valve cusps, 179, 180f
Valvuloplasty, 212
Varicocele, 365
Varicose veins, 165, 178, 179f
Varicosities, 178, 179
Vas deferens, 364, 364f, 368
Vascular, 166, 177
Vascular tunic, 534
Vasectomy, 365, 372, 372f, 373, 397–399
Vasectomy reversal, 373
Vasomotor, 434
Vasomotor center, 434
Vasospasm, 165
Vasovasostomy, 373
Vein, 165, 176, 179
Vena cava, 169
Venereal herpes, 380
Venereal wart, 93
Venous, 165, 195
Ventral, 33, 37, 38
Ventral cavity, 48, 48f
Ventral root, 437
Ventricular, 173
Ventriculotomy, 172
Venule, 178
Verruca, 93, 93f
Vertebra (vertebrae), 495, 501
Vertebral column, 481f, 495, 500–504
Vertebrectomy, 501
Vertebrosternal, 502
Vertical banded gastroplasty, 274, 275f
Vertigo, 553
Vertigo and motion sickness drugs,
    560
Vesicle, 92f
Vesicocele, 294

Vesicovaginal fistula, 353, 353f
Vestibular apparatus, 546
Vestibulocochlear nerve, 546f
Vestibule, 545, 546f
Villus (villi), 246
Visual acuity (VA) test, 555
Vitiligo, 94, 94f
Vitrectomy, 557, 558f
Voiding cystourethrography (VCUG),
    323f
Volvulus, 271
Vomiting, 241, 260
Vulva, 342, 356
Vulvopathy, 345
Vulvouterine, 356

Wall-eye, 551
Wart, 93
Wax emulsifiers, 560
WBC, 82, 87, 171
Weber test, 556
Wedge resection, 128f
Wheal, 92f, 93
Wheezes, 138
White blood cell (WBC, wbc), 82
White matter, 430, 435f
Whooping cough, 142
Wilms tumor, 321
Winter itch, 67
Womb, 349
Word elements, 3–15, 575–584
    combining form, 5–7
    prefix, 13–15, 26–30
    suffix, 7–10, 17–24
    three rules of word building, 10
    word root, 4–5
Word root (WR), 4–5

X-ray, 57
Xanthemia, 82
Xanthocyte, 82
Xanthoderma, 81
Xanthoma, 81, 82
Xanthopia, 537
Xanthosis, 83
Xenograft, 28, 96
Xenophobia, 440
Xeroderma, 68, 79, 81

Rules for Singular and Plural Suffixes

This table presents common singular suffixes, the rules for forming plurals, and examples of each.

Rule		Example	
Singular	*Plural*	*Singular*	*Plural*
-*a*	Retain *a* and add *e*.	pleur*a*	pleur*ae*
-*ax*	Drop *x* and add *ces*.	thor*ax*	thora*ces*
-*en*	Drop *en* and add *ina*.	lum*en*	lum*ina*
-*is*	Drop *is* and add *es*.	diagno*sis*	diagno*ses*
-*ix*	Drop *ix* and add *ices*.	append*ix*	append*ices*
-*ex*	Drop *ex* and add *ices*.	ap*ex*	ap*ices*
-*ma*	Retain *ma* and add *ta*.	carcino*ma*	carcinoma*ta*
-*on*	Drop *on* and add *a*.	gangli*on*	gangli*a*
-*um*	Drop *um* and add *a*.	bacteri*um*	bacteri*a*
-*us*	Drop *us* and add *i*.	bronch*us*	bronch*i*
-*y*	Drop *y* and add *ies*.	deformit*y*	deformit*ies*